Anaesthesia Databook
A CLINICAL PRACTICE COMPENDIUM

Anaesthesia Databook

A CLINICAL PRACTICE COMPENDIUM

Rosemary A. Mason

MB ChB DObst RCOG FFARCS

Consultant Anaesthetist
West Glamorgan Health Authority,
Swansea,
UK

CHURCHILL LIVINGSTONE
EDINBURGH, LONDON, MELBOURNE AND NEW YORK 1990

CHURCHILL LIVINGSTONE
Medical Division of Longman Group UK Limited

Distributed in the United States of America by Churchill
Livingstone Inc., 1560 Broadway, New York, N.Y. 10036,
and by associated companies, branches and
representatives throughout the world.

First published 1990

ISBN 0-443-04120-2

British Library Cataloguing in Publication Data
Mason, Rosemary Anne
  Anaesthesia databook.
  1. Medicine. Anaesthesia — Manuals
  I. Title
617'.96

Library of Congress Cataloging in Publication Data
Mason, Rosemary Anne.
  Anaesthesia databook : a clinical practice compendium / Rosemary Anne Mason.
   p. cm

ISBN 0-443-04120-2
  1. Anesthesia—Handbooks, maunals, etc. I. Title.
  [DNLM: 1. Anesthesia—handbooks. WO 231 M411a]
RD82.2. M36 1989
617'. 96' 0202—dc19
DNLM/DLC
for Library of Congress 89–842 CIP

Produced by Longman Singapore Publishers (Pte) Ltd.
Printed in Singapore

Preface

Year by year, both the scope and complexity of anaesthesia increase. Frequently, and often at short notice, decisions on patient management are required and in which the role of the anaesthetist may be critical. For this advice to be soundly based, it may be necessary, not only to evaluate the appropriateness of a variety of possible anaesthetic techniques, but also to draw together widely disparate pieces of medical knowledge. At a time of increasing specialization, this is and will become progressively more difficult.

I have felt that there are few texts written which lie between the standard textbook and the specialist monograph and which are specifically for the experienced anaesthetist facing awkward problems. My aim therefore has been to attempt to produce a relatively advanced practical reference system for the trained anaesthetist.

This is not a book for beginners. There is no discussion of basic principles or techniques. The information has been collated from a wide range of sources and the bibliography at the end of each topic not only covers the quoted references but also will often provide a guide to more extensive reading. No attempt has been made to provide a didactic manual and, where conflicting opinions exist, these have been recorded so that a balanced judgement can be made in the light of particular circumstances.

To compress the large amount of information into a book of reasonably compact size has meant the adoption of a tight and somewhat indigestible style of writing. However it is envisaged that it will be consulted for specific clinical problems rather than read in continuity.

It is unusual nowadays for a book covering many topics to be written by a single author. However I wished to develop a systematic and unified approach, and it does reflect my personal view on the integration of both medicine in general and anaesthesia.
I hope that this book's niche will prove to be the briefcase or the back of the car and that it might provide a little help in times of crisis!

Swansea 1989   R.A.M

Introduction

This book is laid out as a reference system rather than as a descriptive text. Since the topics are generally covered in an alphabetical manner, a conventional terminal index has deliberately been omitted. Each section reviews a major consideration in anaesthesia though, where necessary, certain subjects are cross referenced between differing sections. An index of contents is however provided at the start of most sections. Where possible, a standardized approach is taken to each topic. The sections appear in the order in which problems may occur, from the initial assessment to the final management of the patient.

Section 1

Covers a range of medical conditions which may present anaesthetic problems. The information, including the bibliography, is self-contained, except where cross references are indicated. Each section describes systematically the preoperative abnormalities, anaesthetic problems and management.

Unlike a standard medical textbook, the space allocated to a particular condition is not necessarily proportional to its frequency of occurrence. Thus, a rare disease producing potentially serious anaesthetic complications may be considered in much more detail than a common condition with fewer associated problems.

Section 2

Reviews potential existing preoperative drug therapy and is divided into three sections. The proprietary and non proprietary lists indicate briefly the nature of a drug, or its action. Those drugs which may have significant interactions are indicated. For these drugs, a reference to further information is made. The third section includes information on important groups of drugs. Pharmacology primarily of specific interest to the anaesthetist is documented.

Section 3

Gives information on drugs which may be particularly required in the perioperative period.

Section 4

Reviews emergency conditions which may present for the first time in the perioperative period. At the request of the publishers, this separate section was created. Inevitably there is some overlap of information with that in section 1.

Section 5

Deals with cardiopulmonary resuscitation, brain death and organ donor management.

Section 6

Normal values.

Appendix

Useful addresses and telephone numbers.

Acknowledgements

The responsibility for the accuracy of the contents of this book remains with myself. However, I owe a large debt of gratitude to my friends and colleagues, who not only were a continuing source of advice and encouragement, but laboured hard to reduce errors to a minimum.

Dr S A D Al-Ismail MB ChB MRCP MRCPath
Consultant Haematologist, West Glamorgan Health Authority, Swansea, South Wales, UK

Dr A C Ames BSc MB BS FRCPath
Consultant Chemical Pathologist, West Glamorgan Health Authority, Swansea, South Wales, UK

Dr J C Mason MA D Phil BM BCh MRCP
Consultant Renal and General Physician, Portsmouth Health District, Portsmouth, England, UK

Mr M C Mason BSc BM BCh FRCS
Consultant Surgeon, West Glamorgan Health Authority, Swansea, South Wales, UK

The entire text was created and edited using the 'Scribe' word processing program designed and marketed by Bucon Limited, Singleton Street, Swansea.

I am particularly grateful to Roy Morgan and Paul Griffiths from the company for their kind, reliable and helpful advice.

List of Abbreviations

ACE	Angiotensin-converting enzyme
ACTH	Adrenocorticotrophic hormone
ADH	Antidiuretic hormone
AF	Atrial fibrillation
AIDS	Acquired immune deficiency syndrome
AIP	Acute intermittent porphyria
ALA	d-Aminolaevulinic acid (synthase)
AMP	Adenosine monophosphate
APTT	Activated partial thromboplastin time
APUD	Amine precursor uptake and decarboxylation
ARDS	Adult respiratory distress syndrome
ASD	Atrial septal defect
AV	Atrioventricular
A–V	Arteriovenous
AVP	Arginine vasopressin
AZT	Zidovudine ('Retrovir')
BBB	Bundle branch block
b.d.	Twice per day
BG	Blood glucose
BMR	Basal metabolic rate
BP	Blood pressure
b.p.m.	Beats per minute
C1	First component of complement
C2	Second component of complement
C4	Fourth component of complement
CABG	Coronary artery bypass graft
CAPD	Continuous ambulatory peritoneal dialysis
ChE	Cholinesterase
CNS	Central nervous system
CPAP	Continuous positive airway pressure
CPB	Cardiopulmonary bypass
CPK	Creatine phosphokinase (creatine kinase)
CPR	Cardiopulmonary resuscitation
CRF	Corticotrophin-releasing factor

CVP	Central venous pressure
CXR	Chest X-ray
DDC	3,5-Dicarbethoxy-1,4-dihydrocolidine
DDAVP	Desmopressin (1-desamino-8-D-arginine vasopressin)
DIC	Disseminated intravascular coagulopathy
DMD	Duchenne muscular dystrophy
DNA	Desoxyribose nucleic acid
DVI	Digital vascular imaging
DVT	Deep venous thrombosis
EBV	Epstein–Barr virus
ECG	Electrocardiogram
ECM	External cardiac massage
EEC	European Economic Community
EMG	Electromyogram
EMLA	Eutectic mixture of local anaesthetics (cream)
ENT	Ear nose and throat
$ETCO_2$	End tidal carbon dioxide
ETT	Endotracheal tube
E_1^f	Fluoride-resistant gene
FBG	Fasting blood glucose
FDA	Food and Drugs Administration (USA)
FDP	Fibrin degradation products
FEV1	Forced expiratory volume in the first second of expiration
FFP	Fresh frozen plasma
FGF	Fresh gas flow
FIO_2	Fractional inspired oxygen
FRC	Functional residual capacity
FSH	Follicle stimulating hormone
G	Gauge
GABA	Gamma amino butyric acid
GFR	Glomerular filtration rate
GH	Growth hormone
GIK	Glucose, insulin, potassium (infusion)
GTT	Glucose tolerance test
G6PD	Glucose-6-phosphate dehydrogenase
HAV	Hepatitis A virus
HBV	Hepatitis B virus
HBcAg	Hepatitis B core antigen
HBeAg	Hepatitis B e antigen
HBsAg	Hepatitis B surface antigen

Hb	Haemoglobin
HbA	Normal adult haemoglobin
HbAS	Sickle cell trait
HbA2	Haemoglobin A2
HbC	Haemoglobin C
HbCO	Carboxyhaemoglobin
HbF	Fetal haemoglobin
HbS	Sickle cell haemoglobin
HbSC	Sickle cell C disease
HbSS	Homozygous sickle cell anaemia
HbThal	Thalassaemia haemoglobin
HC	Hereditary coproporphyria
HELLP	Haemolysis Elevated Liver enzymes and Low Platelet count (syndrome)
HGPRT	Hypoxanthine guanine phosphoribosyl transferase
HIV	Human immunodeficiency virus
HOCM	Hypertrophic obstructive cardiomyopathy
ICP	Intra cranial pressure
IDD	Insulin-dependent diabetes
IgE	Immunoglobulin E
IgG	Immunoglobulin G
IgM	Immunoglobulin M
i.m.	Intramuscular
INR	International normalized ratio
IPPV	Intermittent positive-pressure ventilation
IQ	Intelligence quotient
ISI	International sensitivity index
ITU	Intensive therapy unit
iu	International units
i.v.	Intravenous
JVP	Jugular venous pressure
kPa	Kilopascal
KCCT	Kaolin cephalin clotting time
l	Litre
LA	Local anaesthesia
LAP	Left atrial pressure
LBBB	Left bundle branch block
LFTs	Liver function tests
LSCS	Lower segment Caesarean section
LSD	Lysergic acid diethylamide
LT	Leukotrienes
LVEDP	Left ventricular end diastolic pressure

LVF	Left ventricular failure
MAC	Minimal alveolar concentration
MAO	Monoamine oxidase
MAOI	Monoamine oxidase inhibitor
MAP	Mean arterial pressure
MCV	Mean corpuscular volume
MEN	Multiple endocrine neoplasia
MH	Malignant hyperpyrexia
MHE	Malignant hyperpyrexia equivocal result, consider as MHS
MHN	Malignant hyperpyrexia non-susceptible from proven MH pedigree
MHS	Malignant hyperpyrexia susceptible
mIBG	*Meta*-iodobenzylguanidine
mmHg	Millimetres of mercury
MMR	Masseter muscle rigidity
MPS	Mucopolysaccharidosis
MS	Multiple sclerosis
MSH	Melanocyte-stimulating hormone
MV	Minute volume
MVP	Mitral valve prolapse
MVV	Minute volume ventilation
N	Normal
NANBV	Non-A non-B virus (hepatitis)
NIDD	Non-insulin-dependent diabetes
NMS	Neuroleptic malignant syndrome
NPO	Neurogenic pulmonary oedema
NSAID	Non-steroidal anti-inflammatory drug
$PaCO_2$	Arterial partial pressure of carbon dioxide
PAH	Pregnancy-aggravated hypertension
PAN	Polyarteritis nodosa
PaO_2	Arterial partial pressure of oxygen
PAP	Pulmonary artery pressure
PAWP	Pulmonary artery wedge pressure
PCP	Pulmonary capillary pressure
PCV	Packed cell volume
PCWP	Pulmonary capillary wedge pressure
PDA	Patent ductus arteriosus
PE	Pulmonary embolism
PEEP	Positive end expiratory pressure
PEFR	Peak expiratory flow rate
PIH	Pregnancy-induced hypertension
P mitrale	A prolonged bifid P wave on ECG indicating left atrial enlargement

PP	Pancreatic polypeptide
P pulmonale	A taller than normal P wave on ECG indicating right atrial hypertrophy
PPF	Plasma protein fraction
PPH	Primary pulmonary hypertension
PT	Prothrombin time
PTH	Parathormone
PVC	Polyvinyl chloride
PVR	Pulmonary vascular resistance
q.d.s	Four times per day
Q–Tc	Corrected QT interval
RAP	Right atrial pressure
RBBB	Right bundle branch block
RBC	Red blood corpuscle
RDS	Respiratory distress syndrome
RLF	Retrolental fibroplasia
RR	Respiratory rate
R–R variation	Variations in the intervals between two consecutive R waves (ECG)
RSR1	An initial upward deflection (R) is followed by a downward deflection (S) followed by a second upward deflection (R1) on ECG lead V1
RVEDP	Right ventricular end diastolic pressure
SAP	Systemic arterial pressure
SBE	Subacute bacterial endocarditis
SIADH	Syndrome of inappropriate antidiuretic hormone
SIDS	Sudden infant death syndrome
SLE	Systemic lupus erythematosis
SVC	Superior vena cava
SVT	Supraventricular tachycardia
T3	Tri-iodothyronine
T4	Thyroxine
TCAD	Tricyclic antidepressant
TCT	Thrombin clotting time
t.d.s.	Three times per day
TIA	Transient ischaemic attack
TRH	Thyrotrophin-releasing hormone
TSH	Thyroid-stimulating hormone
TURP	Transurethral resection of the prostate
TV	Tidal volume
u	Unit
UK	United Kingdom

VC	Vital capacity
VF	Ventricular fibrillation
VIP	Vasoactive intestinal peptide
VP	Variegate porphyria
VSD	Ventricular septal defect
VT	Ventricular tachycardia
vWd	von Willebrand's disease
vWF : Ag	von Willebrand factor
WCC	White cell count
WPW	Wolff–Parkinson–White syndrome

Contents

Contents

1

Medical Disorders and Anaesthetic Problems

ACHONDROPLASIA

A type of dwarfism inherited as an autosomal dominant. Cartilage formation at the epiphyses is defective. Bones dependent on cartilage proliferation are thus shortened, whereas periosteal and membranous bones are unaffected. Head and trunk size are normal, but the extremities shortened.

Preoperative abnormalities

1. Individuals are less than 1.4 m tall and of normal intelligence. Hands and feet are short, and the fingers are of equal length. The forehead protrudes, the mandible and tongue are large, but the maxilla is short. There is severe lumbar lordosis, a reduced symphysis pubis to xiphoid distance, and often kyphoscoliosis. The pelvis is small.
2. Spinal canal and foramen magnum stenosis is common and may result in neurological deficits. Anaesthesia may be required for suboccipital craniectomy, laminectomy or ventriculo-peritoneal shunts.
3. Although fertility is low, pregnancy does occur. As a result of the skeletal problems, the fetus remains high, in an intra-abdominal position. This may result in severe respiratory embarrassment in the later stages of pregnancy. The baby is, however, of near normal size, making Caesarean section mandatory.

Anaesthetic problems

1. The larynx is smaller than normal, and its size is related to patient weight rather than to age (Mayhew et al 1986). Intubation problems have been reported due to premature fusion of the bones at the base of the skull. However, in a series of 36 patients (Mayhew et al 1986), no intubation difficulty was experienced.
2. Intravenous access may be a problem, particularly in the infant, due to lax skin and subcutaneous tissues.
3. Sleep apnoea has been reported due to foramen magnum stenosis.
4. Technical difficulties caused by skeletal defects can be experienced during regional anaesthesia (Walts et al 1975). The risk of accidental dural puncture is increased by the narrow epidural space. As neurological problems also often develop spontaneously during the third and fourth decades, such approaches might be better avoided.
5. Neurosurgical operations. Twenty-four patients with achondroplasia undergoing craniectomies were reviewed (Mayhew et al 1986). Out of 16, whose surgery was performed in the sitting position, nine had some degree of air embolism, whereas only one operated on in the prone position had such a problem. The air was usually successfully aspirated, and no patient died. Six other major complications occurred – two patients

had C1 level spinal cord infarction, two had brachial plexus palsies, and one was accidentally extubated. The sixth, after developing severe oedema of the tongue, required tracheostomy. The cause was thought to be extreme flexion of the neck producing venous thrombosis (Mayhew et al 1985).

6. Anaesthesia for Caesarean section may compound all these problems. The supine position in later pregnancy can be associated with severe aortocaval compression and respiratory embarrassment. Successful anaesthetics using both general and epidural techniques have been described (Cohen 1980).

Management

1. It has been suggested that if the sitting position is used, great care should be taken to avoid air embolus (Katz & Mayhew 1985, Mayhew et al 1986). However, no patient died in the series presented. In addition, the prone position may be associated with heavy blood loss, and does not guarantee freedom from air embolism. Whatever position is chosen, air embolism must be anticipated, diagnosed early, and a means of air aspiration be readily available.

2. Possible intubation difficulties should be considered during assessment. A range of endotracheal tubes, of sizes smaller than normal, should be available.

3. Particular care is needed when positioning the patient. Upper limbs should be well supported, and extreme neck flexion avoided.

4. In labour, aortocaval compression must be prevented.

5. Prior to Caesarean section, blood gases should be estimated to assess respiratory function.

BIBLIOGRAPHY

Cohen S E 1980 Anesthesia for Cesarean section in achondroplastic dwarfs. Anesthesiology 52: 264–266
Katz J, Mayhew J F 1985 Air embolism in the achondroplastic dwarf. Anesthesiology 63: 205–207
Mayhew J F, Miner M, Katz J 1985 Macroglossia in a 16 month old child following a craniotomy. Anesthesiology 62: 683–684
Mayhew J F, Katz J, Miner M, Leiman B C, Hall I D 1986 Anaesthesia for the achondroplastic dwarf. Canadian Anaesthetists' Society Journal 33: 216–221
Walts L F, Finerman G, Wyatt G M 1975 Anaesthesia for dwarfs and other patients of pathological small stature. Canadian Anaesthetists' Society Journal 22: 703–709

ACROMEGALY

A rare chronic disease of insidious onset which usually presents in middle life. An increased secretion of growth hormone, most commonly by an adenoma of the eosinophil cells of the pituitary, results in an overgrowth of bone, connective tissue and viscera.

Preoperative abnormalities

1. The head, tongue, jaw, hands and feet are enlarged. Facial features are coarse, and the voice husky.
2. Kyphoscoliosis, muscular weakness, nerve entrapment syndromes, hypertension, acromegalic heart disease (10%), goitre, diabetes mellitus (10–20%), diabetes insipidus, hypercalcaemia, and visual field defects may be present.
3. Enlargement of the sella turcica may be evident on skull X-ray in 90% of cases.
4. Muscle weakness may occur.

Anaesthetic problems

1. Four types of airway problem may present (Southwick & Katz 1979):
    a. Difficulty in obtaining an airtight fit with the mask.
    b. Difficulty in visualizing the larynx – often due to massive hypertrophy of the pharyngeal mucosa.
    c. Difficulty in passing an endotracheal tube due to glottic stenosis or fixation of the vocal cords.
    d. Postintubation, or postoperative obstruction.
Extensive calcification (chondrocalcinosis) of the larynx may also occur (Edge & Whitwam 1981), and decreased cricoid width has been reported (Hassan et al 1976).
2. Increased daytime somnolence and sleep apnoea have been described. Central depression of respiration may be compounded by the residual effects of anaesthetic drugs and result in severe postoperative hypoxia, hypercarbia or respiratory arrest (Kitahata 1971, Ovassapian et al 1981). Sudden deaths, which sometimes occur on return to the ward, may be explicable by a combination of these factors and respiratory obstruction.
3. Hypertension and ischaemic heart disease are frequently present.
4. Acute pulmonary oedema occurring secondary to upper airway obstruction (Goldhill et al 1982).
5. Impaired ulnar artery circulation has been noted in 5 out of 10 acromegalic patients undergoing hypophysectomy (Campkin 1980).

Management

1. Airway problems must be anticipated in advance and a careful history should be directed towards this. X-rays of the neck may indicate overgrowth of pharyngeal tissue, glottic stenosis or chondrocalcinosis. Indirect larygoscopy may be helpful. Airway abnormalities in acromegaly may be classified (Southwick & Katz 1979) as:
    a. No involvement.
    b. Hypertrophied nasal and pharyngeal mucosa, but normal cords.
    c. Glottic stenosis or vocal cord paresis.
    d. Combination of both (b) and (c).

In the presence of either (c) or (d), and especially if there is sleep apnoea, elective tracheostomy should be considered. Intubation, using a fibreoptic bronchoscope, has been claimed to obviate the need for tracheostomy (Venus 1980, Ovassapian et al 1981, Messick et al 1982). However, one patient in whom tracheostomy was avoided, required emergency reintubation on three occasions in the postoperative period – twice for airway obstruction and once for respiratory arrest (Ovassapian et al). Fibreoptic techniques may have transformed the management of difficult intubation as such, but in acromegalics the airway problems are not restricted to the intraoperative period, nor are they solely of a technical nature.

2. Postoperatively, acromegalics should be admitted to an intensive care unit, where respiration and blood gases can be carefully monitored.

3. Ulnar collateral circulation should be tested prior to radial artery cannulation. If doubt exists as to its adequacy, the dorsalis pedis should be used.

BIBLIOGRAPHY

Campkin T V 1980 Radial artery cannulation. Potential hazards in patients with acromegaly. Anaesthesia 35: 1008–1009
Edge W G, Whitwam J G 1981 Chondrocalcinosis and difficult intubation in acromegaly. Anaesthesia 36: 677–680
Goldhill D R, Dalgleish J G, Lake R H N 1982 Respiratory problems and acromegaly. Anaesthesia 37: 1200–1203
Hassan S Z, Matz G J, Lawrence A M, Collins P A 1976 Laryngeal stenosis in acromegaly: a possible cause of airway difficulties associated with anesthesia. Anesthesia and Analgesia 55: 57–60
Kitahata L M 1971 Airway difficulties associated with anaesthesia in acromegaly. British Journal of Anaesthesia 43: 1187–1190
Messick J M, Cucchiara R F, Faust R J 1982 Airway management in patients with acromegaly. Anesthesiology 56: 157
Ovassapian A, Doka J C, Romsa D E 1981 Acromegaly – use of fiberoptic laryngoscopy to avoid tracheostomy. Anesthesiology 54: 429–430
Southwick J P, Katz J 1979 Unusual airway difficulty in the acromegalic patient – indications for tracheostomy. Anesthesiology 51: 72–73
Venus B 1980 Acromegalic patient-indication for fiberoptic bronchoscopy but not tracheostomy. Anesthesiology 52: 100–101

ADDICTION

(see also ALCOHOLISM, AMPHETAMINE ABUSE, COCAINE ABUSE, LSD ABUSE, OPIATE ADDICTION, SOLVENT ABUSE)

The incidence of drug addiction is increasing. Anaesthesia may be required for addicts in either an acute or a chronic state of intoxication. Hazards exist not only for the patient, but for staff in the hospital. Accidental rupture of drug packages concealed in body cavities may result in severe acute absorption.

Individual drugs are dealt with separately, but the following comments are generally applicable.

Anaesthetic problems

1. Increased risk of hepatitis B and HIV.
2. Increased risk of septicaemia, bacterial endocarditis and tetanus, in intravenous drug users.
3. Problems associated with chronic abuse.
4. Problems of acute toxicity.
5. Difficulties with venepuncture.
6. Problems of withdrawal syndrome during a period of illness.
7. Difficulties in obtaining an accurate history.
8. Malnutrition and liver disease.

General management

1. In general, drugs should not be withdrawn in the perioperative period.
2. Patients should be treated as if they were infected with hepatitis B virus.
3. An addiction centre may provide information and advice.

BIBLIOGRAPHY

Caldwell T B 1981 Anesthesia for patients with behavioral and environmental disorders. In: Anesthesia and uncommon diseases. Saunders, Philadelphia
McCammon R L 1986 Anesthesia for the chemically dependent patient. International Anesthesia Research Society Review Course Lectures 47–55
McGoldrick K E 1980 Anesthetic implications of drug abuse. Anesthesiology Review 7: 12–17

ADDISON'S DISEASE
(ADRENOCORTICAL INSUFFICIENCY) (See also Section 4)

Chronic adrenocortical insufficiency is due to a variety of causes. In the commonest form (idiopathic), adrenal autoantibodies are found, and other endocrine deficiencies may be demonstrated. Tuberculosis, secondary carcinoma, and amyloidosis are other causes. Clinically apparent disease occurs only after a 90% loss of adrenocortical tissue. In the majority of patients, Addison's disease will present in a chronic form, and therefore may be difficult to diagnose. Collapse due to classical acute adrenocortical failure is only rarely seen. However, as surgery and anaesthesia are both potent stress factors which require an increased steroid output, this deficiency may become apparent under these circumstances.

Acute adrenocortical insufficiency following sudden withdrawal of long-term steroid therapy, is always a potential problem (Weatherill & Spence 1984).

Preoperative abnormalities

1. Addison's disease can present with weight loss, weakness, infertility,

emotional instability, abdominal pain, and pigmentation of skin and mucous membranes.

2. In mild cases there may be a normochromic, normocytic anaemia, leucocytosis, eosinophilia and a low normal plasma cortisol.

3. In severe cases, hormone output may be undetectable. The characteristic metabolic changes of hyponatraemia, hyperkalaemia, hypoglycaemia, hypercalcaemia and an elevated urea will be present. ECG may be of low voltage with flattening of ST segments. Hypotension or cardiovascular collapse may occur.

Anaesthetic problems

1. A previously undiagnosed Addisonian crisis may be a rare cause of cardiovascular collapse during surgery and anaesthesia (Salam & Davies 1974, Smith & Byrne 1981, Hertzberg & Schulman 1985).
In the majority of these, the diagnosis was made only in retrospect, saline, glucose and steroids having formed part of the general resuscitation of the collapsed patient. Subsequent confirmation of this diagnosis in such patients is potentially hazardous, as withdrawal of the exogenous steroids to test adrenocortical function may put the patient at risk. The author has personal knowledge of a case in which collapse first occurred during anaesthesia for investigation of infertility. Resuscitation with steroids and antibiotics was successful but during the later investigation to exclude Addison's disease, steroids were withdrawn, and sudden death followed. Postmortem examination showed adrenal tuberculosis. This danger can be minimized by the administration of dexamethasone which does not interfere with plasma cortisol estimation (see below).

2. Drugs given during anaesthesia may modify a patient's response to stress.
Etomidate may adversely affect pituitary-adrenal function (Owen & Spence 1984). Increased death rates from infection were reported in patients having intravenous etomidate for sedation in intensive care. Prolonged infusions were shown to produce reversible suppression of adrenocortical response, due to mitochondrial enzyme inhibition. The effect and clinical significance of a single dose of etomidate, or an infusion limited to the duration of anaesthesia alone, is under debate (Owen & Spence 1984, Yeoman et al 1984, Boidin 1986).

Management

1. If the diagnosis is suspected preoperatively, and some adrenal reserve remains, the plasma corticosteroids will tend to be in the low normal range. A plasma cortisol of >600 nmol/l excludes Addison's disease, but a low normal does not prove it, therefore, for confirmation, a stimulation test will be required:

1

Short tetracosactrin test

09.00 a.m.   10 ml heparinized blood for plasma cortisol estimation.
Tetracosactrin 250 μg i.m. given.

09.30 a.m.   Blood taken for plasma cortisol.

Results

Normal: Base-line >200 nmol/l. At 30 minutes an increase of at least 300 nmol/l above this.

Addison's: Low base-line. At 30 minutes, a less than 150 nmol/l increase in response to stimulation.

Normally, no steroids should be administered for 3 days prior to this test. However, if steroids have been given under emergency circumstances, then they should be changed to dexamethasone 0.5 mg b.d. 24 hours before the test starts. Dexamethasone does not register in plasma cortisol assays. An ACTH assay will demonstrate an inappropriate high level in primary adrenocortical insufficiency.

2. Treatment of an Addisonian crisis.

a. Infuse 0.9% saline 1 litre rapidly, then more slowly.

b. Hydrocortisone (hemisuccinate or sodium phosphate) 100 mg i.v. then 6-hourly.

c. Correct hypoglycaemia, if present.

3. Maintenance therapy for Addison's disease.

a. Hydrocortisone 20 mg morning and 10 mg evening, or prednisolone 5 mg morning and 2.5 mg evening.

b. Fludrocortisone acetate 0.1 mg daily is required for primary, but not for secondary hypoadrenalism.

(For equivalent dosages of different steroids, see Section. 2: Corticosteroids)

BIBLIOGRAPHY

Boidin M P 1986 Can etomidate cause an Addisonian crisis? Acta Anaesthesiologica Belgica 37: 165–170

Hertzberg L B, Schulman M S 1985 Acute adrenal insufficiency in a patient with appendicitis during anesthesia. Anesthesiology 62: 517–519

Owen H, Spence A A 1984 Etomidate. British Journal of Anaesthesia 56: 555–557

Salam A A, Davies DM 1974 Acute adrenal insufficiency during surgery. British Journal of Anaesthesia 46: 619–622

Smith M G, Byrne A J 1981 An Addisonian crisis complicating anaesthesia. Anaesthesia 36: 681–684

Weatherill D, Spence A A 1984 Anaesthesia for disorders of the adrenal cortex. British Journal of Anaesthesia 56: 741–749

Yeoman P M, Fellows I W, Byrne A J, Selby C 1984 The effect of anaesthetic induction using etomidate upon pituitary-adrenocortical function. British Journal of Anaesthesia 56: 1291–1292

AIDS
(Acquired Immune Deficiency Syndrome)

A spectrum of disease thought to be caused by infection with a retrovirus, HIV. This may lead to a chronic condition of lymphadenopathy, fever, weight loss and diarrhoea, or to a state of cellular immune deficiency and the development of unusual malignancies or opportunistic infections. It is most common in the homosexual and drug-taking communities, but is found in haemophiliac patients who have received infected blood products prior to antibody screening and heat treatment of Factor VIII concentrates. Some individuals may be carriers, but the full significance of this state and its natural history is not yet known. The virus is transmitted by body fluids, particularly blood and semen, but it would appear that a breach in either skin or mucosa is necessary for infection to occur. Saliva or airborne transmission, where there is intact mucosa, has not yet been demonstrated, but neither has it been disproved. It is probably less infectious than hepatitis B, and present surveys indicate that the risks to health workers are low unless accidental inoculation has occurred (Lee & Soni 1986). However, the recent appearance of this potentially fatal disease has meant that epidemiological studies are, as yet, incomplete. The most recent literature should be consulted. Guidelines for anaesthetists has been produced by the Association of Anaesthetists (1988).

Preoperative abnormalities

1. The patient may either be HIV antibody positive, or show signs of the disease.
2. The neurological manifestations include dementia, peripheral neuropathy, radiculopathy and cranial nerve palsies. Five AIDS patients, one of whom died, had vasovagal episodes associated with lung biopsy. Subsequent investigation suggested a diagnosis of autonomic dysfunction (Craddock et al 1987).
3. The commonest opportunistic infection is *Pneumocystis carinii* pneumonia, but candidal, tuberculous and viral pneumonias occur.
4. Side effects of treatment with antiviral agents may be severe. Zidovudine (Retrovir, AZT) may cause megaloblastic anaemia and neutropenia. It is theoretically possible that interaction with nitrous oxide could occur (Phillips & Spence 1987). Neurological complications of the drug may be difficult to distinguish from those of the disease.

Anaesthetic problems

1. The problems of anaesthesia in the presence of lung disease.
2. Autonomic neuropathy may cause cardiovascular instability.
3. The possibility of transmission of the virus to health-care workers exists, although this is rare (Greene 1986a). Eight health-care workers who had either received a needle stick injury, or who had suffered from dermatitis, were reported as being HIV positive (Weiss 1985).
4. The problems of disposal of contaminated material and the sterilization of equipment.
5. About 20% of patients with AIDS develop parapareses associated

1

with vacuolar degeneration of the spinal cord, and as many as one third develop encephalitis (Greene 1986b). The advisability of spinal and epidural anaesthesia has therefore been questioned.

Management

1. The same precautions should be taken as for hepatitis B. Gown, gloves, mask and eye protection should be worn during anaesthesia. Blood spillage should be avoided. Disposal of needles in a tough disposal bin, without resheathing, is crucial. They should not be passed from one person to another. Care should be taken not to spread blood, sputum or saliva during intubation and extubation. In San Francisco, the problems of identifying each individual HIV carrier has prompted such precautions to be employed for all patients (Arden 1988). In the UK, the wearing of gloves at least is being recommended for all anaesthetics (Association of Anaesthetists 1988).
2. Equipment should be disposable or sterilizable. The virus is destroyed by both heat and chemicals. Reusable equipment should be scrubbed with detergent solution and decontaminated by soaking in glutaraldehyde or sodium hypochlorite solution. Nursing staff should wear goggles during cleaning of equipment. Steam or gas sterilization is also reported to be effective (Arden 1988).

    a. Ventilators. Although HIV infection is not airborne, the use of disposable circuitry and bacterial filters is advisable.

    b. Blood gas machines. The introducer port should be syringed through with 1% sodium hypochlorite and left for 5 minutes. This is followed by two wash cycles and recalibration.

    c. Surfaces should be cleaned with sodium hypochlorite.
3. Only urgent laboratory investigations likely to influence management should be contemplated, to reduce risk to laboratory personnel. Sterilization of any instrument used for the analysis of contaminated blood is mandatory.
4. In view of the poor prognosis, the wisdom of instituting IPPV for respiratory failure should be considered carefully.
5. Before administering regional anaesthesia, a neurological assessment should be performed. Local anaesthetic techniques may be contraindicated if parapareses are already present.

BIBLIOGRAPHY

Arden J 1988 Managing patients with AIDS – update. Anesthesiology 68: 164–165
Association of Anaesthetists 1988 AIDS and hepatitis B. Guidelines for Anaesthetists
Craddock C, Pasvol G, Bull R, Protheroe A, Hopkin J 1987 Cardiorespiratory arrest and autonomic neuropathy in AIDS. Lancet ii: 16–18
Greene E R 1986a AIDS: an overview for anesthesiologists. Anesthesia and Analgesia 65: 1054–1058
Greene E R 1986b Spinal and epidural anesthesia in patients with the acquired immunodeficiency syndrome. Anesthesia and Analgesia 65: 1090–1091

Lee K G, Soni N 1986 AIDS and anaesthesia. Anaesthesia 41: 1011–1016
Phillips A J, Spence A A 1987 Zidovudine and the anaesthetist. Anaesthesia 42: 799–800
Weiss S H 1985 HTLV-III infections among health care workers. Association with needle
    stick injuries. Journal of the American Medical Association 254: 2089–2093

AIR EMBOLISM
(see Section 4)

ALCOHOLISM

Alcoholism has been defined as excessive drinking which results in
impairment of both the subject's health and social activities. If surgical
treatment is required, then three main problems must be considered:

1. The effect of the numerous metabolic and endocrine changes which
occur in longstanding alcoholics.
2. Whether there is acute alcohol toxicity in addition to the above.
3. The problems of alcohol withdrawal, which can occur at any time
between 8 hours and 5 days after abstention.

Preoperative abnormalities

1. Haematological effects. The MCV exceeds 93 fl in 85% of heavy
drinkers. Bone marrow depression can occur, and if liver function is
impaired there may be coagulation defects.
2. Biochemical. Blood alcohol levels:
     80 mg/dl – legal limit for driving (UK)
     200 mg/dl – severe intoxication.
  >400 mg/dl – stupor.
  >500 mg/dl – frequently fatal.
Electrolyte disturbances, particularly hypokalaemia, may exacerbate
delirium tremens.
3. Liver function. Gamma-glutamyltransferase and the
aminotransaminases may be abnormal and the albumin low. Plasma
cholinesterase activity is normal unless hepatic damage is severe. There
may be impaired glucose tolerance after alcohol, followed by
hypoglycaemia occurring between 6 and 24 hours after acute ingestion.
4. Cardiac disease. A dilated cardiomyopathy may occur, and can be
associated with dyspnoea, heart failure, conduction defects, bifid T
waves, digitalis-like ST segments and arrhythmias.
5. Central nervous system effects of Wernicke's disease and Korsakoff's
psychosis and epileptic fits.
6. A peripheral neuropathy may be produced by the combined effect of
alcohol and malnutrition.

1

Anaesthetic problems

1. Acute alcohol toxicity and electrolyte imbalance.
2. Coagulation abnormalities.
3. Possible presence of a full stomach and delayed gastric emptying.
4. Delirium tremens or lesser withdrawal symptoms.
5. Impaired liver metabolism and cirrhosis.
6. Decreased adrenocortical response to stress.
7. Malnutrition and vitamin deficiencies.
8. Dilated cardiomyopathy and arrhythmias.
9. The presence of, or bleeding from, oesophageal varices (Cello et al 1986).
10. Peripheral or autonomic neuropathy.

Management

1. If acute alcohol toxicity is present, then surgery should be delayed if possible (Bruce 1983). Alcohol levels above 250 mg/dl increase surgical morbidity. Correction of dehydration should be tempered by the knowledge that diuresis occurs mainly while the blood alcohol level is rising. Beware of fluid overload. Hypokalaemia may precipitate delirium tremens. Hypoglycaemia may occur 6–24 hours after intake. If i.v. glucose is required, thiamine should be given concurrently.
2. An i.v. preparation of vitamins B and C, such as Parentrovite, is given.
3. Coagulation abnormalities, if present, should be treated with vitamin K1, fresh frozen plasma or platelets.
4. Thiopentone is avoided if a cardiomyopathy is present or there is hypoalbuminaemia. Atracurium is the relaxant of choice if liver function is impaired. Postoperative jaundice frequently occurs several days after operation, irrespective of the anaesthetic agent used. This is due to defective processing of old red blood cells by an impaired liver. The use of halothane is therefore best avoided. A more rational choice would be either enflurane or isoflurane, as they undergo less liver metabolism.
5. Analgesics should be used with caution, and only for pain. Dependence can readily occur.
6. Alcohol withdrawal can be treated with alcohol or chlormethiazole infusions, or benzodiazepines i.v.
   a. Alcohol may be appropriate when surgery is actually required during the phase of withdrawal symptoms. A preoperative infusion of 8% ethanol in isotonic saline at a rate of 0.5 g/kg over 15 minutes is given (Edwards 1985).
   b. Chlormethiazole edisylate 0.8% soln, 320–800 mg (40–100 ml) over 5–10 minutes, then the rate is adjusted. *Note*: Chlormethiazole is dangerous in severe liver disease, or when a patient is acutely intoxicated with alcohol. Severe respiratory depression can result from the combination (McInnes 1987).

c. Delirium tremens can be treated with midazolam 2.5 mg, using additional increments up to a maximum of 10 mg. Diazepam is used in increments up to a total dose of 20 mg.

7. An existing peripheral neuropathy is a contraindication to regional anaesthesia.

8. In the presence of cirrhosis, gastrointestinal bleeding may precipitate hepatic failure. Nasogastric tubes should be inserted cautiously in case oesophageal varices are present.

BIBLIOGRAPHY

Bruce D L 1983 Alcoholism and anesthesia. Anesthesia and Analgesia 62: 84–96.
Cello J P, Crass R A, Grendell J H, Trunkey D D 1986 Management of the patient with hemorrhaging esophageal varices. Journal of the American Medical Association 256: 1480–1484.
Edwards R (ed) 1985 Anaesthesia and alcohol. British Medical Journal 291: 423–424.
Edwards R, Mosher V B 1980 Alcohol abuse, anaesthesia and intensive care. Anaesthesia 35: 474–489.
McInnes G T 1987 Chlormethiazole and alcohol. British Medical Journal 294: 592.

ALDOSTERONISM, PRIMARY
(see CONN'S SYNDROME)

AMNIOTIC FLUID EMBOLISM

Entry of amniotic fluid into the maternal circulation is a rare cause of collapse or sudden haemorrhage in labour or immediately postpartum. The fluid, which contains electrolytes, nitrogenous compounds, lipids, prostaglandins and fetal elements such as squames, hairs, vernix and meconium, enters the maternal venous plexuses via a tear in the amniotic membranes. Fluid entering the pulmonary vascular tree is likely to cause vascular obstruction, pulmonary hypertension and hypoxia, due to ventilation perfusion defects, and cardiac failure. Circulating amniotic fluid has thromboplastic activity and the entry of a significant amount is usually associated with disseminated intravascular coagulation. Abnormal fibrinolysis may occur in addition. There is a mortality in excess of 80% and the diagnosis is often made at postmortem. The condition is largely unpreventable.

Presentation

1. A review of 272 cases (Morgan 1979) showed that 90% occurred during labour, and that 88% were in multiparous patients. Presenting symptoms were respiratory distress with cyanosis (51%), cardiovascular collapse (27%), convulsions (10%), haemorrhage (12%). Associated features can include coagulation abnormalities, coma and pulmonary oedema (Lumley et al 1979, Mainprize & Maltby 1986). Bronchospasm is rare.

2. The onset is often dramatic.

3. One fatal case presented with an asymptomatic fall in oxygen saturation, measured by pulse oximetry, during Caesarean section under epidural anaesthesia (Quance 1988).

Diagnosis

1. Initially, this is made on clinical grounds. The primary concern is that of resuscitation of the collapsed patient; 25% will be dead within the first hour. Of those who survive for more than an hour, the incidence of DIC is 40% (Morgan 1979).

2. The diagnosis may be confirmed if fetal squames are seen on sputum examination, or by the finding of amniotic fluid in a blood sample taken from a CVP line or a pulmonary artery catheter (Shah et al 1986).

Treatment

1. Cardiovascular collapse or even cardiac arrest, may be the initial event. Cardiopulmonary resuscitation is instituted. Hypoxia is treated with oxygen and, if necessary, IPPV and PEEP.

2. Circulatory support with inotropic agents may be required, but needs careful monitoring. In a severe case, in which haemodynamic monitoring was used, left and right heart failure, with high pulmonary wedge and central venous pressures, and a 35% shunt were found (Moore et al 1982). Nitroglycerin has been used to reduce pulmonary artery pressure in a patient who developed amniotic fluid embolism during Caesarean section (Shah et al 1986).

3. Replacement of blood volume may be needed for haemorrhage. Treatment of any bleeding diathesis will require repeated clotting screens and specialist haematological advice. In general, whole blood is followed by fibrinogen 2 g and then the tests are repeated.

4. If there is evidence of massive DIC, then the use of heparin may be considered. Again, haematological advice should be sought.

BIBLIOGRAPHY

Lumley J, Owen R, Morgan M 1979 Amniotic fluid embolism. A report of three cases. Anaesthesia 34: 33–36
Mainprize T C, Maltby J R 1986 Amniotic fluid embolism: a report of four probable cases. Canadian Anaesthetists' Society Journal 33: 382–387
Morgan M 1979 Amniotic fluid embolism. Anaesthesia 34: 20–32
Moore P G, James O F, Saltos N 1982 Severe amniotic fluid embolism: case report with haemodynamic findings. Anaesthesia and Intensive Care 10: 40–44
Quance D 1988 Amniotic fluid embolism: detection by pulse oximetry. Anesthesiology 68: 951–952
Shah K, Karlman R, Heller J 1986 Ventricular tachycardia and hypotension with amniotic fluid embolism during Cesarean section. Anesthesia and Analgesia 65: 533–535

AMPHETAMINE ABUSE

Amphetamines are sympathomimetic amines, which, in the initial stages of intoxication, elevate the mood and increase alertness, thus reducing the need for sleep. They act both directly and indirectly on the sympathetic nervous system, via the peripheral nerve endings. Catecholamines are released within the CNS, and there is prevention of catecholamine re-uptake by adrenergic nerve endings. Tolerance readily occurs. Amphetamine abusers often use other drugs in addition.

Preoperative abnormalities

1. The patient may be suffering from acute toxicity. Initially signs of irritability, with tremor, dilated pupils and sweating may be displayed. Increasing doses cause tachycardia, fever and mild hypertension, with agitation and confusion. Delirium, rising blood pressure, hyperpyrexia and the onset of arrhythmias, precede convulsions, coma and death.
2. In chronic abuse there may be marked tolerance.

Anaesthetic problems

1. Studies on dogs have shown that MAC values for halothane were altered by both acute and chronic amphetamine intake (Johnston et al 1972). Acute intoxication resulted in an increased MAC for halothane, whereas chronic abuse for 7 days decreased the MAC for halothane. Dogs subjected to chronic abuse had a poor response to indirectly acting sympathetic agents.
2. Hazards in anaesthesia, particularly for Caesarean section in chronic amphetamine abusers, have been reported (Samuels et al 1979, Smith & Gutsche 1980). In one patient, a longstanding heroin and amphetamine abuser, epidural anaesthesia was established with lignocaine 2% 10 ml. After transfer to theatre, two successive doses of 12 ml and 6 ml of chloroprocaine 3% did not extend the block, and it was assumed that the catheter had become displaced. General anaesthesia was induced with thiopentone 200 mg and suxamethonium. Cardiac arrest occurred soon after surgery began. Resuscitation with adrenaline, bicarbonate and isoprenaline proved successful. On recovery, the patient admitted to taking amphetamines just prior to admission. It was postulated that chronic users of amphetamines do not respond to stress and may develop a type of autonomic dysfunction. Another patient, also a chronic amphetamine abuser, developed hypotension, tachycardia and peripheral vasoconstriction intraoperatively, for which 500 ml colloid and 1300 ml crystalloid was given. After extubation, pulmonary oedema developed and IPPV, with PEEP, was required for 8 hours. Her rapid recovery was felt to be consistent with the diagnosis of hydrostatic pulmonary oedema, rather than gastric inhalation or septicaemia.

3. Arrhythmias may occur, particularly in the presence of agents which sensitize the heart to the effects of catecholamines (McGoldrick 1980).
4. There may be delayed recovery from anaesthesia (McCammon 1986).

Management

1. A careful history should be taken in an attempt to establish the presence of acute or chronic abuse. Denial or concealment may occur (Samuels et al 1979). Urinary estimations of amphetamines and their metabolites can be performed, but this facility is not usually available in the acute situation.
2. Rehydration may be required when toxicity is present, particularly in those who are pyrexial.
3. ECG, core temperature and blood pressure should be monitored from the induction of anaesthesia.
4. In cases of acute intoxication, chlorpromazine has been recommended. Benzodiazepines are reported as being suitable for the chronic abuser (Caldwell 1981).
5. The management of hypertension may require the use of alpha blockers. Because of its longer action, diazoxide 300 mg (or 5 mg/kg) may be more appropriate than phentolamine (Caldwell 1981).
6. Halothane should be avoided in the presence of amphetamines.
7. Direct-acting vasopressors are recommended to treat hypotension in the chronic abuser (Johnston et al 1972).

BIBLIOGRAPHY

Caldwell T B 1981 Anesthesia for patients with behavioral and environmental disorders. In: Anesthesia and uncommon diseases. Saunders, Philadelphia
McCammon R L 1986 Anesthesia for the chemically dependent patient. International Anesthesia Research Society Review Course Lectures 47–55
McGoldrick K E 1980 Anesthetic implications of drug abuse. Anesthesiology Review 7: 12–17.
Samuels S I, Maze A, Albright G 1979 Cardiac arrest during Cesarean section in a chronic amphetamine abuser. Anesthesia and Analgesia 58: 528–530.
Smith D S, Gutsche B B 1980 Amphetamine abuse and obstetrical anesthesia. Anesthesia and Analgesia 59: 710–711.

AMYLOIDOSIS

Amyloidosis is a general term for a variety of different disease processes involving the deposition of fibrillary material in tissues. This is formed of protein subunits sharing a common beta-pleated sheet structure, but derived from proteins of great chemical diversity. These fibrils are resistant to normal proteolytic digestion and share a common histochemical staining property to Congo red. In the light of advances in the understanding of the structural chemistry of amyloid, the old terms primary and secondary have been replaced (Glenner 1980).

1. Immunocytic (including myeloma associated) amyloidosis predominantly involves mesenchymal tissue. This results in neuropathies, carpal tunnel syndrome, macroglossia, a restrictive cardiomyopathy (90% of cases), skin, gut and kidney lesions.
2. Reactive amyloidosis can occur in association with chronic infective, inflammatory and neoplastic disorders. The most common include rheumatoid arthritis, tuberculosis, Still's, Crohn's and Hodgkin's diseases, ankylosing spondylitis and renal cell carcinoma. Parenchymal tissue tends to be primarily involved, particularly in the kidneys, liver, spleen and thyroid. In over 50% of cases the heart is affected, but less severely so than in the immunocytic form.

Preoperative abnormalities
1. Cardiac involvement may present with a digitalis-resistant heart failure, arrhythmias, and conduction defects.
2. Unusual skin lesions, bullae or non-thrombocytopenic purpura feature in 40% of cases with the immunocytic disease. Macroglossia is common. Neurological lesions may affect any type of nerve including those of the autonomic system.
3. The reactive form may present with the nephrotic syndrome, renal failure, hepatosplenomegaly, adrenal failure or lung disease.
4. Amyloidosis should be suspected when a patient presents with multiple organ involvement. Confirmation is by biopsy of an affected organ. Rectal biopsy is diagnostic in 90% of cases of systemic amyloid.
5. Bleeding occurs frequently, although coagulation studies may be normal. Amyloid infiltration of the blood vessels may be the cause (Yood et al 1983). In a series of 100 patients, 41 had one or more bleeding episodes, three of which resulted in death.

Anaesthetic problems
1. Cardiac failure or arrhythmias may produce hypotension during anaesthesia. Resistant heart failure developed after general anaesthesia for cystoscopy, in a patient who had unusual skin petechiae. The diagnosis of amyloidosis was made subsequently, and death occurred on the 15th postoperative day (Welch 1982).
2. Macroglossia, common in the immunocytic form, may pose difficulties with intubation and potential postoperative airway obstruction.
3. Extreme fragility of the skin may occur. In one patient, haemorrhagic rashes and frank bleeding occurred at all the sites where ECG electrodes and adhesive tape had been placed (Dixon 1987).
4. Coagulation studies are unreliable predictors of the likelihood of bleeding. Of 41 patients who bled, only 20% had an abnormal

1

prothrombin time. Bleeding can follow mild trauma and may require surgical intervention. The gastrointestinal tract was the source in 18, a further eight bled after diagnostic procedures and three had haematuria. Coagulation tests were normal in all eight who bled after diagnostic procedures (Yood et al 1983).

5. In the reactive form, the additional problems are those of the primary associated disease, e.g. rheumatoid arthritis.

Management

1. The diagnosis should be suspected in a patient who has multiple organ involvement, especially in the presence of a disease known to be associated with the reactive form.

2. Careful assessment of the heart, lungs and liver for impairment of function is important. Anaesthetic management should be directed appropriately.

3. Difficulties in intubation should be anticipated in the presence of macroglossia. Postoperatively, the patient should be nursed in an intensive recovery area.

4. Coagulation studies should be performed. A normal result does not guarantee that haemorrhage will not occur.

BIBLIOGRAPHY

Dixon J 1987 Primary amyloidosis and skin damage. Anaesthesia 42: 218
Glenner G G 1980 Amyloid deposits and amyloidosis. New England Journal of Medicine 302: 1283–1292, 1333–1343
Welch D B 1982 Anaesthesia and amyloidosis. Anaesthesia 37: 63–66
Yood R A, Skinner M, Rubinow A, Talarico L, Cohen A S 1983 Bleeding manifestations in 100 patients with amyloidosis. Journal of the American Medical Association 249: 1322–1324

AMYOTROPHIC LATERAL SCLEROSIS
(see MOTOR NEURONE DISEASE)

ANKYLOSING SPONDYLITIS

An inflammatory arthropathy of insidious onset. Granulation tissue infiltrates the bony insertions of ligaments and joint capsules, and the disease progresses variably to fibrosis, ossification and ankylosis. The primary sites of involvement are the sacroiliac joints and the spine, but 50% of patients will have extraspinal joint involvement at some time. It is a systemic disorder and a proportion of the patients will develop non-articular manifestations of the inflammatory process.

Preoperative abnormalities

1. Bone and joints
   a. The inflammatory process usually begins at the sacroiliac joints and spreads upwards to involve the spine and costovertebral joints. A limitation of chest expansion to 2.5 cm or less is one of the criteria contributing to the clinical diagnosis. Ossification of interspinous ligaments and the formation of bony bridges between vertebrae occur in the lumbar spine, while cervical spine involvement varies from a degree of limitation of movement of the neck, to complete ankylosis. Those with advanced disease have an increased risk of sustaining a cervical fracture.
   b. Temporomandibular joint involvement is reported to cause limited mouth opening in 10% of patients, but in longstanding disease the incidence may be as high as 30–40%. Sometimes this progresses to complete ankylosis.
   c. Cricoarytenoid arthritis occurs rarely. Dyspnoea, hoarseness and vocal cord fixation may be present.
2. Non-articular disease
   a. Systemic effects, such as fatigue, weight loss, fever, a high ESR and hypochromic anaemia often occur.
   b. 35% of patients have uveitis, and 85% of male patients have prostatitis at some stage of the disease.
   c. Cardiovascular complications have been reported in 3.5% of patients with a 15-year history, and in 10% of patients having had the disease for 30 years. Scarring of the adventitia and fibrous proliferation of the intima of the aorta and the valve cusps produce aortitis and aortic insufficiency, and occasionally mitral valve disease. Purkinje tissue involvement may result in conduction defects. Occasionally patients present with complete heart block and yet have minimal skeletal symptoms (Bergfeldt et al 1982).
   d. Pulmonary disease may occur. Upper lobe fibrosis is a well-recognized complication. The seriousness of any pulmonary complication will be accentuated by the limited chest expansion.
   e. Neurological effects are protean. Spinal cord compression, cauda equina syndrome, focal epilepsy, vertebrobasilar insufficiency and peripheral nerve lesions have all been described. In addition there is an increased risk of mild trauma causing cervical fractures (Murray & Persellin 1981).

Anaesthetic problems

1. Cervical spine involvement may increase the difficulties of intubation. Forcible neck movements in the presence of muscle relaxation should be avoided because of the possible risk of cervical fracture, or

vertebrobasilar insufficiency. Death from a retropharyngeal abscess, the result of repeated attempts at blind intubation, has been recorded (Hill 1980).

2. Temporomandibular joint involvement may add to intubation difficulties. Ankylosis of this joint further complicating a case of massive haematemesis has been described (Sinclair & Mason 1984).

3. Respiratory problems and limited chest wall expansion increase the pulmonary complication rate and hence the need for postoperative ventilation.

4. Aortic valve disease and conduction defects can occur.

5. Spinal anaesthesia is technically difficult.

6. Epidural and caudal anaesthesia may be contraindicated, if intubation is potentially difficult. Technical difficulties may also increase the risk of complications. Convulsions due to accidental intraosseous injection of bupivacaine 20 ml, during an attempted caudal block (Weber 1985), and a spinal haematoma following epidural analgesia (Gustafsson et al 1988) are recorded.

7. There is a high incidence of gastrointestinal bleeding following treatment with non-steroidal anti-inflammatory agents.

8. External cardiac massage is ineffective in patients with a rigid chest wall.

Management

1. Neck movements should be assessed with radiological screening. If there is limitation, and the patient has a full set of teeth, then intubation difficulties should be anticipated. In such cases, an awake intubation is the safest option. A fibreoptic bronchoscope has been used to perform nasal intubation in a patient whose upper lip was pressed against her chest wall (Ovassapian et al 1983). In this particular case, tracheostomy would have been impossible. However, in some circumstances, for example, surgery for active haematemesis, preliminary tracheostomy under local anaesthesia may be the technique of choice (Sinclair & Mason 1984). In cases where intubation is potentially difficult, epidural and caudal anaesthesia are contraindicated.

2. An ECG is mandatory and cardiovascular complications should be treated appropriately.

3. A cervical support should be used during anaesthesia, especially if there are signs of vertebrobasilar insufficiency.

4. If the vertebrobasilar circulation is compromised, and general anaesthesia absolutely contraindicated, spinal anaesthesia may be possible using radiological control, a 19 gauge needle and the assistance of an orthopaedic drill or hammer.

5. After major surgery, a short period of postoperative ventilation may be required and an admission to an ITU advisable.

BIBLIOGRAPHY

Bergfeldt L, Edhag O, Vedin L, Vallin H 1982 Ankylosing spondylitis. An important cause of severe disturbances of the cardiac conduction system. American Journal of Medicine 73: 187–191
Gustafsson H, Rutberg H, Bengtsson M 1988 Spinal haematoma following epidural analgesia. Anaesthesia 43: 220–222
Hill C M 1980 Death following dental clearance in a patient suffering from ankylosing spondylitis. British Journal of Oral Surgery 18: 73–76
Murray G C, Persellin R H 1981 Cervical fracture complicating ankylosing spondylitis. American Journal of Medicine 70: 1033–1041
Ovassapian A, Land P, Schafer M F, Cerullo L, Zalkind M S 1983 Anesthetic management for surgical corrections of severe flexion deformity of the cervical spine. Anesthesiology 58: 370–372
Sinclair J R, Mason R A 1984 Ankylosing spondylitis. The case for awake intubation. Anaesthesia 39: 3–11
Weber S 1985 Caudal anaesthesia complicated by intraosseous injection in a patient with ankylosing spondylitis. Anesthesiology 63: 716–717

AORTIC REGURGITATION
(INCOMPETENCE)

Regurgitation of blood from the aorta into the left ventricle during diastole may be due to aortic cusp distortion (rheumatic heart disease), cusp perforation (bacterial endocarditis) or to dilatation of the aortic ring (Marfan's syndrome, aortic dissection, connective tissue diseases, etc).

The volume of blood regurgitated depends on the extent of the incompetence, the aortic/left ventricular pressure gradient during diastole, and the diastolic time. The regurgitated volume is added to that entering from the left atrium, so that both left ventricular hypertrophy and dilatation occur. Left ventricular volume overload occurs in a ventricle which is initially distensible, and in some cases the stroke volume may be increased to over 20 l/min. Later the myocardium becomes stiffer, the LVEDP rises, premature mitral valve closure may occur and cardiac failure finally supervenes. Symptoms may appear late, and do not correlate well with the severity of regurgitation or myocardial depression.

Acute lesions, usually in association with endocarditis, may occasionally occur. In these cases of rapid onset, the haemodynamic situation is very different from that in the chronic disease, and many of the signs associated with the chronic lesion are absent.

Preoperative abnormalities

1. Symptoms do not correlate well with signs. Initially reduced exercise tolerance and dyspnoea occurs. Later there are signs of congestive cardiac failure. Chest pain may occur in advanced disease as diastolic coronary artery flow is impaired and coronary flow may be limited to systole.

2. The signs are a large volume, rapid upstroke, collapsing pulse (high systolic, low diastolic), a precordial left ventricular impulse and an early diastolic murmur, maximum on expiration, at the left sternal edge.

3. Increasing left ventricular hypertrophy and cavity dilatation can lead to gross cardiomegaly on CXR, and increased left ventricular voltages with repolarization abnormalities on ECG.

4. The left ventricle is initially compliant, with a large stroke volume and a low LVEDP. Finally, when myocardial structural changes take place, the ejection fraction falls and failure occurs, with signs of increased pulmonary venous pressure, a third heart sound and pulmonary inspiratory crackles.

Anaesthetic problems

These largely depend upon the severity of the regurgitation, and the presence or absence of myocardial failure. In mild or moderate regurgitation there are usually no problems. In the severe case, risks may be high. Anaesthesia can acutely disturb compensatory mechanisms. Factors which oppose these compensatory mechanisms may produce pulmonary oedema, reduced forward cardiac output and myocardial ischaemia.

1. There are significant pathophysiological differences between acute and chronic aortic regurgitation.

In chronic disease, compensation is accomplished by hypertrophy and dilatation of the left ventricle and a reduction in peripheral resistance. A tachycardia prevents overdistension of the ventricle in diastole. Initially, the left ventricle is compliant, and left ventricular filling pressures alter relatively little with volume changes. In these cases, vasoconstriction is likely to increase the regurgitant volume.

In acute lesions however, the normal-sized left ventricle has only a limited capacity for distension, and life-threatening pulmonary oedema occurs early. Compensation for the fall in stroke volume and cardiac output is in part achieved by peripheral vasoconstriction and tachycardia. In such cases, the effect of anaesthetic techniques which produce peripheral vasodilatation is potentially disastrous. A death occurred during epidural anaesthesia for Caesarean section, in a patient who presented with previously undiagnosed aortic regurgitation, systolic and diastolic hypertension and increasing cardiac failure (Alderson 1987).

2. A bradycardia is disadvantageous. It allows overdistension of the ventricles, a rise in left atrial pressure and pulmonary congestion.

3. Inhalation agents may worsen myocardial depression.

Management

1. Mild or moderate regurgitation requires a careful anaesthetic, avoiding volume depletion, myocardial depression and bradycardia.

1

Antibiotic cover should be given. Both regional and general anaesthesia are well tolerated.

2. If there is evidence of decompensation, a detailed cardiological assessment is required. In addition, the differentiation between acute and chronic aortic regurgitation is crucial for the management of the severe case. In either case there may be sensitivity to changes in peripheral vascular resistance.

3. Agents which depress myocardial contractility are avoided.

4. Bradycardia is prevented and a fairly fast heart rate maintained. Pancuronium has been suggested as a suitable agent for producing a mild tachycardia.

5. With severe disease, haemodynamic monitoring is essential. This will enable the effects of drug and fluid therapy to be monitored closely. The response to acute events cannot always be predicted. In the case of chronic aortic regurgitation, vasodilators and sometimes inotropic agents, may be required. The use of epidural anaesthesia, or a drug with mild alpha adrenergic blocking effects, such as droperidol, has been recommended to reduce afterload. Adequate preload must first be achieved.

In acute aortic regurgitation however, techniques which produce an uncontrolled fall in peripheral resistance must be avoided.

6. Catastrophic pulmonary oedema requires intensive therapy. A dilating inotrope such as dobutamine, a reduction of left atrial pressure with diuretics and vasodilators such as glyceryl trinitrate or nitroprusside, and IPPV, may all be required (Stone et al 1980).

BIBLIOGRAPHY

Alderson J D 1987 Cardiovascular collapse following epidural anaesthesia for Caesarean section in a patient with aortic incompetence. Anaesthesia 42: 643–645.
Stone J G, Hoar P F, Calabro J R, DePetrillo M A, Bendixen H H 1980 Afterload reduction and preload augmentation improve the anesthetic management of patients with cardiac failure and valvular regurgitation. Anesthesia and Analgesia 59: 737–742.

AORTIC STENOSIS

Aortic stenosis may be valvular, subaortic or supravalvular. The normal area of the valve is 3 cm^2. Symptoms and signs appear when the area is reduced to about 0.8 cm^2. Unlike hypertension, in which the resistance to left ventricular function is variable and depends upon the state of the peripheral vasculature, the resistance to ejection of blood by the left ventricle in aortic stenosis is fixed. A pressure gradient occurs across the valve. This is increased on tachycardia and exercise. In order to overcome the obstruction, left ventricular hypertrophy occurs and this is associated with a loss of compliance, and without an increase in cavity size. Stroke volume is therefore limited. Ventricular dilatation only occurs in the late stages, or when the valve becomes incompetent. The dangerous feature of this condition is that signs and symptoms appear late in the disease. Once they occur, the prognosis poor. A pulse pressure of <30 mmHg reflects severe disease. Conversely, if systolic blood pressure is >180 mmHg, the disease is not significant. In older patients, coronary artery disease may contribute to symptoms and cardiac dysfunction. Significant aortic stenosis in patients over 40 (a systolic ejection murmur of at least grade II–VI) was identified as a risk factor for life-threatening and fatal cardiac complications in non-cardiac surgical procedures (Goldman et al 1977).

Preoperative abnormalities

1. The onset of symptoms occurs relatively late in the disease and includes dyspnoea, intolerance of exertion, angina and syncope. LVEDP is raised and the occurrence of pulmonary oedema on exertion may be the first sign of decompensation.
2. The pulse is slow rising and of decreased amplitude. There is an ejection systolic murmur, maximal in the aortic area and radiating into the right side of the neck.
3. CXR initially shows normal cardiac size. Left atrial enlargement and dilatation of the aortic root may be seen later.
4. In the presence of significant stenosis, the ECG usually shows left ventricular hypertrophy, but not always. The diagnosis should be considered in elderly patients with LVF. In failure, when the cardiac output is low, the murmur is soft or absent.
5. Sudden death may occur.
6. The diagnosis is rapidly made by echocardiography, and Doppler studies give the pressure gradients.

Anaesthetic problems

In symptomatic aortic stenosis, a number of factors will alter the haemodynamic state and disturb compensatory mechanisms. One or more of the following problems may result.

1. Myocardial ischaemia. The hypertrophied myocardium is very vulnerable to ischaemia. Prolonged tachycardia, hypotension or hypovolaemia may produce myocardial ischaemia. At low heart rates there is an inability to increase stroke volume.
2. Fall in cardiac output. Precipitated by hypovolaemia, myocardial depressants, bradycardias, peripheral vasodilatation and atrial arrythmias.
3. Pulmonary oedema. Interference with atrial function by arrythmias or fluid overload, causes cardiac decompensation.
4. Decreased cerebral blood flow.
5. Resuscitation from a state of asystole is very difficult and once this state is achieved, the prognosis poor.

Management

Management of the symptomatic patient requires careful monitoring with the insertion of an arterial line and CVP. Some authors recommend PAP in addition. All anaesthetic drugs must be given with caution, and therapeutic manoeuvres, such as fluid loading and treatment of adverse heart rates, must be performed with particular care, to avoid wide swings in cardiovascular pressures and myocardial oxygen supply.

1. If the condition is symptomatic, cardiological advice should be obtained. Aortic valve replacement or a balloon valvuloplasty may be more important than the proposed operation.
2. Control of heart rate.
Slow rhythms are treated with atropine and atrial arrhythmias are prevented. Atrial fibrillation with decompensation may be an indication for cardioversion.
3. Prevention of hypotension.
Induction must be slow. High concentrations of myocardial depressants, such as halothane and enflurane, are avoided, and the vascular volume maintained. The exact method of anaesthesia is probably less important than the care with which it is administered and the patient monitored. In the presence of outflow obstruction, a regional technique is probably less controllable than a general anaesthetic. However, opinions vary. Inotropes may be needed.
4. Precordial ECG lead is observed for evidence of myocardial ischaemia.
5. Prophylaxis against SBE.
6. Should cardiac arrest occur, effective cardiac massage can only be obtained after opening the chest.

BIBLIOGRAPHY

Goldman L, Caldera D L, Nussbaum S B et al 1977 Multifactorial index of cardiac risk in non cardiac surgical procedures. New England Journal of Medicine 297: 845–850

APUDOMAS

A group of tumours of neuroectodermal origin, whose cells have common cytochemical characteristics. The name arises from their ability to handle certain amines (Amine Precursor Uptake and Decarboxylation). They can secrete a wide variety of peptides or amine products, a number of which have anaesthetic significance. This section enumerates the differing types of tumour, the normal and ectopic hormones which have been attributed to them, and some of their actions (Whitwam 1977, Bouloux 1987, Weatherill 1988). For specific syndromes reported as having anaesthetic significance, see under the individual names.

1

Tumour	Normal hormones	Some ectopic hormones
Bronchial carcinoid and oat cell carcinoma	(5HT)	ACTH, ADH, MSH, VIP glucagon, calcitonin, insulin, prolactin, GH
Chemodectoma	noradrenaline, dopamine	calcitonin, ACTH
Ganglioneuro-blastoma		noradrenaline, VIP
Gastrointestinal carcinoid	gastrin, VIP, glucagon, enteroglucagon	ADH, ACTH, MSH
Islet cell adenoma	insulin, glucagon, PP	ACTH, MSH, ADH, VIP
Paraganglioma	(adrenaline, noradrenaline, 5HT)	ACTH, MSH, VIP
Phaeochromocytoma	adrenaline, dopamine, noradrenaline	ACTH, insulin
Pituitary adenoma	GH, prolactin, LH, ACTH, MSH	
Thymoma		calcitonin, ACTH
Thyroid medullary carcinoma	calcitonin (5HT)	ACTH, MSH, insulin

Hormones, abbreviations and actions

ACTH:	adrenocorticotrophic hormone – hypokalaemic alkalosis, oedema, pigmentation, diabetes.
ADH:	antidiuretic hormone – water retention, hyponatraemia leading to confusion and fits.
Adrenaline:	intermittent hypertension, headache, sweating and palpitations.
Calcitonin:	Regulates plasma calcium; decreases bone absorption, increases renal calcium and phosphate excretion. Increased calcitonin secretion occurs in thyroid medullary carcinoma, but plasma calcium is usually normal.
Gastrin:	Gross gastric acid hypersecretion, peptic ulceration.
Glucagon:	Hyperglycaemia unresponsive to insulin, weight loss, migratory skin rash, anaemia.
GH:	Growth hormone – acromegaly, hypertension, impaired glucose tolerance.
5HT:	5-hydroxytryptamine – diarrhoea, intermittent hypertension and tachycardia, hyperglycaemia, possibly flushing.
Insulin:	Hypoglycaemic attacks. Often diagnosed as fits, faints, hysteria, drunkenness.
LH:	Luteinizing hormone – ovulatory control and spermatogenesis.
MSH:	Melanocyte stimulating hormone – pigmentation.
Noradrenaline:	Sustained hypertension, headache, sweating and palpitations.
PP:	Pancreatic polypeptide – inhibits pancreatic exocrine secretion, relaxes gall bladder.
Prolactin:	Amenorrhoea, galactorrhoea and infertility.
VIP:	Vasoactive intestinal peptide: watery diarrhoea, hypokalaemia , hypochlorhydria and hypotension.

BIBLIOGRAPHY

Bouloux P-M 1987 Multiple endocrine neoplasia. Surgery 1: 1180–1185.
Weatherill D 1988 Anaesthesia, APUDomas and multiple endocrine neoplasia. Surgery 60: 1437–1439
Whitwam J G 1977 APUD cells and the apudomas. A concept relevant to anaesthesia and endocrinology. Anaesthesia 32: 879–888.

ARTHROGRYPOSIS

Not a distinct entity, but rather a symptom complex, in which there is congenital stiffness of joints, most probably due to immobility of limbs in utero (Dubovitz 1978). The primary cause may be a myopathy or muscle dystrophy, a neurological disorder, or even oligohydramnios. One case occurred after the mother had received tubocurarine in the tenth week of pregnancy for the treatment of tetanus. The joint rigidity is fibrous, not bony, and most marked in distal joints. Frequently the arms are rotated internally and the hips externally, sometimes with dislocation. Talipes and flexion deformities of the wrists are common. Both contractures and muscle atrophy occur secondary to immobility.

Preoperative abnormalities

1. Although the postural deformities are similar, the underlying lesion, and hence the individual prognosis, is very different.
2. EMG and muscle biopsy will distinguish neuropathic from myopathic and dystrophic conditions, and also from the congenital fibre-type disproportion.

Anaesthetic problems

1. This is controversial. An increased incidence of MH has been postulated, but the evidence for this is largely anecdotal. In only one case were the MH criteria convincing (Baudendistel et al 1984). The likelihood of this association was also challenged in a review of 67 patients with arthrogryposis who had undergone a total of 398 anaesthetics (Baines et al 1986). No evidence could be found that an MH episode had occurred in any of them. However, few of the anaesthetic papers have discussed the specific origin of each case of arthrogryposis. It is therefore possible that an MH-like episode could occur in those forms of arthrogryposis associated with congenital muscle dystrophy, but not in the other associated conditions.
2. Severe deformities may cause difficulties in intubation.

Management

1. Elucidation of the cause of the condition may be helpful, if only for the future resolution of anaesthetic risk factors. Conduction studies and EMG may assist in this.
2. Since the risk of MH is unproven, it is suggested that the use of halothane in these patients is justified when alternative agents may place the child at an even greater risk (Baines et al). Certainly, monitoring for the early detection of MH must be impeccable and the means of its

treatment immediately available. A child with an arthrogryposis of myopathic origin requiring a pyelolithotomy, and whose CPK was 880 iu/l, had an uneventful anaesthetic when ketamine and pancuronium were used (Oberoi et al 1987).

BIBLIOGRAPHY

Baines D B, Douglas I D, Overton J H 1986 Anaesthesia for patients with arthrogryposis multiplex congenita. What is the risk of malignant hyperpyrexia? Anaesthesia and Intensive Care 14: 370–372
Baudendistel L, Goudsouzian N, Cote C, Strafford M 1984 End-tidal CO_2 monitoring. Its use in the diagnosis and management of malignant hyperthermia. Anaesthesia 39: 1000–1003
Dubovitz V 1978 Arthrogryposis multiplex congenita. In: Muscle disorders in childhood. Saunders, Philadelphia
Oberoi G S, Kaul H L, Gill I S, Batra R K 1987 Anaesthesia in arthrogryposis multiplex congenita: case report. Canadian Journal of Anaesthesia 34: 288–290

ASTHMA

A condition of hyperreactivity of the tracheobronchial tree, in which a number of exogenous and endogenous stimuli can produce reversible airway obstruction. Histamine and the leukotrienes (LT) are thought to be the most active chemical mediators, while acetylcholine may contribute via a disturbance in autonomic balance (Galant 1987). As obstruction worsens, increasingly smaller airways are affected. Expiration is prolonged, residual volume and functional residual capacity are increased, while vital capacity, inspiratory capacity and expiratory reserve volume are reduced. Widespread ventilation perfusion inequalities may occur to produce hypoxia, at a time when the work of breathing is considerably increased. In addition to bronchospasm, the pathological changes include oedema of the bronchial mucosa, secretion of mucus and epithelial desquamation.

For a more detailed description see Kingston and Hirshman (1984).

Preoperative abnormalities

1. There may be a history of wheezing, dyspnoea, cough, and sputum production. The chest may be hyperresonant and the breath sounds diminished, with prolonged expiration and an audible wheeze. In very severe cases the wheeze disappears.
2. Medication may include parasympatholytics, theophylline derivatives, beta adrenergic stimulants, sodium cromoglycate and steroids.
Increasingly, medication is being given in aerosol form to reduce systemic side-effects.
3. CXR may show an increase in bronchovascular markings and hyperinflation, in the later stages, some degree of emphysema. In the acute case a CXR is essential to exclude pneumothorax.

4. An FEV_1 of less than 1 litre, or an FEV_1/VC ratio of less than 40% and a raised $PaCO_2$, may all indicate the need for postoperative IPPV. A PEFR of less than 120 l/min and an MVV of less than 50% of the predicted level also indicate severe obstruction.
5. There may be an improvement in pulmonary function tests and blood gases after administration of bronchodilators.

Anaesthetic problems

1. An increased incidence of postoperative pulmonary complications.
2. During light anaesthesia there is an increased sensitivity to airway manipulations. Intubation may produce acute bronchospasm. In a computer-aided incidence study of 136 929 anaesthetics, it was found that bronchospasm was usually triggered by mechanical stimuli (Olsson 1987).
3. Cardiac arrhythmias can occur more frequently in the presence of hypoxia and acidosis, or following the overuse of sympathomimetic agents. Sudden spontaneous deaths in asthmatics have been attributed to the combination of nebulized high dose beta$_2$ sympathomimetics and long-acting theophylline derivatives.
4. Halothane can interact with aminophylline to produce serious arrhythmias, even when theophylline levels are within the therapeutic range. This combination was suggested to have been the cause of ventricular fibrillation (Stirt & Sternick 1982) and ventricular tachycardia (Roizen & Stevens 1978). The xanthines are beta adrenergic stimulators which release noradrenaline and inhibit the breakdown of cyclic AMP.
5. Inhalational agents may worsen ventilation perfusion inequalities and increase hypoxia, by reducing hypoxic pulmonary vasoconstriction.
6. Perioperative steroid cover is advisable if steroids have been used within the previous year.
7. In severe cases, postoperative IPPV may be required. It does, however, carry a high risk of complications such as pneumothorax, cardiac arrhythmias, pneumonia and heart failure.

Management

1. Elective surgery should not take place in the presence of infection or untreated bronchospasm. Preoperative preparation will include physiotherapy, bronchodilators, antibiotics and an assessment of the likelihood of the need for IPPV in the postoperative period.
2. Anxiety is often a feature of the asthmatic patient. Care and understanding should be shown at the preoperative visit, and a sedative premedication, such as an antihistamine, is advantageous. The potential seriousness of this disease must not be underestimated.
3. Despite a drying effect on secretions, atropine may be desirable for a smooth induction. It can also improve dilatation in the larger bronchi by blocking vagal constrictor effects. Although pethidine has been

promoted as a bronchodilator, it has recently been shown to be a more common cause of histamine release than morphine. Even when bronchospasm is absent, some form of preoperative bronchodilator therapy is advisable.

4. Even when attacks are infrequent, endotracheal intubation is one of the commonest causes of intraoperative bronchospasm in patients who have any history of asthma. The carina is particularly sensitive to stimulation. Before intubation, it is wise to deepen anaesthesia or apply a local anaesthetic to the vocal cords. There is experimental evidence that reflex bronchospasm is prevented by i.v. lignocaine, but not that due to the release of allergic mediators (Downes et al 1980).

5. Ketamine has been suggested to be a suitable induction agent for emergency anaesthesia in asthmatics, when a rapid sequence induction is required (Hirshman et al 1979). A comparison with thiopentone in dogs showed it to have a protective effect against bronchospasm, which was abolished by beta adrenergic blockers.

6. Halothane, enflurane and isoflurane are all effective at reversing antigen-induced bronchospasm (Hirshman et al 1982). However, halothane sensitizes the heart to the effect of exogenous and endogenous catecholamines. It also interacts with aminophylline to produce arrhythmias, so isoflurane may be the most appropriate choice.

7. Treatment of acute bronchospasm.

　a. If this occurs following intubation, the easiest initial manoeuvre is to try and deepen the anaesthetic using an inhalation agent.

　b. Residual bronchospasm is treated with aminophylline, 5 mg/kg over a period of 10–15 min. If necessary, an infusion of 0.5 mg/kg/h is started. Plasma theophylline levels must be estimated if treatment is prolonged for more than 24 hours. The therapeutic range is 10–20 mg/l but toxic effects such as fits, arrhythmias and cardiac arrest have been described with plasma levels as low as 25 mg/l. Extreme caution is necessary if the patient has already been taking sustained-release theophylline preparations.

　c. Salbutamol infusion, 5 μg/min (5 ml of 1 mg/ml soln added to 500 ml 0.9% saline to give a final concentration of 10 μg/ml).

8. Indications for IPPV in asthmatics

　a. Distress and exhaustion.

　b. Deterioration in arterial blood gases. PaO_2 <6.7 kPa or $PaCO_2$ >6.7 kPa, and increasing metabolic acidosis.

　c. Cardiac arrhythmias or hypotension.

　d. Acute crises such as cardiorespiratory arrest, decreased conscious level due to sedatives, or a collapsed lung.

9. Technique of IPPV in asthmatics.

Inotropes should be available at intubation. Patients should be underventilated and therefore muscle relaxants may be required. Provided life-threatening hypoxia is avoided, it is unnecessary to aim for normal blood gases. Take care to prevent hyperinflation.

BIBLIOGRAPHY

Downes H, Gerber N, Hirshman C A 1980 I.v. lignocaine in reflex and allergic
bronchoconstriction. British Journal of Anaesthesia 52: 873–878
Galant S P 1987 Anaesthesia and asthma. In: Anaesthesia review 4. Churchill Livingstone,
Edinburgh
Hirshman C A, Downes H, Farbood A, Bergman N A 1979 Ketamine block of bronchospasm
in experimental canine asthma. British Journal of Anaesthesia 51: 713–718
Hirshman C, Edelstein G, Peetz S, Wayne R, Downes H 1982 Mechanisms of action of
inhalational agents on airways. Anesthesiology 56: 107–111
Kingston H G G, Hirshman C A 1984 Perioperative management of the patient with asthma.
Anesthesia and Analgesia 63: 844–855
Olsson G L 1987 Bronchospasm during anaesthesia. A computer-aided incidence study of
136, 929 patients. Acta Anaesthesiologica Scandinavica 31: 244–252
Roizen M F, Stevens W C 1978 Multiform ventricular tachycardia due to the interaction of
aminophylline and halothane. Anesthesia and Analgesia 57: 738–741
Stirt J A, Sternick C S 1982 Aminophylline and anesthesia. Anesthesiology 57: 252–253

'ATHLETE'S HEART'

A name given to certain cardiac and ECG changes found in some athletes,
and which most probably represent physiological adaptations of the heart
to endurance sports. When these cardiac abnormalities occur, the main
problem is to differentiate them from pathological heart disease.

Preoperative abnormalities

The patients are usually of an age group, and a degree of fitness, which
would not routinely justify a preoperative ECG. However, an unduly
slow, and sometimes irregular pulse may lead an observant physician to
perform one. The ECG may show large voltages and tall T waves, with
dilatation and hypertrophy of the left ventricle. A sinus bradycardia will
be found in the majority of cases. There may be a range of depolarization
abnormalities including nodal escape, first- and second-degree heart block,
right bundle branch block or ST-segment abnormalities (Pedoe 1983).

Anaesthetic problems

The major problem is that of diagnosis. There have been reports of fit
young patients presenting with unexpected episodes of arrhythmias or
conduction defects during anaesthesia (Bullock & Hall 1985, Abdulatif
et al 1987). The first problem is to exclude causes such as hypercarbia,
hypoxia, inhalational agents, the response to surgical stimuli and the use
of vasoconstrictors. The second is to be aware of rarer causes of
arrhythmias such as malignant hyperpyrexia, solvent abuse, ankylosing
spondylitis, sarcoidosis, mitral valve prolapse and cardiomyopathies.

Management

1. If the pathological abnormalities have been excluded, then treatment is not necessarily indicated. Recent reports have confirmed that patients with 'athlete's heart' remain haemodynamically stable during anaesthesia, and the conduction defects respond to atropine.

2. It is essential that such patients are not labelled as having a pathological cardiac condition. If doubt persists, referral to a cardiologist who is known to be aware of the condition, is advised. Extensive invasive investigations will not usually be appropriate. Unlike patients with coronary artery disease, these individuals should not show progressive abnormalities with exercise ECGs. Echocardiography may demonstrate an increase in left ventricular wall and cavity size, by as much as 20% above the normal for the size of patient.

BIBLIOGRAPHY

Abdulatif M, Fahkry M, Naguib M, Gyamfi Y-A, Saeed I 1987 Multiple electrocardiographic anomalies during anaesthesia in an athlete. Canadian Journal of Anaesthesia 34: 284–287.
Bullock R E, Hall R J C 1985 Athletic dysrhythmias. A case report. Anaesthesia 40: 647–650
Pedoe D T 1983 Sports injuries. Cardiological problems. British Journal of Hospital Medicine 29: 213–220

AUTONOMIC FAILURE

Failure, or dysfunction, of the autonomic nervous system is being increasingly recognized as a complication of a number of disease processes. In familial dysautonomia (Riley–Day syndrome), there is a decrease in all the neuronal populations, as well as a decrease in synthesis of noradrenaline. Dysfunction may be secondary to diabetes, Guillain–Barré syndrome, Parkinson's disease, Shy–Drager syndrome, tetanus, AIDS, postcerebrovascular states, alpha-blocking drugs, and the peripheral neuropathy of amyloid disease.

Autonomic dysfunction can be central or peripheral in origin, and may affect sympathetic or parasympathetic nerves. While autonomic failure will produce widespread disturbance of organ function, it is the cardiovascular and respiratory effects which are of particular concern to the anaesthetist.

Preoperative abnormalities

1. Patients exhibit orthostatic hypotension, and an inability, in response to stress, to produce the normal pressor response which depends on reflex vasoconstriction and tachycardia. There is reversal of the usual diurnal pattern of blood pressure and also of that normally produced by postural changes. A number of clinical features of autonomic dysfunction have been described.

a. Postural hypotension. The blood pressure rises when in the supine position at night, and falls on standing. A fall in the systolic blood pressure of 30 mmHg, on standing, is significant.

b. Abnormal blood pressure response to the Valsalva manoeuvre. This manoeuvre involves taking a maximum inspiration, blowing into a tube connected to a mercury manometer, and elevating the mercury level to 40 mmHg for 10 seconds. A slow blow-off valve in the system requires the subject to blow continuously to maintain the pressure. Four phases of response are described in normal individuals:

    i. A rapid rise in arterial pressure immediately after the onset of straining, as the intrathoracic pressure is added to systemic arterial pressure.

    ii. A fall in blood pressure, with an associated tachycardia due to diminished venous return. Some restoration in pressure occurs later in this phase.

    iii. Following the release in straining, there is a sudden brief reduction in pressure.

    iv. Finally there is a terminal elevation of pressure above control values, associated with a bradycardia. The release of the Valsalva manoevre restores venous pressure and cardiac output at a time when the peripheral vessels are still constricted. The arterial pressure rises above normal, the baroreceptors are stimulated, and a bradycardia occurs until the pressure returns to its normal value.

As a patient with autonomic failure cannot respond with vasoconstriction, the blood pressure continues to fall during the Valsalva manoeuvre. There is no overshoot in blood pressure when the straining is released, with a gradual return to normal. No tachycardia or bradycardia occurs.

In clinical practice this has been difficult to demonstrate without direct arterial monitoring (Brown 1987). However a technique, in which a pulse oximeter is linked to a chart recorder, is now available to show this (Broome & Mason 1988).

2. The R–R variation on the ECG is lost, and there are no heart rate changes on taking six deep breaths.

3. Fluid and electrolyte homeostasis is disturbed, resulting in a failure to concentrate urine at night. There is a nocturnal diuresis and sodium loss (Watson 1987).

Anaesthetic problems

1. Hypotension. Blood pressure is extremely sensitive to changes in extracellular fluid volume, and hypotension may occur on induction of anaesthesia.

2. Arrhythmias and unexpected cardiac arrest have been described.

3. Respiratory arrest and diminished sensitivity to hypoxia and hypercarbia have been reported (Page & Watkins 1978).

4. The response to catecholamines is variable (Stirt et al 1982). In central dysfunction, the response to indirect-acting catecholamines is normal, and there is no sensitivity to those acting directly. With peripheral dysfunction, there may be lesser response to indirect-acting catecholamines, but an exaggerated (denervation hypersensitivity) response to those acting directly.

Management

For the problems of the individual diseases, see Diabetes, Familial dysautonomia, Shy–Drager Syndrome, Guillain–Barré Syndrome, Tetanus, etc. It is important to realize that autonomic dysfunction exists to varying degrees. It is not an all or none phenomenon (Ewing & Clarke 1986).

1. Good management lies in the anticipation of possible problems, close patient monitoring, and the minimization of cardiovascular changes by judicious fluid and drug therapy.
2. ECG and blood pressure should be monitored from the outset of the anaesthetic.
3. All drugs should be given with caution. Hypotension may require treatment with a fluid load and intropic agents.
4. The patient should be ventilated, or respiration closely monitored, particularly in the postoperative period.

BIBLIOGRAPHY

Broome I J, Mason R A 1988 Identification of autonomic dysfunction with a pulse oximeter. Anaesthesia 43: 833–836
Brown M J 1987 The measurement of autonomic function in clinical practice. Journal of the Royal College of Physicians 21: 206–209
Ewing D J, Clarke B F 1986 Autonomic neuropathy: its diagnosis and prognosis. Clinics in Endocrinology and Metabolism 15: 855–888
Page M McB, Watkins P J 1978 Cardiorespiratory arrest and diabetic autonomic neuropathy. Lancet i: 14–16
Stirt J A, Frantz R A, Gunz E F, Connolly M E 1982 Anesthesia, catecholamines and hemodynamics in autonomic dysfunction. Anesthesia and Analgesia 61: 701–704
Watson RDS (ed) 1987 Treating postural hypotension. British Medical Journal 294: 390–391

BUDD–CHIARI SYNDROME

A syndrome caused by obstruction to the hepatic venous outflow. It may be secondary to haematological disorders, malignancy, oral contraceptives, heart failure or constrictive pericarditis. The site of the obstruction may be anywhere from the inferior vena cava to the smaller hepatic veins. The condition may be acute or chronic. Surgery may be required (Gupta et al 1986).

1

Preoperative abnormalities

1. Ascites and hepatomegaly will be present in the majority of cases. Abdominal pain, splenic enlargement or jaundice also occur. When the vena cava is involved there will be dependent oedema.
2. Liver function abnormalities depend on the site and severity of the obstruction.

Anaesthetic problems

1. Hepatic function may be compromised.
2. Surgery may be required for portacaval shunt. This has been described in a patient with paroxysmal nocturnal haemoglobinuria (Taylor et al 1987).

BIBLIOGRAPHY

Gupta S, Blumgart L H, Hodgson H J F 1986 Budd–Chiari syndrome: Long-term survival and factors affecting mortality. Quarterly Journal of Medicine 60: 781–791
Taylor M B, Whitwam J G, Worsley A 1987 Paroxysmal nocturnal haemoglobinuria. Perioperative management of a patient with Budd–Chiari syndrome. Anaesthesia 42: 639–642

BUERGER'S DISEASE

A type of occlusive peripheral vascular disease which occurs predominantly in young men. There is a marked association with smoking. The disease primarily affects small vessels of the feet, legs and hands, and is exacerbated by vasospasm. The aetiology is not fully understood but may have an immunological component. Abnormal responses to type I and III collagen have been demonstrated. The intense inflammation of the early stages progresses to fibrous encasement of the whole neurovascular bundle.

Preoperative abnormalities

1. Raynaud's disease, non-healing ulcers or gangrene of the feet may occur, even in the presence of femoral and popliteal pulses. The hands may be similarly affected. Frequently there is preceding or accompanying phlebitis.
2. Peripheral pulses are reduced or absent. Allen's test may show a poor collateral circulation to the hand.

Anaesthetic problems

1. Intra-arterial cannulation for blood pressure monitoring is not usually recommended, and indirect Doppler methods are advised. However, in

major procedures there may be overriding indications for direct pressure measurements.

2. Analgesia may be needed for peripheral ischaemia.

Management

1. Axillary artery pressure monitoring in a patient with Buerger's disease and an intracranial aneurysm has been described (Yacoub et al 1987). A continuous axillary brachial plexus block weas established prior to cannulation of the axillary artery with a 20 G catheter. Care was taken to maintain the patient's core temperature with a warming blanket and there was minimal reduction in arterial pressure during clipping of the aneurysm.

2. Continuous local anaesthesia via a silastic catheter inserted in the region of the median nerve has been reported (Saddler & Crosse 1988).

BIBLIOGRAPHY

Saddler J M, Crosse M M 1988 Ischaemic pain in Buerger's disease. Anaesthesia 43: 305–306.
Yacoub O F, Bacaling J H, Kelly M 1987 Monitoring of axillary arterial pressure in a patient with Buerger's disease requiring clipping of an intracerebral aneurysm. British Journal of Anaesthesia 59: 1059–1062.

BURNS

For the anaesthetist who is only occasionally involved in the management of patients with thermal injury, two particular aspects are likely to be of concern:

1. The immediate resuscitation of the patient prior to transfer to a specialist unit.

2. The surgical treatment of a previously burned patient at some time after the original incident.

Presenting problems

1. Loss of water, solutes and albumin from the damaged area. The amount will depend upon the area and thickness burned and the time since injury.

2. Airway and lung problems. These may consist of:

a. Heat injury to the upper respiratory tract with possible mucosal oedema.

b. Systemic carbon monoxide poisoning, which may be fatal.

c. Cyanide poisoning.

d. Chemical damage to the lungs due to acid smoke constituents.

e. Sepsis.

3. Provision of adequate analgesia and sedation, in the presence of altered pharmacodynamics.

4. The stress response to burns. Levels of circulating catecholamines and cortisol are raised and the metabolic rate is increased. There is a high incidence of acute gastric erosions and stress ulcers, which develop within the first 72 hours.

5. Vasoactive mediators, released from the burn, increase vascular permeability and cause cell membrane defects which contribute to intracellular swelling. They may also be involved in the development of the respiratory distress syndrome, which may present as late as the fourth day.

6. Bacterial invasion of the burned tissue.

7. Anaesthesia for surgery at some time after the burn incident, with particular reference to the altered response to neuromuscular blocking agents.

Management

1. Resuscitation

Initially, assessment is directed to the extent and thickness of the burns, in order to calculate colloid and crystalloid replacement. The aim is to maintain cardiac output and renal blood flow, but to minimize oedema of burned and non-burned tissue. In general, fluid replacement is required for burns of >15% in adults and of >10% for children. Established protocols are available and should be used.

Disagreement still exists as to whether colloid or crystalloid should be used. A mixture is probably appropriate (Brown 1985). An estimate of the percentage area burned can be calculated by knowing the approximate normal distribution of surface area : thorax 18%, abdomen 18%, legs 18% each, arms 9% each, and the head 9%. This distribution differs in children and particularly in babies.

A number of methods of calculation have been advocated. In the absence of an established protocol, the following may act as a guide prior to transfer.

A = Colloid	1 ml × % burns × wt in kg
B = Crystalloid	1 ml × % burns × wt in kg
C = Metabolic water requirements	1000 ml, or more if needed

For the first day of burn give:

2A + B + C (half of which should be given in the first 8 hours, the other half in the next 16 hours)

The colloid may be albumin solution, Haemaccel or Gelofusine. The aim is to maintain a normal haematocrit and a urine output of more than 50 ml/h, a pulse of <120/min and a sodium excretion of >30 mmol/l.

2. Respiratory problems.

a. If heat injury has occurred, fibreoptic bronchoscopy may be indicated to establish its extent. Occasionally laryngeal oedema occurs.
b. Carbon monoxide combines with haemoglobin to form carboxyhaemoglobin (HbCO). The affinity of carbon monoxide for haemoglobin is such that a concentration of 0.1% can reduce the oxygen-carrying capacity by 50%, and the oxygen dissociation curve is shifted to the left. On admission, 100% oxygen is given and HbCO estimated (Armstrong 1985).
c. Some fatalities have been noted to have high blood cyanide levels which, although difficult to measure in the acute situation, have been reported to correlate well with HbCO levels. If the latter is raised, cyanide poisoning should be considered.
d. Smoke contains carbon particles, gases and vapours which may cause chemical damage to the alveoli. Respiratory parameters, including blood gases, require close monitoring as deterioration may indicate the onset of pulmonary oedema or acute ARDS. A rising respiratory rate, a PaO_2 of <11 kPa on 40% O_2, and a shunt of more than 15% are indicators of the need for endotracheal intubation and PEEP. Tracheostomy should be avoided if possible. Steroids are ineffective and may increase morbidity and mortality.
3. Pain relief is a problem both in the acute stage and later, during changes of dressings.
a. Opiates may be required acutely before transfer. Although initial studies on burned patients have indicated no difference in the pharmacokinetics of morphine when compared with normal subjects, the narcotic requirements are generally increased (Martyn 1986). Fears of addiction are theoretical. In a large US survey, not a single case was discovered.
  Intravenous analgesia is required initially, and patient controlled analgesia may be helpful.
b. Administration of Entonox (by the patient himself) is useful for dressings, analgesia beginning after 20 seconds, with a peak effect between 40 seconds and 2 minutes.
c. Low-dose ketamine. This has been suggested for short-term pain relief. The use of ketamine 0.1% solution in 5% dextrose, by slow i.v. infusion and adjusted according to effect (Ito & Ichiyanagi 1974), or as an i.m. dose of 0.5 mg/kg (Grant et al 1981), has been reported.
4. Antacids and cimetidine 5–6 mg/kg 6-hourly, are given in the first 24 hours.
5. Suxamethonium is well known to release massive amounts of potassium in burned patients from the 20th to 60th day. There is now evidence that this response may last for up to 2 years. It is suggested that, following burns, instead of being present only at the motor end-plates, acetylcholine receptors spread throughout the whole muscle. Since suxamethonium is structurally similar to acetylcholine, then potassium is released from the whole membrane (Demling 1985). In

addition, resistance to non-depolarising relaxants has been noted. A number of mechanisms may be responsible. Neuromuscular monitoring of these patients is essential.

BIBLIOGRAPHY

Armstrong R F 1985 Burns and the inhalation injury. In: Anaesthesia review 3. Churchill Livingstone, Edinburgh
Brown J M 1985 Aspects of thermal injury. In: Recent Advances in Anaesthesia and Analgesia 15. Churchill Livingstone, Edinburgh
Demling R H 1985 Burns. New England Journal of Medicine 313: 1389–1398
Grant I S, Nimmo W S, Clements J A 1981 Pharmacokinetics and analgesic effects of i.m. and oral ketamine. British Journal of Anaesthesia 53: 805–810
Ito Y, Ichiyanagi K 1974 Postoperative pain relief with ketamine infusion. Anaesthesia 29: 222–229
Martyn J 1986 Clinical pharmacology and drug therapy in the burned patient. Anesthesiology 65: 67–75

CARCINOID SYNDROME
(see also Section 4)

Carcinoids are gastrointestinal tumours which arise from the fore, mid and hind gut. Mid-gut tumours are the commonest, 36–46% occurring in the appendix. Less than 25% of tumours produce the carcinoid syndrome, and the symptoms are probably proportional to the amount of secreting tissue present. Serotonin and the bradykinins are the commonest hormones produced. The majority of patients with the syndrome have liver metastases. Exceptions to this are the tumours from which the venous blood passes directly into the systemic circulation (e.g. bronchial and ovarian). In most cases the liver inactivates the hormones, and no symptoms are produced.

Preoperative abnormalities

1. Serotonin can cause diarrhoea, hypertension and tachycardia, mild hyperglycaemia, hypoproteinaemia and possibly flushing.
2. Bradykinin, if secreted, causes flushing, hypotension, bronchospasm and increased capillary permeability. The latter results in oedema and loss of electrolytes from the vascular compartment. A careful history may help to indicate whether significant amounts of bradykinins are being secreted.
3. Other vasoactive peptides such as histamine and prostaglandins may be involved, but their part in the syndrome has not as yet been elucidated.
4. Preoperative investigations should include the urinary 5-hydroxyindole acetic acid levels, which will be raised, and blood glucose, which may be raised. Liver scan and LFTs may be abnormal, with raised liver enzymes and hypoproteinaemia.
5. In some cases there may be tricuspid or pulmonary valve disease secondary to chronic serotonin secretion.

Anaesthetic problems

A small number of patients with carcinoid syndrome have developed serious cardiovascular complications during anaesthesia, thought to be due to secretion of hormones by the tumour, provoked by mechanical, biochemical or pharmacological stimuli.

1. Serotonin is invariably produced, and if secreted in excess during anaesthesia, is thought to cause hyperkinetic states of hypertension and tachycardia (Casthely et al 1986), certain types of flushing, and prolonged recovery.

2. Bradykinins may or may not be secreted. Their possible effects include hypotension (Marsh et al 1987), due to both vasodilatation and increased capillary permeability, flushing and bronchospasm (Miller et al 1980). The bradykinin effects seem to be the most life threatening.

3. Other vasoactive substances, such as prostaglandins, may be secreted but their significance still requires to be elucidated.

Management

1. Treatment of heart failure and hypoproteinaemia, if present.
2. Antiserotonin therapy.
Preoperative:
EITHER   cyproheptadine 4 mg t.d.s. for 3 days and 4 mg with the premedication.
OR   ketanserin 40 mg b.d. for 3 days (if available).
Intraoperative:
In attempts to treat hypertension and tachycardia arising during anaesthesia, numerous differing antiserotoninergic drugs have been used. These have included methotrimeprazine 2.5 mg i.v. (Mason & Steane 1976), cyproheptadine 1 mg i.v. (Solares et al 1987), ketanserin 10 mg given over a period of 3 minutes and then an infusion of 3 mg/h (Fischler et al 1983). The choice is often governed by the availability of the drug.

3. Somatostatin analogues have been found to inhibit the release of active mediators from carcinoid tumours. Octreotide (Sandostatin, Sandoz SMS 201–995) 50–100 μg i.v. has been used both prophylactically (Roy et al 1987), and for emergency treatment of a carcinoid crisis (Marsh et al 1987).

4. Specific antibradykinin therapy has included aprotinin (an infusion of 200 000 kiu, set up 1 hour prior to surgery and continued 4-hourly) and corticosteroids. However, reports of their effectiveness in treating complications have been mixed.

5. The role of histamine is uncertain. The flushing in a patient with a gastric carcinoid was blocked by a combination of H_1 and H_2 antagonists (Roberts et al 1979).

6. Anaesthetic drugs. Morphine should be avoided because of histamine

release. Suxamethonium fasciculations may increase intra-abdominal pressure and release tumour hormones. D-tubocurarine and alcuronium cause undesirable hypotension. Pancuronium or vecuronium are probably the most appropriate muscle relaxants.

7. Vasopressors of the catecholamine type, or those which act by the release of catecholamines, may activate tumour kallikrein which is the inactive precursor of bradykinin.

8. Regional anaesthesia does not block the effect of the hormones on the receptors, and hypotension may precipitate a bradykininergic crisis.

BIBLIOGRAPHY

Casthely P A, Jablons M, Griepp R B, Ergin M A, Goodman K 1986 Ketanserin in the preoperative and intraoperative management of a patient with carcinoid tumour undergoing tricuspid valve replacement. Anesthesia and Analgesia 65: 809–811.
Fischler M, Dentan M, Westerman M N, Vourc'h G, Freitag B 1983 Prophylactic use of ketanserin in a patient with carcinoid syndrome. British Journal of Anaesthesia 55: 920
Marsh H M, Martin J K, Kvols L K et al 1987 Carcinoid crisis during anaesthesia: successful treatment with a somatostatin analogue. Anesthesiology 66: 89–91
Mason R A, Steane P A 1976 Carcinoid syndrome: its relevance to the anaesthetist. Anaesthesia 31: 228–242
Miller R, Boulukos P A, Warner R R P 1980 Failure of halothane and ketamine to alleviate carcinoid syndrome-induced bronchospasm during anesthesia. Anesthesia and Analgesia 59: 621–623
Roberts L J II, Marney S R Jr, Oates J A 1979 Blockade of the flush associated with metastatic gastric carcinoid by combined histamine H1 and H2 receptor antagonists. New England Journal of Medicine 300: 236–238.
Roy R C, Carter R F, Wright P D 1987 Somatostatin, anaesthesia and the carcinoid syndrome. Anaesthesia 42: 627–632
Solares G, Blanco E, Pulgar S, Diago C, Ramos F 1987 Carcinoid syndrome and intravenous cyproheptadine. Anaesthesia 42: 989–992

CARDIAC TAMPONADE
(see also Section 4)

This can occur when a pericardial effusion (or a collection of blood within the pericardial cavity) restricts cardiac filling during diastole, by the effect of external pressure. When the pericardium becomes no longer distensible, small volume increases produce a rapid increase in pericardial pressure. There is a fixed decreased diastolic volume of both ventricles. In inspiration, the right ventricle fills at the expense of the left, and the left ventricular stroke volume falls producing pulsus paradoxicus, a cardinal sign. A tachycardia and peripheral vasoconstriction will initially compensate for the fall in cardiac output. Signs of respiratory distress then supervene and sudden cardiac arrest may occur.

Malignant disease is the commonest cause; infection, trauma, postcardiac surgery, pacemaker or CVP line insertion, intracardiac injection and anticoagulants are others. The long-term prognosis is related to the cause.

Preoperative abnormalities

1. A raised CVP, rapid low volume pulse, hypotension, and reflex peripheral arterial and venous vasoconstriction. The fixed low cardiac output may be aggravated by straining at stool, or on the assumption of the supine position. Straining may cause syncope (Keon 1981).
2. Pulsus paradoxicus. Normally on inspiration there is a slight fall in systolic pressure. In cardiac tamponade this fall is accentuated, usually to greater than 10 mmHg, and sometimes to even more than 20 mmHg. Pulsus paradoxicus is easily detected by palpation, but may be measured by an auscultation method (Lake 1983). Using a sphygmomanometer, the cuff pressure should first be reduced until the sound is intermittent, then deflation continued until all the beats are heard. The difference between the two pressures is then measured.
3. Respiratory distress occurs, especially when lying down.
4. If the collection of fluid is greater than 250 ml, the CXR may show an enlarged, globular cardiac outline, the left border of which may be straight or even convex. The right cardiophrenic angle will be less than 90°. The lung fields are clear. The diagnosis can be confirmed by echocardiography (Horgan 1987).

Anaesthetic problems

Anaesthesia in the presence of cardiac tamponade may be fatal. Abolition of the vasoconstrictor compensation will cause cardiovascular collapse. Cardiac arrest and death during a halothane induction in a 9-year-old boy who was due to have a cervical node biopsy has been reported (Keon 1981). The patient had a mild degree of respiratory distress, worse in the supine position, and prior to admission, an episode of loss of consciousness with peripheral cyanosis had occurred while straining at stool. Postmortem examination showed a large malignant lymphoma which enveloped the heart and infiltrated the pericardium.

Management

1. Monitor direct arterial and central venous pressures.
2. Minimise the factors which worsen the haemodynamic situation. These are:
   a. An increase in intrathoracic pressure. If ventilation is already being undertaken, for example after cardiac surgery, then PEEP should be avoided. This further reduces cardiac output, especially at slow rates of ventilation (Mattila et al 1984). Otherwise, the maintenance of spontaneous respiration until relief of the tamponade is imminent has been recommended (Moller et al 1979).
   b. Low intravascular volume. The blood volume must be maintained with i.v. fluids according to the haemodynamic responses.
   c. Decreased myocardial contractility. Dopamine has been reported as having had a favourable effect on haemodynamics, even in the

presence of severe tamponade (Mattila et al 1984). If general anaesthesia is essential, diazepam has been recommended to prevent the reduction in ventricular filling pressure caused by thiopentone.
3. Relief of tamponade. If possible, needle pericardiocentesis, with or without catheter insertion should be performed under local anaesthesia (Stanley & Weidauer 1973, Horgan 1987). ECG and radiological screening should be used, with facilities for emergency thoracotomy available. A subxiphoid approach can be used in which the needle enters the angle between the xiphisternum and the left costal margin, and is aimed towards the left shoulder (Cobbe 1980). A Seldinger technique with insertion of a soft catheter should be used. Continuous gentle aspiration assists identification of the pericardial sac. Safety may be increased by the use of a sterile ECG lead attached to the needle. An alternative apical approach can be made through the fifth intercostal space on the left side.

BIBLIOGRAPHY

Cobbe S M 1980 Pericardial effusions. British Journal of Hospital Medicine 23: 250–255
Horgan J H 1987 Cardiac tamponade. British Medical Journal 295: 563
Keon T P 1981 Death on induction of anesthesia for cervical node biopsy. Anesthesiology 55: 471–472
Lake C L 1983 Anesthesia and pericardial disease. Anesthesia and Analgesia 62: 431–443
Mattila I, Takkunen O, Mattila P, Harjula A, Mattila S, Merikallio E 1984 Cardiac tamponade and different modes of artificial ventilation. Acta Anaesthesiologica Scandinavica 28: 236–240
Moller C T, Schoonbee C G, Rosendorff C 1979 Haemodynamics of cardiac tamponade during various modes of ventilation. British Journal of Anaesthesia 51: 409–415
Stanley T H, Weidauer H E 1973 Anesthesia for the patient with cardiac tamponade. Anesthesia and Analgesia 52: 110–114

CARDIOMYOPATHIES

A group of diseases of unknown aetiology, affecting cardiac muscle. There are three main pathophysiological groups, diagnosed by echocardiography (Oakley 1987):

1. Dilated (congestive) cardiomyopathy, in which there is a decrease in contractile force in the left or right ventricle, resulting in systolic failure. It may be associated with a number of conditions including those of toxic (e.g. alcohol), metabolic, neurological and inflammatory origins.
Peripartum cardiomyopathy is a dilated form specifically associated with late pregnancy or the first 5 months of the puerperium.
2. Hypertrophic (obstructive) cardiomyopathy (HOCM) is an autosomal dominant inherited condition in which there is often massive ventricular hypertrophy and impaired diastolic function.
3. In restrictive cardiomyopathy there is a loss of ventricular distensibility, either due to endocardial or myocardial problems. There is a restriction to diastolic filling, resembling constrictive pericarditis. This is a rare form.

1

Preoperative abnormalities

1. Dilated cardiomyopathy (Johnson & Palacios 1982)
There is a marked reduction in ejection fraction (often <0.4 when heart
failure supervenes). The heart becomes dilated and there is often increased
peripheral resistance to compensate. Vasodilators and ACE inhibitors
therefore form part of the treatment, which aims to reduce the myocardial
work. Systemic embolism can occur, and when arrhythmias supervene the
patient should be anticoagulated indefinitely.

2. Hypertrophic cardiomyopathy (HOCM, idiopathic hypertrophic
subaortic stenosis)
The hypertrophy and fibrosis mostly affects the septum, but may
involve the whole of the left ventricle. There is resistance to inflow, and
therefore diastolic failure is the main problem in advanced disease. The
patient may present with dyspnoea, dizziness, syncope, angina or
arrhythmias. Sudden death can occur. While sinus rhythm is usual, the
late onset of atrial fibrillation is ominous. An apical and left sternal edge
systolic murmur may occur. The patient may be on beta blockers to
prevent tachycardias, or calcium channel blockers to improve myocardial
relaxation and hence pressure/volume relationships (Lorell et al 1982).
Again the risks of systemic embolism may necessitate anticoagulation.

The ECG shows left ventricular hypertrophy, and often Q waves and
ST and T wave changes. CXR usually shows slight cardiomegaly.

3. Restrictive cardiomyopathy
The main feature of this rare form is the loss of ventricular distensibility
due to rigidity imposed by endocardial or myocardial disease. One type is
associated with marked eosinophilia. In this there is a reduction in the
ventricular cavity size and distortion of the AV valves. Again there are
diastolic filling problems, with a picture resembling constrictive
pericarditis. The endocardial disease may produce thromboembolic
problems.

SUMMARY:

	Dilated	Hypertrophic	Restrictive
PRIMARY PROBLEM	systolic	diastolic	diastolic
PRESENTS WITH	heart failure arrhythmias systemic embolism	dyspnoea syncope angina arrhythmias	eosinophilia heart failure
PRINCIPLE TREATMENT	diuretics anticoagulants vasodilators ACE inhibitors	amiodarone anticoagulants beta blockers Ca antagonists	steroids cytotoxics
AVOID	myocardial depressants	digoxin beta stimulators vasodilators or hypotensives	morphine

Anaesthetic problems

In advanced cases of these three disease types, the pathophysiology is extremely variable and the effect of anaesthesia unpredictable. If the diagnosis is known in advance, then expert cardiological assessment is essential. However, in many cases, the condition mimics ischaemic or hypertensive heart disease, or may be unrecognized until an anaesthetic causes decompensation. More detailed advice should be obtained from the references, but a broad outline is described.

1. Dilated cardiomyopathy
   a. Myocardial depressants may precipitate acute cardiac failure. Two cases of unexpected peripartum cardiomyopathy each presented with acute pulmonary oedema at Caesarean section (Malinow et al 1985). One occurred during spinal anaesthesia, the other after a general anaesthetic. Postoperative echocardiography showed dilated, hypokinetic ventricles, which subsequently returned to normal. The prognosis in the dilated form is, in general, poor. The peripartum disease is variable. Some patients die in the acute phase, some have chronic cardiac problems, while others will make a complete recovery, but may relapse in subsequent pregnancies (O'Connell et al 1986). If cardiomegaly persists at the onset of the next pregnancy, the mortality may be as high as 60%.
   b. Arrhythmias are common and sudden death can occur.
2. Hypertrophic cardiomyopathy (HOCM)
   a. Tachycardias due to emotion, exercise and pain, and drugs such as digoxin and beta stimulators, will all increase the outflow tract gradients and may considerably reduce the cardiac output to essential organs, such as the myocardium and brain. Patients are often already on beta blockers to prevent tachycardias.
   b. Hypotension due to blood loss, regional anaesthesia, or vasodilator drugs, cause similar reductions in cardiac output and can worsen obstruction. A series of 52 general and four spinal anaesthetics in patients with HOCM was reviewed (Thompson et al 1985). One of the patients having a spinal anaesthetic sustained a myocardial infarction and subsequently died. Severe bradycardia and hypotension has been reported in patients with hypertrophic cardiomyopathy during spinal anaesthesia (Baraka et al 1987) and epidural anaesthesia (Loubser et al 1984).
   c. A systolic murmur may be present that increases in intensity when blood loss occurs, and decreases when intravascular volume is increased (Lanier & Prough 1984). These authors believe that HOCM should be considered in any elderly patient who develops a systolic murmur during longstanding hypertension.
   d. Arrhythmias. The patient may already be taking amiodarone for these.
   e. Anticoagulant therapy.

3. Restrictive cardiomyopathy
a. A fall in intravascular volume will decrease the ventricular filling pressure and accentuate the existing restriction to diastolic filling.
b. Changes in heart rate in either direction will impair diastolic filling.
c. Frequently the systolic function is normal. In some cases there is an additional impairment of ventricular function. In these, myocardial depressants may cause cardiovascular collapse.

Management

In advanced cases, careful cardiological assessment is required. The presence of cardiac failure will necessitate the monitoring of direct arterial blood pressure and ventricular filling pressures. Facilities for temporary pacing should be immediately available. The anaesthetist should understand the pathophysiology of the condition and the cardiovascular effects of the drugs and anaesthetic agents used.

1. Dilated cardiomyopathy
a. Myocardial depressants such as thiopentone, halothane and enflurane should be avoided. A nitrous oxide, oxygen, narcotic, benzodiazepine, relaxant technique is best.
b. The ECG should be carefully observed for ventricular arrhythmias and heart block, so that treatment can be rapidly instituted.
c. Regional anaesthesia may be considered for appropriate surgical procedures, provided the filling pressures are well controlled and there is no myocardial ischaemia. An epidural anaesthetic given for hip replacement, to a patient with severe dilated cardiomyopathy due to alcohol, has been reported (Amaranath et al 1986). PAP was measured, and the only complication was an episode of pulmonary hypertension after insertion of the femoral prosthesis. Epidural anaesthesia has also been reported for a Caesarean section in which an impedance cardiograph was used for haemodynamic monitoring (Gambling et al 1987). Two episodes of hypotension were treated with ephedrine.
d. Patients in heart failure require diuretics, and may need dobutamine or dopamine if there is a perioperative low cardiac output state. Occasionally isoprenaline may be necessary. Sodium nitroprusside can improve cardiac output by reducing the ventricular afterload.

2. Hypertrophic cardiomyopathy
The obstruction is dynamic (Maron et al 1987). Management should aim to decrease the obstruction, by decreasing myocardial contractility, and increasing preload and afterload.
a. A tachycardia from premedication, intubation, too light anaesthesia, ketamine, or cardiac stimulants must be avoided. Preoperative beta blockers should be maintained.
b. Drugs and techniques which cause vasodilatation and hypotension must not be used. Blood loss should be replaced promptly. An intraoperative diagnosis of hypertrophic cardiomyopathy was made

during hip replacement in a patient with a history of hypertension (Lanier & Prough 1984). Blood loss was associated with a sudden increase in intensity of her systolic murmur and the appearance of a systolic click. Postoperative echocardiography confirmed the diagnosis.

Regional anaesthesia is contraindicated. As isoflurane and morphine produce marked venodilatation, halothane or enflurane, and fentanyl should be used in preference. Provided the pulse is slow and the vascular volume maintained, halothane will minimize the severity of the obstruction by decreasing the force of ventricular contraction.

c. Hypotension should be treated by restoring vascular volume. If vasopressors are required, an alpha$_1$ agonist such as phenylephrine or methoxamine is the most suitable.

3. Restrictive cardiomyopathy

Maintenance of the compensatory mechanisms for the impaired diastolic filling are essential.

a. Adequate ventricular filling. Blood volume is maintained, and morphine and isoflurane avoided because of venous dilatation.

b. Adequate heart rate. Pancuronium may be advantageous.

c. Myocardial contractility. In severe disease, fentanyl, ketamine and benzodiazepines should be used rather than thiopentone, halothane and enflurane.

BIBLIOGRAPHY

Amaranath L, Esfandiari S, Lockrem J, Rollins M 1986 Epidural analgesia for total hip replacement in a patient with dilated cardiomyopathy. Canadian Anaesthetists' Society Journal 33: 84–88.
Baraka A, Jabbour S, Itani I 1987 Severe bradycardia following epidural anesthesia in a patient with idiopathic hypertrophic subaortic stenosis. Anesthesia and Analgesia 66: 1337–1338
Gambling D R, Flanagan M L, Huckell V F, Lucas S B, Kim J H K 1987 Anaesthetic management and non-invasive monitoring for Caesarean section in a patient with cardiomyopathy. Canadian Journal of Anaesthesia 34: 505–508.
Johnson R A, Palacios I 1982 Dilated cardiomyopathies of the adult. New England Journal of Medicine 307: 1051–1058
Lanier W, Prough D S 1984 Intraoperative diagnosis of hypertrophic obstructive cardiomyopathy. Anesthesiology 60: 61–63
Lorell B H, Paulus W J, Grossman W, Wynne J, Cohn P F 1982 Modification of abnormal left ventricular diastolic properties by nifedipine in patients with hypertrophic cardiomyopathy. Circulation 65: 499–507
Loubser P, Suh K, Cohen S 1984 Adverse affects of spinal anesthesia in a patient with idiopathic hypertrophic subaortic stenosis. Anesthesiology 60: 228–230
Malinow A M, Butterworth J F, Johnson M D 1985 Peripartum cardiomyopathy presenting at Cesarean delivery. Anesthesiology 63: 545–547
Maron B J, Bonow R O, Cannon R O, Leon M B, Epstein S E 1987 Hypertrophic cardiomyopathy. New England Journal of Medicine 316: 780–790, 844–852
Oakley C M 1987 Cardiomyopathies. In: Oxford textbook of medicine. Oxford Scientific Publications, Oxford
O'Connell J B, Constanzo-Nordin M R, Subramanian R, Robinson J A, Wallis D E, Scanlon P J, Gunnar R M 1986 Peripartum cardiomyopathy: clinical hemodynamic, histologic and prognostic characteristics. Journal of the American College of Cardiology 8: 52–56
Thompson R C, Liberthson R R, Lowenstein E 1985 Perioperative anesthetic risk of noncardiac surgery in hypertrophic obstructive cardiomyopathy. Journal of the American Medical Association 254: 2419–2421

1

CAROTID BODY TUMOUR
(see also APUDOMAS)

A tumour of ectodermal origin. One of a group known as the paraganglionomas, which are associated with the sympathetic nervous system. The cells of the carotid body normally act as chemoreceptors, but in common with other APUD cells, can secrete a variety of amines and peptides. Most carotid body tumours are non-functional, but occasionally they secrete noradrenaline, dopamine, calcitonin or ACTH. They may be malignant and can metastasize.

Preoperative abnormalities

1. The tumour usually presents as a mass in the neck.
2. Arteriography or DVI is essential to delineate the blood supply.
3. Radioisotope scans may show tumours elsewhere.
4. Clinical and biochemical signs of catecholamine secretion should be sought.

Anaesthetic problems

1. Those of catecholamine secretion if the tumour is functional. Episodes of severe hypertension and tachycardia during anaesthesia for biopsy of undiagnosed neck masses have been recorded (Clarke et al 1976, Newland & Hurlbert 1980). Both patients were found to have raised catecholamine levels, and were treated as for phaeochromocytoma during their subsequent tumour resection.
2. Blood loss may be brisk and heavy.
3. Reflex bradycardia, and occasionally cardiovascular collapse, due to carotid sinus stimulation has been reported (Kraayenbrink & Steven 1985).
4. Postoperative neurological complications are not uncommon (Wright et al 1979).

Management

1. See management of phaeochromocytoma.
2. Atropine may be required for bradycardias, although this may not protect the patient from cardiovascular collapse even when the carotid sinus is only lightly stimulated. A technique has been proposed (Boyd 1980), in which the dissection to expose the carotid bifurcation is performed in such a manner as to avoid pressure on the sinus. Lignocaine is then irrigated locally, prior to infiltration with further lignocaine.

BIBLIOGRAPHY

Boyd C H 1980 Anaesthesia for carotid body tumour resection. Anaesthesia 35: 720
Clarke A D, Matheson H, Boddie H G 1976 Removal of catecholamine-secreting
   chemodectoma. Anaesthesia 31: 1225–1230
Kraayenbrink M A, Steven C M 1985 Anaesthesia for carotid body tumour resection in a
   patient with the Eisenmenger syndrome. Anaesthesia 40: 1194–1197
Newland M C, Hurlbert B J 1980 Chemodectoma diagnosed hypertension and tachycardia
   during anesthesia. Anesthesia and Analgesia 59: 388–390
Wright D J, Pandya A, Noel F 1979 Anaesthesia for carotid body tumour resection.
   Anaesthesia 34: 806–808

C1 ESTERASE INHIBITOR DEFICIENCY
(ACQUIRED)

This may be a familial (see Hereditary angioneurotic oedema) or, less
commonly, an acquired disorder involving the complement system. The
acquired form is mostly associated with a B-lymphocyte malignancy, and
antibodies have been detected against abnormal immunoglobulins present
on the malignant B-cells. Reaction between the two cause C1 activation,
which in turn produces a secondary reduction in the concentrations of C1,
C2 and C4 esterase inhibitors (Geha et al 1985).

Preoperative abnormalities

1. As with hereditary angioneurotic oedema there is a low level of C1
esterase inhibitor, and sometimes life-threatening episodes of oedema of
the upper airway may develop in response to stress or local trauma.
However, attacks of oedema may occur without any obvious reason.
2. Adrenaline, antihistamines and steroids are known to be ineffective as
prophylaxis and treatment for these attacks.
3. The two conditions may be distinguished by the fact that in the
acquired form the onset is late, no family history is elicited, and the
underlying malignancy may already have been diagnosed.

Anaesthetic problems

1. Intubation and manipulation of the upper airway may precipitate local
angioneurotic oedema for which treatment with adrenaline, steroids or
antihistamines is ineffective.
2. Although tranexamic acid has been advocated to prevent attacks in
both forms, venous thrombosis has been reported after its prophylactic use
during surgery in the acquired disease (Razis et al 1986).

Management

1. Danazol is a progestogen derivative which probably increases the hepatic synthesis of C1 esterase inhibitor. Its prophylactic value in the acquired and hereditary disorders has been reported (Razis et al 1986). Danazol 200 mg t.d.s. should be given preoperatively, but may take several days to become effective.

2. Tranexamic acid should probably be avoided in the acquired form, especially in the presence of a thrombocytosis.

3. The preoperative prophylactic use of fresh frozen plasma, and C1 inhibitor concentrate has been reported (Plenderleith et al 1988).

BIBLIOGRAPHY

Geha R S, Quinti I, Austen K F, Cicardi M, Sheffer A, Rosen F S 1985 Acquired C1 inhibitor deficiency associated with anti-idiotypic antibody to monoclonal immunoglobulins. New England Journal of Medicine 312: 534–540
Plenderleith J L, Algie T, Whaley K 1988 Acquired C1 esterase inhibitor deficiency. Anaesthesia 43: 246–247
Razis P A Coulson I H, Gould T R, Findley I L 1986 Acquired C1 esterase inhibitor deficiency. Anaesthesia 41: 838–840

CHERUBISM

A familial condition which may present during childhood with mandibular, and sometimes maxillary enlargement. It usually regresses spontaneously during adolescence, but sometimes facial or incidental surgery is required prior to this.

Preoperative abnormalities

The mandible is enlarged and X-ray shows multilocular cysts. The maxilla may be similarly affected.

Anaesthetic problems

Intubation difficulties have been encountered. A case has been described in which the enlargement of the mandible had encroached on the displacement area of soft tissue bounded by the mandible, such that visualization of the cords was impossible (Maydew & Berry 1985).

Management

Difficult intubation should be anticipated. An awake intubation technique is the safest but, if the patient refuses, spontaneous respiration should be maintained during induction and intubation. Facilities must be available for an immediate tracheostomy, should it be required.

BIBLIOGRAPHY

Maydew R P, Berry F A 1985 Cherubism with difficult laryngoscopy and tracheal intubation. Anesthesiology 62: 810–812

CHRISTMAS DISEASE (HAEMOPHILIA B)
see HAEMOPHILIA A

COARCTATION OF THE AORTA, ADULT

A congenital narrowing of the aorta which may be pre- or post-ductal. The pre-ductal form is usually a long narrow segment and is associated with other cardiac defects. This type usually presents with heart failure before the age of one and requires treatment in a paediatric cardiac surgical unit. It will not be considered further here. The post-ductal form, however, is often asymptomatic and the patient may present in later life for surgery of some other condition, or for correction of the coarctation itself (Branthwaite 1980).

Preoperative abnormalities

1. There may be moderate hypertension, the arm blood pressure being higher than that in the leg. If the left subclavian artery arises at or below the constriction there may be an absent or reduced left radial pulse. If both radial and femoral pulses are felt together, the small volume of the femoral pulse, and the delay in pulsation, will be obvious.
2. Collateral circulation develops in the internal mammary, intercostal and subscapular arteries. The latter may be seen if the scapula is illuminated from the side.
3. A systolic murmur is usually heard along the left sternal edge radiating up into the neck. 25% of patients with coarctation have a bicuspid aortic valve and there may be some aortic incompetence.
4. CXR may show notching of the undersides of the ribs due to intercostal artery dilatation. There may be pre- and post-stenotic dilatation of the aorta.
5. Occasionally cerebral berry aneurysms may occur. In such cases the incidence of subarachnoid haemorrhage is increased, because of the high arterial pressure.
6. Angina or left ventricular failure may present late in untreated adult coarctation, but this is unusual. If it does occur there may be other contributing factors.

Anaesthetic problems

If, prior to elective surgery, a previously undiagnosed coarctation is found, then treatment of the coarctation may be considered to be the priority.

1. Upper body hypertension. The control of arterial pressure, both above and below the lesion, may be a problem during resection of the coarctation. The less severe the coarctation and the fewer the collaterals, then the more the rise in blood pressure on cross clamping the aorta is likely to be. This hypertension responds poorly to hypotensive agents as there is little variable peripheral resistance available proximal to the coarctation.

Hypertension occurred in a 16-year-old during anaesthesia with halothane, and prior to aortic clamping (Wilkinson & Clark 1982). It was resistant to sodium nitroprusside and other vasodilators. This may have been due to involvement of the renin-angiotensin system. Preoperative treatment with an angiotensin I converting enzyme inhibitor, such as captopril, might be appropriate.

2. Any operation in the area of the dilated collateral vessels may result in heavy bleeding, especially when the chest is opened.

3. Hypoperfusion of the spinal cord. This may cause paraplegia, and is more likely in those patients with few collaterals.

4. Susceptibility to bacterial endocarditis.

5. If there are left subclavian abnormalities, then the left arm cannot be used for blood pressure monitoring.

6. Postoperative hypertension (for more than 12 hours), associated with high plasma noradrenaline levels due to sympathetic overactivity. The magnitude of the rise has been found to relate to the preoperative level of the pressure gradient across the coarctation (Benedict et al 1978). This hypertension can cause bleeding, aortic dilatation or intracranial haemorrhage. Plasma noradrenaline may still be significantly raised 6 months postoperatively.

7. Some adults with coarctation also have aortic incompetence. Acute LVF and cardiac arrest occurred immediately after correction of a coarctation in one patient with severe aortic incompetence. This was thought to be secondary to an acute decrease in coronary perfusion (Rufilanchas et al 1977).

Management

1. Antihypertensive therapy should be used until the day of operation. Beta blockers may reduce intubation hypertension.

2. Appropriate prophylaxis for endocarditis should be given.

3. Resection of coarctation.

   a. Cannulation of the right radial artery, and insertion of an internal jugular venous line are required. Aortic pressure measurement distal to the lesion is more difficult, but can be monitored via a needle inserted by the surgeon (Fisher & Benedict 1977), or by femoral arterial cannulation using a Seldinger technique (Branthwaite 1980).

   b. Moderate induced hypotension is required to reduce bleeding. However, a mean arterial pressure of less than 50 mmHg is not only difficult to achieve, but may compromise perfusion to structures, such as the spinal cord, below the lesion. A short-acting drug, such as sodium nitroprusside or trimetaphan, can be tried, so that it can be discontinued just prior to aortic cross-clamping.

c. Careful monitoring to detect and to vigorously treat postoperative hypertension (usually within 72 hours) is needed. A combination of alpha and beta blockade may be required.

BIBLIOGRAPHY

Branthwaite M 1980 Coarctation of the aorta. In: Anaesthesia for cardiac surgery and allied procedures. Blackwell Scientific, Oxford
Benedict C R, Grahame-Smith D G, Fisher A 1978 Changes in plasma catecholamines and dopamine beta-hydroxylase after corrective surgery for coarctation of the aorta. Circulation 57: 598–602
Fisher A, Benedict C R 1977 Adult coarctation of the aorta: anaesthesia and postoperative management. Anaesthesia 32: 533–538
Rufilanchas J J, Villagra F, Maronas J M, Tellez G, Agosti J, Juffe A, Figuera D 1977 Coarctation of the aorta and severe aortic insufficiency: what to repair first? American Journal of Surgery 134: 428–430
Wilkinson C, Clark H 1982 Refractory hypertension during coarctectomy. Anesthesiology 57: 540–542

COCAINE ABUSE

Cocaine is an alkaloid present in the shrub, *Erythroxylon coca*. It produces CNS stimulation, euphoria and hallucinations. As a sympathetic stimulant, it acts by preventing the uptake of catecholamines into sympathetic nerve endings. While there is evidence that it has been used as a euphoriant in the Central Amazon from as early as the ninth century, the past 15 years has seen a notable increase in its use. It has been said to produce emotional, but not physical dependence. However, more recently, the use of chemically modified forms (paste, crack and freebase) for inhalation or smoking, has resulted in higher blood concentrations. These forms appear to be producing dependence. The taking of cocaine for recreational purposes has been more prevalent in the USA than in the UK. The greatly increased production and illicit trade from South America may soon change this (Gossop 1987).

Toxic effects of cocaine are marked. A series of 68 deaths associated with its illicit use has been reported in Florida (Wetli & Wright 1979). Analysis of the cases showed that the effects after i.v. use included immediate respiratory collapse and death, or death after up to 3 hours in coma. After nasal or oral ingestion a delay of up to an hour occurred before convulsions and death. Average blood levels were highest in those with oral intake (average 0.92 mg/dl), lowest in those after i.v. (0.3 mg/dl) and intermediate after use of the nasal route (0.44 mg/dl). Oral ingestion is an uncommon route for those seeking euphoria. The majority of deaths were deliberate, or accidental when packages of cocaine which were swallowed for concealment (body packing) burst in the gut. That cocaine is potentially dangerous even when given non-intravenously, has been confirmed (Isner et al 1986). Seven patients had acute cardiac events which bore a temporal relationship to intranasal cocaine use. These included myocardial infarction, ventricular tachycardia and fibrillation, myocarditis and two sudden deaths. Existing heart disease was not a prerequisite. Large doses of cocaine were not essential, and fits did not necessarily occur before cardiac toxicity. A further 19 case reports were analysed. Cocaine is frequently taken in combination with other drugs. Anaesthetists may be involved with anaesthesia for chronic users, or in the resuscitation of those with acute toxicity.

Presenting problems

1. The cardiovascular effects of cocaine are biphasic. An initial rise in blood pressure and a tachycardia, due to sympathetic stimulation, precedes the marked depression of the CNS. Sweating, vomiting and restlessness may occur. Sympathetic vasoconstriction may be intense, with increased metabolism, hyperpyrexia, hypoxia and convulsions. Ventricular fibrillation or asystole has occurred with doses as low as 30 mg.
2. Toxic doses produce an initial tachypnoea and increased depth of respiration. This may be rapidly followed by central respiratory depression.
3. When taken nasally, the vasoconstrictor effects on the mucosa may eventually lead to nasal ulceration and septal perforation.
4. A greatly increased risk of endocarditis in i.v. cocaine users (Chambers et al 1987).
5. Smoking or inhalation of hot cocaine fumes may cause pulmonary damage, as may the chemicals used in the processing (Gossop 1987).
6. I.v. users have an increased risk of contracting hepatitis B and AIDS.
7. Plasma cholinesterase is essential for the metabolism of cocaine. Individuals with enzyme abnormality or deficiency are at risk from sudden death (Cregler & Mark 1986).

Management

1. Beta blockers have been used to counteract the sympathetic effects of cocaine, but an alpha adrenergic blocker, such as phentolamine, should be available in case of marked hypertension. Regimens have included propranolol (1 mg i.v. each minute up to a total of 8 mg) to obtain a decrease in heart rate within 1–3 minutes (Gay et al 1976). It is, however, now suggested that beta blockade alone may worsen hypertension by unopposed alpha stimulation (Gay & Loper 1988). Labetalol (20 mg i.v. stat followed by an infusion of 60 mg/h) may be more appropriate. That the beta effects of labetalol are much more marked than the alpha effects must not be overlooked. The use of calcium antagonists for arrhythmias has also been suggested (Cregler & Mark 1986).

2. For the treatment of convulsions, either a benzodiazepine or incremental doses of thiopentone are indicated. Immediate attention should be paid to oxygenation and control of the airway. A profound metabolic acidosis occurs in association with convulsions, and their immediate control might decrease the cardiac effects of cocaine (Jonsson et al 1983).
3. Restlessness or agitation in the chronic cocaine abuser can be treated with benzodiazepines. Increasing the usual dosage by 50% has been recommended (Gay et al 1976).
4. Phenothiazines are contraindicated because they potentiate cerebral depressant drugs.

BIBLIOGRAPHY

Chambers H F, Morris D L, Tauber M G, Modin G 1987 Cocaine use and the risk for endocarditis in intravenous drug users. Annals of Internal Medicine 106: 833–836
Cregler L L, Mark H 1986 Medical complications of cocaine abuse. New England Journal of Medicine 315: 1495–1500
Gay G R, Inaba D S, Rappolt R T, Gushue G F, Perkner J J 1976 Cocaine in current perspective. Anesthesia and Analgesia 55: 582–587
Gay G R, Loper K A 1988 Control of cocaine induced hypertension with labatolol. Anesthesia and Analgesia 67: 92
Gossop M 1987 Beware cocaine. British Medical Journal 295: 945
Isner J M, Estes N A, Thompson P D et al 1986 Acute cardiac events temporally related to cocaine abuse. New England Journal of Medicine 315: 1438–1443
Jonsson S, O'Meara M, Young J B 1983 Acute cocaine poisoning. Importance of treating seizures and acidosis. American Journal of Medicine 75: 1061–1064
Wetli C V, Wright R K 1979 Death caused by recreational cocaine use. Journal of the American Medical Association 241: 2519–2522

CONN'S SYNDROME (PRIMARY ALDOSTERONISM)

Excess aldosterone production may be due to an adrenal adenoma, adrenal hyperplasia or a carcinoma. Aldosterone is a mineralocorticoid secreted by the zona glomerulosa of the adrenal cortex. It promotes sodium reabsorption and potassium exchange mainly in the renal tubules, but to a lesser extent in the intestine, salivary and sweat glands. The final stage of aldosterone secretion is controlled by the renin-angiotensin system. Activation of this system occurs in response to sodium or water depletion.

Preoperative abnormalities

1. The main features are hypertension, hypokalaemia and alkalosis. Symptoms, should they occur, are usually secondary to the hypokalaemia and may include muscle weakness, polyuria, polydipsia and tetany. A patient who presented with a flaccid quadriparesis, had the condition reversed by a potassium infusion (Gangat et al 1976).
2. Urinary potassium is high despite a low total body potassium, and the

serum sodium may be in the upper range of normal or be slightly elevated.

3. Plasma renin levels are low and plasma aldosterone is elevated.

4. Tumours must be distinguished from bilateral adrenal hyperplasia, with radionuclide imaging, or occasionally adrenal vein sampling. In adrenal hyperplasia, surgery is inappropriate.

5. The ECG may show T-wave flattening and U waves.

6. Glucose tolerance may be abnormal in up to 50% of patients.

Anaesthetic problems

1. Hypertension and sodium retention. Hypertensive peaks may occur at intubation.

2. Low total body and plasma potassium levels cause muscle weakness and increased sensitivity to non-depolarizing muscle relaxants. Intraoperative arrhythmias may also be produced. A patient in whom tonic muscle contractions occurred during induction and whose subsequent potassium balance studies suggested that the potassium stores had been depleted by 30–40%, has been described (Gangat et al 1976).

Management

1. Hypertension must be controlled preoperatively. An aldosterone antagonist, such as spironolactone 100 mg t.d.s., should be included as both the hypertension and potassium loss will be improved.

2. A potassium infusion is required both pre- and intra-operatively. Total body potassium is depleted, and ECG and plasma potassium levels are both unreliable guides (Gangat et al 1976).

3. Preoperative beta blockers may reduce the hypertension on intubation (Shipton & Hugo 1982).

4. Normocapnoea should be maintained to prevent potassium returning to the cells (Weatherill & Spence 1984). An initial period of postoperative ventilation may be required to counteract the compensatory respiratory acidosis.

5. Following removal of the tumour, the reversal of the electrolyte abnormalities occurs earlier than the correction of hypertension.

6. Glucocorticoid replacement should not be required if the other adrenal is intact.

BIBLIOGRAPHY

Gangat Y, Triner L, Baer L, Puchner P 1976 Primary aldosteronism with uncommon complications. Anesthesiology 45: 542–544
Shipton E A, Hugo J M 1982 An aldosterone-producing adrenal cortical adenoma. Anaesthesia 37: 933–936
Weatherill D, Spence A A 1984 Anaesthesia and disorders of the adrenal cortex. British Journal of Anaesthesia 56: 741–749

CREUTZFELDT-JAKOB DISEASE

A rare encephalopathy of late middle age causing widespread progressive neurological signs and symptoms, including presenile dementia. Death usually occurs within 6 months. It is caused by a virus which can be isolated from the brain, spinal cord and many other tissues, and can be experimentally transmitted to animals. There is no detectable immune reaction. The virus is difficult to destroy by either physical or chemical methods, and there have been reports involving iatrogenic transmission of the virus in two neurosurgical procedures, a corneal graft (MacMurdo et al 1984) and the use of growth hormone from cadaveric pituitaries. The incubation period was about 18 months.

Preoperative abnormalities

1. Dementia of rapid onset, and focal or generalized epilepsy are two prominent features, although other focal neurological signs occur. Deterioration to decerebrate or decorticate states is usually rapid.
2. EEG is non-specific but there are often periodic discharges of slow waves and spikes.
3. Diagnosis can only be confirmed by brain biopsy.

Anaesthetic problems

1. Any tissue or body fluid should be considered as potentially infectious, although in reality the main danger probably lies in accidental inoculation.
2. Occasionally patients may have autonomic dysfunction.
3. Rarely, there are abnormalities of liver function.

Management

1. Particular care should be taken during brain biopsies in undiagnosed cases of presenile dementia (du Moulin & Hedley-Whyte 1983). The anaesthetist should wear gown, gloves and mask.
2. Equipment should preferably be disposable. Linen and instruments should be soaked in 1% sodium hypochlorite before being bagged (du Moulin & Hedley-Whyte 1983).
3. The virus is difficult to destroy by physical and chemical means. Experiments have shown that soaking in 0.5% sodium hypochlorite for 1 hour, autoclaving for 1 hour at 121°C (103.4 kPa) or a combination of these, will inactivate it (Brown et al 1982). Hands should be washed (not scrubbed) with aqueous povidone iodine if penetration of the skin has occurred. Equipment surfaces should be washed with sodium hypochlorite.

BIBLIOGRAPHY

Brown P, Gibbs C J, Amyx H L, Kingsbury D T, Rohwer R G, Sulima M P, Gajdusek D C 1982 Chemical disinfection of Creutzfeldt–Jakob disease virus. New England Journal of Medicine 306: 1279–1282
du Moulin G C, Hedley-Whyte J 1983 Hospital-associated viral infection and the anesthesiologist. Anesthesiology 59: 51–65
MacMurdo S D, Jakymec A J, Bleyaert A L 1984 Precautions in the anesthetic management of a patient with Creutzfeldt–Jakob disease. Anesthesiology 60: 590–592

CRI DU CHAT SYNDROME

A chromosomal abnormality due to short arm deletion on the number 5 chromosome. It is associated with a number of characteristic features. Most patients die in childhood.

Preoperative abnormalities

1. The infant has microcephaly, micrognathia, hypertelorism, severe mental retardation, epicanthic folds and a cat-like cry.
2. There may be a number of other abnormalities, including congenital heart disease.

Anaesthetic problems

1. Difficulties in intubation have been reported (Yamashita et al 1985). Although the characteristic cry may be partially neurogenic in origin, a number of upper airway abnormalities have been described. These include a small, narrow larynx, a long floppy epiglottis, and retrognathia.
2. The babies are hypotonic and may be sensitive to non-depolarizing muscle relaxants.
3. A tendency to pulmonary aspiration may lead to chronic respiratory infections.

Management

1. Awake intubation or inhalation induction should be performed.
2. Minimal doses of relaxants, or controlled ventilation without relaxation may be wise.
3. Care with nursing and feeding may reduce aspiration problems.

BIBLIOGRAPHY

Yamashita M, Tanioka F, Taniguchi K, Matsuki A, Oyama T 1985 Anesthetic consideration in Cri du Chat syndrome. A report of three cases. Anesthesiology 63: 201–202

CUSHING'S SYNDROME AND CUSHING'S DISEASE

Cushing's syndrome is the general term used for a disorder caused by excess circulating glucocorticoid. Cushing's disease specifies one of its causes; that of pituitary-dependent adrenal hyperplasia, secondary to ACTH secretion. This accounts for about 70–80% of cases of Cushing's syndrome. Other important causes are adrenal cortical tumour (5–10%) and ectopic ACTH-producing tumours (5–10%).

Preoperative abnormalities

1. A review of 31 patients with Cushing's disease has shown that the commonest clinical features, in order of frequency, were weakness, thin skin, obesity, easy bruising, hypertension, menstrual disorders, hirsutism, impotence, striae, proximal muscle weakness, oedema, osteoporosis, mental disorders, diabetic GTT, backache, acne, hypokalaemia and fasting hyperglycaemia (Urbanic & George 1981). Fractures occur, and wound healing is poor.
2. Biochemical abnormalities include hypokalaemic alkalosis, sodium and water retention, hyperglycaemia, lack of diurnal variation in plasma cortisol with its failure to decrease at night, and increased urinary free cortisol.
3. Patients have an increased incidence of infections.

Anaesthetic problems

1. Venous access may be difficult due to fragility of veins.
2. Hypertension, with or without heart failure, may be present.
3. Hypokalaemia. There may be severe depletion of potassium stores.
4. Diabetes mellitus.
5. Muscle weakness may contribute to postoperative respiratory failure.
6. There is an increased risk of deep vein thrombosis.

Management

1. Hypertension and heart failure, if present, must be treated.
2. Diabetes must be controlled.
3. Hypokalaemia requires identification and correction.
4. In florid cases, drug control of adrenocortical function with metyrapone, an 11-beta-hydroxylase inhibitor, may be advisable before operation (Montgomery & Welbourn 1978).
5. Careful positioning of the patient to avoid fractures of osteoporotic bone is required.
6. Steroids should be maintained during and after surgery (Weatherill & Spence 1984).

1

BIBLIOGRAPHY

Montgomery D A D, Welbourn R B 1978 Cushing's syndrome: 20 years after adrenalectomy. British Journal of Surgery 65: 221–223
Urbanic R C, George J M 1981 Cushing's disease – 18 years' experience. Medicine 60: 14–24
Weatherill D, Spence A A 1984 Anaesthesia and disorders of the adrenal cortex. British Journal of Anaesthesia 56: 741–749

CYSTIC FIBROSIS

An autosomal recessive syndrome primarily involving the exocrine glands and producing a variable pattern of the disease. Glandular secretions are relatively concentrated, with excess electrolytes and altered mucous glycoproteins. This leads to abnormal mucociliary transport, although ciliary function is normal (Rutland & Cole 1981). As a result, gland ducts become blocked. This predisposes to infection, hyperplasia and hypertrophy. The patient may develop progressive chronic respiratory problems in childhood, malabsorption and cirrhosis of the liver. Progressive lung damage can lead to pulmonary hypertension and right heart failure. Advances in the management of the disease has extended life-expectancy, therefore more patients are likely to present for surgery. The operative mortality has dropped dramatically during the past 20 years. In a review of 77 patients undergoing 126 procedures, of which 86% were operations directly related to the disease itself, no evidence was produced that anaesthesia had any deleterious effect on lung function (Lamberty & Rubin 1985).

Preoperative abnormalities

1. Sweat test. High sodium (>60 mmol/l in infants, >65 mmol/l suggestive, >90 mmol/l diagnostic in children), and high chloride levels.
2. Viscous secretions, defective mucociliary transport and altered lung mechanics produce severe chest infections. Bronchiectasis, pulmonary fibrosis and emphysema follow.
3. Pulmonary hypertension, secondary to hypoxia, may develop in advanced lung disease. Cor pulmonale finally supervenes.
4. Abnormal liver function due to cirrhosis.
5. Pancreatic insufficiency occurs in 80–90% of patients. Malabsorption, hypoproteinaemia and low body weight result. Prothrombin time may be prolonged due to loss of fat-soluble vitamins.
6. Nasal polyps are present in 10–15% of cases.
7. Pneumothorax, which is difficult to treat, is common in adults. A study of 243 adults showed that 46 (18.9%) had at least one pneumothorax, from which seven had died (Penketh et al 1982). This complication is much less frequent in children (2–7%).

Anaesthetic problems

1. Despite the improvement in prognosis, when lung disease is severe, the mortality is increased.

2. Gaseous induction is both slow, due to low ventilation perfusion ratios, and stormy.

3. The endotracheal tube is easily blocked by secretions.

4. There is a high incidence of perioperative respiratory complications. These include pneumothorax, pneumonia, airway obstruction, atelectasis, respiratory failure and arrest.

5. Bronchoscopy and lung washout is associated with episodes of profound hypoxia (Harnik et al 1983).

6. Periods of oxygen desaturation during sleep may occur postoperatively.

7. Nasal polyps can cause airway obstruction.

8. There is a high sodium loss, especially when hot.

Management

1. Respiratory and cardiovascular function must be carefully assessed.

2. Regular, intensive physiotherapy is mandatory.

3. Infections, especially with pseudomonas, require treatment with an aminoglycoside and penicillin combination.

4. Parenteral vitamin K will be needed if the prothrombin time is prolonged.

5. Nebulized bronchodilator drugs will reduce bronchospasm.

6. Local anaesthesia should be employed if possible.

7. Sedative premedication should be avoided. Anti-sialogogues may be used if essential, but perhaps prior to induction.

8. Inhalational induction can be stormy, and should be avoided.

9. All patients require endotracheal intubation to facilitate aspiration of secretions, oxygenation and ventilation.

10. Anaesthetic gases must be humidified and tracheal secretions aspirated regularly during the operation.

11. The viscidity of secretions is reduced by keeping the patient well hydrated.

12. The role of bronchial washouts in the management of cystic fibrosis is controversial. Its benefit in some patients has been supported (Harnik et al 1983). Repeated aliquots of up to 20 ml 5% acetylcysteine in saline were instilled into the main divisions of the bronchial tree, to a total volume of 200–300 ml, over a period of 20–30 minutes. Concomitant monitoring with a transcutaneous oxygen monitor enabled oxygenation to be restored before dangerous hypoxia occurred.

13. Pneumothorax in the adult, treated by simple drainage, is associated with a high incidence of recurrence (Penketh et al 1982). A persistent leak for 7 days was suggested as an indication for surgical intervention.

Subsequently it has been found that recurrence of a pneumothorax within 6 months of surgery denotes a very poor prognosis (Robinson & Branthwaite 1984).

BIBLIOGRAPHY

Harnik E, Kulczycki L, Gomes M N 1983 Transcutaneous oxygen monitoring during bronchoscopy and washout for cystic fibrosis. Anesthesia and Analgesia 62: 357–362
Lamberty J M, Rubin B K 1985 The management of anaesthesia for patients with cystic fibrosis. Anaesthesia 40: 448–459
Penketh A, Knight R K, Hodson M E, Batten J C 1982 Management of pneumothorax in adults with cystic fibrosis. Thorax 37: 850–853
Robinson D A, Branthwaite M A 1984 Pleural surgery in patients with cystic fibrosis. Anaesthesia 39: 655–659
Rutland J, Cole P J 1981 Nasal mucociliary clearance and ciliary beat frequency in cystic fibrosis compared with sinusitis and bronchiectasis. Thorax 36: 654–658

DEMYELINATING DISEASES

A general name for a group of neurological diseases involving myelin sheath abnormalities. The myelin surrounding an axon may develop normally and then be lost later, to leave the axon itself preserved. Alternatively there may be some defect in the original formation of myelin as a result of an error of metabolism. The commonest presentation is in multiple sclerosis (MS), whose aetiology is unknown, but is probably multifactorial. Susceptibility to MS may be genetically determined. Viral and immune factors are possibly involved. Plaques of demyelination are scattered throughout the nervous system, usually in the optic nerve, brainstem and spinal cord. The peripheral nerves are not involved. Only the problems of multiple sclerosis will be discussed further.

Preoperative abnormalities

1. The diagnosis is made on clinical grounds, when neurological lesions are disseminated both in time and space. Consequently the clinical picture is highly variable.
2. The commonest presenting symptoms, in order of frequency, are limb weakness, visual disturbances, paraesthesiae and incoordination. Legs are more commonly involved before the arms, with signs of spasticity and hyperreflexia. Urinary symptoms may occur.
3. Progression, with remissions and relapses, is very variable. Infection, trauma or stress may be associated with relapses.
4. A small rise in body temperature can cause a definite deterioration in neural function.
5. Mild dementia and dysarthria may appear as the disease progresses.

Anaesthetic problems

Reports of anaesthetics given to patients with MS are both numerous and conflicting. The advice with regard to the avoidance of particular drugs or techniques is inconsistent and often based on small numbers of patients. Major difficulty exists in the separation of drug effect from surgery, pyrexia or stress as a cause of a relapse. An analysis of 88 general anaesthetics given to 42 patients did not show a relapse rate greater than that which would have been expected to have occurred spontaneously (Bamford et al 1978).

1. Both experimentally and clinically, an increase in body temperature has been shown to cause a deterioration in nerve conduction and neurological signs.

2. Spinal anaesthesia. A review of the medical literature, and a limited personal experience, led one group to the conclusion that spinal anaesthesia was associated with an increased incidence of neurological complications (Bamford et al 1978).

3. Epidural anaesthesia. A combined experience of 57 epidural anaesthesics in MS patients, without complications, but also regrettably without details, has been claimed by five anaesthetists from four different countries (Crawford et al 1981). Temporary neurological deficits have, however, been reported. One patient developed localised paraesthesiae lasting 7 hours and 7 weeks respectively following two epidurals, in consecutive labours (Warren et al 1982). The longer deficit followed a total dose of bupivacaine of 562.5 mg during a 15 hour period. It was postulated that neurotoxicity might have followed the diffusion of the anaesthetic into the dural space. Nothing definite exists in the literature to suggest that patients be denied the benefits of an epidural anaesthetic, should it be considered necessary.

4. Local anaesthesia. 1000 procedures performed under local anaesthesia in 98 patients did not significantly increase the relapse rate (Bamford et al 1978). There is, however, evidence that local anaesthetics can cross the blood–brain barrier more readily in MS, and toxicity is more likely to occur.

5. Muscle relaxants. Resistance to atracurium, in association with an abnormally high concentration of skeletal muscle acetylcholine receptors, has been reported in a patient with MS and spastic paraparesis (Brett et al 1987).

6. There is an increased incidence of epilepsy in MS patients.

Management

1. It is vital to know, either from the notes or from staff, whether or not the patient is aware of the precise diagnosis. Appropriate discussions will take place with the patient in the light of this knowledge.

2. Elective surgery should not be undertaken in the presence of fever.

3. Spinal anaesthesia should be avoided (Bamford et al 1978).

4. If a regional block is required, then epidural anaesthesia is preferable and should not be denied. Accurate documentation of the existing signs and symptoms, and a full discussion with the patient is essential.

5. The maximal dose of local anaesthetic should be reduced below that normally recommended (Jones & Healy 1980). Techniques which require large doses should not be used.

BIBLIOGRAPHY

Bamford C, Sibley W, Laguna J 1978 Anesthesia in multiple sclerosis. Le Journal Canadien des Sciences Neurologiques 5: 41–44

Brett R S, Schmidt J H, Gage J S, Schartel S A, Poppers P J 1987 Measurement of acetylcholine receptor concentration in skeletal muscle from a patient with multiple sclerosis and resistance to atracurium. Anesthesiology 66: 837–839

Crawford J S, James F M, Nolte H, van Steenberge A, Shah J L 1981 Regional analgesia for patients with chronic neurological disease and similar conditions. Anaesthesia 36: 821

Jones R M, Healy T E J 1980 Anaesthesia and demyelinating disease. Anaesthesia 35: 879–884

Warren T M, Datta S, Ostheimer G W 1982 Lumbar epidural anesthesia in a patient with multiple sclerosis. Anesthesia and Analgesia 61: 1022–1023.

DERMATOMYOSITIS/POLYMYOSITIS COMPLEX

A group of autoimmune inflammatory conditions primarily affecting muscle and skin, although there may be multisystem involvement. The related diseases include primary idiopathic polymyositis, primary idiopathic dermatomyositis, dermatomyositis associated with malignancy, a childhood form of dermatomyositis, and a form of the complex which is associated with other collagen diseases (Bellamy et al 1984).

Preoperative abnormalities

1. The myositis may present with muscle pain, tenderness and weakness, involving proximal and distal muscles and the axial skeleton. Contractures and muscle atrophy may occur later.

2. A violaceous appearance of the eyelids and upper part of the face is caused by the cutaneous lesions.

3. An underlying malignancy is not uncommon, particularly when the complex presents in older men.

4. There may be patchy infiltration of the lungs, peripheral oedema, and soft-tissue calcification.

5. Muscle enzyme levels may be raised and the patient anaemic.

6. Attendance at an ENT department is a common method of presentation (Metheny 1978). Voice changes, and upper oesophageal dysphagia were found to be the most frequent problems. Laryngo-oesophageal tone is reduced, with dysfunction of the tongue and soft palate. Saliva pools in

the pyriform fossa, and regurgitation and aspiration leading to pneumonia, may occur.
7. Necrotising vasculitis and cardiac involvement may appear in the childhood form.
8. The patient may be on steroids or immunosuppressives.

Anaesthetic problems

1. An underlying malignancy will be present in up to 20% of patients.
2. The myositis may result in sensitivity to muscle relaxants. An abnormal response to suxamethonium was reported in a young child. Before muscle relaxation occurred, fasciculations were followed by a short period of muscle contraction (Johns et al 1986). However, neuromuscular monitoring in two patients receiving atracurium (Ganta et al 1988), and one having vecuronium (Saarnivaara 1988) did not reveal an abnormal response or sensitivity.
3. Swallowing and vocal cord dysfunction may cause pooling of secretions and aspiration of gastric contents (Metheny).
4. Pneumonia and postoperative respiratory insufficiency may occur.

Management

1. A careful assessment of the systems involved in the disease, and in particular for signs of malignancy.
2. Monitoring of neuromuscular function is essential.
3. In view of the problems with swallowing and pooling of secretions, intubation has been recommended (Eisele 1981).

BIBLIOGRAPHY

Bellamy N, Kean W F, Buchanan W W 1984 Connective tissue diseases. The dermatopolymyositis complex. Hospital Update 10: 74–76
Eisele J A 1981 Connective tissue diseases. In: Anaesthesia and uncommon diseases. Saunders, Philadelphia
Ganta R, Campbell I T, Mostafa S M 1988 Anaesthesia and acute dermatomyositis/polymyositis. British Journal of Anaesthesia 60: 854–858
Johns R A, Finholt D A, Stirt J A 1986 Anaesthetic management of a child with dermatomyositis. Canadian Anaesthetists' Society Journal 33: 71–74
Metheny J A 1978 Dermatomyositis: a vocal and swallowing disease entity. Laryngoscope 88: 147–161
Saarnivaara L H M 1988 Anesthesia for a patient with polymyositis undergoing myomectomy of the cricopharyngeal muscle. Anesthesia and Analgesia 67: 701–702

DIABETES INSIPIDUS

The result of a failure of vasopressin secretion by the posterior part of the pituitary. In the presence of low levels of ADH, the kidney is unable to conserve water, and large volumes of dilute urine are excreted. It may be

1

secondary to pituitary or hypothalamic surgery, head injury and tumour. Diabetes insipidus is also common in brain-dead patients. Lithium treatment may rarely be associated with a mild diabetes insipidus-like syndrome.

Preoperative abnormalities

1. Polyuria and polydipsia. The urine volume may reach 24 l/day.
2. Hypovolaemia and hypernatraemia.
3. Urinary osmolality is low (50–100 mOsm/kg), and there is an increased plasma osmolality.

Anaesthetic problems

1. If the patient does not increase his fluid intake, there will be dehydration, hypernatraemia and plasma hyperosmolality.
2. Electrolyte imbalance.
3. Severe hypovolaemia associated with diabetes insipidus in cadaveric organ donors will require treatment. If vasopressin is used, and its administration continued until the kidneys are removed, there is an increase in the incidence of tubular necrosis and graft failure in the recipient (Graybar & Tarpey 1987). An analogue, desmopressin, has no vasoconstrictor effects.

Management

1. Desmopressin nasally 10–20 μg b.d., or 0.5–2 μg i.v., increases water reabsorption from the renal tubules.
2. The urine output and serum osmolality is monitored. If the osmolality is >290 mOsm/kg, then i.v. fluids and desmopressin are required.

BIBLIOGRAPHY

Graybar G B, Tarpey M 1987 Kidney transplantation. In: Anesthesia and organ transplantation. Saunders, Philadelphia

---

DIABETES MELLITUS

In insulin-dependent diabetes (IDD, type I), the insulin deficiency means that catabolism exceeds anabolism, and in the absence of treatment a state of hyperosmolar ketoacidosis will progress to hypokalaemia, dehydration, coma and death. In non-insulin-dependent diabetes (NIDD, type II) the pancreas still secretes insulin, but supply may not meet demand and under certain circumstances, such as surgical stress, there is insulin resistance and gluconeogenesis. The metabolic changes produced by surgery will worsen the state of diabetes.

Surgery should not be undertaken in diabetics who are out of control. Conversely, hypoglycaemia may be undetectable, and therefore dangerous, during anaesthesia. The increased insulin requirements must therefore be monitored closely and balanced with a supply of glucose and potassium.

Preoperative abnormalities

1. Diagnosis
A fasting venous or capillary whole blood glucose of >6.7 mmol/l, or a venous plasma level of >7.8 mmol/l. This can then be confirmed with a second FBG or a value after a glucose load. In symptomatic patients a random glucose of 11.1 mmol/l or more is usually diagnostic (Alberti & Hockaday 1987).
2. Metabolic
In the absence of insulin there is increased lipid metabolism with fatty acid release, increased ketone production such that the supply exceeds utilization, and increased gluconeogenesis and glycogenolysis. The net result is acidaemia, ketoacidosis, and hyperglycaemia. This hyperosmolar state leads to polyuria, which in turn causes urinary loss of sodium, potassium, calcium, phosphate and magnesium. The acidosis results in loss of cellular potassium and the deficiency of insulin prevents cellular uptake of potassium. Sodium is also lost with the urinary excretion of ketoacids.
3. Cardiovascular disease
Large vessel disease leads to atherosclerosis and myocardial disease. The microangiopathy, which affects particularly renal, retinal and digital vessels, appears to be related to the high levels of blood glucose. There is a high mortality from myocardial and peripheral vascular disease.
4. Resistance to infection and wound healing are both impaired.
5. Renal failure is a common complication of diabetes, and the mortality from renal transplantation is two to four times greater than in non-diabetic patients.
6. Peripheral and autonomic neuropathies, which may be related to high levels of sorbitol, are common.

Anaesthetic problems

1. There is a higher morbidity and mortality in diabetic than in non-diabetic patients. Myocardial disease and infection are chiefly responsible for this.
2. Surgery and stress worsen the state of diabetes and may be accompanied by some degree of insulin resistance. In addition, insulin resistance occurs in association with severe infection, obesity, liver disease, steroid therapy and cardiopulmonary bypass.
3. Hypoglycaemia can occur suddenly during anaesthesia. The usual warning signs are absent and brain damage can ensue.

4. While a mild elevation of blood glucose is acceptable during surgery, it should be maintained between 6 and 13 mmol/l. The renal threshold for glucose is 10 mmol/l. At levels greater than this, the glycosuria causes an osmotic diuresis, with loss of water and electrolytes.

5. The administration of lactate-containing solutions may increase blood glucose, or may exacerbate lactic acidosis when this occurs in hyperglycaemic states.

6. Ketosis may produce insulin resistance and alter the metabolism of anaesthetic agents. It also increases potassium loss from the body. Hypokalaemia may induce cardiac arrhythmias during anaesthesia.

7. Ketoacidosis is associated with gastric atony and ileus, which increases the risk of inhalation of gastric contents.

8. Autonomic neuropathy may be responsible for cardiovascular and respiratory complications during anaesthesia. Five cases were reported in which episodes of cardiorespiratory arrest occurred in association with anaesthesia, in diabetics (Page & Watkins 1978). It was suggested that autonomic neuropathy could reduce the respiratory responses to hypoxia and hypercarbia. There is also an impaired ability to respond to stress by vasoconstriction and tachycardia (see Autonomic failure).

Management

1. General assessment
A thorough assessment of the degree of multiorgan involvement by the diabetic process is required. In particular the presence of cardiovascular and renal diseases, or autonomic neuropathy (see Autonomic failure) must be determined. If there is autonomic failure, then there should be close respiratory and cardiovascular monitoring throughout the perioperative period.

2. Assessment of diabetic control
This includes estimations of FBG levels, glucose test strips and urinalysis. There are variations in level dependent on the method of sampling. Whole blood glucose values are 10–15% less than plasma values, and fasting capillary is 7% greater than venous values.

3. Management of diabetes during elective surgery
In theory, diabetics should be admitted 2–3 days in advance of surgery and appear first on a morning operating list. Long-acting oral hypoglycaemics should be discontinued 2 days in advance, or changed to short-acting ones. Similarly, long-acting insulins should be changed to either Actrapid or other short-acting insulin. In practice the anaesthetist is often presented with diabetic patients the evening before operation, in which none of these conditions have been met!

   a. Diet controlled and patients with NIDD
      i. Minor surgery
      May need no treatment, but the latter should be monitored closely for hypoglycaemia.

ii. Major surgery
(or in NIDD patients with a FBG >10 mmol/l on the morning of operation)
Treat with an insulin infusion as for IDD.
b. Insulin-dependent diabetics
Various methods of administering insulin have been described. A short-acting insulin may be given subcutaneously 4-hourly, continuously i.v. by syringe pump, or mixed with glucose and potassium.

A currently accepted method is a glucose/insulin/potassium (GIK) infusion (Alberti & Thomas 1979, Bowen et al 1984). Despite past fears of insulin absorption into the container and tubes, if the first 50 ml are washed through, 75–90% of the insulin is delivered. Should the infusion run too fast or stop, all the constituents are similarly affected. In addition, if the infusion is started when the morning insulin would have been due, the need for early morning surgery is less urgent. The main disadvantage is the wasted solutions if the insulin dose has to be altered frequently.

Technique
   i. Preoperative FBG should be <13 mmol/l. Cancellation may be considered if levels are higher than this. The aim should be to maintain a BG of 5–10 mmol/l.
   ii. Infuse Actrapid 10 u + KCl 10 mmol + 10% glucose 500 ml, at a rate of 100 ml/h.
   iii. Repeat BG in 2–3 hours; if >10 mmol/l increase insulin to 15 u and check BG in further 2 hours. If <5 mmol/l then no insulin should be given.
   iv. BG should be measured 2-hourly, and serum potassium twice on the day of infusion.
However, there is still no clear evidence that the GIK regimen is superior to a regimen using a half to one-third of the patient's normal insulin, given s.c., with i.v. glucose, 5–10 g/h (Hall & Desborough 1988).

An alternative method is to use a syringe pump to administer the insulin, starting at 2–3 u/h, separately from the glucose and potassium.
4. The ketoacidotic diabetic
a. In young diabetics severe ketoacidosis may cause abdominal pain. If the vomiting starts before the pain, the cause is more likely to be ketoacidosis, whereas pain preceding vomiting is more likely to be surgical.
b. If severe ketoacidosis is present and conditions permit, surgery should be delayed for 4–5 hours. Without prior control of the diabetes, the mortality is high.
c. Treatment of severe diabetic ketoacidosis (adult).
   i. Investigations
Glucose, sodium, potassium, urea, serum osmolality, blood gases.

ii. Monitoring

BP, pulse, respiration, urine output, CVP measurement

iii. Rehydration

0.9% saline 1 litre is given in 30 minutes, then 1 litre per hour for 2 hours, followed by 500 ml hourly until a total of 5–7 litres has been given. 500 ml is then infused 2–4-hourly.

When a BG of 10–14 mmol/l has been achieved, change to 5% glucose 4-hourly.

If sodium >146 mmol/l then, after second litre 0.9% saline, substitute sodium chloride 0.18% and glucose 4%.

iv. Insulin therapy

Give 6 u i.v. stat, then using hourly glucose test strips, regulate the rate on a sliding scale.

v. Potassium

Immediately following the first dose of insulin, give potassium chloride 13 mmol/h in the saline. Monitor serum potassium:

K+ <3 mmol/l	give 39 mmol/h
K+ 3–4 mmol/l	give 26 mmol/h
K+ 4–6 mmol/l	give 13 mmol/h
K+ >6 mmol/l	stop potassium

vi. Acidosis

pH = <7.0, give sodium bicarbonate 100 mmol and KCl 20 mmol in the first 30 minutes.

pH = 7.0–7.1, give sodium bicarbonate 50 mmol and KCl 10 mmol.

5. Insulin resistance

In a number of circumstances insulin resistance occurs. Normally the ratio of insulin to glucose required is 10 u insulin to 500 ml 10% dextrose. In patients with severe infection, obesity, liver disease, on steroid therapy or undergoing cardiopulmonary bypass, the dose of insulin may have to be increased by up to four times the normal ratio.

6. Impaired conscious level in diabetics

Causes include hypoglycaemia, diabetic ketoacidosis, hyperglycaemic hyperosmolar non-ketotic coma, and lactic acidosis.

Typical laboratory findings are (Alberti & Hockaday 1987):

a. Hypoglycaemia

BG <2 mmol/l

b. Severe diabetic ketoacidosis

BG >15 mmol/l	Ketones + to +++
Dehydration +++	Hyperventilation +++

c. Hyperglycaemic, hyperosmolar, non-ketotic coma

BG >15 mmol/l	Ketones 0 to +
Dehydration ++++	No hyperventilation

d. Lactic acidosis

BG variable	Ketones 0 to +
Dehydration 0 to +	Hyperventilation +++

Other non-diabetic causes should not be forgotten.

BIBLIOGRAPHY

Alberti K G M M, Hockaday T D R 1987 Diabetes mellitus. In: Oxford Textbook of Medicine.
    Oxford University Press, Oxford
Alberti K G M M, Thomas D J B 1979 The management of diabetes during surgery. British
    Journal of Anaesthesia 51: 693–710
Bowen D J, Daykin A P, Nancekievill M L, Norman J 1984 Insulin-dependent diabetic
    patients during surgery and labour. Anaesthesia 39: 407–411
Hall G M, Desborough J P 1988 Diabetes and anaesthesia – slow progress. Anaesthesia 43:
    531–532
Page M McB, Watkins P J 1978 Cardiorespiratory arrest and diabetic autonomic neuropathy.
    Lancet i: 14–16

DOWN'S SYNDROME

This well-known syndrome with characteristic morphological features and
mental retardation, results from the chromosomal abnormality, trisomy 21.
Mortality is increased at any stage of life, but improved medical and
nursing care means that many more individuals are surviving into
adulthood and may present for surgery. 60–70% patients now survive
beyond 10 years of age.

Preoperative abnormalities

1. Cardiac abnormalities occur in 50–60% of patients and are usually
responsible for the initial mortality in infancy. The commonest lesions are
septal defects, Fallot's tetralogy and patent ductus arteriosus.
2. A defect in the immune system results in an increased incidence of
infection. Granulocyte abnormalities, decreased adrenal responses and
defects in cell-mediated immunity have all been identified.
3. Skeletal abnormalities occur. Atlantoaxial instability has only recently
been recognized as a problem, just at a time when these children are
being encouraged to participate in gymnastics! In one survey, 18% of 85
Down's children had C1/C2 articulation abnormalities. 12% had
subluxation alone and 6% were associated with odontoid peg
abnormalities (Semine et al 1978). The cause is still uncertain, but poor
muscle tone, ligamentous laxity and abnormal development of the
odontoid peg may act in concert.
4. Biochemical abnormalities have been found and may involve serotonin,
catecholamine and amino acid metabolism.
5. Thyroid hypofunction is common in adults. A child with Down's
syndrome with a thyrotoxic crisis which mimicked malignant hyperpyrexia
has also been described (Peters et al 1981).
6. Sleep-induced ventilatory dysfunction has been reported.
7. Institutionalized Down's patients have an increased incidence of
hepatitis B antigen.

Anaesthetic problems

The incidence of significant abnormalities is high. In a review of 100 cases of Down's syndrome requiring surgery, 44 patients had lesions requiring cardiac surgery and 41 others had abnormalities or diseases with anaesthetic implications (Kobel et al 1982).

1. Cervical spine abnormalities increase the risk of dislocation of certain cervical vertebrae on intubation, or when the patient is paralysed with muscle relaxants. Atlantoaxial subluxation and spinal cord compression were discovered in two children, after anaesthesia for surgical procedures. In neither case had cervical spine screening been carried out, nor had precautions been taken during intubation (Moore et al 1987, Williams et al 1987).
2. A smaller endotracheal tube size is required than would be anticipated for the age of the patient (Kobel et al 1982).
3. Airway and intubation difficulties sometimes occur, due to a combination of anatomical features. These include a large tongue, a small mandible and maxilla, a narrow nasopharynx and irregular teeth.
4. Postoperative stridor after prolonged nasal intubation has been reported (Sherry 1983). Congenital subglottic stenosis occurs occasionally.
5. Obstructive sleep apnoea is common in Down's syndrome (Silverman 1988). Chronic episodes of hypoxia and hypercarbia may lead to pulmonary hypertension and congestive heart failure. Airway patency depends upon both the anatomical structure of the upper respiratory tract, and the normal functioning of the pharyngeal muscles. Abnormalities of either or both may occur.
6. A higher incidence of atelectasis and pulmonary oedema was reported after surgery for congenital heart disease (Morray et al 1986). Those with Down's syndrome and ventricular septal defects were predisposed to pulmonary vascular obstruction.

Management

1. Lateral X-rays of the neck in full flexion and extension positions are required to detect atlantoaxial instability. This may show as an increase in the distance between the posterior surface of the anterior arch of the atlas and the anterior surface of the odontoid process (Hungerford et al 1981). If instability is present, great care should be taken to immobilize the neck during intubation and muscle relaxation.
2. An endotracheal tube should be used which is 1–2 sizes smaller than would be expected from the patient's age.
3. If prolonged nasotracheal intubation is required, steroids should be given prior to extubation. The child should receive humidification and be observed carefully for signs of stridor. There may be an indication for respiratory stimulants.
4. Close observation is required in the perioperative period to detect episodes of obstructive apnoea. A pulse oximeter may be useful.

1

BIBLIOGRAPHY

Hungerford G D, Akkaraju V, Rawe S E, Young G F 1981 Atlanto-occipital and atlanto-axial dislocations with spinal cord compression in Down's syndrome: a case report and review of the literature. British Journal of Radiology 54: 758–761

Kobel M, Creighton R E, Steward D J 1982 Anaesthetic considerations in Down's syndrome. Canadian Anaesthetists' Society Journal 29: 593–599

Moore R A, McNicholas K W, Warran S P 1987 Atlantoaxial subluxation with symptomatic spinal cord compression in a child with Down's syndrome. Anesthesia and Analgesia 66: 89–90

Morray J P, MacGillivray R, Duker G 1986 Increased perioperative risk following repair of congenital heart disease in Down's syndrome. Anesthesiology 65: 221–224

Peters K R, Nance P, Wingard D W 1981 Malignant hyperthyroidism or malignant hyperthermia? Anesthesia and Analgesia 60: 613–615

Semine A A, Ertel A N, Goldberg M J, Bull M J 1978 Cervical spine instability in children with Down's syndrome. Journal of Bone and Joint Surgery 60A: 649–652

Sherry K M 1983 Post-extubation stridor in Down's syndrome. British Journal of Anaesthesia 55: 53–55

Silverman M 1988 Airway obstruction and sleep disruption in Down's syndrome. British Medical Journal 296: 1618–1619

Williams J P, Somerville G M, Miner M E, Reilly D 1987 Atlanto-axial subluxation and trisomy-21: another perioperative complication. Anesthesiology 67: 253–254

DROWNING AND NEAR DROWNING

Drowning is one of the commonest causes of accidental death in young people and is potentially remediable if appropriate treatment is instituted without delay. Early animal experiments led to undue emphasis being placed on the differences between salt and fresh water, the accompanying osmotic changes, and in fresh water, the possibility of massive haemolysis. In practice, the inhaled volumes are much less than those induced experimentally, the haemolysis is not significant, and in large series of patients reaching hospital the electrolyte and blood values showed no significant difference between the two (Golden 1980). In general therefore, the management of drowning depends on the clinical state, not the medium. Of more importance is the diagnosis of incidents possibly contributing to the clinical state such as alcohol intoxication, head and neck injury, abdominal injury, epilepsy or myocardial infarction. One of the crucial factors affecting survival from near drowning is the institution of prompt effective CPR at the site of the incident, and prior to hospital admission.

Presentation

1. Respiration may be adequate, inadequate or absent. In a review of 130 cases, those with adequate respiration on arrival in hospital had an excellent prognosis (Simcock 1986).
2. If aspiration of water has occurred, then hypoxia may be present, due to washing out of surfactant, and intrapulmonary shunting. Signs of inhalation may not be immediately evident.
3. Circulatory changes are complex. In the most serious group, asystole

1

or VF may be present. Severe vasoconstriction may make it difficult to determine whether there is cardiac output or not (Modell 1986). In the less severe case there may be hypovolaemia and poor peripheral perfusion.

4. Hypothermia is common. At 26–28°C it may be difficult to reverse VF or asystole. Above 30°C the problem is less urgent. A moderate degree of hypothermia has a cerebral protectant effect.

5. Secondary drowning has been described, in which pulmonary oedema may develop at any time up to 3 days after the event. In children, secondary drowning in salt water has been found to have a worse prognosis than that after fresh-water incidents (Pearn 1980).

Investigations

1. After the initial resuscitation, monitoring of blood gases, CXR and base deficit will indicate whether there is further development, or resolution, of any respiratory complications.

2. ECG may show arrhythmias, especially on rewarming. The CVP will indicate hypovolaemia and urine output helps to guide therapy.

3. Core temperature monitoring.

4. Determinations of haemoglobin, haematocrit, electrolytes and urea levels are required. These will give baseline values in case of subsequent complications, but changes are usually small and rarely need therapy.

Management

1. If there is still no evident cardiac output on admission to hospital, then ECM should be continued until the nature of the cardiac rhythm is established on ECG.

2. An attempt is made to maintain the PaO_2 above 8 kPa with up to 50% oxygen. If this is impossible and there is significant intrapulmonary shunting, IPPV with PEEP will be needed. Should hypotension result, expansion of the vascular volume will be required.

3. Treatment of any circulatory failure should be monitored with a CVP. Hypovolaemia occurs commonly, particularly in salt-water drowning. PPF may be required. If crystalloid is needed then dextrose 5% should be used in salt-water drowning, and saline in fresh water. If pH is <7.2, partial correction of the acidosis is advisable.

4. Unless the body temperature is less than 30°C, in which case serious cardiac arrhythmias may occur, rapid treatment of the hypothermia is unnecessary and possibly dangerous. Sudden vasodilatation may cause hypotension, and increases the hazard of cold acidotic blood returning to the heart. Moderate hypothermia is of positive benefit in reducing hypoxic brain damage, especially in children. Successful resuscitation has been achieved after total immersion for 25 minutes at 4°C in a child (Theilade 1977). If the temperature is below 30°C then warmed peritoneal dialysis should be considered.

1

5. The use of steroids is controversial. Despite this, many authors admit to giving high-dose methylprednisolone, 30 mg/kg for two doses.
6. Antibiotic therapy depends on the likely water pollution. Ampicillin is commonly used prophylactically.

Complications

1. Cerebral oedema.
2. Pulmonary infection.
3. Renal failure has been reported.

BIBLIOGRAPHY

Simcock A D 1986 Treatment of near drowning – a review of 130 cases. Anaesthesia 41: 643–648
Golden F StC 1980 Problems of immersion. British Journal of Hospital Medicine 23: 371–383
Modell J H 1986 Near drowning. Circulation 74: (suppl IV) 27–28
Pearn J H 1980 Secondary drowning in children. British Medical Journal 281: 1103–1105
Theilade D 1977 The danger of fatal misjudgement in hypothermia after immersion. Anaesthesia 32: 889–892

DUCHENNE MUSCULAR DYSTROPHY
(DMD)

An X-linked recessive, severe muscular dystrophy which usually presents with proximal lower limb and pelvic muscle weakness. The weakness, which is progressive and varies between muscles, is due to a decrease in the total number of muscle fibres. The young child, on attempting to rise, will use its arms to 'climb' up its own legs. Cardiac muscle disease occurs with characteristic ECG changes and a hypertrophic cardiomyopathy. The condition steadily progresses to involve other muscles until finally death, from respiratory failure (75% of cases), pneumonia or cardiac disease, occurs between the ages of 10 and 20.

Preoperative abnormalities

1. Varying degrees of muscle weakness are present, with initial involvement of the thighs and pelvis. The calf muscles are enlarged with fatty tissue (pseudohypertrophy) and if the shoulder girdle is affected there is winging of the scapulae. Progressive scoliosis usually occurs. The child is often obese and eventually becomes confined to a wheelchair.
2. Vital capacity falls progressively, and when below 700 ml the risk of death is high. Diaphragmatic weakness occurs and blood gases may show hypoventilation and hypoxia in the later stages of the disease.
3. Serum CPK can be grossly raised, the highest levels often occurring in the early stages of the disease. An EMG will confirm the presence of a myopathy.

4. Clinical signs of a hypertrophic cardiomyopathy, with diastolic failure due to left ventricular inflow obstruction, may exist. The ECG shows abnormalities in over 90% of patients. Characteristic changes are a tall R wave and an RSR1 in lead V1, a deep Q wave in leads V3–6, a prolonged PR interval, and a sinus tachycardia. Echocardiography will demonstrate mitral valve prolapse in 25% of patients. Sudden death can occur.

Anaesthetic problems

Although many apparently uneventful anaesthetics have been given to patients with DMD (Richards 1972), there are now sufficient reports of serious intraoperative or postoperative complications that extreme care should be taken for the whole perioperative period. While the respiratory complications usually occurred with advanced disease, this is not necessarily the case with acute cardiac events. The occurrence of cardiac arrest during anaesthesia was sometimes the first indication that the child had a muscle dystrophy (Seay et al 1978).

1. Tachycardia, ventricular fibrillation and cardiac arrest have all been reported during induction of anaesthesia (Genever 1971, Linter et al 1982, Smith & Bush 1985, Buzello & Huttarsch 1988). Most reports have involved the use of suxamethonium and may therefore have been associated with acute hyperkalaemia. However, a case in which a rise in temperature and cardiac arrest occurred after 11 minutes of an inhalation induction (assisted ventilation) with halothane alone, has been reported in a child with a CPK of 14 000 iu, who was to undergo muscle biopsy (Sethna & Rockoff 1986).

2. It has been suggested that DMD is associated with an increased incidence of MH (Brownell et al 1983, Rosenberg & Heiman-Patterson 1983, Wang & Stanley 1986). Cases have been reported which have some, and occasionally all, of the clinical features of MH, but few papers present in vitro or electron microscopic evidence of MH. One paper reported an abnormal contraction to halothane, but not to caffeine, in muscle taken from a 4-year-old boy with DMD (Rosenberg & Heiman-Patterson 1983). Another showed abnormal responses to both tests in a 5-year-old child, who had suffered cardiac arrest, metabolic acidosis and acute rhabdomyolysis following suxamethonium (Brownell et al 1983). Whether or not MH and DMD regularly coexist is debatable. However, from a clinical point of view, in either condition, suxamethonium or halothane may be the triggering agents for a variety of non-specific complications, which can occur and are associated with acute disruption of muscle. These include pyrexia, tachycardia, acidosis, hyperkalaemia, asystole, VF, muscle spasm, acute rhabdomyolysis and a high CPK. All of these complications have been reported, either singly, or in various combinations, in some patients with DMD.

3. If asystole or VF occurs, then the cardiomyopathic heart may be resistant to resuscitation measures (Sethna et al 1988).

4. The response to non-depolarizing agents may be abnormal. This cannot be predicted in advance. The stage of the disease and the muscles monitored will presumably have some bearing on this. Cumulative 50% and 90% blocking doses of vecuronium were determined in two 4-year-old boys (Buzello & Huttarsch 1988). Although the authors found no increase in sensitivity to vecuronium, the recovery time from 75% to 25% block of twitch tension was three to nearly six times that of normal.

5. It has been suggested, on theoretical grounds, that the accumulation of acetylcholine at the motor end-plate caused by the administration of neostigmine might trigger rhabdomyolysis (Buzello & Huttarsch 1988). This has not been confirmed clinically.

6. Postoperative respiratory insufficiency. There are a number of reports of 'uneventful' anaesthetics using a barbiturate, suxamethonium and halothane, but in which delayed respiratory insufficiency occurred from 5 to 36 hours postoperatively (Smith & Bush 1985). Difficulty in swallowing, breathing and clearing secretions all featured in the pattern of deterioration. Despite intubation and IPPV, a number of the children subsequently had cardiac arrests from which they could not be resuscitated.

7. Isolated myoglobinuria following adenoidectomy was the first indication of DMD in a 5-year-old boy (Rubiano et al 1987).

Management

1. Assessment of respiratory function is helpful, if the child is old enough to cooperate. Diaphragmatic involvement suggests serious impairment. A difference in vital capacity of more than 25% between the erect and supine positions is indicative of diaphragmatic weakness (Heckmatt 1987). In the later stages of DMD, arterial blood gases will show impending respiratory failure. Assessment is particularly important when major elective surgery, such as scoliosis correction, is contemplated (Milne & Rosales 1982). It has been suggested that, for scoliosis surgery, the patient should have a VC of at least 20 ml/kg (or 30% of predicted) and an inspiratory capacity of 15 ml/kg.

2. Evidence of cardiac involvement should be sought. This may vary from ECG changes alone to diastolic failure.

3. If advanced disease is present, the wisdom and possible benefits of surgery should be weighed against the risks. If the assessment is misjudged, elective surgery may hasten death, or commit a patient with a progressive and ultimately fatal disease to a period of prolonged ventilation.

4. Consideration should be given to the use of a local anaesthetic technique.

5. Suxamethonium should not be used in patients with DMD as, at present, it does not appear possible to predict which patients might develop hyperkalaemia, cardiac arrest, rigidity, rhabdomyolysis or

1

postoperative respiratory failure, all of which complications have been attributed to its use.

6. In view of the variability of response, neuromuscular monitoring and incremental dosages should be employed when non-depolarizing muscle relaxants are used. Vecuronium has been suggested as being suitable, although there may be a prolonged duration of action. Responses in the peripheral muscles do not always reflect those in respiratory muscles, and the evoked EMG may recover faster than the actual mechanical response (Buzello & Huttarsch 1988).

7. Although many patients have been safely anaesthetized with halothane, its use has been challenged, particularly when the CPK is very high. The report of cardiac arrest occurring during an inhalational induction with halothane is of concern (Sethna & Rockoff 1986). So also is the critical review condemning the use of halothane in patients with DMD and a high CPK (Roizen 1987). The cause of the arrest cannot be accurately determined, but it is easy to visualize how a serious arrhythmia might occur in a myopathic heart with a combination of even mild respiratory obstruction, light anaesthesia and halothane. That halothane given alone is capable of producing muscle breakdown is demonstrated by the report of myoglobinuria following an anaesthetic in which suxamethonium was not used (Rubiano et al 1987).

8. Those authors who have described complications clinically similar to malignant hyperthermia, suggest that a non-MH-triggering anaesthetic should be given to patients with DMD. On the contrary, halothane has been used safely in many cases and it can be argued that it is easier and hence safer to use in young children.

Whichever technique is chosen, ECG, temperature and ETCO$_2$ should be monitored from the start of the anaesthetic and dantrolene must be immediately available.

9. Observation in a high dependency area for the first 24–48 hours after anaesthesia will assist in the early detection of pulmonary insufficiency. If doubt arises, it is much safer to ventilate the patient until all drugs have been eliminated.

BIBLIOGRAPHY

Brownell A K W, Paasuke R T, Elash A, Fowlow S B, Seagram C G, Diewold R J, Friesen C 1983 Malignant hyperthermia in Duchenne muscular dystrophy. Anesthesiology 58: 180–182

Buzello W, Huttarsch H 1988 Muscle relaxation in patients with Duchenne's muscular dystrophy. British Journal of Anaesthesia 60: 228–231

Genever E E 1971 Suxamethonium induced cardiac arrest in unsuspected pseudohypertrophic muscular dystrophy. British Journal of Anaesthesia 43: 984–986

Heckmatt J Z (Editorial) 1987 Respiratory care in muscular dystrophy. British Medical Journal 295: 1014–1015

Linter S P K, Thomas P R, Withington P S, Hall M G 1982 Suxamethonium associated hypertonicity and cardiac arrest in unsuspected pseudohypertrophic muscular dystrophy. British Journal of Anaesthesia 54: 1331–1333

Milne B, Rosales J K 1982 Anaesthetic considerations in patients with muscular dystrophy undergoing spinal fusion and Harrington rod insertion. Canadian Anaesthetists' Society Journal 29: 250–254

Richards W C 1972 Anaesthesia and serum creatine phosphokinase levels in patients with Duchenne's pseudohypertrophic muscular dystrophy. Anaesthesia and Intensive Care 1: 150–153

Roizen M F 1987 Comment. Survey of Anesthesiology 31: 232–233

Rosenberg H, Heiman-Patterson T 1983 Duchenne's muscular dystrophy and malignant hyperthermia: another warning. Anesthesiology 59: 362

Rubiano R, Chang J-L, Carroll J, Sonbolian N, Larson C E 1987 Acute rhabdomyolysis following halothane anesthesia without succinylcholine. Anesthesiology 67: 856–857

Seay A R, Ziter F A, Thompson J A 1978 Cardiac arrest during induction of anesthesia in Duchenne muscular dystrophy. Journal of Pediatrics 93: 88–90

Sethna N F, Rockoff M A 1986 Cardiac arrest following inhalation induction of anesthesia in a child with Duchenne's muscular dystrophy. Canadian Anaesthetist's Society Journal 33: 799–802

Sethna N F, Rockoff M A, Worthen H M, Rosnow J M 1988 Anesthesia related complications in children with Duchenne muscular dystrophy. Anesthesiology 68: 462–465

Smith C L, Bush G H 1985 Anaesthesia and progressive muscular dystrophy. British Journal of Anaesthesia 57: 1113–1118

Wang J M, Stanley T H 1986 Duchenne muscular dystrophy and hyperthermia: two case reports. Canadian Anaesthetists' Society Journal 33: 492–497

DYSTROPHIA MYOTONICA
(AND OTHER MYOTONIC SYNDROMES)

Dystrophia myotonica, myotonia congenita and paramyotonia, are three distinct diseases of autosomal dominant inheritance, in which myotonia occurs. Myotonia is a persistence of muscle contraction beyond the duration of the voluntary effort or stimulation. In myotonia congenita (Thomsen's disease), the generalized myotonia is enhanced by cold and resting, but may be improved by exercise. Subjects with paramyotonia have attacks of muscle weakness resembling those in periodic paralysis, to which it may be related. Again, the myotonia is provoked by cold. Dystrophia myotonica (Steinert's disease), to which this section refers, is a syndrome in which there is myotonia and dystrophic changes in certain muscles, associated with other clinical features. The site of the abnormality is the muscle fibre, as myotonia persists after the administration of neuromuscular blocking agents, local anaesthetics, and neural section.

Preoperative abnormalities

1. Clinical features

a. Infancy. The baby may present with feeding difficulties or respiratory insufficiency. There is generalized hypotonia, facial diplegia and mental retardation. There may be thin ribs, high diaphragm and peripheral oedema. Myotonia is not a feature. Usually one parent has the disease.

b. Adult form. This usually presents in the third and fourth decades. Myotonia is associated with weakness and muscle wasting. Unlike most other myopathies, it predominantly involves the distal and cranial muscles. After a handshake, the patient cannot relax, and percussion myotonia may be demonstrated, particularly in the tongue or thenar eminence. Frontal baldness, ptosis and facial weakness, cataracts, hypogonadism, cardiomyopathy and conduction abnormalities, and a low IQ, are other features of the condition. There is an increased CPK. Death may occur in middle age from respiratory or cardiac complications.

2. EMG shows electrical after-discharge.

Anaesthetic problems

1. There may be chronic underventilation and respiratory muscle weakness. Vital capacity, expiratory reserve volume, maximum breathing capacity and maximal inspiratory pressure are all markedly reduced, due to abnormalities in the respiratory muscles. It has been suggested that central nervous system disease may contribute to the poor respiratory reserve. Somnolence and prolonged apnoea can occur, and respiration is readily depressed by barbiturates, inhalation agents, benzodiazepines and opiates (Aldridge 1985).

2. It may be difficult to prevent myotonia from occurring during surgical manipulation and diathermy, as it is not necessarily abolished by muscle relaxants, local or regional anaesthesia. Depolarizing relaxants can produce a prolonged contraction which outlasts the duration of effect. Non-depolarizing relaxants may or may not produce relaxation. In one case, masseter spasm and shivering occurred for 4 minutes after the administration of fentanyl (Paterson et al 1985). Hypothermia, shivering and potassium may all cause generalized myotonia.

3. There may be cardiovascular disease. Arrhythmias, including AF and conduction defects, cardiomyopathy, mitral valve prolapse and heart failure have been reported.

4. Disordered oesophageal contraction may predispose to pulmonary aspiration.

5. There is an increased incidence of postoperative problems (Moore & Moore 1987). A 32-year-old man had a stormy course after thymectomy (Mudge et al 1980). Complications included pneumonia, pulmonary emboli and cardiac arrhythmias.

6. Although pregnancy is rare, if it occurs it may be associated with an increase in myotonic symptoms (Paterson et al 1985).

Management

1. A detailed clinical examination for the distribution of muscle weakness and myotonia.

2. If the respiratory muscles are involved, lung function tests and blood gases will give some indication of the severity of the restrictive lung defect.

3. Arrhythmias should be diagnosed and treated. Occasionally a temporary pacemaker may be required.

4. Induction agents should be given in small doses. The anaesthetist should be prepared to treat the apnoea which often follows.

5. The use of suxamethonium should be avoided. Intubation may be possible using thiopentone and an inhalational agent alone.

6. Non-depolarizing relaxants can be used, but they do not guarantee muscle relaxation. There are conflicting reports concerning the reliability of neostigmine as an antagonist. Incomplete reversal of neuromuscular blockade is common and there are reports of a second dose of neostigmine worsening the situation. The problem may be avoided by ventilating the patient postoperatively until all drugs have been excreted and respiration is adequate.

7. The use of local or regional techniques will avoid some of the problems associated with drugs used for general anaesthesia (Bray & Inkster 1984). Successful epidural anaesthesia has been reported in a patient for Caesarean section (Paterson et al 1985), and a caudal epidural was used in a 2-year-old child (Alexander et al 1981). However, these techniques will not always guarantee surgical muscle relaxation.

8. A number of measures have been tried in attempts to reduce myotonia. Severe uterine spasm, occurring during Caesarean section under spinal anaesthesia, was relieved by the application of bupivacaine 30 ml 0.5% to the cut surface of the myometrium (Cope & Miller 1986). However, administration of dantrolene failed to produce muscle relaxation in a patient undergoing cholecystectomy (Phillips et al 1984).

9. Measures to prevent pulmonary aspiration, prompt attention to respiratory inadequacy and the use of antibiotics, may all help to prevent the occurrence of pneumonia and lung abscess.

10. The operating theatre should be kept warm and measures taken to avoid shivering.

BIBLIOGRAPHY

Aldridge M 1985 Anaesthetic problems in myotonic dystrophy. British Journal of Anaesthesia 57: 1119–1130

Alexander C, Wolf S, Ghia J N 1981 Caudal anesthesia for early onset myotonic dystrophy. Anesthesiology 55: 597–598

Bray R J, Inkster J S 1984 Anaesthesia in babies with congenital dystrophia myotonica. Anaesthesia 39: 1007–1011

Cope D K, Miller J N 1986 Local and spinal anesthesia for Cesarean section in a patient with myotonic dystrophy. Anesthesia and Analgesia 65: 687–690

Moore J K, Moore A P 1987 Postoperative complications of dystrophia myotonica. Anaesthesia 42: 529–533

Mudge B J, Taylor P B, Vanderspek A F L 1980 Perioperative hazards of myotonic dystrophy. Anaesthesia 35: 492–495

Paterson R A, Tousignant M, Skene D S 1985 Caesarean section for twins in a patient with myotonic dystrophy. Canadian Anaesthetists' Society Journal 32: 418–421

Phillips D C, Ellis F R, Exley K A, Ness M A 1984 Dantrolene sodium and dystrophia myotonica. Anaesthesia 39: 568–573

1

EATON–LAMBERT SYNDROME

A myasthenic-like syndrome associated with carcinomas, usually of the lung, which sometimes precedes the tumour by as much as 2 years. Muscle weakness and fatiguability often involve the thigh and pelvic muscles primarily. There appears to be a failure of release of acetylcholine quanta at the neuromuscular junction, although each quantum released is normal. Animal studies using IgG from affected patients would appear to indicate that autoantibodies are involved.

Preoperative abnormalities

1. Muscles are fatiguable, as in myasthenia gravis, but the proximal limbs and trunk are initially affected rather than the eye muscles. In contrast to myasthenia, although the patient complains of fatiguability, the muscle power may actually increase after brief exercise. Lower limb reflexes are reduced or absent, but may be enhanced by prior voluntary contraction, whereas in true myasthenia, reflexes are preserved. Neostigmine produces little or no improvement in the weakness.
2. EMG shows an increase in amplitude of action potentials in response to stimulation at high rates.
3. Patients tend to be older than those with myasthenia.
4. Associated lung carcinomas are usually oat cell in type, and are often small and less aggressive than normal.
5. Some improvement may be obtained with guanidine, steroids or plasma exchange.

Anaesthetic problems

1. Prolonged paralysis can occur with depolarizing or non-depolarizing relaxants. Inadequate reversal may occur with neostigmine. An improvement in evoked action potential has been reported after treatment with 4-aminopyridine (Agoston et al 1978).

Management

1. Muscle relaxants should, if possible, be avoided. If essential, the effects of small doses should be monitored carefully. A local anaesthetic technique may be appropriate.
2. Respiratory insufficiency should be treated with postoperative IPPV.

BIBLIOGRAPHY

Agoston S, van Weerden T, Westra P, Broekert A 1978 Effects of 4-aminopyridine in Eaton Lambert syndrome. British Journal of Anaesthesia 50: 383–385

EBSTEIN'S ANOMALY

A rare congenital cardiac abnormality. The septal and posterior cusps of
the tricuspid valve are displaced downwards and are elongated, such that
a varying amount of the right ventricle effectively becomes part of the
atrium. Its wall is thin and it contracts poorly. The remaining functional
part of the right ventricle is therefore small. The foramen ovale is patent
or defective in 80% of cases.
The degree of abnormality of right ventricular function, and the size of the
ASD, are probably the main determinants of the severity of the condition.
The right ventricular systolic pressure is low, and the RVEDP is elevated.
Tricuspid incompetence can occur. There may be a right to left shunt, with
cyanosis, on effort, and pulmonary hypertension and right heart failure
may supervene. However, the natural history of the disease is very
variable. 50% of cases present in infancy with cyanosis. In some adults,
symptoms may be precipitated by the onset of arrhythmias, or by
pregnancy. A few patients remain asymptomatic, even as adults.

Preoperative abnormalities

1. There may be dyspnoea and cyanosis at rest, on moderate exertion, or
the patient may be asymptomatic.
2. Episodes of tachyarrhythmias occur in 25% of patients. Some provoke
syncopal attacks.
3. ECG may show varying abnormalities, including large peaked P waves,
a long P–R interval, Wolff–Parkinson–White syndrome, RBBB and right
heart strain.
4. CXR may show cardiomegaly, with a prominent right heart border and
poorly perfused lung fields.
5. Paradoxical systemic embolism and subacute bacterial endocarditis may
occur.

Anaesthetic problems

These will depend upon the anatomical abnormality, the degree of right
to left shunt and the presence or absence of right heart failure.

1. Prolonged anaesthetic induction times, due to pooling of drugs in the
large atrial chamber, have been reported (Elsten et al 1981, Halpern et al
1985).
2. The use of intracardiac catheters may be hazardous as serious cardiac
arrhythmias can be provoked.
3. Air entering peripheral venous lines may cause paradoxical air
emboli.

4. Tachycardia is poorly tolerated because of impaired filling of the functionally small right ventricle.

5. Hypotension may increase the right to left shunt, if present.

6. Hypoxia causes pulmonary vasoconstriction, which also increases a right to left shunt.

7. There is a risk of bacterial endocarditis, especially if there is a CVP line in situ.

8. Deterioration may occur in pregnancy (Linter & Clarke 1984), or with the onset of arrhythmias.

Management

1. The severity of the lesion must be assessed.

2. Heart failure and arrhythmias require treatment.

3. Antibiotic prophylaxis against SBE should be given.

4. If a CVP is used for monitoring, its tip should be kept within the SVC. The use of intracardiac catheters should probably be avoided.

5. Techniques should aim to minimize tachycardia and hypotension.

6. Oxygen therapy increases pulmonary vasodilatation.

7. A number of anaesthetic techniques have been reported. A two-catheter epidural technique was used for vaginal delivery, to minimize hypotension (Linter & Clarke 1984). Caesarean section has been reported under general anaesthesia, preceded by fentanyl (Halpern et al 1985), and a neurolept analgesic technique was described for hysterectomy (Bengtsson et al 1977).

BIBLIOGRAPHY

Bengtsson I M, Magno R, Wickstrom I 1977 Ebstein's anomaly – anaesthetic problems. British Journal of Anaesthesia 49: 501–503

Elsten J L, Kim Y D, Hanowell S T, Macnamara T E 1981 Prolonged induction with exaggerated chamber enlargement in Ebstein's anomaly. Anesthesia and Analgesia 60: 909–910

Halpern S, Gidwaney A, Gates B 1985 Anaesthesia for Caesarean section in a preeclamptic patient with Ebstein's anomaly. Canadian Anaesthetists' Society Journal 32: 244–247

Linter S P K, Clarke K 1984 Caesarean section under extradural analgesia in a patient with Ebstein's anomaly. British Journal of Anaesthesia 56: 203–205

ECLAMPSIA AND SEVERE PRE-ECLAMPSIA

Pre-eclampsia is a syndrome of unknown aetiology which is associated with pregnancy. It affects a wide variety of organs and therefore produces diverse manifestations. The main presenting feature is hypertension, with either proteinuria or oedema, or both. Maternal complications include eclampsia, cerebral haemorrhage, cerebral oedema, renal failure and left ventricular failure.

Eclampsia, a cerebral complication, is marked by the onset of convulsions. Cerebral haemorrhage and cerebral oedema are the most frequent causes of death in pre-eclampsia. Deaths from pre-eclampsia nearly equal those from eclampsia, and together they are the most important obstetric cause of maternal mortality in the Western world (Redman 1988).

Occasionally an intracranial aneurysm may rupture during pregnancy. The presentation will share some of the features of eclampsia and severe pre-eclampsia – an acute severe headache and neurological signs, with or without a period of unconsciousness. It is crucial that this is distinguished from pre-eclampsia. It has been suggested that early diagnosis and surgery will improve the morbidity and mortality of this condition (Giannotti et al 1986).

A small group of patients have been described with the HELLP syndrome which comprises pre-eclampsia, in association with haemolysis, elevated liver enzymes and a low platelet count.

Presentation

1. Severe pre-eclampsia is associated with a BP of 160/110 or more on at least two occasions 6 hours apart, and proteinuria of >5 g in 24 hours (Wright 1983).
2. Whilst pre-eclampsia is common in the young primiparous patient, there appears to be a subgroup for whom the maternal and fetal risks are particularly high (Connell et al 1987). The patient with pre-eclampsia at special risk is the older (>25 years), multiparous patient, and particularly the one who develops an impairment in her level of consciousness.
3. The onset of convulsions denotes eclampsia. It may be associated with cerebral haemorrhage or diffuse oedema.
4. The HELLP syndrome may present with bleeding due to thrombocytopenia, a fall in haemoglobin due to haemolysis and abnormal LFTs (Duffy 1988).

Problems

1. Hypertension, which may be complicated by cerebral oedema, haemorrhage or heart failure. Both pre-eclampsia, and pregnancy-aggravated hypertension, are associated with exaggerated pressor responses to accelerated labour, or to noxious stimuli such as endotracheal intubation or extubation. The hypertensive response to intubation has provoked cerebral haemorrhage (Fox et al 1977). In a study of pre-eclamptics undergoing Caesarean section, it has been shown that even in those receiving a conventional antihypertensive regimen, intubation was associated with an average increase in SAP of 54.4 mmHg (Connell et al 1987). In some patients, increases of over 70 mmHg occurred. It is recognized that, in normotensive patients, mean arterial pressures exceeding 130–150 mmHg may be associated with a loss of protective cerebral autoregulation (Wright 1983, Richards et al 1986).

2. Impaired renal function which may progress to anuria. Even in mild pre-eclampsia, the GFR is decreased by 25%. Renal failure accounts for about 10% of deaths from eclampsia.

3. Plasma volume may be decreased by up to 40% in severe cases. Despite sodium and water retention, the CVP is low. This is in part due to increased vascular permeability causing loss of fluid and protein from the circulation.

4. Maternal systemic blood flow is reduced secondary to vasoconstriction, increased peripheral resistance and raised blood viscosity. Diminished placental blood flow results in placental infarction and separation, which leads to decreased fetal growth and sometimes death. Maternal vessels become very sensitive to the effects of exogenous catecholamines.

5. A coagulopathy may occur, which is probably consumptive in origin. The number and quality of platelets commonly decrease and the thrombin time becomes prolonged. Prothrombin time, partial thromboplastin time and fibrinogen abnormalities may occur.

6. Pulmonary oedema, which can be vascular or neurogenic in origin, may produce cyanosis and respiratory distress.

7. Headache, epigastric pain, visual disturbances, hyperreflexia or cerebral irritability may be warning signs of impending eclampsia. Delayed recovery of consciousness following an eclamptic fit may indicate the occurrence of cerebral oedema or intracranial haemorrhage.

8. Not all fits occurring during pregnancy and labour are due to eclampsia. Eclamptic fits must be distinguished from those due to hyponatraemia associated with the concomitant administration of oxytocics and dextrose-containing fluids, a ruptured intracranial aneurysm, or other intracranial pathology.

9. Pulmonary aspiration and airway obstruction are both more likely to occur in oversedated or unconscious patients.

10. Rarely, severe pre-eclampsia is associated with abnormal liver function and hepatic damage.

11. Occasionally, laryngeal oedema may occur unexpectedly, and cause intubation problems (Seager & MacDonald 1980).

Management of severe pre-eclampsia

This is a potentially lethal condition which should be managed in a high dependency area. Monitoring and treatment requires close cooperation between obstetrician, anaesthetist and paediatrician, whether or not operative delivery is required. General anaesthesia may be particularly hazardous in some patients, and additional precautions should be taken to prevent hypertensive peaks during intubation and extubation.

Management of the severe pre-eclamptic, throughout the peripartum period, should be directed towards:

1. Monitoring
CVP, ECG, arterial pressure and urine output is monitored, as is neuromuscular function if general anaesthesia is required.
2. Control of maternal blood pressure by arteriolar dilatation
A number of different methods of controlling blood pressure prior to delivery have been described. The care with which it is monitored and controlled, is probably of more importance to maternal and fetal welfare than the exact method of control.
  a. Epidural analgesia. This has the dual therapeutic advantages of providing both vasodilatation and analgesia in pre-eclampsia. Provided that no coagulation defect is present, it is the method of choice for operative delivery. Platelet count should be $>100 \times 10^9/l$ and prothrombin time and partial thromboplastin time normal.
  b. Hydralazine 5–10 mg increments i.v., or by infusion.
  c. Diazoxide in 30 mg increments to a total of 300 mg i.v.
  d. Magnesium sulphate, which is used more commonly in the USA than in the UK, is both a vasodilator and a sedative. Magnesium sulphate 2 g stat and 2 g/h, via an infusion.

Magnesium (Mg) levels	
Normal serum	0.7–1.0 mmol/l
Therapeutic anticonvulsant levels	2–3 mmol/l
Loss of patellar reflex	5 mmol/l
Skeletal muscle relaxation	6 mmol/l
Respiratory paralysis	6–7.5 mmol/l
Cardiac asystole	>12 mmol/l

Accidental high levels can be treated by Ca gluconate 1 g slowly.
  e. Trimetaphan, as an infusion, has been used for fine control of blood pressure prior to induction (Lawes et al 1987).
3. Restoration of vascular volume and vasodilatation
This should take place synchronously, preferably using plasma protein fraction or a colloid. The CVP should be maintained around 6–8 cmH$_2$O, with reference to the mid-axillary line. Prevention of vasoconstriction and restoration of blood volume has the additional benefit of improving renal function and uteroplacental blood flow.
4. Prophylaxis against eclamptic fits
Diazepam, magnesium sulphate or chlormethiazole can be used to produce sedation.
5. Protection against acid aspiration syndrome
Sedated patients are particularly at risk.

6. Operative intervention

This should preferably be performed under epidural anaesthesia. In the very severe case, or if epidural anaesthesia is contraindicated, general anaesthesia may be required, but it carries additional risks. A careful technique should aim to modulate the hypertensive peaks provoked by intubation and extubation and to prevent sudden uncontrolled reductions in blood pressure. The latter can, however, be produced by either general or regional anaesthesia. It has been suggested that drugs which will help modify the hypertensive response to intubation, should be given before induction. These are given in addition to the preoperative antihypertensive regimen (Lawes et al 1987). As yet, there appears to be no technique which guarantees protection in every patient. The use of the following drugs has been reported:

a. Lignocaine 1 mg/kg i.v., prior to induction, to reduce haemodynamic responses (Connell et al 1987). Lignocaine has been shown to prevent intracranial hypertension during endotracheal suction in comatose head injury patients (Donegan & Bedford 1980).

b. Practolol in 2 mg increments, to a maximum dose of 0.2 mg/kg, has been found to modify tachycardia in response to intubation if the patient's pulse rate is >120/min (Connell et al 1987). It has been suggested that higher doses than this should not be used, as it may impair heart rate responses, in the event of haemorrhage.

c. An additional bolus of trimetaphan 2.5 mg before induction.

d. A bolus of hydralazine 6.25–12.5 mg i.v. before induction.

e. Fentanyl and droperidol have been used, in addition to conventional antihypertensive therapy (Lawes et al 1987). During preoxygenation, droperidol 5 mg and fentanyl 100 μg were given. After 5 minutes a further 100 μg of fentanyl was added. If the SAP was >170 mmHg, or the MAP >130 mmHg, trimetaphan 2.5 mg was also given. Induction of anaesthesia was only started when these pressure limits were not exceeded. It is essential to have an experienced person available to resuscitate the baby. However this technique was claimed not to have produced significant respiratory depression in unasphyxiated neonates (Lawes et al 1987).

f. Nitroglycerin has been shown to modify the hypertensive response to intubation in severe pre-eclamptics (Hood et al 1985). During preoxygenation, an infusion of nitroglycerin 200 μg/ml was given until the BP was reduced by 20%. The MAP was then maintained at this level during Caesarean section. However, as nitroglycerin is a cerebral vasodilator and increases intracranial pressure, it should not be used in eclampsia, or where there is a possibility of cerebral oedema.

g. Alfentanil 10 μg/kg has been shown to modify the hypertensive response to intubation in the non-hypertensive pregnant patient (Dann et al 1987).

1

Management of eclampsia

1. Convulsions should be controlled with diazepam 5–20 mg, the airway secured and oxygenation maintained. Endotracheal intubation, blood gas estimation and IPPV may be required.
2. Care should be taken to ensure that the diagnosis of eclampsia is correct. If a convulsion is not associated with hypertension, and either oedema or proteinuria, or if the history and signs are atypical, then other causes must be eliminated. If an intracranial aneurysm is suspected, a CT scan should be performed.
3. For control of hypertension, see above.
4. The only ultimate control of the eclampsia is by termination of the pregnancy, either by rapid vaginal delivery or by Caesarean section.
5. If an eclamptic patient remains unconscious 4–6 hours postpartum, neurosurgical advice should be sought. A CT scan will distinguish cerebral oedema from intracranial haemorrhage. It has been suggested that the combination of diffuse white matter oedema and basal cisternal effacement is an indication for intracranial pressure monitoring (Richards et al 1986). A high intracranial pressure (N = 10–15 mmHg) may require specific treatment.

Postdelivery care

Eclampsia may still occur in the postpartum period. In the severe case, intensive monitoring and treatment should continue for 24–72 hours.

BIBLIOGRAPHY

Connell H, Dalgleish J G, Downing J W 1987 General anaesthesia in mothers with severe preeclampsia/eclampsia. British Journal of Anaesthesia 59: 1375–1380
Dann W L, Hutchinson A, Cartwright D P 1987 Maternal and neonatal responses to alfentanil administered before induction of general anaesthesia for Caesarean section. British Journal of Anaesthesia 59: 1392–1396
Donegan M F, Bedford R F 1980 Intravenously administered lidocaine prevents intracranial hypertension during endotracheal suctioning. Anesthesiology 52: 516–518
Duffy B L 1988 HELLP syndrome and the anaesthetist. Anaesthesia 43: 223–225
Fox E J, Sklar G S, Hill C H, Villanueva R, King B D 1977 Complications related to the pressor response to endotracheal intubation. Anesthesiology 47: 524–525
Giannotta S L, Daniels J, Golde S H, Zelman V, Bayat A 1986 Ruptured intracranial aneurysms during pregnancy. Journal of Reproductive Medicine 31: 139–147
Hood D D, Dewan D M, James F M, Floyd H M, Bogard T D 1985 The use of nitroglycerin in preventing the hypertensive response to tracheal intubation in severe preeclampsia. Anesthesiology 63: 329–332
Lawes E G, Downing J W, Duncan P W, Bland B, Lavies N, Gane G A C 1987 Fentanyl/droperidol supplementation of rapid sequence induction in the presence of severe pregnancy induced and pregnancy aggravated hypertension. British Journal of Anaesthesia 59: 1381–1391
Morison D H 1987 Anaesthesia and pre-eclampsia. Canadian Journal of Anaesthesia 34: 415–421
Redman C W G 1988 Eclampsia still kills. British Medical Journal 296: 1209–1210

Richards A M, Moodley J, Graham D I, Bullock M R R 1986 Active management of the
    unconscious eclamptic patient. British Journal of Obstetrics and Gynaecology 93: 554–562
Seager S J, MacDonald R 1980 Laryngeal oedema and preeclampsia. Anaesthesia 35:
    360–362
Wright J P 1983 Anesthetic considerations in eclampsia-preeclampsia. Anesthesia and
    Analgesia 63: 590–601

EHLERS–DANLOS SYNDROME

A group of conditions, of varying inheritance, in which there is a defect in
collagen. Eleven different subtypes have been identified, each showing a
wide spectrum of effects, from mild to very severe (Duvic & Pinnell 1986).
The clinical picture is one of multiple skin and musculoskeletal
abnormalities. Cardiac defects have also been described.

Preoperative abnormalities

1. The whole group is characterized by a hyperextensible and sometimes
fragile skin, hypermobile joints, and a tendency to bruise and bleed
without definite coagulation abnormalities.
2. The ecchymotic form, which involves abnormalities in type III collagen
synthesis, is the most severe. As the predominant collagen of blood
vessels and the gastrointestinal tract is Type III, complications therefore
include aneurysmal dilatation, rupture of blood vessels, and visceral
rupture. Aortic dissection, similar to that in Marfan's syndrome, may
occur. Pregnancy carries a 25% mortality, and the complications of
surgery can be disastrous.
3. Mitral valve prolapse, RBBB, and left anterior hemi-block have been
described in association with some forms of Ehlers–Danlos (Cabeen &
Kovik 1977).

Anaesthetic problems

1. The ecchymotic form may present with uncontrollable haemorrhage or
visceral rupture. Death occurred secondary to a postpartum haemorrhage
in a patient with normal coagulation tests (Dolan et al 1980). Widespread
bleeding from very fragile vessels and a ruptured splenic artery aneurysm
were found at exploratory laparotomy. In this group of patients, the use of
arterial and central venous lines for monitoring can be accompanied by
severe bleeding.
2. Spinal or epidural anaesthesia may be complicated by an epidural
haematoma.
3. Milder forms may have postoperative wound dehiscence.
4. Venous access can be technically difficult due to the hyperextensible
skin. Displacement of the cannula from a vein may remain undetected.
5. If conduction defects such as RBBB and left anterior hemi-block are

present, it is possible that the patient could progress to complete heart block under anaesthesia.

6. There is an increased risk of pneumothorax.

Management

1. If the condition is suspected and time permits, genetic advice should be obtained to assess the type and severity.
2. Blood should be cross-matched and coagulation defects excluded.
3. Intramuscular injections and regional anaesthesia should not be given.
4. Good peripheral venous access or a cutdown should be done. The use of central venous monitoring via a large cannula, at a site where bleeding cannot be controlled by pressure, should be avoided. If essential, a small needle should be used, and a peripheral site selected.
5. Particular care should be taken when endotracheal or nasogastric tubes are inserted.
6. During ventilation, low airway pressures should be used to reduce the risk of a pneumothorax.
7. If conduction defects are present, the temporary insertion of a pacemaker should be considered.
8. Antibiotic prophylaxis is required if there is mitral valve prolapse.

BIBLIOGRAPHY

Cabeen W R, Kovick R B 1977 Mitral valve prolapse and conduction defects in Ehlers–Danlos syndrome. Archives of Internal Medicine 137: 1227–1231
Dolan P, Sisko F, Riley E 1980 Anesthetic considerations for Ehlers–Danlos syndrome. Anesthesiology 52: 266–269
Duvic M, Pinnell S R 1986 Ehlers–Danlos syndrome. In: Pathogenesis of skin disease. Churchill Livingstone, Edinburgh

EISENMENGER'S SYNDROME

A rare syndrome of pulmonary hypertension associated with a reversed or bidirectional cardiac shunt, occurring through a large communication between the left and right heart. The defect may be interventricular, interatrial or aortopulmonary. The development of Eisenmenger's syndrome from the initial left to right shunt is usually a gradual process. Contributory factors to the pulmonary hypertension are hypoxia, high pulmonary blood flow and high left atrial pressure. Irreversible structural changes take place in the small vessels, causing pulmonary vascular obstruction and a reduction in the size of the capillary bed. The pulmonary artery pressure is the same as, or sometimes exceeds, the systemic arterial pressure. The incidence of this syndrome is decreasing because of the more vigorous approach to diagnosis and treatment of congenital heart disease in childhood.

Preoperative abnormalities

1. Presenting symptoms include dyspnoea, tiredness, episodes of cyanosis, syncope or chest pain. Haemoptysis may occur.
2. The direction of the shunt, and hence the presence or absence of cyanosis, depends on a number of factors. These include hypoxia, the pulmonary and systemic blood pressure differences, and the intravascular volume. It can also be affected by certain drugs.
3. CXR shows right ventricular hypertrophy, and ECG indicates varying degrees of right ventricular hypertrophy and strain.
4. Cerebral abscess may occur secondary to clot embolism.

Anaesthetic problems

1. Lowering of systemic arterial pressure by myocardial depression or loss of sympathetic tone is potentially dangerous. Reversal of the shunt may occur, and sudden death has been reported. Hypovolaemia and dehydration are very poorly tolerated.
2. Sinus tachycardia occurs due to exercise or emotion, and episodes of SVT are common after the age of 30. The onset of atrial fibrillation is associated with a marked deterioration in the condition of the patient.
3. Pregnancy carries considerable risks and is contraindicated. Maternal mortality rates of 30% have been reported (Devitt et al 1982). A Caesarean section may increase the mortality to over 60%. Even termination of pregnancy may be hazardous.
4. Complications from the insertion of pulmonary artery catheters for monitoring have included systemic and pulmonary emboli, pulmonary artery rupture and arrhythmias (Robinson 1983). One patient died during removal of a catheter on the fourth day after Caesarean section (Devitt et al 1982). It has been argued that the risks of pulmonary artery catheters in Eisenmenger's syndrome outweigh the benefits (Robinson 1983).
5. Patients are at risk from paradoxical air or clot embolism.

Management

1. Maintenance of an adequate circulating blood volume is essential. Myocardial depressants and peripheral vasodilators should be used with caution. Bradycardia must be prevented.
2. It is unclear as to whether oxygen can cause pulmonary vasodilatation. Although the pulmonary vascular resistance was believed to be fixed in pulmonary hypertension, a high oxygen concentration has been shown to reduce it during Caesarean section (Spinnato et al 1981).
3. Alpha adrenergic vasopressors such as methoxamine or phenylephrine have been recommended for treatment of hypotension on induction of anaesthesia (Foster & Jones 1984). Prophylactic treatment with metaraminol has been suggested (Lumley et al 1977), but, in common with other vasopressors, it also produces pulmonary

vasoconstriction. Bradycardia and a worsening of cyanosis have been associated with its use.

4. IPPV should be used with low inflation pressures.

5. Air must be completely eliminated from all intravenous lines.

6. Appropriate antibiotics are given to prevent bacterial endocarditis.

7. Low-dose heparin may reduce the risk of emboli.

8. Patients are usually advised against pregnancy. If anaesthesia is required either for termination of pregnancy or operative delivery, intensive cardiac care is indicated. Successful epidural anaesthesia has been reported for Caesarean section (Spinnato et al 1981).

BIBLIOGRAPHY

Devitt J H, Noble W H, Byrick R J 1982 A Swan-Ganz catheter related complication in a patient with Eisenmenger's syndrome. Anesthesiology 57: 335–337
Foster J M G, Jones R M 1984 The anaesthetic management of the Eisenmenger syndrome. Annals of the Royal College of Surgeons of England 66: 353–355
Lumley J, Whitwam J G, Morgan M 1977 General anesthesia in the presence of Eisenmenger's Syndrome. Anesthesia and Analgesia 56: 543–547
Robinson S 1983 Pulmonary artery catheters in Eisenmenger's syndrome: many risks, few benefits. Anesthesiology 58: 588–589
Spinnato J A, Kraynack B J, Cooper M W 1981 Eisenmenger's syndrome in pregnancy: epidural anesthesia for elective Cesarean Section. New England Journal of Medicine 304: 1215–1217

ENDOCARDITIS
(see SUBACUTE BACTERIAL ENDOCARDITIS)

EPIDERMOLYSIS BULLOSA
(RECESSIVE DYSTROPHIC)

Epidermolysis bullosa refers to a spectrum of genetic diseases in which the primary feature is the formation of bullae in the skin or mucous membranes, either spontaneously or in response to mechanical injury (Bauer 1986). The individual types can be distinguished by genetic, clinical and pathological features. Recessive dystrophic epidermolysis bullosa, which presents at birth or in infancy, is one of the severe forms.

Preoperative abnormalities

1. Frictional or other trauma causes the formation of bullae in the dermis and mucous membranes. When healing takes place, scarring occurs. There appears to be a decreased number, or an absence, of anchoring fibrils in the dermis, together with an increase in collagenase activity in the blistered skin.

2. The scarring may result in flexion contractures of the limbs, fusion of digits, contraction of the mouth, fixation of the tongue and oesophageal strictures.

3. Protein loss from the skin results in growth failure, anaemia and malnutrition. Teeth are malformed and nails are shed. Dehydration and sepsis are additional problems.

4. Drug treatment may include steroids, phenytoin and vitamin E.

5. There is an increased incidence of amyloidosis and porphyria.

Anaesthetic problems

1. The face mask may cause bullae on the chin, nose and cheek.

2. Intubation may produce bullae in the mouth which can bleed and rupture (Pratilas & Biezunski 1975). Surprisingly however, there are no reports of laryngeal or tracheal bullae forming as a result of endotracheal intubation. This may be because the epithelium of the larynx and trachea is of the ciliated columnar type, and not squamous. It appears to be more resilient. There have been two reports of laryngeal stenosis, but neither patient had ever been intubated.

3. Oral airways have been reported to produce massive bullae in the mouth.

4. Existing oropharyngeal scarring can cause intubation problems.

5. Bullae may occur at the sites of a BP cuff, ECG electrodes or adhesive tape. Shearing forces are mechanically the most damaging to the skin.

6. There is an increased risk of regurgitation and aspiration due to oesophageal strictures.

Management

1. Care should be taken to avoid shearing stresses to the skin while the patient is under anaesthesia. If feasible, the patient should be allowed to position himself on the operating table.

2. The decision whether to use a mask or intubation technique is governed by factors such as the estimated duration of the operation and the pressure required to maintain the mask in position. A review of 131 intubated cases provided no evidence that careful intubation caused laryngeal problems (James & Wark 1982). More commonly, bullae in the mouth have arisen from trauma due to an oral airway, the laryngoscope or by the surgeon. Bullae have also occurred on the face due to pressure from the mask. If the patient is to be intubated, a well-lubricated, smaller size of tube than is normal, should be used. IPPV and muscle relaxation is advisable under these circumstances, to reduce frictional damage due to the patient coughing and straining against the tube (Tomlinson 1983).

3. All instruments should be well lubricated. Petroleum jelly gauze is placed around the mask and where the anaesthetist's fingers support the chin.

4. Modifications to monitoring attachments, in an attempt to reduce skin damage, have been suggested (Kelly et al 1987). Moist gauze was placed underneath the BP cuff, ECG pads had their adhesive trimmed and the gel electrodes were placed under the patient's back. Adhesive tape causes shearing stresses and should be avoided if possible. Where invasive monitoring is necessary, adhesive attachments can be dispensed with. CVP and arterial lines were sutured into place in a patient having a resection of oesophageal stricture (Milne & Rosales 1980).

5. The use of ketamine to avoid both mask anaesthesia and intubation has been proposed.

6. Brachial plexus anaesthesia has been reported for surgery of pseudosyndactyly (Kelly et al 1987, Hagen & Langenberg 1988).

7. Regional anaesthesia may be appropriate on occasions. Epidural and spinal anaesthesia have been reported (Spielman & Mann 1984, Broster et al 1987). The epidural catheters were not secured.

BIBLIOGRAPHY

Bauer E A 1986 Epidermolysis bullosa. In: Pathogenesis of skin diseases. Churchill Livingstone, Edinburgh
Broster T, Placek R, Eggers G W N 1987 Epidermolysis bullosa: anesthetic management for Cesarean section. Anesthesia and Analgesia 66: 341–343
Hagen R, Langenberg C 1988 Anaesthetic management in patients with epidermolysis bullosa dystrophica. Anaesthesia 43: 482–485
James I, Wark H 1982 Airway management during anesthesia in patients with epidermolysis bullosa dystrophia. Anesthesiology 56: 323–326
Kelly R E, Koff H D, Rothaus K O, Carter D M, Artusio J F 1987 Brachial plexus anesthesia in eight patients with recessive dystrophic epidermolysis bullosa. Anesthesia and Analgesia 66: 1318–1320
Milne B, Rosales J K 1980 Anaesthesia for correction of oesophageal stricture in a patient with recessive epidermolysis bullosa. Canadian Anaesthetists' Society Journal 27: 169–171
Pratilas V, Biezunski A 1975 Epidermolysis bullosa manifested and treated during anesthesia. Anesthesiology 43: 581–583
Spielman F J, Mann E S 1984 Subarachnoid and epidural anaesthesia for patients with epidermolysis bullosa. Canadian Anaesthetists' Society Journal 31: 549–551
Tomlinson A A 1983 Recessive dystrophic epidermolysis bullosa. Anaesthesia 38: 485–491

EPIGLOTTITIS
(ACUTE)

An acute inflammation and swelling of the epiglottis, usually due to *Haemophilus influenzae* Type B. It occasionally results in total laryngeal obstruction, and death due to hypoxia. Although primarily a paediatric disorder whose peak incidence arises between the ages of 1 and 4 years, adults can also be affected. However, they present with slightly different clinical pictures. In both, the treatment of choice is short-term nasotracheal intubation, until the swelling has subsided.

Presentation

1. The illness usually is of sudden onset, with high fever, stridor and the development of a muffled voice. The child often leans forward,

drooling saliva. Boys are more frequently affected than girls. In children less than 2 years old, the presentation may be atypical (Blackstock et al 1987).

2. The child may present with increasing respiratory distress and cyanosis. Total airway obstruction can be sudden and without warning. Occasionally, cardiorespiratory arrest can occur before hospital admission.

3. There is a high leucocyte count, and *H. influenzae* is often subsequently grown from blood culture or swabs. A lateral X-ray of the neck may show a swollen epiglottis. However, if epiglottitis is suspected, the patient must only be sent to X-ray accompanied by an experienced member of staff, in case sudden respiratory obstruction occurs.

4. Adults are more likely to present with sore throat and dysphagia. However, there is the same risk of sudden airway obstruction. Of 56 adult cases of epiglottitis, death occurred in four. Two of these were in hospital under observation; they died before airway intervention had been undertaken (Mayosmith et al 1986).

Anaesthetic problems

1. The distinction between acute epiglottitis and acute laryngotracheobronchitis, the other more common cause of stridor, can frequently be made on clinical grounds, although occasionally the diagnosis is difficult.

2. In children, examination of the mouth and throat, or even the distress caused by insertion of an intravenous infusion, may precipitate complete upper airway obstruction.

3. The induction of anaesthesia may abolish accessory respiratory muscle movement, and also cause obstruction.

4. Perioperative complications include cardiorespiratory arrest, accidental extubation, endotracheal tube blockage, pulmonary oedema and pneumothorax. A report of 161 cases of epiglottitis revealed 45 complications in 34 patients and five deaths (Baines et al 1985). Complications included 18 episodes of cardiorespiratory arrest, 10 incidents involving accidental extubation, three cases of pneumothorax, and three episodes of pulmonary oedema following relief of the obstruction.

Management

1. Acute epiglottitis represents a serious emergency which should be attended by an experienced anaesthetist whenever the diagnosis is suspected. In any child with stridor a high index of suspicion must be maintained. Investigation should not be allowed to delay the treatment of life-threatening obstruction (Love et al 1984).

2. In children, no examination of the throat should be made, except under an anaesthetic given by an experienced anaesthetist, and preferably with an ENT surgeon present (Breivk & Klaastad 1978). In adults, it has been suggested that indirect larygoscopy or fibreoptic bronchoscopy may be performed without the risk of precipitating complete obstruction (Love et al 1984), although this is controversial.

3. Inhalation anaesthesia with halothane and oxygen, with or without nitrous oxide, is indicated. An airway should be secured first with an oral tube. This can be replaced at leisure with a suitably sized nasotracheal tube.

4. The tube must be firmly secured and an intravenous infusion set up to prevent dehydration. Bandaging of the hands will reduce the risks of extubation and decannulation.

5. One of the most difficult problems is that of providing sufficient humidification to prevent crusting of the tube. Examination under anaesthetic at 24 hours is advisable. Even if extubation is not possible at that stage, the tube should be changed. In the small child, partial blockage of the tube by secretions is almost invariably found. The mean duration of intubation in one series was 36 hours (Rothstein & Lister 1983). Direct observation of the epiglottis was found to be the only reliable way to determine the stage at which the tube was no longer necessary.

6. The patient should receive a sedative, but not a respiratory depressant. Accidental extubation and endotracheal tube blockage are serious complications which can prove fatal if respiration is depressed.

7. About 80% of *H. influenzae* infections will be sensitive to ampicillin. For the remainder, chloramphenicol is the drug of choice.

8. The use of steroids is controversial. A retrospective non-controlled comparison between one area using them routinely and one only using them occasionally, showed no difference in outcome (Welch & Price 1983). However, in practice, steroids are often given.

9. Short-lived pulmonary oedema occasionally occurs after relief of the obstruction, and should be treated with IPPV.

BIBLIOGRAPHY

Baines D B, Wark H, Overton J H 1985 Acute epiglottitis in children. Anaesthesia and Intensive Care 13: 25–28
Blackstock D, Adderley R J, Steward D J 1987 Epiglottitis in young infants. Anesthesiology 67: 97–100
Breivk H, Klaastad O 1978 Acute epiglottitis in children. British Journal of Anaesthesia 50: 505–510
Love J B, Phelan D M, Runciman W B, Skowronski G A, Turnidge J D 1984 Acute epiglottitis in adults. Anesthesia and Intensive Care 12: 264–269
Mayosmith M J, Hirsch P J, Wodzinski S F, Schiffman F J 1986 Acute epiglottitis in adults. New England Journal of Medicine 314: 1133–1139
Rothstein P, Lister G 1983 Epiglottitis – duration of intubation and fever. Anesthesia and Analgesia 62: 785–787
Welch D B, Price D G 1983 Acute epiglottitis and severe croup. Experience in two English regions. Anaesthesia 38: 754–759

1

FALLOT'S TETRALOGY

A congenital cardiac abnormality. The primary defects are pulmonary infundibular stenosis and a VSD. The VSD is sufficiently large for the pressure in both ventricles to be equal to that of the aorta. The tetralogy is completed by two secondary features, a variable degree of overriding of the aorta, and right ventricular hypertrophy. Dynamic right ventricular outflow obstruction may occur (infundibular spasm), which is increased by sympathetic stimulation. The fraction of the right to left shunt depends upon the relative resistances between the pulmonary (or right ventricular) and systemic outflows.

Preoperative abnormalities

1. Dyspnoea may occur on exertion and is hypoxia related. Cyanosis and finger clubbing are variable, depending on the degree of pulmonary stenosis and the size of the shunt. Polycythaemia is common. There is a pulmonary stenotic murmur, but no murmur from the VSD because of the size of the defect. Squatting is thought to reduce the fraction of the shunt, due to an increase in systemic vascular resistance produced by kinking of large arteries. This is commonly seen in children.
2. ECG shows right atrial and right ventricular hypertrophy, right axis deviation and right bundle branch block.
3. CXR shows right ventricular hypertrophy and oligaemic lungs.
4. Initial surgery may have been undertaken to anastomose a systemic to a pulmonary artery, to improve the pulmonary blood flow and reduce cyanosis.
5. There is an increased risk of bacterial endocarditis, emboli, cerebral abscess, syncope and cyanotic attacks.

Anaesthetic problems

1. The right to left shunt, and hence the cyanosis, is increased by a fall in systemic vascular resistance produced by peripheral vasodilatation. This may be caused by factors such as hypovolaemia, drugs or pyrexia.
2. Cyanosis is also worsened by an increase in pulmonary vascular resistance or spasm of the right ventricular infundibulum. Infundibular spasm is produced by increases in catecholamine output, or the administration of drugs with positive inotropic effects. Anxiety, pain, hypercarbia, hypoxia and acidosis are all precipitating factors. These cyanotic attacks, which can occur when awake or under anaesthesia, may initiate a cycle of increasing hypoxia which can result in cerebral damage or death. Propranolol i.v. was successfully used to treat an attack occurring during cardiac catheterization under local anaesthetic (Kam 1978).

1

3. Dehydration in the presence of polycythaemia and raised plasma viscosity increases the incidence of cerebral thrombosis. Polycythaemia may be associated with coagulation defects.

Management

1. Antibiotic cover as prophylaxis against SBE.
2. A good premedication to prevent excitement and anxiety.
3. Measures aimed to reduce the right to left shunt. These include 100% oxygen to decrease PVR, pressor agents such as phenylephrine to increase systemic vascular resistance, and propranolol to decrease outflow tract obstruction.
4. Techniques should avoid hypoxia and hypercarbia, and minimize vasodilatation and sudden increases in cardiac output.
5. Hydration is maintained in the perioperative period, and if there is severe polycythaemia, venesection may be necessary.

BIBLIOGRAPHY

Kam C A 1978 Infundibular spasm in Fallot's tetralogy. Anaesthesia and Intensive Care 6: 138–140

FAMILIAL DYSAUTONOMIA
(RILEY–DAY SYNDROME)

A rare autosomal recessive neurological disease presenting from birth. Although most of the nervous system is involved, the autonomic and peripheral neuronal elements are of most concern to the anaesthetist. A decrease in sympathetic, parasympathetic and sensory neurones, a decrease in synthesis of noradrenaline (but with a normal adrenal medulla) and a sensitivity to exogenous catecholamines, have been shown. The IQ is normal. Patients may present for fundoplication, gastrostomy or orthopaedic procedures.

Preoperative abnormalities

1. There is a decreased sensitivity to pain and temperature, muscle hypotonia, incoordination and reduced tendon reflexes. Scoliosis is common, presumably due to inadequate muscle tone and impaired muscle proprioception.
2. Features include autonomic dysfunction with postural hypotension, increased vagal reflexes, swallowing difficulties with drooling of saliva, absent sweating and impaired temperature control.
3. Dysautonomic and emotional crises can occur. Nausea and vomiting is accompanied by hypertension.

Anaesthetic problems

1. Emotion and fear may precipitate a dysautonomic crisis.
2. Patients can develop lung disease secondary to episodes of pulmonary aspiration.
3. Chronic dehydration is common due to dysphagia for fluids.
4. Respiratory responses to hypercarbia and hypoxia are impaired.
5. Autonomic nervous system dysfunction, apparently due to reduced endogenous catecholamine release, means that the patient is unable to respond to hypovolaemia and to drugs causing myocardial depression (Meridy & Creighton 1971, Foster 1983). Several cases in which either cardiac arrest or severe hypotension occurred during general anaesthesia have been reported (Kritchman et al 1959, Axelrod et al 1988).
6. Successful control of intraoperative hypotension with both adrenaline and dopamine infusions have been reported (Stenqvist & Sigurdsson 1982). Exaggerated responses to noradrenaline have occurred and therefore any catecholamines should be administered with caution.
7. The use of atropine is controversial. Reports exist of sensitivity to anti-cholinergic agents, and conversely, of pronounced reactions to vagal stimulation. Both its cautious use and its avoidance have been advocated.
8. Profound vomiting may occur in the perioperative period.
9. Temperature variations can take place.
10. Major problems have occurred in the postoperative period (Meridy & Creighton 1971, Axelrod et al 1988). Complications have included fever, pulmonary atelectasis or infection, aspiration, cardiovascular instability and vomiting crises. An analysis of 127 procedures in 81 patients was reported (Axelrod et al 1988). A high incidence of postoperative atelectasis after gastric surgery prompted a policy of elective ventilation.

Management

1. Intravenous fluid therapy should be started preoperatively to prevent dehydration. Anxiety should be treated. Diazepam has been found to be effective in controlling dysautonomic crises. Cimetidine reduces gastric secretions. Premedication with both drugs has been suggested (Axelrod et al 1988). Opiates and anticholinergics should be avoided.
2. Monitoring of arterial pressure and temperature should preferably be started prior to induction of anaesthesia. Vascular access is facilitated by the relative sensory deficit.
3. The uneventful use of both depolarizing and non-depolarizing relaxants have been reported. However, the presence of hypotonia reduces the requirement for relaxants, and residual neuromuscular blockade may necessitate IPPV in the postoperative period.
4. Blood and fluid loss must be replaced promptly.
5. A dopamine or an adrenaline infusion may be needed if problems

1

occur with intraoperative hypotension. However, catecholamines must be given with care, as sensitivity to their effects has been reported. Close monitoring is required, so that the blood pressure is raised, but an unacceptable tachycardia prevented.

6. IPPV is required, even for short cases, because of the impaired response to hypoxia and hypercarbia.

7. Postoperative analgesia is required for abdominal surgery. It has been suggested in these cases that IPPV should be continued postoperatively until analgesics are no longer required (Axelrod et al 1988).

8. Vomiting crises should be treated with gastric decompression, diazepam and cimetidine.

BIBLIOGRAPHY

Axelrod F B, Donenfeld R F, Danziger F, Turndorf H 1988 Anesthesia in familial dysautonomia. Anesthesiology 68: 631–635
Foster J M G 1983 Anaesthesia for a patient with familial dysautonomia. Anaesthesia 38: 391
Kritchman M M, Schwartz H, Papper E M 1959 Experiences with general anaesthesia in patients with familial dysautonomia. Journal of the American Medical Association 170: 529–533
Meridy H W, Creighton R E 1971 General anaesthesia in eight patients with familial dysautonomia. Canadian Anaesthetists' Society Journal 18: 563–570
Stenqvist O, Sigurdsson J 1982 The anaesthetic management of a patient with familial dysautonomia. Anaesthesia 37: 929–932

FAMILIAL PERIODIC PARALYSIS

There are two principal types, both of which are autosomal dominant:

1. Hypokalaemic periodic paralysis.
2. Hyperkalaemic periodic paralysis.

HYPOKALAEMIC PERIODIC PARALYSIS

A rare disease which usually starts in teenagers. Episodes of flaccid paralysis are precipitated by stress, cold, trauma, surgery, infections and high carbohydrate meals. Attacks may last from several hours to 2 days. Certain muscle groups are likely to be involved more than others. It is associated with hypokalaemia but the exact mechanism for its periodic nature and its skeletal and cardiac effects is not known. Increased potassium excretion from the body is not involved. There does however seem to be an increased uptake of potassium by the cells. The cell membrane potential has been found to be reduced during attacks, making the muscle inexcitable. Insulin and glucose, steroids, thyroxine and beta stimulation can all increase cellular potassium uptake and worsen an existing hypokalaemia.

Preoperative abnormalities

1. Attacks of paralysis are most likely to involve the arms, legs, trunk and neck, but usually in an asymmetric manner. Proximal muscles are mainly affected. Death may occasionally occur during an attack due to respiratory failure or aspiration. Fortunately however, the diaphragm and cranial muscles are not usually involved. The patients are more sensitive than normal to a reduction in serum potassium, such that muscle weakness may start at a level of 3 mmol/l and may become profound when <2.5 mmol/l (Ellis 1980).

2. Patients are usually taking oral potassium. Symptoms may be improved by acetazolamide. This probably acts by producing a metabolic acidosis, thus reducing potassium uptake by the cells. Spironolactone can be used prophylactically.

3. Hypokalaemia, which can be as low as 1.6 mmol/l, may be accompanied by ECG changes such as T-wave flattening, U waves, arrhythmias, and bradycardias.

4. During an attack, the EMG shows action potential lengthening, progressing into electrical silence.

5. Thyrotoxic periodic paralysis may produce a similar picture (Fozard 1983, Robson 1985).

Anaesthetic problems

1. Attacks of paralysis can be precipitated by administration of glucose and insulin, sodium bicarbonate, diuretics, a heavy carbohydrate meal, undue stress, hypothermia, or a salt load.

2. Although patients with spontaneous attacks rarely require respiratory support, this is not always so in the postoperative period. Most case reports have shown uneventful intraoperative courses with a wide range of anaesthetic techniques employed. However, the incidence of postoperative paralysis, often developing some hours later, is about 25%. Most of these episodes have been associated with hypokalaemia (Siler & Discavage 1975, Rollman et al 1985).

3. Hypokalaemia during surgery may be accompanied by ECG changes out of proportion to the measured serum potassium.

4. The effect of muscle relaxants may be difficult to distinguish from the paralysis itself. One family had a total of 21 anaesthetics. The three patients who received muscle relaxants were the only ones who had postoperative paralyses (Horton 1977).

Management

1. Stress and anxiety should be reduced by using adequate premedication. Treatment with beta blockers has been reported, but only during anaesthesia.

2. Core temperature should be monitored and the theatre warmed.

Precautions should be taken against heat loss during prolonged surgery.
3. ECG should be closely observed throughout the operation for the changes of hypokalaemia.
4. Glucose infusions should be minimized and large sodium loads, particularly bicarbonate, avoided. Serum potassium must be monitored and hypokalaemia treated.
5. Muscle relaxants may not be required. If they are necessary, small increments can be given and the effects assessed with a nerve stimulator. The problems of distinguishing the effects of relaxants from those of the disease itself may be reduced by stimulating the facial nerve which supplies rarely affected muscles. However, even this may be unreliable. Atracurium has been used without complication in a patient with periodic paralysis and a cardiomyopathy (Rooney et al 1988).
6. The patient's ventilation, and his serum potassium, should be closely monitored postoperatively on an intensive care unit.

BIBLIOGRAPHY

Ellis F R 1980 Inherited muscle disease. British Journal of Anaesthesia 52: 153–164
Fozard J R 1983 Anaesthesia and familial hypokalaemic periodic paralysis. Anaesthesia 38: 293–294
Horton B 1977 Anesthetic experiences in a family with hypokalaemic periodic paralysis. Anesthesiology 47: 308–310
Melnick B, Chang J, Larson C, Bedger R 1983 Hypokalemic familial periodic paralysis. Anesthesiology 58: 263–265
Robson N J 1985 Emergency surgery complicated by thyrotoxicosis and thyrotoxic periodic paralysis. Anaesthesia 40: 27–31
Rollman J E, Dickson C M 1985 Anesthetic management of a patient with hypokalemic familial periodic paralysis for coronary artery bypass surgery. Anesthesiology 63: 526–527
Rooney R, Shanahan E, Sun T, Nally B 1988 Atracurium and hypokalemic familial paralysis. Anesthesia and Analgesia 67: 782–783
Siler J N, Discavage W J 1975 Anesthetic management of hypokalaemic periodic paralysis. Anesthesiology 43: 489–490

HYPERKALAEMIC PERIODIC PARALYSIS

A similar, but separate, inherited disease. The serum potassium may rise by 20% during an attack, and paralysis may occur with serum levels no greater than 4 mmol/l. Changes in membrane potential and release of potassium from muscle have both been demonstrated. Administration of potassium can precipitate an attack although the serum potassium may remain normal. Changes in potassium alone cannot account for the problem. An abnormality of the sarcolemma causing spontaneous depolarization has been postulated.

Preoperative abnormalities

1. Attacks of paralysis usually last for less than 2 hours. They are shorter than in the hypokalaemic form, and may be precipitated by hunger, cold and exercise. Mild paralysis may occur with a serum potassium >4 mmol/l and may become severe when >7 mmol/l (Ellis 1980).

2. The distribution of paralysis is similar, but the facial and tongue muscles may be involved. Percussion myotonia may be marked in an attack, which can be precipitated by giving potassium.
3. EMG shows increased spontaneous activity and myotonic discharges.
4. ECG may show peaking of the T waves, even prior to the episode of paralysis.

Anaesthetic problems

1. Anaesthesia may precipitate paralysis, which can continue for some hours into the postoperative period (Egan & Klein 1959).

Management

1. Dextrose should be infused during the period of fasting prior to anaesthesia.
2. Hyperkalaemia will respond to calcium gluconate or dextrose and insulin, which move potassium back into the cells. Thiazide diuretics are used prophylactically.
3. Sodium-containing, potassium-free, intravenous fluids should be used.
4. As with the hypokalaemic form, monitoring of serum potassium, ECG and neuromuscular function, is essential. The possible need for postoperative ventilation should be anticipated.

BIBLIOGRAPHY

Ellis F R 1980 Inherited muscle disease. British Journal of Anaesthesia 52: 153–164
Egan T J, Klein R 1959 Hyperkalemic familial periodic paralysis. Pediatrics 24: 761–773

FAT EMBOLISM

A syndrome most often associated with long bone fractures, in which fat particles, possibly from the marrow, embolize to different organs. Emboli to the pulmonary capillaries are of particular clinical significance. Local endothelial damage and small vessel obstruction occur, probably due to a combination of interactions between marrow fat, free fatty acids and platelets (Gossling & Donohue 1979). The resulting increase in capillary permeability produces ventilation perfusion abnormalities and hypoxia. While fat emboli probably occur in the pulmonary vessels in the majority of cases of long bone fracture, only a small proportion develop the classical syndrome.

Presenting problems

1. Signs and symptoms may occur immediately following injury but are often delayed for up to 48 hours.

1

2. A petechial rash, particularly over the upper half of the body, in the retina and the conjunctivae, appears in 50–60% of cases. This rash is diagnostic of the syndrome.

3. An interstitial pneumonitis may present with tachycardia, dyspnoea, pyrexia, cyanosis, and frothy sputum. CXR may show bilateral pulmonary infiltrates. Florid pulmonary oedema has been reported (Hagley 1983). Respiratory failure may ensue.

4. An altered conscious level, with confusion and restlessness, are usually signs of cerebral hypoxia. Coma may follow.

5. A fall in haemoglobin, hypoxia, acidosis and thrombocytopenia can all occur. Three fatal cases were reported in which disseminated intravascular coagulation was a prominent feature (Hagley 1983).

6. In severe cases the mortality may be from 10% to 45%. Pulmonary involvement is the predominant cause of death.

Diagnosis

1. Initially diagnosis is made on clinical grounds by the occurrence of some or all of the features, appearing within 48 hours of a long bone fracture. The femoral shaft or neck, the pelvis and the tibia, are the bones most commonly involved.

2. Examination of the sputum and urine may show fat globules. These may also be seen in retinal vessels, if the patient is sufficiently cooperative during ophthalmic examination.

Management

1. Respiratory management is the most important task. Continual assessment of the clinical situation, including blood gases, is essential. Hypoxia should be initially treated with oxygen, and if necessary, with IPPV and PEEP.

2. Fractures must be stabilized.

3. Early administration of corticosteroids may reduce the mortality. A series of 64 high-risk patients with isolated long bone injuries, but with no other injuries which might predispose to ARDS, were studied (Schonfeld et al 1983). Methylprednisolone 7.5 mg/kg, 6-hourly for 12 doses, was given to 21 patients. None developed the fat embolism syndrome, whereas in the placebo group nine out of the 41 did. Six cases were severe and three were mild.

4. Cardiovascular support may be required.

BIBLIOGRAPHY

Gossling H R, Donohue T A 1979 The fat embolism syndrome. Journal of the American Medical Association 241: 2740–2742
Gossling H R, Pellegrini V D 1982 Fat embolism syndrome. Clinical Orthopaedics and Related Research 165: 68–82
Hagley S R 1983 Fulminant fat embolism syndrome. Anaesthesia and Intensive Care 11: 162–166

Schonfeld S A, Ploysongsang Y, DiLisio R, Crissman J D, Miller E, Hammerschmidt D E, Jacob H S 1983 Fat embolism prophylaxis with corticosteroids. A prospective study in high-risk patients. Annals of Internal Medicine 99: 438–443

FRIEDREICH'S ATAXIA

A hereditary ataxia in which degeneration of the pyramidal and spinocerebellar tracts, and atrophy of the dorsal root ganglia, result in ataxia and combined upper and lower motor neurone lesions. Cardiac lesions are frequently associated. The condition usually presents between the ages of 5 and 15 years. A metabolic defect has been postulated.

Preoperative abnormalities

1. This usually presents with gait ataxia. Later the upper limbs become clumsy, with intention tremor. The cerebellar lesion causes nystagmus and dysarthria. The dorsal root lesion is associated with sensory impairment and depressed reflexes. The corticospinal tract degeneration causes progressive weakness and extensor plantars. Pes cavus is often present.
2. Cardiac abnormalities are present in over 90% of patients. These may consist of asymptomatic ECG or echocardiographic changes. However, up to 50% have clinical cardiac disease, which includes hypertrophic cardiomyopathy and conduction defects. Sudden death may occur.
3. Disability progressively increases. The development of scoliosis and the need for a wheelchair are closely associated. Scoliosis occurs in 80% of patients and surgery may be required for its correction (Bird & Strunin 1984, Bell et al 1986). Chest infections are common.
4. Diabetes has been found in 18% of patients and a diabetic glucose tolerance curve in 40%.
5. EMG is usually normal, but motor nerve conduction velocities are decreased.

Anaesthetic problems

1. Although sensitivity to non-depolarizing relaxants has been reported, this is not always so. Suggestions of a myasthenic-like response were not confirmed when a nerve stimulator was used (Bell et al 1986). However, as different muscles are affected to a variable degree, the response may depend both on the progression of the disease and the muscle group being monitored.
2. If cardiac disease is present, there is a risk of arrythmias and heart failure. A patient having scoliosis surgery developed heart failure on the 34th postoperative day, possibly due to pulmonary emboli in addition to longstanding cardiomyopathy (Bell et al 1986). This subsequently proved fatal.

1

3. As the degree of scoliosis increases, or if diaphragmatic weakness develops, cardiopulmonary failure becomes a significant problem (see also Scoliosis). Chest infections readily occur.

Management

1. Assessment of respiratory reserve, and vigorous treatment of chest infections with physiotherapy and antibiotics.
2. Assessment, monitoring and treatment of cardiac lesions as appropriate.
3. Neuromuscular monitoring should be instituted, preferably prior to induction of anaesthesia. The monitoring of more than one muscle group may be necessary.

BIBLIOGRAPHY

Bell C F, Kelly J M, Jones R S 1986 Anaesthesia for Friedreich's ataxia. Anaesthesia 41: 296–301
Bird T M, Strunin L 1984 Hypotensive anesthesia for a patient with Friedreich's ataxia and cardiomyopathy. Anesthesiology 60: 377–380
Campbell A M, Finley G A 1989 Anaesthesia for a patient with Friedreich's ataxia and cardiomyopathy. Canadian Journal of Anaesthesia 36: 89–93

GILBERT'S DISEASE
(IDIOPATHIC UNCONJUGATED HYPERBILIRUBINAEMIA)

An autosomal dominant, benign condition, in which there is a mildly elevated unconjugated bilirubin, without either structural liver disease or haemolytic anaemia. It is possibly due to difficulty in uptake and conjugation of bilirubin.

Preoperative abnormalities

1. Serum unconjugated bilirubin is raised, but usually to a level <50 μmol/l, and clinical jaundice is barely detectable. However, fluctuating mild jaundice may occur, particularly in the presence of stress, infection, starvation or surgery.
2. Other liver function tests are normal, and there is no haemolytic anaemia.

Anaesthetic problems

1. The condition itself is of no significance. However, the appearance of jaundice postoperatively may suggest more serious problems, and therefore the confirmation of Gilbert's syndrome as the cause is useful (Taylor 1984).
2. Starvation may elevate the bilirubin level.
3. The metabolism of morphine may be delayed.

1

Management

1. If Gilbert's disease is suspected, the administration of nicotinic acid 50 mg i.v will double or treble the plasma unconjugated bilirubin within 3 hours. In normal patients, or in those with other liver disease, the rise will be less marked.
2. Morphine should be used with caution.
3. Early morning surgery and a dextrose infusion will reduce the increase in bilirubin produced by starvation.

BIBLIOGRAPHY

Taylor S 1984 Gilbert's syndrome as a cause of postoperative jaundice. Anaesthesia 39: 1222–1224

GLOMUS JUGULARE TUMOUR

A rare, slow-growing, vascular tumour of the glomus bodies, usually arising from the dome of the jugular bulb. It is one of the paraganglionic tumours, related to the branchial arches. The symptoms, which are various, will depend in part on local extension or invasion by the tumour. The mode of presentation includes a swelling in the neck, middle ear disease, or symptoms indicative of involvement of the cerebellum, brainstem or skull base. Although normally non-functional, it occasionally produces catecholamines. It must be distinguished from glomus tumours, which arise from the tympanic plexus. Surgical removal is either through the auditory canal or via a mastoid approach.

Preoperative abnormalities

1. Pulsatile tinnitus, hearing loss and facial paralysis can occur when the middle ear is involved.
2. Clinical signs of IX, X, XI and XII cranial nerve lesions denote extension of the tumour into the base of the skull.
3. Intracranial extension may give V and VI nerve lesions.
4. Occasionally, functioning tumours can produce catecholamines.
5. Invasion of the jugular vein or internal carotid artery may occur.
6. Ten per cent of patients will have another paraganglionic tumour.
7. The tumours can be visualized using carotid angiography or digital vascular imaging. Vascularity and collateral circulation may be assessed.

Anaesthetic problems

1. Excision may require extensive surgery involving different surgical disciplines. Combined or two-stage procedures may be necessary.

2. Blood loss may be heavy (Ghani et al 1983). The blood supply usually comes from the external carotid, but extensive tumours may also be supplied by collateral circulation from the internal carotid.
3. Occasionally the tumour may actually involve the internal carotid artery itself or invade the jugular vein to give tumour emboli.
4. Surgery has been reported as lasting for up to 17 hours, therefore heat loss can be a problem.
5. The problems of any neurosurgical procedure, including that of air embolism.
6. Ligation of the internal carotid artery may be necessary (Braude et al 1986).

Management

1. A two-stage operation may be planned if the tumour is very extensive and involves two different surgical fields (Mather & Webster 1986).
2. Hypotensive anaesthesia may be required to reduce blood loss.
3. Prior radiological embolization of the tumour to reduce haemorrhage may be required.
4. If carotid artery ligation is contemplated, adequacy of the collateral circulation must be assessed.
5. Hypothermia and cerebral protection may be required in tumours involving the carotid artery. A technique has been described in which moderate hypothermia, normocarbia, normotension and thiopentone infusion provided successful cerebral protection for resection of an extensive tumour which involved the internal carotid (Braude et al 1986).

BIBLIOGRAPHY

Braude B M, Hockman R, McIntosh W A, Hagen D 1986 Management of a glomus jugulare tumour with internal carotid artery involvement. Anaesthesia 41: 861–865
Ghani G A, Sung Y-F, Per-Lee J H 1983 Glomus jugulare tumours – origin, pathology and anesthetic considerations. Anesthesia and Analgesia 62: 686–691
Mather S P, Webster N R 1986 Tumours of the glomus jugulare. Anaesthesia 41: 856–860

GLUCAGONOMA

A rare glucagon-secreting tumour of the alpha cells of the pancreatic islets. One of the group of tumours classified as APUDomas. Glucagon causes glycogenolysis, release of insulin and catecholamines, protein breakdown, lipolysis and ketogenesis. In addition, it is known to have positive inotropic and chronotropic effects, which are not prevented by beta blockers.

Preoperative abnormalities

1. The patient may present with a bullous skin condition, known as necrolytic migratory erythema.
2. Glucose tolerance tests may show mild or frank diabetes.
3. Basal plasma glucagon level is raised.
4. Pancreatic polypeptide is also often raised.

Anaesthetic problems

1. Wide fluctuations in plasma glucagon levels have been reported to occur during handling of the tumour (Nicholl & Catling 1985). The levels recorded were, however, less than those needed to produce pharmacological effects, and no cardiovascular changes were seen.
2. Fluctuations of blood sugar also occurred, but were not of clinical significance.
3. Other neuroendocrine hormones can be produced (see Apudomas).

Management

Evidence of secretion of other neuroendocrine hormones should be sought.

BIBLIOGRAPHY

Nicoll J M V, Catling S J 1985 Anaesthetic management of glucagonoma. Anaesthesia 40: 152–157

GLUCOSE-6-PHOSPHATE DEHYDROGENASE DEFICIENCY

A sex-linked hereditary abnormality in which the activity or stability of the enzyme glucose-6-phosphate dehydrogenase (G6PD) is markedly diminished. It is most commonly found among blacks and people of Mediterranean origin. It is also found in North European and South-east Asian populations. G6PD is an essential enzyme for glucose metabolism in the pentose phosphate pathway within the RBC. This pathway is ultimately involved in the production of reduced glutathione, and the reduction of methaemoglobin within the RBC. When G6PD activity is impaired, the accumulation of methaemoglobin and a deficiency of reduced glutathione alter cell integrity. Globin precipitates, known as Heinz bodies, are produced and the RBCs become more prone to haemolysis. Several variants of the A and B G6PD subtypes have been described, resulting in different clinical severity.

Preoperative abnormalities

1. With rare exceptions, the only clinical manifestation of G6PD deficiency is haemolytic anaemia. Usually the anaemia is episodic and is associated with stress, most notably drug administration, infection, the newborn period, and in certain individuals, exposure to fava beans (favism). Drugs known to cause haemolysis in G6PD deficiency subjects include the antimalarials, primaquine and chloroquine, the sulphonamides, tolbutamide, nitrofurantoin, the sulphones, methylene blue, nalidixic acid, high-dose aspirin, vitamin C, vitamin K, phenacetin and nitrates. Chloramphenicol, quinidine and quinine affect those with the Mediterranean form of the condition only. Two to five days after ingestion of one of these drugs, there may be abdominal pain and jaundice associated with a fall in haemoglobin level. Heinz bodies appear in the blood during this period.
2. Chronic non-spherocytic haemolytic anaemia, with jaundice, and splenomegaly may be seen occasionally. The anaemia is not usually severe, but in some instances, frequent transfusions have been reported.
3. There is an increased incidence of cataracts and vitreous haemorrhage.

Anaesthetic problems

1. Drug-induced haemolysis can occur after administration of any of the above drugs.
2. The appearance of postoperative jaundice may cause confusion as to its origin (Shapley & Wilson 1973).
3. G6PD-deficient individuals may be sensitive to overdoses of prilocaine and sodium nitroprusside, not as a result of methaemoglobinaemia as sometimes stated, but because of the concurrent production of oxidizing chemicals which can produce haemolysis (Smith & Snowden 1987). If clinically significant methaemoglobinaemia occurs in a G6PD patient, methylene blue is ineffective in treatment, and may cause haemolysis (Smith & Snowden).
4. Malignant hyperthermia was reported to have occurred in a patient with G6PD deficiency (Younker et al 1984). However, there was no mention of confirmation of the diagnosis of MH, with in vivo or in vitro tests.

Management

1. Elective surgery should not be undertaken during a haemolytic episode.
2. Agents known to produce haemolysis should be avoided. Particular care should be taken not to exceed the maximum safe doses of sodium nitroprusside or prilocaine (Smith & Snowdon 1987).
3. A folic acid supplement may be required.

1

BIBLIOGRAPHY

Shapley J M, Wilson J R 1973 Post-anaesthetic jaundice due to glucose-6-phosphate
  dehydrogenase deficiency. Canadian Anaesthetists' Society Journal 20: 390–392
Smith C L, Snowdon S L 1987 Anaesthesia and glucose-6-phosphate dehydrogenase
  deficiency. Anaesthesia 42: 281–288
Younker D, DeVore M, Hartlage P 1984 Malignant hyperthermia and glucose-6-phosphate
  dehydrogenase deficiency. Anesthesiology 60: 601–603

GLYCOGEN STORAGE DISEASES

A group of genetic diseases in which there are defects in enzymes
concerned with either the breakdown or the branching of glycogen.
The Cori classification is:

I = von Gierke's		V = McArdle's
II = Pompe's		VI = Her's
III = Cori's, Forbes		VII = Thompson
IV = Andersen's		VIII = Tarin

Type	Enzyme deficiency	Affected organs
I	glucose-6-phosphatase	liver and kidneys
II	alpha-1,4 glucosidase	skeletal and cardiac muscle
III	amylo-1,6 glucosidase	liver, skeletal and cardiac muscle and blood cells
IV	amylo-1,4 to 1,6-transglucosidase	liver, skeletal and cardiac muscle and blood cells
V	muscle phosphorylase	muscle
VI	liver phosphorylase	liver and white blood cells
VII	phosphoglucomutase	muscle
VIII	muscle fructokinase	muscle and red blood cells

The commoner of the diseases are dealt with under the individual
names.

BIBLIOGRAPHY

Casson H 1975 Anaesthesia for portacaval bypass in patients with metabolic disease. British
  Journal of Anaesthesia 47: 969–975
Cox J M 1968 Anesthesia and glycogen-storage disease. Anesthesiology 29: 1221–1225
Edelstein G, Hirshman C A 1980 Hyperthermia and Ketoacidosis during anesthesia in a child
  with glycogen storage disease. Anesthesiology 52: 90–92
Ellis F R 1980 Inherited muscle disease. British Journal of Anaesthesia 52: 153–164

GOODPASTURE'S SYNDROME

A general term applied to a combination of glomerulonephritis and lung
haemorrhage, which may be caused by a variety of diseases processes
(Holdsworth et al 1985). It is usually, but not invariably, rapidly

1

progressive. It is typically associated with antibodies to glomerular basement membrane (anti-GBM), detectable in plasma by radioimmunoassay and by immunofluorescence techniques on muscle biopsy. These cross-react with alveolar basement membrane, although those with lung haemorrhage are usually smokers, and those with isolated anti-GBM nephritis are non-smokers. Systemic vasculitides such as PAN and Wegener's granulomatosis may also cause lung haemorrhage and renal failure.

Preoperative abnormalities

1. Usually presents with cough, dyspnoea, haemoptysis which may be massive, and anaemia.
2. The pulmonary lesions proceed to interstitial fibrosis and haemosiderin deposits. Lung function tests show a restrictive type of abnormality.
3. Glomerulonephritis, which usually follows or coincides with pulmonary lesions, may produce proteinuria, haematuria and casts. The end-result is renal failure.

Anaesthetic problems

1. Poor respiratory function with hypoxaemia, respiratory alkalosis and lung haemorrhage.
2. Impaired renal function and sometimes renal failure.
3. Hypochromic anaemia and a high ESR.
4. Patients may be on immunosuppressives or steroids, or undergoing plasma exchange, with the aim of reducing the antibody titre.

Management

1. Preoperative assessment of lung function and, in particular, blood gases. Elective pulmonary surgery should not be undertaken during active haemorrhage.
2. Assessment of renal function and appropriate management.

BIBLIOGRAPHY

Holdsworth S, Boyce N, Thomson N M, Atkins R C 1985 The clinical spectrum of acute glomerulonephritis and lung haemorrhage (Goodpasture's syndrome). Quarterly Journal of Medicine 55: 75–86

GUILLAIN–BARRÉ SYNDROME

An acute ascending polyneuropathy in which motor involvement predominates. It probably has an immunological basis. Infection, surgery and immunizations have all been implicated in its development. Its progress is variable and the mortality is 5–20%. The anaesthetist may be involved in treatment of respiratory insufficiency, or for surgery.

Preoperative abnormalities

1. Muscle weakness usually starts in the legs and progresses upwards, at a variable rate. Up to 50% of cases have bulbar involvement. There may be respiratory insufficiency requiring IPPV, and an inability to clear secretions.
2. Mild sensory disturbances and loss of tendon reflexes occur.
3. Autonomic dysfunction may produce cardiovascular instability and an impairment of normal compensatory vasoconstrictor responses (Lichtenfeld 1971). Changes of position can be accompanied by marked reductions in blood pressure. Attacks of sweating, tachycardia and hypertension may occur. Brady- and tachyarrhythmias may necessitate pacemaker insertion. Sudden deaths have occurred, probably due to arrhythmias. It has been suggested that the lack of respiratory variation in heart rate, which is characteristic of autonomic dysfunction, occurs more often in the group of patients with respiratory muscle weakness, who require IPPV (Oakley 1984).
4. The CSF protein content is raised, with no increase in cell count.

Anaesthetic problems

1. If the intercostal muscles are affected, respiration and sputum clearance may be compromised. Bulbar weakness may result in pulmonary aspiration and segmental collapse.
2. Autonomic dysfunction can produce postural variations in blood pressure and marked hypotension on induction of anaesthesia. Cardiovascular collapse has been reported, occurring immediately after the administration of a spinal anaesthetic (Perel et al 1977). This was thought to be caused by a combination of hypotension due to the spinal, and a 30° head-up tilt.
3. Administration of suxamethonium may be associated with transient severe hyperkalaemia. In one patient, asystole after suxamethonium was subsequently followed by rhabdomyolytic renal failure (Hawker et al 1985).
4. Hyponatraemia may occasionally occur, due to inappropriate ADH secretion.

Management

1. In the presence of decreasing respiratory function, IPPV may be required. Vital capacity should be measured 4-hourly during the phase of deterioration. The use of accessory muscles of respiration, and the reduction of vital capacity to 1 litre (or 15 ml/kg), presages respiratory

failure (Ferner et al 1987). Facial weakness is an ominous sign. The institution of IPPV may be accompanied by hypotension. Tracheostomy is required when prolonged ventilation is anticipated.

2. In patients who require IPPV, continuous cardiac monitoring is required. It has been suggested that regularity of the heart rate, measured by minimal R–R interval variation on deep breathing, may indicate autonomic failure and the possibility of sudden death due to arrhythmia (Oakley 1984) (see Autonomic failure). Pacemaker insertion may have to be considered.

3. General care includes:

    a. Physiotherapy for the chest, with passive movements for the limbs.

    b. Nasogastric feeding. Constipation should be anticipated, with the use of stool softeners or enemas.

    c. Psychological management. The patient may be very frightened, and constant reassurance is needed. Depression is a frequent problem in the later stages.

4. Reports of the efficacy of plasma exchange are variable. On balance plasmapheresis appears to be safe. It has been shown to accelerate recovery and shorten the ventilation time, particularly if it is instituted early (Hughes 1985).

5. Steroids are now not recommended.

6. If general anaesthesia is required, suxamethonium should be avoided.

BIBLIOGRAPHY

Ferner R, Barnett M, Hughes R A C 1987 Management of Guillain–Barré syndrome. British Journal of Hospital Medicine 38: 525–530
Hawker F, Pearson I Y, Soni N, Woods P 1985 Rhabdomyolytic renal failure and suxamethonium. Anaesthesia and Intensive Care 13: 208–209
Hughes R A C 1985 Plasma exchange for Guillain–Barré syndrome. British Medical Journal 291: 615–616
Lichtenfeld P 1971 Autonomic dysfunction in the Guillain–Barré syndrome. American Journal of Medicine 50: 772–780
Oakley C M 1984 The heart in the Guillain–Barré syndrome. British Medical Journal 288: 94
Perel A, Reches A, Davidson J T 1977 Anaesthesia in the Guillain–Barré syndrome. Anaesthesia 32: 257–260

HAEMOGLOBINOPATHIES
(see also THALASSAEMIA)

Normal haemoglobin (HbA) consists of a colourless protein, globin, which is made up from two alpha and two beta polypeptide chains, and four haem radicals. The haem radical is a porphyrin structure, at the centre of which is a hexavalent iron atom. Four of the valencies are occupied by the nitrogen atoms of pyrrole rings, and the fifth, by one of the globin polypeptide chains. The last one is therefore free for haemoglobin to transport oxygen, in a reversible combination.

1

The haemoglobinopathies result from inherited structural alterations in one of the globin chains. The thalassaemias, on the other hand, result from inherited defects in the rate of synthesis of one or more of the globin chains.

Types of haemoglobinopathies

1. Sickle cell disease and allied disorders.
2. Haemoglobinopathies producing cyanosis.
3. Haemoglobinopathies associated with unstable haemoglobin.
4. Haemoglobinopathies producing polycythaemia.

Types of normal haemoglobin

HbA   Normal adult haemoglobin. Has two alpha and two beta chains. Ninety-eight per cent of adult molecule is in this form.

HbF   Fetal haemoglobin. Has two alpha and two gamma chains. Is gradually replaced during the first 6 months of life, but varying amounts may persist in the haemoglobinopathies and modify the disease severity.

HbA2   Forms 2.5% of adult haemoglobin. Has two alpha and two delta chains.

SICKLE CELL DISEASE

A genetic abnormality of haemoglobin synthesis involving the substitution of valine for glutamic acid at the sixth amino acid position in the beta chain of the globin molecule. It occurs most frequently in blacks of African origin and in some Mediterranean races. Resistance to malaria occurs.

Sickle cell disease   A general term encompassing all abnormal combinations in which HbS forms a part, e.g. HbSS, HbSC, HbSThal.

Sickle cell anaemia   Refers to HbSS only.

Sickle cell trait   Refers to HbAS.

The homozygous form (HbSS, sickle cell anaemia) affects 0.25% of the UK black population, while the heterozygous form (HbAS, sickle cell trait) affects up to 10%. In HbAS, the red blood cells contain 20–45% HbS, whereas in HbSS the content is 85–95% HbS.

The solubility of deoxygenated HbS is much lower than that of HbA and it has a tendency to gel. A lowered oxygen tension within the red cells is associated with stacking of the haemoglobin molecules into long crystals. The cell membrane is deformed by these molecular changes, and the red cell takes on a sickle shape. Dehydration promotes this tendency, and sickling increases the blood viscosity. Once initiated the process can be self perpetuating. Obstruction of blood vessels to organs may occur, and results in tissue infarction. Oxygenation can reverse the sickling process in the initial stages, but when repeated episodes have taken place, cell membrane changes tend to make it irreversible.

Haemolytic anaemia and jaundice occur as a result of premature destruction of these abnormal RBCs. The mean red cell life will depend on the percentage of abnormal haemoglobin within an individual cell. Cells with a majority of abnormal haemoglobin can have their life reduced from 120 days to less than 20.

In sickle cell anaemia, variable increases in fetal haemoglobin of up to 20% can occur. The levels may be genetically determined. High levels of HbF are advantageous, as its mixture with HbS will increase the solubility of the reduced haemoglobin, and thus decrease the severity of the disease.

Preoperative abnormalities

1. Sickle cell screening (Sickledex) is a rapid diagnostic test which detects the presence of HbS, but does not distinguish HbSS from HbAS or HbSC. For elective procedures the genotype should be determined by haemoglobin electrophoresis.
2. Patients with HbSS have a severe haemolytic anaemia, whereas those with HbAS usually have a normal haemoglobin. The clinical severity of HbSC varies. Some individuals with HbSC are virtually asymptomatic, but half of them will develop symptoms during childhood and most others become symptomatic in adolescent or adult life.
3. Sickle cell disease is associated with small vessel occlusion and episodes of infarction in affected organs. These may involve bone, bone marrow, liver, spleen, brain and lung. The episodes cause pain, pyrexia and tachycardia. Reduced oxygen tension and acidosis cause sickling of red cells. The increased viscosity encourages stasis and sludging, which in turn produce occlusion, ischaemia and infarction. Further hypoxia and acidosis perpetuate the cycle.
4. Renal problems may occur both in HbAS and HbSS. Papillary necrosis and haematuria can develop due to sickling in the juxtamedullary glomeruli. The concentrating capacity of the kidney is reduced and at least 2 litres of fluid per day are required to excrete the normal osmolar load.
5. In HbSS, varying crises can occur.
   a. The vaso-occlusive problems have been described.
   b. Sequestration crises occur particularly in infants and young children, and result from massive sudden pooling of red cells, especially in the spleen. It is the main cause of infant death in the first year of life.

c. An aplastic crisis is due to sudden marrow depression, and is generally associated with infection, especially viral.

d. Haemolytic crises sometimes occur in association with glucose-6-phosphate dehydrogenase deficiency following drug therapy.

6. Infants less than 6 months old have high percentages of HbF, and therefore may not require transfusion.

Anaesthetic problems

1. Sickling of red blood cells may be precipitated by hypoxia, acidosis, cold and hyperosmolality. Organ infarction, ischaemia and further hypoxia may result. The postoperative period is often the most hazardous time. Increased sickling of red blood cells occurs, with progressive decreases in the saturation of haemoglobin with oxygen.

In HbSS:
a. 100% saturation – some sickling occurs.
b. 65% saturation – 75% of cells are sickled.
c. 50% saturation – all cells are sickled.
d. The critical PaO_2 for irreversible sickling is 5.5 kPa.

In HbAS:
a. If 40% HbS, sickling starts at 40% saturation.
b. The critical PaO_2 for irreversible sickling is 2.7 kPa.

2. Sickle cell trait does carry a small risk. Sudden deaths during exercise, and splenic infarcts at altitude have been reported in the US forces literature. Despite statements to the contrary, anaesthesia for those with the sickle cell trait has not been entirely free from complications.

Adequate oxygenation cannot always be guaranteed during anaesthesia and recovery.

Failure to detect airway obstruction and cyanosis in the recovery room resulted in hypoxic fits, cerebral infarction and subsequent death, in a patient with HbAS (personal communication). In another case cardiac arrest and subsequent maternal death occurred during Caesarean section (Anaesthetic Advisory Committee to the Chief Coroner of Ontario 1987). It was postulated that aortocaval compression had occurred, and its relief at delivery allowed the sudden return of hypoxic, acidotic and sickled blood to the heart.

3. Patients with sickle cell states who are shocked, hypoxic and acidotic are difficult to resuscitate.

4. The reduced concentrating capacity of the kidney, which tends to be progressive, means that the patient cannot compensate for dehydration.

5. Some cases of von Willebrand's disease have been reported in association with HbSS and HbAS in patients presenting with haematuria.

6. Children less than 3 years old are at risk from sepsis.

Management

1. Diagnosis
Sickle cell screening should be done in at-risk populations prior to anaesthesia, even when the Hb is normal. A normal haemoglobin can also occur in patients with HbSC, and yet severe sickling take place.

2. Manoeuvres to prevent sickling of red blood cells:

a. Hypoxia in both the arterial and venous sides of the circulation must be avoided. Monitoring of both arterial and central venous PO_2 may be useful. Transcutaneous PO_2 measurement has been suggested, but does not always reflect arterial, or regional PO_2 (Dhamee et al 1982).

b. Acidosis must not occur. A mild respiratory alkalosis can be maintained by IPPV. Alkalinization with sodium bicarbonate has been suggested, although significant degrees of alkalosis may impair oxygen release (see e.).

c. Body temperature is maintained. Hypothermia increases sickling and blood viscosity, which result in stasis.

d. Local circulatory stasis is prevented. Increased oxygen extraction, possibly producing dangerously low venous PO_2 levels despite a normal PaO_2, is avoided. Vasopressors should not be used, and a tourniquet only if essential, although its use has been reported in 21 patients with few complications (Stein & Urbaniak 1980). During labour, precautions against aortocaval compression are essential. Epidural anaesthesia was reported to have improved a sickle cell crisis involving the extremities, in a patient in active labour (Finer et al 1988).

e. Dehydration, which increases sickling, has to be avoided. The decreased concentrating capacity of the kidney accentuates the problem. To prevent dehydration, in the immediate preoperative period, 10 ml/kg/h of Hartmann's solution, with 44–50 mmol sodium bicarbonate added to each litre, has sometimes been recommended. This also maintains a mild alkalosis, but not all authorities agree that this is either necessary or effective.

f. Elective surgery should not take place in the presence of infection, as a crisis may be precipitated.

3. Measures to reduce the amount of HbS
These are controversial. The complexity of each technique has tended to vary inversely with the number of patients reported. As the highest incidence of the disease occurs in countries where facilities may be limited, this is perhaps not surprising. Series of 505 (Oduro & Searle 1972) and 284 (Homi et al 1979) general anaesthetics given to patients with various haemoglobinopathies, have been published. Six patients died in each group. All deaths occurred in the postoperative period, and in only two was there any suggestion that the anaesthetic management might have contributed. One patient, who had an elective procedure in spite of a preoperative pyrexia, died of pneumonia. The second, a man with a head injury, received sedation during a carotid angiogram. It should not

1

be overlooked that in one of the series (Homi et al 1979) only 21% of the 202 patients with HbSS received a preoperative blood transfusion.

In contrast, transfusion as a means of reducing the relative amounts of HbS prior to, or during, surgery has been advocated. It has been suggested that for major surgery, the aim should be a reduction of HbS to 30%, in the presence of a haematocrit of 36% (Esseltine et al 1988). Each technique has its indications, advantages and disadvantages.

a. Preoperative transfusion only if the haemoglobin is below a certain level (Homi et al 1979).

b. Preoperative transfusion of 15–20 ml/kg packed red cells, 1–2 days before elective, or immediately prior to emergency surgery (Janik & Seeler 1980).

c. Serial transfusions during a 10–15-day preoperative period.

d. Exchange transfusion either pre- or intraoperatively (Riethmuller et al 1982).

If operative transfusion is required, fresh blood, which has high 2,3-diphosphoglycerate levels is preferable.

BIBLIOGRAPHY

Anaesthesia Advisory Committee to the Chief Coroner of Ontario 1987 Intraoperative death during Caesarean section in a patient with sickle cell trait. Canadian Journal of Anaesthesia 34: 67–70
Dhamee M S, Whitesell R C, Munshi C 1982 Towards safer anaesthesia in sickle cell states. Anaesthesia 37: 94–95
Esseltine D W, Baxter M R N, Bevan J C 1988 Sickle cell states and the anaesthetist. Canadian Journal of Anaesthesia 35: 385–403
Finer P, Blair J, Rowe P 1988 Epidural analgesia in the management of labour pain and sickle cell crisis. Anesthesiology 68: 799–800
Homi J, Reynolds J, Skinner A, Hanna W, Sergeant G 1979 General anaesthesia in sickle cell disease. British Medical Journal 1: 1599–1601
Janik J, Seeler R A 1980 Perioperative management of children with sickle haemoglobinopathy. Journal of Pediatric Surgery 15: 117–120
Oduro K A, Searle J F 1972 Anaesthesia in sickle cell states: a plea for simplicity. British Medical Journal 4: 596–598
Riethmuller R, Grundy E M, Radley-Smith R 1982 Open heart surgery in a patient with homozygous sickle cell disease. Anaesthesia 37: 324–327
Stein R E, Urbaniak J 1980 Use of the tourniquet during surgery in patients with sickle cell haemoglobinopathies. Clinical Orthopaedics and Related Research 151: 231–233

HAEMOLYTIC URAEMIC SYNDROME

A syndrome of thrombocytopenia, haemolytic anaemia, renal vascular injury and renal failure. It occurs most commonly in infants and young children. In adults it tends to be associated with viral toxins, immunosuppressive drugs, oral contraceptives or postpartum. There is widespread vascular endothelial damage with deposition of fibrin, and intravascular haemolysis. All organs are affected, although the kidney is primarily involved. The prognosis in children is reasonably good, whereas in adults the renal failure is usually irreversible.

Preoperative abnormalities

1. In young children the presenting problem is usually gastroenteritis with bloody diarrhoea.
2. Progression occurs to haemolytic anaemia and renal failure. The exact mechanism and sequence of events is not known. However, the primary lesion appears to be one of renal vascular endothelial injury, possibly due to lipid peroxidation (Neild 1987). Factor VIII is released from the endothelium, and platelet aggregation, with subsequent thrombosis and necrosis, occurs. A deficiency of prostacyclin has also been demonstrated. The oxidant injury may also damage the red cells, which then become more susceptible to destruction. A consumptive coagulopathy is well recognized.
3. In adults, there may be a relevant drug history. Mitomycin C, 5-fluorouracil and oral contraceptives have all been implicated. The syndrome can occur postpartum, and occasionally there may be a family history.
4. Hepatosplenomegaly may be present.
5. There is widespread organ involvement and the condition merges imperceptibly with thrombotic, thrombocytopenic purpura. Cardiac, neurological, and hepatic problems have been described.

Anaesthetic problems

1. Anaesthesia may be required for the creation of arteriovenous shunts for renal dialysis (Johnson & Rosales 1987).
2. Haematological problems include anaemia, thrombocytopenia and occasionally coagulation abnormalities.
3. Cardiovascular complications include hypertension, pericardial effusion and heart failure.
4. Neurological complications include fits, unconsciousness and hemiplegia.
5. Hepatic dysfunction may occur.

Management

1. Most of the patients are children, therefore peritoneal dialysis is the treatment of choice. If fluid overload and hyperkalaemia are already present, haemodialysis may be needed prior to the administration of a general anaesthetic.
2. Fresh frozen plasma may be of benefit.
3. Control of hypertension and fluid and electrolyte balance may be needed.
4. During anaesthesia, a technique using IPPV, isoflurane and atracurium, with neuromuscular monitoring, has been suggested (Johnson & Rosales 1987). Postoperative IPPV may be required.
5. Steroids are not indicated. Heparin is sometimes used.

BIBLIOGRAPHY

Johnson G D, Rosales J K 1987 The haemolytic uraemic syndrome and anaesthesia. Canadian Journal of Anaesthesia 34: 196–199
Neild G 1987 The haemolytic uraemic syndrome: a review. Quarterly Journal of Medicine 63: 367–376

HAEMOPHILIA A
(and HAEMOPHILIA B)

Haemophilia A is a sex-linked recessive inherited coagulation disorder, associated with reduced levels of factor VIII. Males are affected, while females are the carriers. Occasional instances of female deficiency have been described where the mother is a carrier and the father has haemophilia A. Haemophilia A is clinically indistinguishable from haemophilia B (Christmas disease), which is a rarer condition associated with a deficiency of factor IX. Haemophilia A will be dealt with in detail, but the principles of the anaesthetic management of haemophilia B are similar.

Preoperative abnormalities

1. The clinical severity is related to factor VIII levels as measured by clotting assay. The factor level can be expressed as iu/ml, or as a percentage of normal. The normal range is 50–200 iu/ml, or 50–200%

Factor level (%)	Clinical severity	Type of bleeding
<1	Severe	frequent spontaneous bleeding
2–5	Moderate	variable – some spontaneous bleeding; severe bleeding after trauma
6–15	Mild	bleeding on trauma
>15	Very mild	bleed only after severe trauma or major surgery

2. Spontaneous bleeding affects mainly joints and muscles. Inadequately treated, recurrent joint bleeds can lead to ankylosis and permanent joint deformities.
3. Coagulation tests detect the abnormality in intrinsic pathway with prolongation of partial thromboplastin generation. Whole blood clotting time is usually normal except in the most severe cases. Bleeding time is normal. Definite diagnosis by factor VIII : C assay.
4. Treatment is by replacement of deficient factor VIII.
5. Complications of treatment include production of factor VIII antibodies in 6–10% of patients, allergic reactions, transmission of viruses, especially NANB hepatitis, hepatitis B and HIV.

Anaesthetic problems

1. High risk of transmitting hepatitis B or NANB hepatitis.
2. Need to avoid i.m. injections and regional anaesthesia. Special care is required during laryngoscopy and endotracheal intubation.
3. Problems of venous access.

Management

1. Advice of a haematologist, and knowledge of an individual patient's history, is essential.
2. Source of factor VIII concentrate.
   a. Cryoprecipitate. Average factor VIII content is about 2 iu/ml. It is only suitable for treatment in children or mild haemophiliacs.
   b. Human freeze-dried factor VIII. Both NHS and commercial preparations are available. All preparations are now heat treated to eliminate HIV infections.
   c. Animal freeze-dried factor VIII. Commercially produced bovine and porcine with high potency of animal factor VIII. The material is highly antigenic and is indicated for patients with high titre factor VIII antibodies.

$$\text{Dose in units of factor VIII} = \frac{\% \text{ rise needed} \times \text{patients weight in kg}}{1 \cdot 5 - 2}$$

3. Prior to major surgery, patients should be tested to exclude factor VIII antibodies, and assess the response to factor VIII infusion.
4. During surgery, the infusion therapy should be controlled by specific factor assay. The amount and duration of treatment depends on the response to factor VIII infusion, and its half-life (between 7 and 22 hours, with an average of 12 hours). It also depends on the nature of the operation and the time taken for the wound to heal.

In severe haemophilia A it is usual to give an immediate preoperative dose of 50 iu/kg of factor VIII, and on the evening of operation a second dose of 25 iu/kg. The pre- and postinfusion factor VIII level should be measured for the first dose. On the second day 25 iu/kg is given twice daily and continued for 7–10 days. A safe objective is to keep the postinfusion factor VIII near 100% and the pre-infusion level near 50% for the first week postoperatively. Therefore daily assay is needed for the first week, then less frequent assays can be done. After 7–10 days it is usually safe to reduce the frequency of doses from twice to once daily. If factor VIII level is found to be particularly low in individual patients, then more frequent administration of factor VIII is needed.
5. In mild haemophiliacs undergoing minor surgery or dental extraction, the i.v. infusion of desmopressin in a dose of 0.3 μg/kg in 50 ml saline 0.9% will give a short-term rise in factor VIII. Water retention may occur. Stimulation of the fibrinolytic system necessitates the simultaneous use of tranexamic acid.

6. Dental surgery may be achieved using a single dose of factor VIII, 25–30 iu/kg. Tranexamic acid 10 mg/kg i.v. is given initially, then 15 mg/kg t.d.s. orally is continued for 10 days. Postoperatively, infection predisposes to bleeding, so prophylactic antibiotics are needed.

7. The presence of factor VIII antibody is a contraindication to surgery, except where life saving. Under such circumstances large doses may have to be given (Rizza 1984).

8. In three large retrospective studies of surgery in haemophilia and related disorders, individual problem cases were discussed (Sampson et al 1979, Kasper 1985, Kitchens 1986). The safety of elective surgery performed in large centres was emphasized. However, the incidence of postoperative bleeding varied from 5% (Sampson et al 1979) to 23% (Kasper 1985). A range of factor VIII levels were achieved, but the minimum level required to prevent postoperative bleeding is still to be determined. Average trough levels of about 30% in the first 5 days have been recorded and have led to the suggestion that the previously recommended levels were not necessary (Sampson et al 1979). On the contrary, there are cases in which postoperative bleeding occurred despite adequate levels of factor VIII (Kasper et al 1985). Increasing factor VIII doses threefold, from 600 to 2000 iu/kg/operation, to raise the trough levels from 37% to 70%, did not reduce the incidence of postoperative bleeding. It was concluded that factor VIII levels could not be the only determinant of bleeding in haemophilia.

9. Analgesia must be carefully managed. In the above series, persistence of bleeding was sometimes related to the inadvertent use of aspirin-containing compounds or NSAIDs. Mild pain should be treated with paracetamol, pentazocine, dihydrocodeine or buprenorphine. Opiate analgesics should be used with caution to prevent addiction.

HAEMOPHILIA B
(*CHRISTMAS DISEASE*) (*see also HAEMOPHILIA A*)

A sex-linked recessive inherited coagulation disorder associated with reduced levels of factor IX.

Preoperative abnormalities

1. For clinical features and severity see Haemophilia A.

2. Coagulation tests detect the abnormality in intrinsic pathway and the definitive diagnosis is made on factor IX assay.

Anaesthetic problems

See Haemophilia A.

Management

1. The principles of treatment for major surgery and dental extraction are the same as in haemophilia A. However, desmopressin is not effective in factor IX deficiency.

2. Treatment is by replacement with factor IX concentrates (both NHS and commercial
The recovery of factor IX is less than in factor VIII, so the dose required is greater:

$$\text{Dose in units of factor IX} = \frac{\% \text{ rise needed} \times \text{patients weight in kg}}{0.9}$$

BIBLIOGRAPHY

Kasper C K, Boylen A L, Ewing N P, Luck J V Jr, Dietrich S L 1985 Hematologic management of hemophilia A for surgery. Journal of the American Medical Association 253: 1279–1283
Kitchens C S 1986 Surgery in hemophilia and related disorders. Medicine 65: 34–45
Rizza C R 1984 Haemophilia A and B. Prescribers' Journal 24: 71–78
Sampson J F, Hamstra R, Aldrete J A 1979 Management of hemophiliac patients undergoing surgical procedures. Anesthesia and Analgesia 58: 133–135

HEART BLOCK
(see also SICK SINUS SYNDROME)

A patient may present for surgery either with a permanent pacemaker in situ, or with a bradyarrhythmia which may require the insertion of a temporary transvenous pacemaker for the perioperative period. Increasing numbers of pacemakers are being implanted, and in some cases increasingly complex electronic devices are being used.

Preoperative abnormalities

1. Heart block may be congenital or acquired, and the latter either acute or chronic.
Congenital heart block may occur alone, or in association with other cardiac abnormalities. As an isolated phenomenon it is relatively benign, as the block to conduction is at the level of the AV node. The ventricular pacemaker is proximal to the bifurcation of the bundle of His, so the QRS complexes are narrow, and the ventricular conduction system intact. The rate is relatively high and can vary from 40 to 80 per minute, and may increase with exercise. However, sudden death may occasionally occur.

In chronic acquired heart block the defect is more distal in the conducting system. The AV junction or bundle branches are usually involved, the QRS complexes are wide, the heart rate is lower and not increased by exercise. The prognosis is generally worse, but ultimately depends on the underlying cause.

2. Heart block can be divided into three types:

a. First-degree AV block:

P–R interval prolonged beyond 0.21 seconds.

b. Second-degree AV block:

i. Type I   Progressive P–R lengthening until a complete failure of conduction and a beat is dropped (Wenkebach phenomenon).

ii. Type II   Intermittent failure of AV conduction without preceding prolongation of P–R interval. This type is of more serious significance than type I, and often progresses to third degree AV block.

c. Third degree AV block:

Complete dissociation of the atria and ventricles due to failure of atrial impulses to be transmitted.

3. Patients may present with syncopal (Stokes–Adams) attacks, fatigue, angina or heart failure.

Anaesthetic problems

1. Patients with second-degree heart block, particularly type II, may progress to complete heart block under anaesthesia, due to interference with cardiac conduction.

2. Those with complete heart block may be unable to compensate for a fall in cardiac output by increasing their ventricular rate. Organ blood flow may be dramatically reduced. When increases in stroke volume can no longer compensate for slow heart rates, cardiac failure occurs.

3. When patients with heart block are anaesthetized, there is no method of monitoring the adequacy of cerebral blood flow and hence there is the risk of cerebral damage.

4. The problems of the underlying cause. The commonest cause of third-degree AV block in the elderly is idiopathic fibrosis. However, other causes include coronary artery disease, cardiomyopathy, drugs and cardiac surgery.

5. The use of surgical diathermy in the presence of pacemakers may produce complications:

a. With an older type of pacemaker, ventricular fibrillation has been reported rarely (Titel & El Etr 1968).

b. Inhibition of demand pacemaker function (Wajszczuk et al 1969) or interference with AV sequential pacemaker (Dressner & Lebowitz 1988).

c. 'Phantom' reprogramming of a programmable pacemaker (Domino & Smith 1983).

d. Idiosyncratic responses in multiprogrammable pacemakers. In one case, interference with the quartz crystal clock was interpreted as impending battery failure and the pacemaker went into a slow back-up mode aimed at preserving battery life (Shapiro et al 1985).

6. In order to prevent pacemaker inhibition during diathermy, the placement of a strong magnet over the pulse generator has been advocated (Simon 1977). This is said to change a demand pacemaker to an asynchronous one. In certain models, however, this manoeuvre may allow the electromagnetic waves of the diathermy to reprogramme and change the firing rate of the pacemaker.
7. Pacemaker failure may occur during surgery. This may be due to loose connections, battery failure, displacement of a lead or a change in pacemaker threshold.
8. Halothane raises the pacing threshold and should be avoided.

Management

1. The indications for insertion of a transvenous pacemaker prior to surgery are sometimes controversial, but may include:
   a. Sinoatrial node dysfunction producing a brady/tachyarrhythmia syndrome.
   b. Second- or third-degree AV block.
   c. LBBB and first-degree heart block.
   d. Bifascicular block. RBBB in combination with posterior fascicular block often progresses to third-degree heart block. It has therefore been suggested that bifascicular block is an indication for a temporary pacemaker. However, some authors believe this to be unneccessary (Rooney et al 1976). No complications occurred during epidural anaesthesia in patients with RBBB and left anterior fascicular block who were asymptomatic (Coriat et al 1981).
It has also been suggested that a temporary pacemaker is unnecessary in congenital complete heart block, especially in children, as the rate is usually relatively high and the prognosis good. However, should problems occur, temporary transvenous cardiac pacing takes time to institute. In a prospective survey of 153 insertions, the median time was found to be 20 minutes (Donovan & Lee 1984).
2. If a permanent pacemaker is already in situ, information on its mode of function should be sought (Horgan 1984). All patients with pacemakers are regularly reviewed in a pacemaker clinic. The pacemaker markings, date of insertion and battery life should be checked.
   a. Pacemaker markings
      I Chamber paced:
         V = ventricle, A = atrium, D = double.
      II Chamber sensed:
         V = ventricle, A = atrium, D = double, O = none.
      III Mode of response:
         T = triggered, I = inhibited, D = double, O = none.
      IV Programmable functions:
         P = simple programmable, M = multiprogrammable,
         C = communicating, O = none.

V Special anti-tachyarrhythmic functions:
B = bursts of impulses, N = normal rate competition,
S = scanning response, E = externally activated.

b. Pacemaker type and function

The most common type of pacemaker in use is VVI. The chamber paced is the ventricle, as is the chamber sensed, and the pacemaker is inhibited by spontaneous ventricular activity.

A programmable pacemaker is one in which certain parameters such as rate, sensitivity, output and refractory period, can be changed non-invasively. This is done with a programmer, which sends electromagnetic coded signals to the pacemaker. Some of the multiprogrammable ones have very complex functions to treat difficult arrhythmias and to anticipate problems such as battery failure.

Although VVI will be the most frequently encountered, other types of pacemaker may be needed on occasions, to cope with individual requirements or pacing problems (Shaw & Whistance 1986):

i. Maintenance of atrial transport. Atrial demand pacemakers (AAI) are useful in sick sinus syndrome, when atrioventricular conduction is intact. It is haemodynamically advantageous if atrial synchrony is maintained, as an atrial contribution to ventricular filling may improve the cardiac output by up to 30%, as compared with that produced by VVI pacemakers. This may be important for patients with ventricular pacing, who are experiencing symptoms suggestive of the pacemaker syndrome. Dizziness or syncope may result from hypotension due to loss of atrioventricular synchrony, or to retrograde ventriculoatrial conduction.

ii. Rate responsiveness to exercise. Dual-chamber pacemakers (e.g. DDD) can stimulate both chambers in sequence, and if atrial activity is normal they allow a 'physiological' response to exercise. Where there is sinus disease, other variables, such as respiratory rate will have to be used to assess body activity.

iii. Antitachycardia pacemakers. These have been designed to detect tachycardias, then terminate them by breaking the re-entrant circuit.

c. Pacemaker threshold

If possible, a cardiologist should be asked to check the pacing threshold which is the minimum voltage necessary for the pacing stimulus to capture the ventricles consistently. Pacemaker function depends on both electrical and non-electrical factors. The threshold for capture is dependent upon cellular factors such as acid-base balance, hypoxia, potassium and drugs. If the threshold increases, there may be intermittent failure of pacing. If the threshold decreases there is a risk of inducing ventricular fibrillation.

d. Detection of pacemaker dysfunction.

The occurrence of syncope may suggest pacemaker dysfunction. A 10% decrease in heart rate in a fixed rate pacemaker may indicate impending battery failure. An irregular heart rate in a VVI pacemaker means that R waves are not being sensed.

3. The use of diathermy

Advice is still usually given that this should only be used if really necessary. Although many of the modern pacemakers are said to be safe with diathermy, problems have been encountered. As pacemakers have become more complex, with programmes both to detect and eliminate external electrical interference, and to provide back-up for programme or battery failure, so idiosyncratic complications may arise. Two cases of apparent pacemaker malfunction have been reported, which were a direct result of the complex back-up functions of the pacemaker (Shapiro et al 1985).

If diathermy is needed:

a. Place the indifferent electrode of the diathermy on the same side as the operating site and as far away from the pacemaker as possible.

b. Limit its frequency and duration of use, and keep the diathermy current as low as possible.

c. Use a bipolar rather than a unipolar diathermy.

d. Check the patient's pulse for inhibition of pacemaker function. If this occurs, and provided its use is not contraindicated in the pacemaker literature, then the use of a magnet may be tried. This usually converts a demand to a fixed rate pacemaker, whatever the intrinsic rhythm. However, with certain programmable pacemakers, this may cause phantom reprogramming.

e. With a programmable pacemaker, it might be helpful to have the programmer itself available in theatre, so that the programming could be checked at the end of the operation. However, in many cases this is not feasible.

4. Pacemaker failure (Donovan & Lee 1984)

Whenever a pacemaker is in situ, atropine, adrenaline and isoprenaline should be available, for use in the event of pacemaker failure.

If failure to pace occurs with a temporary pacemaker:

a. Try reversing the polarity.

b. Try increasing the output to maximum.

c. Change to VOO (asynchronous) mode.

d. Check that the connections are intact.

e. Change the whole unit, or the batteries.

f. If using a bipolar lead, try each as unipolar.

g. Turn the patient into the left lateral position to improve electrode contact.

h. Change the pacing lead.

5. Monitoring of pulse and blood pressure

Blood pressure should be carefully monitored. If the ECG is susceptible to diathermy influence, then other methods of pulse observation, such as palpation or an oesophageal stethoscope, should be used to detect pacemaker inhibition. Direct arterial monitoring is advisable in major cases.

BIBLIOGRAPHY

Coriat P, Harari A, Ducardonet A, Tarot J P, Viars P 1981 Risk of advanced heart block during extradural anaesthesia in patients with right bundle branch block and left anterior hemiblock. British Journal of Anaesthesia 53: 545–548

Domino K B, Smith T C 1983 Electrocautery-induced reprogramming of a pacemaker using a precordial magnet. Anesthesia and Analgesia 62: 609–612

Donovan K D, Lee K Y 1984 Indications for and complications of temporary transvenous cardiac pacing. Anaesthesia and Intensive Care 13: 63–70

Dressner D L, Lebowitz P W 1988 Atrioventricular sequential pacemaker inhibition by transurethral electrosurgery. Anesthesiology 68: 599–601

Horgan J H 1984 Cardiac pacing. British Medical Journal 288: 1942–1944

Rooney S-M, Goldiner P L, Muss E 1976 Relationship of right bundle branch block and marked left axis deviation to complete heart block during general anaesthesia. Anesthesiology 44: 64–66

Shapiro W A, Roizen M F, Singleton M A, Morady F, Bainton C R, Gaynor R L 1985 Intraoperative pacemaker complications. Anesthesiology 63: 319–322

Shaw D B, Whistance A W T 1986 Clever pacemakers. Hospital Update 12: 843–852

Simon A B 1977 Perioperative management of the pacemaker patient. Anesthesiology 46: 127–131

Titel J H, El-Etr A A 1968 Fibrillation resulting from pacemaker electrodes and electrocautery during surgery. Anesthesiology 29: 845–846

Wajszczuk W J, Mowry F M, Dugan N L 1969 Deactivation of a demand pacemaker by transurethral electrocautery. New England Journal of Medicine 280: 34–35

HEPATITIS (VIRAL)

A number of different viruses cause individual types of hepatitis:

    a. Hepatitis A virus (HAV).
    b. Hepatitis B virus (HBV).
    c. Non-A non-B hepatitis virus (NANBV).
    d. Epstein–Barr virus (EBV: in infectious mononucleosis).
    e. Cytomegalovirus.
    f. Herpes simplex virus.

HEPATITIS A

Usually occurs in children and has an incubation period of between 15 and 40 days. Spread is primarily gastrointestinal. Serological diagnosis depends on finding antibody in the IgM plasma fraction in the acute stage and subsequently in the IgG fraction, which indicates immunity. Gamma globulin is of prophylactic value. HAV accounts for only about 20% of adult hepatitis.

HEPATITIS B

Is of particular interest to the anaesthetist and is considered in some detail.

Epidemiology

Hepatitis B has a long incubation period of 2–6 months, and was initially thought to be spread only by the parenteral route. Until the 1960s, HAV and HBV infections were clinically indistinguishable, other than by inference from a history of blood transfusion, the incubation period, or by epidemiological studies.

Studies on institutionalized mentally retarded children, not only confirmed the differences in incubation period between the two diseases, but unexpectedly showed that both viruses could be transmitted either orally or parenterally. HBV could therefore be transmitted by close physical contact and actual skin penetration was not essential. Differentiation between the two diseases by inference, from a history of parenteral transmission, was therefore no longer reliable.

Australia antigen

An antibody was discovered in a haemophiliac which reacted with the serum of an Australian aborigine. This new antigen was therefore named the Australia antigen. It was later found to be only associated with serum hepatitis. Subsequent widespread testing for the Australia antigen revealed that particular populations had a higher incidence of the antigen than others. Amongst these were leukaemics, haemophiliacs, institutionalized patients, drug abusers, patients with chronic renal failure on dialysis, those of Central African origin and paid blood donors in the USA.

Australia antigen and renal dialysis units

Patients with renal failure proved to be a particular problem. They often had a mild form of hepatitis and readily became asymptomatic carriers. The widespread contact with blood and dialysis patients on haemodialysis units facilitated HBV transmission, so that in the late 1960s many dialysis units had epidemics of hepatitis. Screening of all blood donors, barrier techniques, and the provision of separate facilities for infected patients, has resulted in HBV no longer being epidemic in British renal units after 1973. However this is not so with all units abroad, so any relaxation of strict screening of patients may still have serious effects.

Serological markers (Tedder 1980)

The Australia antigen is now known as hepatitis B surface antigen (HBsAg) and denotes current HBV infection. Antibody (antiHBs) means past infection and present immunity. If HBV is treated with detergent, the core structure with its antigen HBcAg is released. AntiHBc is normally present in excess and therefore free HBcAg is never detected in serum. The presence of AntiHBc indicates past or present infection and levels may be very high in carriers. A further antigen (HBeAg) is detectable in the early stages of infection and in some carriers.

NON-A NON-B HEPATITIS

This is the commonest type of hepatitis associated with blood transfusion and is a diagnosis by exclusion. Despite the fact that blood-carrying HBV has been screened out by the blood transfusion services, hepatitis still occurs. There may be more than one virus involved in NANBH.

Anaesthetic problems of hepatitis B

1. There is a small risk of infection from a patient with HBV. Transmission can occur by accidental inoculation, by splashing infected material into the eye, or occasionally by ingestion of virus-containing material.
2. If infection occurs and the anaesthetist is not immune, acute hepatitis may manifest itself after 2–6 months. Occasionally it is fatal. The majority of patients will be normal afterwards and the antigen usually disappears from the serum within 4 weeks. A few patients may develop chronic liver disease.
3. After infection, some apparently healthy people become carriers of the antigen and therefore are potentially dangerous to other people.
4. HBV is resistant to destruction by physical methods.

Management

1. Selective patient screening
Patients admitted to hospital who fall into one of the increased risk categories should be screened. These may include drug addicts, haemophiliacs, homosexuals, renal patients, those with tattoos, and patients who have had recent jaundice. Elective surgery should be delayed in patients with acute hepatitis until they are no longer infectious.
2. A carrier state is confirmed when at least two specimens over a period of a few months have similar HBeAg levels. Carriers are divided into 'simple', who are of low infectivity, and 'super' carriers who are highly infectious. These can be distinguished serologically (Tedder 1980).
3. The DHSS has now advised that certain hospital staff, including those working in operating theatres, should be vaccinated against HBV. Guidelines on hepatitis B and AIDS have been issued by the Association of Anaesthetists (1988).
4. If accidental inoculation of a member of staff occurs from a HBsAg patient, screening of that member should be immediately performed. If there is evidence of immunity, nothing more need be done. If not, passive immunization with HB immunoglobulin should be carried out within 24–48 hours and again at 1 month. Active immunization can be given at the same time. The recently introduced genetically engineered vaccines (e.g. Engerix B) are probably now preferable to those from human sources.

1

5. Operating theatre management of HBsAg-positive patients.
   a. The patient should be last on the theatre list.
   b. Minimize the number of staff in theatre.
   c. Staff should wear gown, gloves, masks and visors.
   d. Attempt to use only disposable linen and instruments.
   e. Meticulous attention must be paid to prevention of needle stick injuries. Accidents should be reported.
   f. Surfaces will require decontamination with sodium hypochlorite.
   g. Metal should be treated with glutaraldehyde.
6. Blood samples and pathological specimens.
   a. Specimens should be taken by qualified staff.
   b. Do not squirt blood or sheath needles.
   c. Specimens and needle disposal box should be labelled 'hepatitis risk'. Check that the specimen tube is intact.
   d. Keep tests to a minimum and if suspected, screen first.
   e. Seal the tube inside a plastic bag; do not use staples; attach forms to the outside.
   f. Simply wash blood off unbroken skin and clean surfaces with sodium hypochlorite.
   g. If skin is pierced, clean, allow to bleed, then seal.
   h. Consider giving hepatitis immunoglobulin.
   i. The patient should be followed up.

BIBLIOGRAPHY

Association of Anaesthetists 1988 AIDS and hepatitis B. Guidelines for Anaesthetists
Browne R A, Chernesky M A 1984 Viral hepatitis and the anaesthetist. Canadian Anaesthetists' Society Journal 31: 279–286
du Moulin G C, Hedley-Whyte J 1983 Hospital-associated viral infection and the Anesthesiologist. Anesthesiology 59: 51–65
Oxman M N 1984 Hepatitis-B vaccination of high-risk hospital personnel. Anesthesiology 60: 1–3
Tedder R S 1980 Hepatitis B in hospitals. British Journal of Hospital Medicine 23: 266–279

HEPATORENAL SYNDROME

A loosely applied term, often used wherever hepatic and renal problems coincide. It initially referred to the renal failure which occasionally follows surgery for obstructive jaundice, particularly if the serum bilirubin is >145 μmol/l. Some hepatologists feel it should only be used for unexplained renal failure complicating hepatic cirrhosis (Hishon 1981). The prevention of renal failure after surgery in jaundiced patients is considered. The references cover wider aspects.

Presenting problems

1. Jaundice is produced by obstruction of the biliary tree usually by stones, tumour or stricture. Conjugated bilirubin fails to reach the gut.

1

Alkaline phosphatase levels frequently exceed 210 iu/l.
2. Hepatocellular damage inevitably occurs if the obstruction has been present for any length of time. Serum transaminases may be moderately raised.
3. Pruritus and bradycardia may accompany severe jaundice.
4. An absence of bile salts from the gut impairs the absorption of vitamin K and causes a prolonged prothrombin time.

Management

1. Preoperative prophylactic measures will reduce the incidence of postoperative renal failure in jaundiced patients. Initially, the problem was thought to be due to anoxia and the toxic effects of bilirubin. The protective function of i.v. mannitol has been demonstrated (Dawson 1965, Baum et al 1969). Adequate preoperative hydration is required. This is followed by mannitol 10%, 0.5–1 g/kg to promote a urine output of at least 50 ml/h. It may not be universally successful in preventing renal problems.
2. The renal problems have been linked with endotoxaemia. Portal endotoxaemia has been demonstrated, at operation, in patients with obstructive jaundice (Bailey 1976). Those who additionally had a peripheral endotoxaemia developed a significant fall in creatinine clearance. It has also been suggested that the absence of bile salts allows endotoxin to be absorbed from the gut. Oral administration of sodium taurocholate, 1 g t.d.s. for 48 hours, has been shown to be protective (Evans et al 1982). In patients with serum bilirubin levels above 145 μmol/l, it was recommended that a combination of mannitol with fluids, antibiotics and bile salts be used.

BIBLIOGRAPHY

Bailey M E 1976 Endotoxins, bile salts and renal function in obstructive jaundice. British Journal of Surgery 63: 774–778
Baum M, Stirling G A, Dawson J L 1969 Further study into obstructive jaundice and ischaemic renal damage. British Medical Journal 2: 229–231
Dawson J L 1965 Postoperative renal function in obstructive jaundice: effect of a mannitol diuresis. British Medical Journal 1: 82–86
Evans H J R, Torrealba V, Hudd C, Knight M 1982 The effect of preoperative bile salt administration on postoperative renal function in patients with obstructive jaundice. British Journal of Surgery 69: 706–708
Hishon S 1981 The hepatorenal syndrome. Hospital Update 7: 1027–1035

HEREDITARY ANGIONEUROTIC OEDEMA
(see also C1 ESTERASE INHIBITOR DEFICIENCY)

A symptom complex of intermittent painless, non-itching, swelling of subcutaneous tissue, respiratory mucosa and intestinal walls. Acute attacks may be precipitated by trauma or stress, and can last from a few hours up to 4 days. Often presenting in adolescence, it is an autosomal dominant condition in which there is a deficiency or abnormality of the inhibitor of the activated first component of complement (C1 inhibitor). Complement, whose major function is to eliminate antigen, is present in serum and a number of other body fluids, and is a mediator of immunological tissue damage (Powell 1984). The complement system is a cascade resembling the clotting sequence, in which a series of normally inactive proteins sequentially activate each other. The complement cascade is initially activated by either the classical or alternate pathways. It is normally kept under control by inhibitors, or when activated, by the spontaneous decay of the active component. The kinin-generating and fibrinolytic systems are also involved and the oedema appears to be due to generation of a peptide which causes increased capillary permeability.

Preoperative abnormalities

1. Attacks of angioneurotic oedema can be precipitated by trauma or stress, or there may be no obvious cause. Serious effects occur if the oedema involves the airway or leads to intestinal obstruction. The oedema does not respond to treatment with steroids, antihistamines or adrenaline.
2. A family history of the disease is usually elicited. In the past, the development of acute laryngeal oedema has carried a high mortality.
3. Plasma C1 inhibitor levels are below normal. During attacks there is a low C4 and often a low C2. Levels remain normal in 15% of cases, but a functional abnormality exists (Powell 1984).

Anaesthetic problems

1. Patients may present with acute upper airway obstruction due to oedema. Emergency tracheostomy may be needed (Hamilton et al 1977).
2. Surgery involving tooth extraction or endotracheal intubation carries a risk of initiating an attack.
3. Attacks of abdominal pain may occur due to intestinal oedema. Unless the diagnosis is made, patients may be submitted to unnecessary operations (Beck et al 1973).
4. The use of epsilon aminocaproic acid, a fibrinolytic inhibitor, as a prophylactic measure, has been associated with the development of deep venous thrombosis (Hamilton et al 1977).

Management

1. Attacks of glottic oedema can be treated with FFP, which contains C1 inhibitor. A single transfusion will maintain the level for between 1 and 4 days. Clinical improvement has been seen within 40 minutes. There is a theoretical risk that an attack may be worsened, due to the C2 and C4 content of FFP.

1

2. In patients presenting with acute abdominal pain, the diagnosis of intestinal oedema may be confirmed by a barium meal and follow-through examination. Administration of FFP has been shown to relieve symptoms within 2–3 hours (Beck et al 1973).
3. If elective or emergency surgery is required, prophylaxis can be achieved with FFP (Hopkinson & Sutcliffe 1979, Poppers 1987). Preferably, 2 units of FFP should be given 24 hours in advance. C1 inhibitor levels are increased for up to 4 days.
4. For prophylaxis, either danazol (a progestogen) 200 mg t.d.s., or stanozolol (an anabolic steroid) 2.5–10 mg daily, can also be given. Danazol increases the plasma levels of C1 esterase inhibitor and C4 (Gelfand et al 1976), probably by influencing hepatic synthesis of the inhibitor. It starts to act within 24 hours, and is at a maximum at 1–2 weeks. If possible, 10 days' treatment should be given before surgery. Tranexamic acid, 1.5 g t.d.s., can be added to the regimen, if necessary.
5. Facilities for tracheostomy should be available in life-threatening conditions.
6. For severe cases, purified C1 esterase inhibitor can be obtained from the Scottish Blood Transfusion Service, or from Immuno Limited (Rye Lane, Dunton Green, Sevenoaks, Kent TN14 5HB, UK).

BIBLIOGRAPHY

Beck P, Wills D, Davies G T, Lachmann P J, Sussman M 1973 A family study of hereditary angioneurotic oedema. Quarterly Journal of Medicine 42: 317–339
Gelfand J A, Sherins R J, Alling D W, Frank M M 1976 Treatment of hereditary angioedema with danazol. New England Journal of Medicine 295: 1444–1448
Hamilton A G, Bosley A R J, Bowen D J 1977 Laryngeal oedema due to hereditary angioedema. Anaesthesia 32: 265–267
Hopkinson R B, Sutcliffe A J 1979 Hereditary angioneurotic oedema. Anaesthesia 34: 183–186
Poppers P J 1987 Anaesthetic implications of hereditary angioneurotic oedema. Canadian Journal of Anaesthesia 34: 76–78
Powell R J 1984 Serum complement levels. British Journal of Hospital Medicine 32: 104–110

HEREDITARY SPHEROCYTOSIS

A familial haemolytic anaemia of autosomal dominant inheritance in which premature destruction of intrinsically abnormal erythrocytes occurs in the spleen.

Preoperative abnormalities

1. Small spherocytic red blood cells are present in the peripheral blood. The surface to volume ratio is altered and the normal discoid shape is lost. Cells have an increased osmotic fragility, their survival time is reduced and there is marrow hyperplasia.
2. Splenomegaly, mild haemolytic anaemia and acholuric jaundice.

3. A raised reticulocyte count of up to 20%.
4. An increased incidence of gallstones and leg ulcers.
5. RBC survival times are improved by splenectomy.

Anaesthetic problems

Splenectomy is needed in the majority of patients. Cholecystectomy may also be required.

Management

Prophylactic pneumococcal vaccine may be required if splenectomy is undertaken.

HERS' DISEASE, CORI TYPE VI GLYCOGEN STORAGE DISEASE

One of the glycogen storage diseases in which there is a reduced amount of alpha-1,4-glucan phosphorylase present in the liver and white blood cells (Howell & Williams 1983). It is similar to type I, von Gierke's disease, but is less severe.

Preoperative abnormalities

1. Hepatomegaly occurs due to increased glycogen stores in the liver.
2. There is a tendency to hypoglycaemia and a variable response to glucagon and adrenaline (Cox 1968).
3. Children may present with failure to thrive.
4. Tends to be less severe than type I disease. In a series of patients having portacaval shunt surgery for metabolic diseases, the single type VI case was the only one not to require parenteral nutrition (Casson 1975).

Anaesthetic problems

Hypoglycaemia and acidosis can occur after starvation.

Management

A dextrose infusion, to prevent an acidosis at the beginning of surgery, should be given during the period of preoperative starvation.

BIBLIOGRAPHY

Casson H 1975 Anaesthesia for portocaval bypass in patients with metabolic diseases. British Journal of Anaesthesia 47: 969–975
Cox J M 1968 Anesthesia and glycogen storage disease. Anesthesiology 29: 1221–1225
Howell R R, Williams J C 1983 The glycogen storage diseases. In: The metabolic basis of inherited disease. McGraw-Hill, New York

1

HOMOCYSTINURIA

One of the aminoacidurias, this autosomal recessive metabolic disease results from a deficiency of cystathionine B synthetase, which catalyses the reaction of homocystine and serine to produce cystathionine (Watts 1983). Large amounts of homocystine and methionine are found in the blood and the urine. Excess homocystine causes a loss of endothelial cells from the intima of blood vessels, exposing collagen and allowing platelet thrombi to form on the surface. There is platelet consumption, and a reduction in platelet count. The decrease in cystine, which is an important constituent of the cross-linkages in collagen, produces a weakened collagen. There is fragmentation of elastic tissue of large arteries (Carson et al 1965).

Preoperative abnormalities

1. Abnormalities include lens dislocation, ligamentous laxity, elongated extremities similar to Marfan's syndrome, but without the hyperextensiblity of joints, kyphoscoliosis, and brittle, light-coloured hair. If the condition is not diagnosed and treated early, mental retardation occurs.

2. Homocystine, which is not normally present in the urine, occurs in large amounts, as does methionine. Its irritant effect on the vascular endothelium causes platelet aggregation and subsequent thromboembolism. Major thromboembolic episodes occurred in five out of a series of ten patients (Carson et al 1965).

3. Treatment consists of a diet which is low in methionine but contains cystine supplements. Pyridoxine, dipyramidole and acetylsalicylic acid may be used to decrease platelet adhesion. Vitamin B12 and folic acid are also given.

Anaesthetic problems

1. Thomboembolism, which can be fatal, may occur in association with surgery.

2. Patients may have increased insulin levels resulting in hypoglycaemia.

3. Regional anaesthesia has certain theoretical disadvantages. Penetration of a large epidural blood vessel might initiate thrombosis, as may the accompanying venous stasis of the lower limbs.

4. Anaesthesia for the surgery of lens dislocation is most frequently reported (Frost 1980, Grover et al 1979, Parris & Quimby 1982).

Management

1. Dehydration must be avoided, and a good cardiac output and peripheral perfusion maintained.

2. Blood viscosity and platelet adhesiveness can be reduced by dextran, and the prior administration of pyridoxine.
3. Dextrose infusion will prevent hypoglycaemia.
4. Early mobilization and low-dose heparin therapy decreases the chance of postoperative thromboembolism.

BIBLIOGRAPHY

Carson N A J, Dent C E, Field C M B, Gaull G E 1965 Homocystinuria. Journal of Pediatrics 66: 565–583
Frost P M 1980 Anaesthesia and homocystinuria. Anaesthesia 35: 918–919
Grover V K, Malhotra S K, Kaushik S 1979 Anaesthesia and homocystinuria. Anaesthesia 34: 913–914
Parris W C V, Quimby C W 1982 Anesthetic considerations for the patient with homocystinuria. Anesthesia and Analgesia 61: 708–710
Watts R W E 1987 Inborn errors of metabolism. In: Oxford textbook of medicine. Oxford Scientific Publications, Oxford

HUNTER'S SYNDROME
(see HURLER'S and MUCOPOLYSACCHARIDOSES)

HUNTINGTON'S CHOREA

A degenerative neurological disorder inherited as an autosomal dominant. Progressive degradation and death of neurones is accompanied by a decrease in the levels of many neurotransmitters (Martin & Gusella 1986). The onset occurs between 30 and 45 years and death frequently follows within 10–15 years of the first symptoms.

Preoperative abnormalities

1. Clinical features are progressive and include choreiform movements, ataxia, dysarthria and dementia. Sleep and anaesthesia usually abolish the chorea, which may not return until several hours following the anaesthetic.
2. The chorea may be preceded by several years of gradually increasing personality changes and mental deterioration.
3. Patients with the clinical disease may be taking a variety of drugs to improve the chorea, including the butyrophenones, phenothiazines and tetrabenazine.

Anaesthetic problems

1. Of the 15 cases, using a variety of agents, reported in the anaesthetic literature, four were accompanied by prolonged apnoea or recovery (Davies 1966, Gualandi & Bonfanti 1968, Blanloeil et al 1982). Barbiturate (Davies 1966) and suxamethonium (Gualandi & Bonfanti 1968) sensitivities have been suggested as the likely causes. Plasma cholinesterase measurement was not mentioned. Subsequent papers have, however, reported successful anaesthetics in which one or both of these agents were given (Farina & Raucher 1977, Browne & Cross 1981, Costarino & Gross 1985), while others used alternative agents (Lamont 1979, Johnson & Heggie 1985, Rodrigo 1987). Assessment of the possible causative factors for either prolonged apnoea or delayed recovery from anaesthesia, must take account of:

a. A higher than expected incidence of atypical plasma cholinesterase (the fluoride-resistant gene, E_1^f) has been confirmed in patients with Huntington's chorea (Whittaker 1980).

b. These patients are often receiving a variety of powerful psychotropic drugs including phenothiazines and butyrophenones, and tetrabenazine, a drug which depletes stores of cerebral biogenic amines. Any of these may interact with anaesthetic agents.

c. In advanced cases, there are gross atrophic changes in the cerebral cortex and basal ganglia.

d. Patients are frequently wasted and of poor nutritional status.

Management

1. Plasma cholinesterase investigations should be carried out prior to an anaesthetic, even if the use of suxamethonium is not intended. Their documentation may be of subsequent value. Should suxamethonium be required in the absence of the results, or if non-depolarizing agents are used, neuromuscular monitoring is essential.

2. The dosages of all anaesthetic agents should be kept to a minimum, bearing in mind the pathology of the disease itself, preoperative drugs, and the general nutrition of the patient.

BIBLIOGRAPHY

Blanloeil Y, Bigot A, Dixneuf B 1982 Anaesthesia in Huntington's chorea. Anaesthesia 37: 695–696

Browne M G, Cross R 1981 Huntington's chorea. British Journal of Anaesthesia 53: 1367

Costarino A, Gross J B 1985 Patients with Huntington's chorea may respond normally to succinylcholine. Anesthesiology 63: 570

Davies D D 1966 Abnormal response to anaesthesia in a case of Huntington's chorea. British Journal of Anaesthesia 38: 490–491

Farina J, Rauscher L A 1977 Anaesthesia and Huntington's chorea. British Journal of Anaesthesia 49: 1167–1168

Gualandi W, Bonfanti G 1968 Un caso di apnea prolungata in corea di Huntington. Acta Anaesthesiologica (Padova) 19: 235–238

Johnson M K, Heggie N M 1985 Huntington's chorea: a role for the newer anaesthetic agents. British Journal of Anaesthesia 57: 235–236

Lamont A M S 1979 Brief report: anaesthesia and Huntington's chorea. Anaesthesia and Intensive Care 7: 189–190

Martin J B, Gusella J F 1986 Huntington's disease. Pathogenesis and management. New England Journal of Medicine 315: 1267–1276

Rodrigo M R C 1987 Huntington's chorea: midazolam, a suitable induction agent? British Journal of Anaesthesia 59: 388–389

Whittaker M 1980 Plasma cholinesterase variants and the anaesthetist. Anaesthesia 35: 174–197

1

HURLER, HURLER–SCHEIE, SCHEIE AND HUNTER SYNDROMES
(see also MUCOPOLYSACCHARIDOSES)

The mucopolysaccharidoses (MPS) are a group of inherited connective tissue syndromes which result from enzyme deficiencies.

Mucopolysaccharides are constituents of normal connective tissue and are composed of repeating disaccharide units connected to protein. They are normally broken down in the cell lysosomes to monosaccharides and amino acids. In the absence of certain enzymes, intermediate products of degradation accumulate. Cell size increases and cell function is impaired. The effects depend upon the enzyme defect and the specific organs involved. Hurler, Hurler–Scheie and Scheie syndromes are all type I MPS. Hunter's, type II, is similar to Hurler's, but less severe and with no mental retardation. All four are considered together here because they produce similar anaesthetic problems, and are the most difficult of the MPS types with which the anaesthetist might have to deal.

Anaesthesia is most likely to be required for ENT procedures, the repair of inguinal or umbilical herniae, and, more recently, amnion transplant (King et al 1984).

Preoperative abnormalities

Hurler's syndrome (type IH: gargoylism)
Craniofacial:
   Coarse features, irregular teeth, gum hypertrophy, macroglossia, corneal opacities, mouth breathing and frequent respiratory infections.
Cardiac:
   Coronary artery disease due to intimal deposition of mucopolysaccharides, valvular lesions and cardiac failure.
Skeletal:
   Dwarfing, short neck, kyphoscoliosis and claw hand.
   Atlanto-axial instability has been described.
Mental status:
   Subnormal.
Other organs:
   Hepatosplenomegaly, umbilical and inguinal herniae.

Scheie (type IS)
Craniofacial:
   Corneal clouding, prognathism and macroglossia.
Cardiac:
   Aortic incompetence.
Skeletal:
   Normal stature, short neck, deformity of hands and feet.

Mental status:
   Normal.
Other organs:
   Glaucoma, herniae and carpal tunnel syndrome.

Hurler–Scheie (type IH/S)
(Intermediate between Hurler and Scheie)

Hunter's (type II)
X-linked recessive, similar to Hurler's but less severe. There is evidence
of two distinct groups, mild and severe. This distinction is based on the
presence or absence of progressive mental retardation (Young & Harper
1982).

Craniofacial:
   Coarse facies, deafness and papilloedema.
Skeletal:
   Dwarfism, claw hands and stiff joints.
Cardiac:
   Coronary intimal thickening, valvular disease and heart failure. Heart
   disease is the commonest cause of death.
Mental status:
   Normal in the mild form, progressive retardation in the severe.
Other organs:
   Hepatosplenomegaly. The majority of patients have either umbilical
   or inguinal herniae.

Anaesthetic problems

1. Airway maintenance and induction difficulties. Reviews of patients
with MPS have noted that over 50% had airway-related problems (Baines
& Keneally 1983, Kempthorne & Brown 1983, King et al 1984, Herrick
& Rhine 1988). The majority were either Hurler or Hunter MPS.
Difficulties in airway maintenance appear in part to stem from
obstruction by soft-tissue deposits in the mouth, the tongue and the
pharyngeal tissues, and in part from excess tracheobronchial secretions.
2. Intubation difficulties were again reported in over 50% of cases. The
above problems are compounded by the large head and hypertelorism.
Complete failure to intubate occurred in three patients, another had a
hypoxic cardiac arrest (Kempthorne & Brown 1983) but was resuscitated,
and one died (Young & Harper 1982). It has been noted that the larynx
is often smaller than anticipated.
3. Venous access may be a problem (King et al 1984).
4. Atlanto-occipital instability may occur on occasions, and a spastic
quadriplegia has been reported in Hurler's (Brill et al 1978).
5. Fatal postoperative respiratory obstruction has been reported
secondary to glottic oedema in an abnormal larynx (Hopkins et al 1973).
Emergency tracheostomy proved difficult because of hard, thickened
cartilage.

Management

1. A drying agent is essential, and sedatives best avoided in these patients.
2. Cardiological assessment is required.
3. Cervical spine should be screened to detect atlanto-axial instability.
4. It has been claimed that inhalation inductions are difficult, and intravenous agents are dangerous (Herrick & Rhine 1988). Muscle relaxants should not be used until the airway is ensured.
5. A nasal airway has been suggested as being more effective than an oral one (Brown 1984). Lateral X-rays in two patients have shown that an oral airway pushes the epiglottis down and backwards to occlude the laryngeal inlet, whereas a nasal airway keeps it forward. Preoperative tracheostomy has been reported in patients with known failed intubation (Baines & Keneally). Secretions may still block the tube.
6. Local anaesthetic techniques should be considered. Spinal anaesthesia has been reported in a patient with a previous failed intubation (Sjögren & Pedersen 1986).

BIBLIOGRAPHY

Baines D, Keneally J 1983 Anaesthetic implications of the mucopolysaccharidoses. Anaesthesia and Intensive Care 11: 198–202
Brill C B, Rose J S, Godmilow L, Sklower S, Willner J, Hirschhorn K 1978 Spastic quadriparesis due to C1–C2 subluxation in Hurler syndrome. Journal of Pediatrics 92: 441–443
Brown T C K 1984 The airway in mucopolysaccharidoses. Anaesthesia and Intensive Care 12: 178
Herrick I A, Rhine E J 1988 The mucopolysaccharidoses and anaesthesia: a report of clinical experience. Canadian Journal of Anaesthesia 35: 67–73
Hopkins R, Watson J A, Jones J H, Walker M 1973 Two cases of Hunter's syndrome. The anaesthetic and operative difficulties in oral surgery. British Journal of Oral Surgery 10: 286–299
Kempthorne P M, Brown T C K 1983 Anaesthesia and the mucopolysaccharidoses. Anaesthesia and Intensive Care 11: 203—207
King D H, Jones R M, Barnett M B 1984 Anaesthetic considerations in the mucopolysaccharidoses. Anaesthesia 39: 126–131
Sjögren P, Pedersen T 1986 Anaesthetic problems in Hurler–Scheie syndrome. Report of 2 cases. Acta Anaesthesiologica Scandinavica 30: 484–486
Young I D, Harper P S 1982 Mild form of Hunter's syndrome: clinical delineation based on 31 cases. Archives of Disease in Childhood 57: 828–836

HYDATID DISEASE

Hydatid cysts are the larval stage of the tapeworm, *Echinococcus granulosus*. Dogs are the main hosts. Man and sheep are intermediate hosts. Hydatid disease is not uncommon among the mid-Wales farming communities and up to 26% of farm dogs in this area have *E. granulosus* (Morris 1981). If the ova are ingested by man, embryos are released when the chitinous coat is digested. These enter the liver by the portal vein. They may be destroyed or they may develop into a cyst. In man, the cysts are found in the liver (65%), lung (25%), muscles (5%), bone (3%) and brain (1%).

Each cyst is two layered and contains straw-coloured fluid in which there are free scolices, brood capsules containing scolices, and daughter cysts. Around the cyst is an area of compressed host tissue and fibrosis known as the pericyst. In 5–10% of cases the cyst will die, and calcification may occur (Lewis et al 1975).

Preoperative abnormalities

1. Hepatic cysts occur most frequently in the right lobe. Bacterial infection may result in a liver abscess. Rupture into a bile duct, or bile duct obstruction may occur and produce biliary colic. There may be jaundice. The number and location of the cysts can be shown on CT scan or ultrasound.
2. Pulmonary cysts can present with haemoptysis, dyspnoea, cough or chest pain. CXR may show a variety of appearances including an oval opacity, evidence of bronchial fistula formation, or rupture of the cyst with the development of a fluid level.
3. Eosinophilia occurs in about 30% cases. The Casoni skin test is still used for screening. Immunoelectrophoresis is the most specific test. Complement fixation test is positive in up to 80% of cases. Haemagglutination test detects a specific antibody.

Anaesthetic problems

1. Pulmonary hydatid cysts can cause bronchial obstruction and occasionally they may rupture into the airway. If this happens, flooding of the lungs occurs, with widespread dissemination of the scolices.
2. Hydatid fluid is highly antigenic, and rupture of a cyst has occasionally produced sudden death from an anaphylactic reaction (Jakubowski & Barnard 1971).
3. Cerebral cysts can produce raised intracranial pressure.

Management

1. Surgical removal is indicated, except in older patients with small cysts. Meticulous care must be taken to avoid rupture and spread of the fertile scolices.
2. Relatively new drugs, such as mebendazole, are being tested as scolicidal agents.
3. Pulmonary cysts. Protective formalin-soaked packs are placed round the wound, an incision is made through the pericyst and the cyst is carefully extruded by the anaesthetist, using gentle hand ventilation (Saidi 1977).
4. Due to the risk of an anaphylactic reaction, the need for the

immediate availability of adrenaline, metaraminol, isoprenaline and steroids has been stressed (Lewis et al 1975).

BIBLIOGRAPHY

Jakubowski M S, Barnard D E 1971 Anaphylactic shock during operation for hydatid disease. Anesthesiology 34: 197–199
Lewis J W, Koss N, Kerstein M D 1975 A review of echinococcal disease. Annals of Surgery 181: 390–396
Morris D L 1981 The management of hydatid disease. British Journal of Hospital Medicine 25: 586–595
Saidi F 1977 A new approach to the surgical treatment of hydatid cyst. Annals of the Royal College of Surgeons 59: 115–118

HYPERCALCAEMIA

When artefactual causes of a raised serum calcium have been excluded, the commonest causes of hypercalcaemia are malignancy and hyperparathyroidism. Sarcoidosis, thyrotoxicosis and vitamin D toxicity are uncommon. Other causes are extremely rare. Occasionally a patient with hypercalcaemia may present for anaesthesia. Severe hypercalcaemia (>3.2 mmol/l) may be dangerous and, in consultation with a physician, urgent lowering of the level may be required.

Preoperative abnormalities

1. Any malignancy with destructive bone metastases can produce hypercalcaemia, by releasing calcium into the plasma. The commonest causes are breast carcinoma and myeloma.
2. Hypercalcaemia and a raised parathyroid hormone level (PTH) is diagnostic of hyperparathyroidism. However, PTH levels may take several weeks to obtain and treatment may be required before the result is available.
3. Carcinoma of the lung or a renal cell carcinoma may rarely release a parathormone-like substance, leading to hypercalcaemia.
4. Symptoms of hypercalcaemia may be vague. They include general muscle weakness, apathy, gastrointestinal complaints such as nausea, vomiting and constipation, weight loss, thirst, polyuria and mental disturbances, progressing to unconsciousness. Renal stones may form. Symptoms do not usually occur until the serum calcium is >3.2 mmol/l. ECG may show an abnormally short Q–T interval.

Anaesthetic problems

1. A hypercalcaemic patient may be severely dehydrated.
2. Hypercalcaemia may precipitate fatal arrythmias.
3. Digitalis toxicity is exacerbated by a high serum calcium.

1

Management

1. Replacement of extracellular fluid by rehydration is the first and most important manoeuvre. A diuresis causes excretion of calcium in the urine. An infusion of 1 litre of sodium chloride 0.9% 3–4-hourly for 24 hours should reduce the serum calcium by 0.5 mmol/l. Loop diuretics can be added, but not until adequate fluid repletion is achieved. Thiazide diuretics should not be used as they increase tubular reabsorption of calcium. Fluid balance and serum potassium levels require careful monitoring.

2. Corticosteroids can be used, although there is some question about their efficiency. Calcitonin (100–400 iu s.c. 8-hourly) reduces mobilization of calcium from bone and will also produce an early, but transient effect (48–72 hours) on calcium levels.

3. The use of diphosphonates (e.g. etidronate), which may reduce osteoclastic bone resorption, is being investigated (Stevenson 1985).

4. Mithramycin, a cytotoxic antibiotic, has hypocalcaemic properties, but its action is delayed and myelosuppression, hepatic and renal toxicity are a problem (Brada & Horwich 1986).

BIBLIOGRAPHY

Brada M, Horwich A 1986 Oncological emergencies. Hospital Update 12: 799–812
Stevenson J C 1985 Malignant hypercalcaemia. British Medical Journal 291: 421–422

HYPERTENSION
(ACUTE EMERGENCY see also Section 3)

Patients on antihypertensive medication frequently present for surgery and the need for the continuance of therapy in the perioperative period is well recognized. The principle drugs and their side effects are described in Section 2. Recent articles have reviewed the current management of hypertension, and discussed the benefits and limitations of long-term therapy (Smith & Littler 1987, Heagerty 1988).

The management of patients presenting with untreated hypertension depends upon the level of the diastolic blood pressure and the surgical circumstances. For elective surgery, as long as the diastolic pressure does not exceed 110 mmHg, there is no evidence of increased cardiac complications (Goldman & Caldera 1979). Patients with persistent diastolic levels above this should be referred to a physician for leisurely treatment.

Urgent surgery may be required in patients with diastolic blood pressures of 110–120 mmHg. A number of drugs given before or during anaesthesia have been reported to attenuate, although not necessarily abolish, untoward haemodynamic and arrhythmic responses to noxious stimuli such as laryngoscopy and intubation. These include a benzodiazepine premedication, beta blockers, moderate to high doses of fentanyl or alfentanil, droperidol and lignocaine. These have been administered either individually, or in varying combinations (Donegan & Bedford 1980, Prys-Roberts 1984, Dann et al 1987, Lawes et al 1987).

The occurrence of severe untreated hypertension (a diastolic pressure >130 mmHg) in the perioperative period is known to be associated with an increased morbidity and mortality. Potential complications include cerebral haemorrhage, hypertensive encephalopathy, left ventricular failure, renal failure and vascular damage to the eyes.

A number of agents exist for the treatment of the acute hypertension. The choice depends on the cause, the accompanying pathology, monitoring facilities and familiarity with the use of the drug. Therapy should be extremely cautious, as restoration of normal blood pressure has been associated with myocardial infarction, stroke, and blindness. This is particularly true in the elderly. There are probably few occcasions where the blood pressure needs to be reduced more quickly than over a number of hours, and probably days.

Acute treatment of severe hypertension may be required:
  a. If there is a need for urgent surgery.
  b. If uncontrolled hypertension arises in the perioperative period.
  c. For specific clinical problems such as phaeochromocytoma, pre-eclampsia, acute aortic dissection and left ventricular failure.

Drugs used in the more urgent treatment of hypertension

Nifedipine

A calcium channel blocker which relaxes smooth muscle. Produces tachycardia, headache, flushing and sweating.
  a. Route: sublingual or oral.
  b. Dose: 10 mg.
  c. Onset: 5 minutes (sublingual), 20 minutes (oral).
  d. Max. effect: 30 minutes (sublingual), 40 minutes (oral).
  e. Duration: 3 hours (sublingual), 8–12 hours (oral).

Hydralazine (see also Section 3)

A direct dilator of arterioles. Produces tachycardia and an increase in cardiac output. Should therefore be avoided in myocardial ischaemia or LVF.
  a. Route: i.v., i.m. or by infusion.
  b. 5–20 mg, given slowly over 20 minutes. Can repeat after 30 minutes.
  c. Onset: 3–6 minutes.
  d. 3–6 hours (i.v.), 4–8 hours (i.m.).

Diazoxide (see also Section 3)

A direct dilator of arterioles. Causes sodium and water retention. Tachycardia and increased cardiac oxygen consumption means that it is contraindicated in myocardial ischaemia and LVF.

    a. Route: i.v.
    b. 30–300 mg i.v. incremental doses in a supine patient. Can be repeated up to three times in 24 hours.
    c. Onset: 3–5 minutes.
    d. Max. effect: 20–40 minutes.
    e. Duration: 4–12 hours.

Minoxidil

A potent orally active vasodilator. Direct dilator of arterioles, with little effect on capacitance vessels. A reflex tachycardia and fluid retention means that beta blockers and diuretics must be given in addition. For severe hypertension when other drugs have failed.

    a. Route: oral.
    b. 2.5 mg b.d., increasing by 5–10 mg each 3 days up to maximum of 25 mg b.d.
    c. Onset: 20 minutes.
    d. Max. effect: 2–3 hours.
    e. Duration: half-life 3 hours but effects may persist beyond 24 hours.

Labetalol

A combined alpha and beta adrenergic blocker. The beta effects are three to seven times more powerful than the alpha effects. It is not very effective if the patient is already taking antihypertensives. Potentially dangerous in phaeochromocytoma.

    a. Route: i.v., i.m. or infusion.
    b. Dose: 10–50 mg i.v.; infusion 2 mg/min to a maximum of 200 mg.
    c. Onset: i.v. 5–20 minutes.
    d. Duration: 3–4 hours.

Sodium nitroprusside (see also Section 3)

Direct-acting vasodilator. Increases coronary artery blood flow and decreases pulmonary artery pressure. Unstable in solution in the light therefore requires covering with aluminium foil. Must be discarded if blue. Direct arterial monitoring is required.

For acute use, the maximum safe dose is 1.5 mg/kg. If used long term, cyanide and thiocyanate levels must be monitored. With toxic levels there is severe metabolic acidosis and progressive hypotension. If accidental overdose occurs, sodium thiosulphate (25 ml 50% soln over 10 minutes)

or dicobalt edetate (300 mg over 10 minutes then 50 ml 50% glucose) is given.
  a. Route: by infusion only.
  b. Dose: 50 mg in 500 ml gives 100 μg/ml; titrate by effect, starting at 0.5 μg/kg/min.
  c. Onset: 1–5 minutes.
  d. Duration: 2–5 minutes.

Trimetaphan

A ganglion blocking agent and direct peripheral vasodilator. Causes tachycardia, tachyphylaxis and pupillary dilatation. Maximum dose 1 g.
  a. Route: by infusion only.
  b. Dose: 500 mg in 500 ml, start at 3–4 mg/min.
  c. Onset: 1–5 minutes.
  d. Duration: 5–10 minutes.

Phentolamine

An alpha adrenergic receptor blocker and direct vasodilator. Used specifically for hypertensive crises associated with phaeochromocytoma or adrenaline overdose.
  a. Route: i.v. or infusion.
  b. 2.5–5 mg each 5 minutes (i.v.), 5–60 mg over 10–30 minutes at a rate of 0.1–2 mg/min (infusion).
  c. Onset: 2–5 minutes (i.v.).
  d. Duration: 10–15 minutes.

Clonidine

A centrally acting alpha stimulant which reduces sympathetic outflow from the brain stem vasomotor centre. May produce a drop in cerebral blood flow. Use with caution in cerebrovascular disease.
  a. Route: i.m. or i.v.
  b. Dose: 300 μg i.m., 150–300 μg i.v. over 5–10 minutes, to a maximum of 750 μg in 24 hours.
  c. Onset: 5 minutes (i.m.), immediate (i.v.).
  d. Duration: 5–6 hours (i.m.), 3–4 hours (i.v.).

BIBLIOGRAPHY

Dann W L, Hutchinson A, Cartwright D P 1987 Maternal and neonatal responses to alfentanil administered before induction of general anaesthesia for Caesarean section. British Journal of Anaesthesia 59: 1392–1396
Donegan M F, Bedford R F 1980 Intravenously administered lidocaine prevents intracranial hypertension during endotracheal suctioning. Anesthesiology 52: 516–518
Goldman L, Caldera D L 1979 Risks of general anesthesia and elective operation in the hypertensive patient. Anesthesiology 50: 285–292

Heagerty A M 1988 Recent advances in therapy for hypertension. British Journal of Anaesthesia 61: 360–364

Lawes E G, Downing J W, Duncan P W, Bland B, Lavies N, Gane G A C 1987 Fentanyl/droperidol supplementation of rapid sequence induction in the presence of severe pregnancy-induced and pregnancy aggravated hypertension. British Journal of Anaesthesia 59: 1381–1391

Prys-Roberts C 1984 Anaesthesia and hypertension. British Journal of Anaesthesia 56: 711–724

Smith S A, Littler W A 1987 Drugs used in the treatment of hypertension. In Anaesthesia review 4. Churchill Livingstone, Edinburgh

Walters B N J 1984 Urgent treatment of acute hypertension. British Journal of Hospital Medicine 10: 49–52

HYPONATRAEMIA

Occurs in about 10% of the hospital population (Flear et al 1981). Plasma sodium levels <120 mmol/l, which are considered to be dangerous, are found in only 0.2% of patients. Chronic levels lower than this may be tolerated surprisingly well. However, in the acute situation, levels between 120 and 125 mmol/l have sometimes produced fits.

Hyponatraemia is usually due to water overload, and may occur preoperatively as a result of some underlying illness or therapy, or postoperatively secondary to enthusiastic overhydration with non-salt-containing fluids. After operation most patients have been shown to have raised plasma levels of ADH. In addition, a number of drugs possess antidiuretic properties. The administration of large amounts of simple dextrose solutions can therefore cause fluid retention and hyponatraemia.

If possible, the primary cause should be determined. Therapeutic measures, if required, differ markedly, and depend on the aetiology. In many cases an underlying illness may simply require treatment, while water intake should be restricted where appropriate.

Rapid intravenous correction of hyponatraemia in the presence of postoperative water intoxication has been associated with death and cerebral damage. Rapid changes in brain hydration due to osmotic gradients may be responsible (Arieff 1986, Swales 1987). It is illogical to treat an excess of water with more water and salt.

Causes

1. Dilutional hyponatraemia
   a. Excess water intake
   Water retention can occur due to the perioperative infusion of large volumes of non salt containing glucose solutions. Oxytocin and opiates, which both have antidiuretic properties, given during labour or prostaglandin termination of pregnancy, can compound the problem (Feeney 1982). In patients treated with beta adrenergic stimulants to

suppress premature labour, retention of water is thought to be one of the contributing factors towards the rare development of pulmonary oedema (Hawker 1984). Surgery is normally associated with raised ADH levels. The use of certain drugs, such as vasopressin, DDAVP and steroids, will tend to exacerbate the situation. The features of the TURP syndrome (see Section 4) are in part due to hyponatraemia, secondary to absorption of glycine from the prostatic venous sinuses during prostatectomy.

b. Decreased water clearance

May be due to appropriate, or inappropriate secretion of ADH. The syndrome of inappropriate ADH (SIADH) is said to occur with a variety of conditions. It may be associated with a tumour, most frequently bronchial carcinoma, thoracic disease, IPPV, the Guillain–Barré syndrome and a variety of cerebral problems such as injury, meningitis or primary tumours. However, it has been suggested that the hyponatraemia associated with CNS lesions is iatrogenic, occurring secondary to excessive administration of fluids (Bouzarth & Shenkin 1982).

2. Loss of body solutes

a. Loss of sodium

Causes include diuretics, gastrointestinal losses, renal disease, adrenal insufficiency, withdrawal of steroid therapy, salt depletion and severe hypothyroidism.

Further causes of solute loss have been suggested (Flear et al 1981), but there is controversy about their significance.

b. Loss of intracellular anions and potassium

If solute is lost, cells become hypo-osmolar. To prevent cell shrinkage, the plasma osmolality falls and hyponatraemia is produced.

c. Membrane defects result in leakage of cellular contents. This is suggested to occur in sick cell syndrome, associated, for example, with heart failure.

d. In cachexia, the catabolic state results in impaired production of intracellular anions.

Doubt has been cast on the concept of sick cell syndrome (Leaf 1974, Bichet & Schrier 1982), as the leakage of intracellular solute into the extracellular fluid should be capable of being demonstrated by a positive osmolal gap (measured minus calculated osmolality) and a normal serum osmolality. Some studies have failed to confirm this.

3. Increase in solute in plasma

Results in a redistribution of water to maintain osmotic balance. Can occur in:

a. An infusion of mannitol.

b. Sudden hyperglycaemia.

c. The sick cell syndrome (see above)

It is suggested that serious illness may cause cell membrane defects which result in loss of intracellular solutes into the extracellular fluid, which in turn pulls out intracellular water. Hyponatraemia occurs, but if this theory is correct, the plasma osmolality should remain normal, and an osmolal gap should be shown.

4. Excess of large paraprotein or lipid molecules

May decrease the fractional water content of plasma and give a falsely low sodium level (pseudohyponatraemia).

5. Reduction of plasma proteins

At physiological pH these contribute to the anions. A reduction may result in a compensatory fall in sodium.

Problems

1. Cerebral complications. A decreased conscious level and fits may occur. The level at which this appears is variable, often depending on the rapidity with which the hyponatraemia has developed. Fits can occur when plasma sodium levels are <123 mmol/l.

2. Pulmonary oedema may occur.

3. Complications during correction. Although severe hyponatraemia in itself may be dangerous, it has been suggested that its rapid correction may be even more so (Arieff 1986, Sterns et al 1986).

This view has, however, been challenged (Narins 1986). In the proponents' series (Arieff 1986, Sterns et al 1986), retrospective studies of 15 and six patients respectively seemed to indicate that correction of hyponatraemia with i.v. saline appeared to be associated with sudden deterioration, brain damage and death. This deterioration, which usually took place after correction of the plasma levels, has been termed 'osmotic demyelination syndrome' (Sterns et al 1986). In one of the studies, data over a 15-year period had been collected on 15 previously healthy women who developed severe hyponatraemia after elective surgery (Arieff 1986). The average preoperative sodium of 138 mmol/l fell to 108 mmol/l about 48 hours after surgery. Fits and respiratory arrest occurred in all patients, 27% died, 13% had limb paralyses and 60% remained in a persistent vegetative state. The presenting picture was one of SIADH, and a number of the patients had received drugs with antidiuretic properties. Significantly, the original hypotonic state was entirely iatrogenic. All patients had been given large volumes of only dextrose containing fluids and were in an average net positive fluid balance of 7.5 litres. After the diagnosis of hyponatraemia had been made, sodium chloride in a variety of concentrations was given. Some patients recovered consciousness as the serum sodium rose, only to lapse into coma subsequently.

Diagnosis

A number of investigations may be required for the evaluation of hyponatraemia, although in many cases not all are necessary.

a. Plasma electrolytes, urea, creatinine and glucose.
b. Plasma osmolality.
c. Urine osmolality and urinary sodium, 24 hours if possible.
d. Serum proteins.
e. Plasma cortisol.
f. Serum lipids.
g. Body weight changes.

1. Dilutional hyponatraemia
May be diagnosed on history alone. During prostaglandin termination
of pregnancy or in labour, the administration of more than 3.5 litres of
dextrose 5% with oxytocin has been associated with water intoxication
and fits (Feeney 1982). Postoperative hyponatraemia may be a
combination of dilution with 5% dextrose and an elevated ADH level.
   Hyponatraemia, low plasma osmolality, a urine osmolality of about
3–4 times that of the plasma, and a high urinary sodium is highly
suggestive of SIADH. Causes of SIADH should be sought.
2. Loss of body solutes
Where there is sodium depletion, the urinary sodium excretion may be
<20 mmol/24 h, or a single sample concentration may be <10 mmol/l. In
renal disease or heart failure these measurements may not be reliable.
   Hypokalaemia and alkalosis may indicate total body potassium
depletion.
3. Increase in solute in plasma
Iso-osmotic redistribution of water takes place when there is a sudden
increase in a solute. This may occur in hyperglycaemia, and possibly in
the sick cell syndrome. When the integrity of the cell membrane is
impaired, some leakage of organic solutes is allowed into the extracellular
fluid. The movement of solute is accompanied by water. If this happens,
hyponatraemia should be accompanied by a normal plasma osmolality
and an osmolal gap.
4. Pseudohyponatraemia
Hyponatraemia in the presence of a normal plasma osmolality may also
indicate a paraproteinaemia or high serum triglyceride levels. If these are
removed during estimation, the sodium concentration will be found to
be normal.
5. Decrease in serum cations or increase in anions
Hypoproteinaemia or paraproteinaemia may alter the electrochemical
balance resulting in a compensatory reduction in serum sodium.

Management

1. Dilutional hyponatraemia
Prevention is important, as usually there is an iatrogenic cause.
   a. Excess water intake
   Large quantities of dextrose 5% should not be administered
   perioperatively when antidiuretic factors may be operating. If oxytocin

is required, sodium chloride 0.9% may be used as an alternative vehicle. Should an electrolyte solution be contraindicated, a syringe pump may be used, or the total volume of dextrose 5% limited to 2 litres in 24 hours.

Water restriction should be used as the primary management. Should intravenous correction be required, caution is advisable. In severe symptomatic hyponatraemia, a correction rate of 2 mmol/l/h to achieve a level of between 120 and 130 mmol/l has been proposed as being safe (Narins 1986). Others, however, believe that the serum sodium should be corrected at a rate of less than 12 mmol/l/24 h (Sterns et al 1986). Diuretic therapy has also been advocated.

b. Inappropriate ADH secretion
Water is restricted and potassium given. If unsuccessful, demeclocycline 0.9–1.2 g/day is given in divided doses reducing to a daily maintenance dose of 600–900 mg/day. The renal excretion of water is enhanced by blocking the renal tubular effect of ADH.

2. Loss of body solutes
a. Loss of sodium. Treatment of the underlying illness is usually sufficient. Intravenous saline 0.9% may be required. Hypertonic solutions should be avoided because of the risk of producing sudden osmotic gradients.

b. Diuretics must be discontinued if hypokalaemia is suspected.

3. Increase in solutes in plasma
Treatment of diabetes, if present. If a diagnosis of sick cell syndrome is confirmed, the underlying disease should be treated. Occasionally the use of glucose, insulin and potassium may assist the cell membrane to return to normal. Initially 100 ml 50% dextrose, 20 units soluble insulin and potassium chloride should be used. Subsequent dosage will depend on blood glucose and potassium.

4. Pseudohyponatraemia
There is an osmolar gap, which is the difference between the calculated and measured plasma osmolalities. Osmolality is a measure of the total solute content of body fluids (or the number of particles in a given weight of solvent). As most of the measured osmolality in healthy patients comes from urea, glucose, sodium and its anions, attempts have been made to find the best formula for the calculated osmolality, in order to detect an unmeasured osmolar component, such as alcohol, glycine, trichloroethane, hyperproteinaemia or hyperlipidaemia (Worthley et al 1987). Comparing varying types of patients and five different formulae, the most appropriate was:

$$\text{Calculated osmolality} = 2 \times \text{Na} + \text{urea} + \text{glucose}$$

BIBLIOGRAPHY

Arieff A I 1986 Hyponatraemia, convulsions, respiratory arrest and permanent brain damage after elective surgery in healthy women. New England Journal of Medicine 314: 1529–1535

Bichet D, Schrier R W 1982 Evidence against concept of hyponatraemia and 'sick cells'. Lancet i: 742
Bouzarth W F, Shenkin H A 1982 Is 'cerebral hyponatraemia' iatrogenic? Lancet 1: 1061–1062
Feeney J G 1982 Water intoxication and oxytocin. British Medical Journal 285: 243
Flear C T G, Gill G V, Burn J 1981 Hyponatraemia: mechanisms and management. Lancet ii: 26–31
Hawker F 1984 Pulmonary oedema associated with beta 2 sympathomimetic treatment of premature labour. Anaesthesia and Intensive Care 12: 143–151
Leaf A. Hyponatraemia. Lancet 1974; i: 1119–1120
Narins R G 1986 Therapy of hyponatraemia. New England Journal of Medicine 314: 1573–1575
Sterns R H, Riggs J E, Schochet S S Jr 1986 Osmotic demyelination syndrome following correction of hyponatraemia. New England Journal of Medicine 314: 1535–1542
Swales J D 1987 Dangers in treating hyponatraemia. British Medical Journal 294: 261–262
Worthley L I G, Guerin M, Pain R W 1987 For calculating osmolality, the simplest formula is the best. Anaesthesia and Intensive Care 15: 199–202

HYPOTHYROIDISM

Hypothyroidism may be primary, or secondary to pituitary or hypothalamic disease. Autoimmune thyroiditis is the commonest primary cause, while the sequelae of surgical or radioiodine treatment of thyroid disease are also common. Deficiency of circulating thyroid hormone results in retardation of all body functions.

The condition may be subclinical, mild or severe. It affects all systems of the body and the presentations are protean. Mild disease may be unnoticed preoperatively, but can be responsible for delayed recovery from anaesthesia.

After successful treatment, both TSH and T4 levels should be normal. Replacement therapy must be cautious so as not to precipitate myocardial ischaemia or heart failure. In severe, untreated hypothyroidism, elective surgery must be postponed. If emergency surgery has to be undertaken, the mortality is high. However, in the case of patients with severe angina who require coronary artery surgery, the surgery may have to take precedence. The management of cardiac bypass surgery in patients with hypothyroidism has been described (Finlayson & Kaplan 1982). Thyroxine was not given until after myocardial revascularization. Reduced doses of diazepam and opiates were used for anaesthesia. Digoxin and steroids were also given during operation.

Preoperative abnormalities

1. Delay in the relaxation phase of reflexes, dry skin, a husky voice, loss of the outer part of the eyebrows and weight gain. In severe disease there is lethargy, bradycardia, hypothermia and respiratory depression. Deposition of a mucinous substance causes thickening of the subcutaneous tissues producing a non pitting oedema. Myxoedematous infiltration of the vocal cords and tongue can occur.

Cardiovascular complications include ischaemic heart disease, bradycardia, pericardial effusion and cardiac failure. Neurological complications include carpal tunnel syndrome, polyneuritis, myopathy and cerebellar syndrome. Psychiatric disturbances may be marked.
2. A raised TSH, and reduced T4 and sometimes T3. It should be remembered that depression of T4 alone often occurs in ill patients who are not hypothyroid. Acute hypothyroidism has been described in a severely ill surgical patient (Mogensen & Hjortso 1988).
3. Anaemia, which may be microcytic or macrocytic, hyponatraemia, lactic and respiratory acidosis, inappropriate ADH secretion and hypoglycaemia are features of myxoedema coma.
4. The ECG is of low voltage with flattened or inverted T waves.
5. Associated diseases include diabetes mellitus, pernicious anaemia and Addison's disease.

Anaesthetic problems

1. Severe hypotension, and even cardiac arrest, has been reported after induction of anaesthesia (Abbott 1967, Levelle et al 1985).
2. There is marked sensitivity to anaesthetic agents, narcotics and analgesics (Kim & Hackman 1977).
3. Anaesthesia may precipitate hypothyroid coma.
4. Hypothermia readily occurs under anaesthesia (Abbott 1967).
5. Respiratory responses are impaired. Muscle weakness may predispose to respiratory failure.

An obese patient with undiagnosed myxoedema had severe hypotension on induction, and postoperative respiratory failure. Difficulty occurred in weaning her off the ventilator, and only on the sixth day, when it was noticed that the oxygen consumption index was very low, was the diagnosis of myxoedema made and confirmed biochemically (Levelle et al 1985).
6. Adrenocortical insufficiency may occur in association.
7. Large goitres may cause tracheal narrowing.
8. In the presence of a low BMR, IPPV readily results in hypocapnoea which decreases cerebral blood flow. As cerebral oxygen consumption is not reduced, a relative reduction in cerebral oxygenation may result.

Management

1. In severe hypothyroidism, elective surgery should be cancelled while treatment is instituted. Patients with angina requiring coronary artery bypass surgery may be an exception to this rule (Finlayson & Kaplan 1982, Drucker & Borrow 1985). With milder forms of the disease, the case for cancellation is less clear. In a study of 59 patients with mild or moderate hypothyroidism (with matched controls), the authors found no

evidence to justify deferring surgery until the hypothyroidism had been corrected (Weinberg et al 1983).

2. Adequate treatment of hypothyroidism, using 100–200 μg l-thyroxine daily, takes time to achieve. Particular caution is required in the elderly, or in those with cardiac disease. In these patients, the dose should be reduced to 25 μg per day, increasing only at 3 to 4-weekly intervals. With overt hypothyroidism, it may take 6 months to restore metabolism to normal. A normal T4 and TSH signals adequate treatment. The half-life of 1-thyroxine is 1–2 weeks.

3. Severe hypothyroidism requiring urgent surgery, and myxoedema coma, are probably the only indications for intravenous thyroid replacement.

a. A single dose of lyothyronine sodium 50 μg slowly then 25 μg 8-hourly. ECG control should be used.

b. Hydrocortisone 100 mg 6-hourly and intravenous fluids, including dextrose, may also be required.

4. If urgent surgery is needed in severe disease, careful cardiovascular monitoring is essential. There is minimal reserve. Dehydration and fluid overload are poorly tolerated. Inotropic agents may produce severe arrhythmias and myocardial ischaemia.

5. Controlled ventilation with CO_2 monitoring to avoid hypocapnoea. Postoperative IPPV may be needed.

6. Core temperature should be monitored. A warming blanket, high theatre temperature and use of an infusion warmer will reduce hypothermia.

7. All drugs should be administered with caution.

BIBLIOGRAPHY

Abbott T R 1967 Anaesthesia in untreated myxoedema: report of two cases. British Journal of Anaesthesia 39: 510–514

Drucker D J, Burrow G N 1985 Cardiovascular surgery in the hypothyroid patient. Archives of Internal Medicine 145: 1585–1587

Finlayson D C, Kaplan J A 1982 Myxoedema and open heart surgery: anaesthesia and intensive care unit experience. Canadian Anaesthetists' Society Journal 29: 543–549

Kim J M, Hackman L 1977 Anesthesia for untreated hypothyroidism: report of 3 cases. Anesthesia and Analgesia 56: 299–302

Levelle J P, Jopling M W, Sklar G S 1985 Perioperative hypothyroidism: An unusual postanesthetic diagnosis. Anesthesiology 63: 195–197

Mogensen T, Hjortso N-C 1988 Acute hypothyroidism in a severely ill surgical patient. Canadian Journal of Anaesthesia 35: 74–75

Murkin J M 1982 Anesthesia and hypothyroidism. Anesthesia and Analgesia 61: 371–383

Weinberg A D, Brennan M D, Gorman C A, Marsh H M, O'Fallon W M 1983 Outcome of anesthesia and surgery in hypothyroid patients. Archives of Internal Medicine 143: 893–897

INFECTIOUS MONONUCLEOSIS

A common viral infection caused by the Ebstein–Barr virus which produces a variety of clinical patterns and spectrum of severity. Two rare complications of the disease may occasionally involve the anaesthetist:

1. Acute upper airway obstruction.
2. Guillain–Barré syndrome and bulbar paralysis.

Preoperative abnormalities

1. The three main types are:
   a. Anginose: pharyngitis and adenitis.
   b. Glandular: predominantly lymphadenopathy and mild fever.
   c. Febrile: a prolonged generalized illness with fever.
2. Diagnosis may be confirmed by the Monospot test and specific serology, as well as the presence of a lymphocytosis, with atypical lymphocytes on blood film.
3. Rare complications include thrombocytopenia and acute splenic rupture.

Anaesthetic problems

1. There have been several reports of upper airway obstruction due to lymphoid hyperplasia of Waldeyer's ring and oedema of the faucial arch, epiglottis and aryepiglottic fold (Wolfe & Rowe 1980). Cardiac arrest has been reported during tracheostomy (Lee 1969) and fatalities have occurred (Carrington & Hall 1986).
2. Liver function may be impaired.
3. Infectious mononucleosis is occasionally complicated by the Guillain–Barré syndrome and bulbar palsy. Deaths have been associated with respiratory failure, aspiration and pneumonia.
4. Acute mucosal bleeding may occur, sometimes associated with thrombocytopenia (Johnsen et al 1984).

Management

1. Although upper airway obstruction may be a feature in patients requiring hospital admission, it is generally mild and responds to conservative treatment. The use of a soft nasopharyngeal airway has been suggested, and in 25 cases of airway obstruction thus treated, only one patient required tracheostomy (Snyderman & Stool 1982). However, occasionally severe airway obstruction develops. It is therefore recommended that patients with even slight respiratory embarrassment be observed in a place with ENT and anaesthetic facilities (Johnsen et al 1984).
2. Some surgeons consider 'hot' tonsillectomy to be the treatment of choice. If an anaesthetic is required for adenotonsillectomy, facilities for immediate tracheostomy must be available. A case of stridor was described in which an attempted awake visualization of the pharynx under local anaesthetic precipitated tonsillar bleeding. Immediate tracheostomy was performed under local anaesthesia, followed by a

general anaesthetic for tonsillectomy (Catling et al 1984). Cardiac arrest has also been reported during tracheostomy under local anaesthesia (Lee 1969).

3. Bulbar paralysis may be another indication for tracheostomy (Wolfe & Rowe 1980).

BIBLIOGRAPHY

Carrington P, Hall J I 1986 Fatal airway obstruction in infectious mononucleosis. British Medical Journal 292: 195
Catling S J, Asbury A J, Latif M 1984 Airway obstruction in infectious mononucleosis. Anaesthesia 39: 699–702
Johnsen T, Katholm M, Stangerup S-E 1984 Otolaryngological complications in infectious mononucleosis. Journal of Laryngology and Otology 98: 999–1001
Lee M D 1969 Respiratory obstruction in glandular fever. Journal of Laryngology and Otolaryngology 83: 617–622
Snyderman N L, Stool S E 1982 Management of airway obstruction in children with infectious mononucleosis. Otolaryngology and Head and Neck Surgery 90: 168–170
Wolfe J A, Rowe L D 1980 Upper airway obstruction in infectious mononucleosis. Annals of Otology, Rhinology and Laryngology 89: 430–433

INSULINOMA

A rare insulin-secreting pancreatic islet cell tumour, which may be benign or malignant. Malignancy occurs in about 10% of cases.

Preoperative abnormalities

1. The symptoms, caused by episodic hypoglycaemia, may be suggestive of central nervous system disease, hysteria, epilepsy, sympathetic overactivity, behavioural problems or intoxication. Patients may complain of sweating, hunger, palpitations, or exhibit various focal neurological deficits coinciding with cerebral hypoglycaemia. Symptoms are either spontaneous, or induced by an overnight fast or controlled insulin infusion. They frequently occur before breakfast or during vigorous exercise.
2. Elevated fasting plasma insulin, and C-peptide levels in the presence of hypoglycaemia confirm the diagnosis.
3. Medical control of insulin secretion may be achieved by diazoxide, somatostatin analogue or streptozotocin.
4. A small percentage of insulinomas form part of a multiple endocrine neoplasia syndrome (MEN I).

Anaesthetic problems

1. Hypoglycaemia under anaesthesia
Permanent neurological damage may be caused, but the approach to management of the blood sugar during surgery remains controversial. To

prevent hypoglycaemia, the administration of dextrose 25% via a central venous infusion, whilst checking the plasma glucose at regular but unspecified intervals, has been suggested (Chari 1977). A contrary view is that surgery should only take place in hospitals equipped with an artificial pancreas (Roizen 1986). This device performs on-line glucose estimations and automatically administers glucose/insulin i.v. as necessary (Pulver et al 1980). Others have withheld glucose except when the blood glucose fell below 3 mmol/l (Lamont 1978). This was based on the premise that a rebound hyperglycaemia after insulinoma resection indicated complete removal of the tumour. Thus, if glucose were to be given, the sign would be masked. The reliability of this sign has, however, been questioned. Records of 38 operations for insulinoma in which glucose had not been given were studied (Muir et al 1983) to establish:

a. whether intermittent, as opposed to continuous, sampling of glucose protected the patient from hypoglycaemia?

b. whether the maintenance of moderate hypoglycaemia to subsequently establish complete removal was safe?

c. whether rebound hyperglycaemia was consistent and indicative of complete surgical removal?

It was concluded that

a. provided the glucose was above 3.3 mmol/l, intermittent sampling at 15-minute intervals was safe.

b. the deliberate withholding of intraoperative glucose was potentially dangerous.

c. although rebound hyperglycaemia often occurred, it was of no predictive value during the operation.

2. Hyperglycaemia may occur for the first few postoperative days as a result of persistent high levels of hormones with hyperglycaemic effects.

3. A possible interaction between diazoxide and thiopentone has been suggested (Burch & McCleskey 1981). Two patients on diazoxide infusions developed hypotension on induction of anaesthesia. Diazoxide inhibits insulin release, has peripheral vasodilator effects, and is strongly protein bound. Mechanisms associated with competition for binding sites between the two drugs were postulated.

Management

1. As hyperglycaemic rebound is not predictive of complete removal of the insulinoma during operation, moderate hypoglycaemia would appear to be both unnecessary, and potentially dangerous (Muir et al 1983). Maintenance of a plasma glucose level between 5.5 and 8.5 mmol/l, with estimations at 15-minute intervals, is recommended.

2. Care must be taken to avoid either hyper- or hypoglycaemia. In patients treated with diazoxide, rapid infusion of dextrose 5% was found to produce high glucose levels (Burch & McCleskey 1981). It was suggested that the rate be limited to 2 ml/kg/h.

3. Close cardiovascular monitoring during induction of anaesthesia is essential, especially in patients on diazoxide infusions, when hypotension may be a problem.

BIBLIOGRAPHY

Burch P G, McCleskey C H 1981 Anesthesia for patients with insulinoma treatment with oral diazoxide. Anesthesiology 55: 472–475
Chari P, Pandit S K, Kataria R N, Singh H, Baheti D K, Wig J 1977 Anaesthetic management of insulinoma. Anaesthesia 32: 261–264
Lamont A S M, Jones D 1978 Anaesthetic management of insulinoma. Anaesthesia and Intensive Care 6: 261
Muir J J, Endres S M, Offord K, van Heerden J A, Tinker J H 1983 Glucose management in patients undergoing operation for insulinoma removal. Anesthesiology 59: 371–375
Pulver J J, Cullen B F, Miller D R, Valenta L J 1980 Use of the artificial beta cell during anesthesia for surgical removal of insulinoma. Anesthesia and Analgesia 59: 950–952
Roizen M F 1986 Preoperative evaluation of patients with diseases that require special preoperative evaluation and intraoperative management. In: Anesthesia. Churchill Livingstone, Edinburgh

KEARNS–SAYER SYNDROME

A rare syndrome in which external ophthalmoplegia is associated with neural, retinal and cardiac abnormalities.

Preoperative abnormalities

1. Progressive ophthalmoplegia develops in early adulthood.
2. Retinal pigmentation occurs.
3. There may be proximal limb muscle weakness, and sometimes bulbar involvement and cerebellar ataxia.
4. The incidence of cardiac conduction defects increases with age and syncope or sudden death may occur in the fourth decade.

Anaesthetic problems

1. Conduction defects, including bundle branch block and complete heart block, have been described.
2. In the presence of muscle weakness, an abnormal response to muscle relaxants might be anticipated. However, neuromuscular studies using both suxamethonium and pancuronium have been performed in a patient. There was a normal response to both relaxants, and no significant hyperkalaemia occurred after suxamethonium (D'Ambra et al 1979).

Management

1. Conduction defects may necessitate preoperative transvenous pacemaker insertion.
2. Neuromuscular monitoring is advisable.

1

BIBLIOGRAPHY

D'Ambra M N, Dedrick D, Savarese J J 1979 Kearns–Sayer syndrome and pancuronium-succinylcholine-induced neuromuscular blockade. Anesthesiology 51: 343–345

KLIPPEL–FEIL SYNDROME

An inherited autosomal dominant condition in which skeletal abnormalities, particularly in the cervical spine, may be associated with genitourinary and cardiac anomalies.

Preoperative abnormalities

1. A short webbed neck, with restricted movement and undescended, winged scapulae. Several cervical vertebrae may be fused or reduced in number. The base of the skull may be flattened (platybasia) and the thoracic vertebrae occasionally involved. Kyphoscoliosis and spinal cord anomalies may occur. The syndrome has been classified according to the pattern of vertebral fusion:

Type I   Block fusion of all cervical and some upper thoracic vertebrae

Type II   Fusion of one or two parts. Often C2/3 and C5/6

Type III Types I and II combined with lower thoracic or lumbar involvement

2. Significant genitourinary abnormalities were found in 64% of patients in one series (Moore et al 1975). Problems included renal agenesis, ectopia and malrotation, and penile hypospadias.

3. An incidence of congenital heart disease of 4–14% has been reported. Lesions include patent ductus arteriosus, coarctation of the aorta and mitral valve prolapse.

4. Maxillofacial abnormalities may occur.

Anaesthetic problems

1. A short neck and fused cervical vertebrae may contribute to difficulties in intubation.

2. If cervical instability is present, there is a risk of spinal cord injury.

3. Sleep apnoea has been reported.

Management

1. X-rays of the cervical spine will indicate the types of cervical anomaly, and flexion and extension views, the presence of any instability.

2. Examination for possible intubation difficulties must be done. Awake intubation may be considered appropriate. This was used in a patient for Caesarean section who had Klippel–Feil syndrome, congenital hydrocephalus and pre-eclampsia (Burns et al 1988). An inhalation induction was described in a neonate with coincidental Klippel–Feil and a craniocervical encephalocele (Naguib et al 1986).

3. If cardiac defects are diagnosed, prophylactic antibiotic therapy should be given.

BIBLIOGRAPHY

Burns A M, Dorje P, Lawes E G, Neilsen M S 1988 Anaesthetic management of Caesarean section for a mother with pre-eclampsia, the Klippel–Feil syndrome and congenital hydrocephalus. British Journal of Anaesthesia 61: 350–354
Moore W B, Matthews T J, Rabinowitz R 1975 Genitourinary anomalies associated with Klippel–Feil syndrome. Journal of Bone and Joint Surgery 57A: 355–357
Naguib M, Farag H, Ibrahim A E W 1986 Anaesthetic considerations in Klippel–Feil syndrome. Canadian Anaesthetists' Society Journal 33: 66–70

LARYNGEAL PAPILLOMATOSIS

Benign warty tumours of the larynx which occur in children and are probably viral in origin. They arise most commonly on the true cords with extension onto the ventricles. Frequently recurrent, they may be present in other parts of the respiratory tract.

Preoperative abnormalities

1. Usually presents in early childhood with hoarseness, cough, respiratory distress, or stridor due to upper airway obstruction. Of 90 patients whose symptoms presented between birth and age 11, nearly half occurred before the age of 2, 90% had a voice change, 44% airway obstruction and 39% stridor (Cohen et al 1980).
2. Chronic airway obstruction may lead to pulmonary hypertension, right ventricular hypertrophy, cor pulmonale and polycythaemia (Hawkins & Udall 1979).
3. Regression may occur at puberty.
4. Tracheal involvement is more frequent than was previously thought (Weiss & Kashima 1983).

Anaesthetic problems

1. Upper respiratory tract obstruction in young infants.
2. Multiple anaesthetics may be required. In one series, 66% of the patients had multiple diffuse disease and each required an average of 15.9 anaesthetics (Cohen et al 1980).
3. Tracheostomy (and possibly intubation) may seed papillomas and cause distal spread of the disease.

4. Tracheobronchial papillomatosis has been reported to occur in 2–26% of cases of laryngeal papillomatosis. A case was reported in which an absence of ventilation of the right lung was noticed during resection of laryngeal papillomata in a 10-year-old child. At bronchoscopy a large papilloma was found to be occluding the right main bronchus. Tracheostomy had been performed in this child at an earlier stage (Callander 1986).

Management

1. Endoscopy and resection or laser excision may be required regularly. A rigid bronchoscope should be available in case of sudden obstruction of the airway by a papilloma.

2. Tracheostomy should be avoided unless life saving. A low incidence of tracheobronchial papillomata (3.3%) in one series was suggested to be due to the low incidence of tracheostomy (4%) in that hospital when compared with that (10%) in the cases referred from elsewhere (Cohen et al 1980).

3. If avoidance of endotracheal intubation may reduce the chance of spread, a technique using inhalation anaesthesia, local anaesthetic spray, or insufflation of halothane and oxygen (or air in the case of laser surgery) can be commended. In a series, less than one-third of the 1047 anaesthetics were given through an endotracheal tube or a tracheostomy (Cohen et al 1980). The avoidance of a Venturi technique has also been suggested (Weiss & Kashima 1983).

4. Postoperative humidification of oxygen is recommended.

5. Perioperative corticosteroids have been proposed to reduce postoperative oedema but their use is arguable. Laser techniques are increasingly being used for laryngeal lesions and seem to be associated with less postoperative complications.

6. If severe obstructive symptoms are present, the airway must be secured before general anaesthesia is given.

7. Airway manipulation in small children is often complicated by coughing, excess secretions and laryngeal spasm. An infusion of procaine (2% soln in 5% dextrose) 1 mg/kg/min i.v. was found to produce much smoother operating conditions when compared with identically anaesthetized matched controls. Recovery was more rapid and there were no signs of toxicity (Lawson et al 1979).

BIBLIOGRAPHY

Callander C C 1986 Tracheobronchial papillomatosis: anaesthetic implications. Anaesthesia and Intensive Care 14: 201–202

Cohen S R, Geller K A, Seltzer S, Thompson J W 1980 Papilloma of the larynx and tracheobronchial tree in children. Annals of Otology, Rhinology and Laryngology 89: 497–503

Hawkins D B, Udall J N 1979 Juvenile laryngeal papillomas with cardiomegaly and polycythemia. Pediatrics 63: 156–157

Lawson N W, Rogers D, Seifen A, White A, Thompson D 1979 Intravenous procaine as a

1

supplement to general anesthesia for carbon dioxide laser resection of laryngeal papillomas in children. Anesthesia and Analgesia 58: 492–496

Weiss M D, Kashima H K 1983 Tracheal involvement in laryngeal papillomatosis. Laryngoscope 93: 45–48

LESCH–NYHAN SYNDROME

An X-linked recessive disorder of purine metabolism in which there is an absence of hypoxanthine guanine phosphoribosyl transferase (HGPRT) activity. There is primary purine overproduction with hyperuricaemia, gout and choreoathetoid spasticity.

Preoperative abnormalities

1. Mental retardation, choreoathetoid movements, spasticity and bizarre episodes of self mutilation.
2. Hyperuricaemia results in a nephropathy and urinary tract calcification. Death frequently results from renal failure in the third decade.
3. Arthritis and gouty tophi occur.
4. A B-lymphocyte immune deficiency may result in an increased susceptibility to infection.
5. Urinary uric acid is always raised and serum urate usually so.

Anaesthetic problems

1. Self mutilation may result in scarring of the mouth region.
2. Patients are susceptible to aspiration pneumonitis.
3. Abnormal adrenergic responses and decreased monoamine oxidase activity has been reported (Larson & Wilkins 1985).

Management

1. Teeth extraction may be required to reduce the trauma from self mutilation.
2. It has been suggested that the use of suxamethonium be avoided (Larson & Wilkins 1985).

BIBLIOGRAPHY

Larson L O, Wilkins R G 1985 Anesthesia and the Lesch–Nyhan Syndrome. Anesthesiology 63: 197–199

LYSERGIC ACID DIETHYLAMIDE (LSD) ABUSE

LSD is a psychedelic drug, which can either be synthesized, or obtained naturally from the seeds of *Rivea corymbosa* (morning glory), or ergot fungus on rye. Its effect is almost entirely on the CNS and it rapidly produces tolerance. Intoxicated patients are liable to injure themselves and be unaware of it. Respiratory depression has been reported.

Preoperative abnormalities

1. The onset of CNS effects occurs 40 minutes after an oral dose. Hallucinations may last for 2 hours and the biological half-life is 3 hours (Caldwell 1981).

Effects (Caldwell 1981):

0.5–1 μg/kg	Euphoria and a degree of visual, auditory or tactile disturbances
1 μg/kg	Increases sensory distortion
2 μg/kg	Alarming hallucinations
0.2 mg/kg	Possible lethal threshold

2. Central autonomic stimulation occurs, probably mediated via the hypothalamus. Parasympathetic and sympathetic effects include tremors, tachycardia, hypertension, fever, piloerection, mydriasis, lacrimation and hyperreflexia.
3. LSD has analgesic properties.
4. Tolerance to both autonomic and psychic effects is produced rapidly, but dependence does not occur.
5. LSD produces EEG changes.

Anaesthetic problems

1. Injury may be sustained without the patient being aware of it.
2. Hypertension, tachycardia and fever occur with toxic doses.
3. Interaction with belladonna alkaloids may occur.
4. Some inhibition of cholinesterase activity has been reported and theoretically it may prolong the action of suxamethonium.
5. Exaggerated responses to other sympathomimetic amines may occur.
6. Increased toxicity of ester-type local anaesthetics has been suggested (McGoldrick 1980).

Management

1. Heart rate, blood pressure and temperature should be monitored continuously.
2. Persistent sympathetic effects during general anaesthesia can be treated with alpha and beta blockers:

Phentolamine 1–2 mg and repeat, or infusion of 0.1–2 mg/min.
Propranolol 0.5 mg at 10-min intervals to a maximum of 5 mg.
Metoprolol 1–2 mg/min up to 5 mg. Repeat at 5-min intervals to a total of 10–15 mg.

3. If sedatives are required, a benzodiazepine or chlorpromazine have been suggested as being suitable.

4. Anticholinergics should be avoided if the patient shows signs of toxicity, as they may enhance the effects of LSD.

5. If the effects of LSD are still present, less analgesia will be needed. Opiates should be used cautiously in case of respiratory depression (McCammon 1986).

6. The concomitant use of other sympathomimetics should be avoided.

BIBLIOGRAPHY

Caldwell T 1981 Anesthesia for patients with behavioral disorders. In: Anesthesia and uncommon diseases. WB Saunders, Philadelphia
McCammon R L 1986 Anesthesia for the chemically dependent patient. International Anesthesia Research Society Review Course Lectures 47–55
McGoldrick K E 1980 Anesthetic implications of drug abuse. Anesthesiology Review 7: 12–17

MALIGNANT HYPERPYREXIA

A rare pharmacogenetic condition, or possibly a spectrum of conditions, of complex inheritance. Malignant hyperpyrexia (MH) usually presents during general anaesthesia with a syndrome indicative of greatly accelerated muscle metabolism. The exact defect is unknown. Dysfunction of the sarcoplasmic reticulum and abnormalities of intracellular ionic calcium are thought to play an important role, with the secondary, and possibly synergistic effects of the sympathetic nervous system (Gronert et al 1988). The primary release of calcium is normal, but there is thought to be an enhanced calcium-induced release of calcium from the sarcoplasmic reticulum, by agents known to induce MH (Fletcher 1987). Studies on erythrocytic membranes suggest that there may be a generalized membrane permeability defect.

The cardinal signs include hyperpyrexia, respiratory and metabolic acidosis, with or without muscle rigidity. It can be precipitated by a number of drugs, known as 'trigger' agents. Until recently the mortality was high but it has now been dramatically reduced from about 70% to 24% (Ellis et al 1986), although this decrease is less than had been predicted. The reduction has been achieved by:

1. An increased awareness of the condition.

2. More intensive patient monitoring for sensitive indicators, such as $ETCO_2$, which assist early diagnosis.

3. Availability of an i.v. form of dantrolene sodium, a drug which has played an important role in the treatment of MH. In the past, the diagnosis has been made too readily on clinical grounds alone. In retrospect, a number of cases previously thus identified in the literature may well not have been true MH. In 1984 the European MH Group (Ellis et al 1984) agreed a protocol for the diagnosis of the condition. This was subsequently modified (European MH Group 1985). It is hoped that the standardization of in vitro tests and diagnostic classification will allow further elucidation of the precise defect. Case reports should now only be given credence when the diagnosis has been confirmed according to these criteria.

Is MH associated with other conditions?

During anaesthesia, patients with a number of other disorders have developed clinical syndromes which have certain features in common with MH, and as a result have been labelled as being 'associated with an increased risk of MH'.

These assertions may prove not to be true. For example, certain other neuromuscular conditions may be associated with acute rhabdomyolysis, a high CPK, mild pyrexia and acidosis, and yet in vitro testing may show the patient not to be MH susceptible. In addition, investigation of six survivors of the neuroleptic malignant syndrome (NMS) revealed that five were negative for MH, and one result was equivocal (Krivosic-Horber et al 1987). This would suggest that NMS is a distinct entity, but sharing with MH common clinical features, and a response to dantrolene. The suggestions of an association between sudden infant death syndrome (SIDS) and MH have also been disputed (Ellis et al 1988).

Presentation

1. A family history of MH may be elicited. Confirmatory tests may or may not have been performed. According to standard criteria agreed by members of the European MH Group (1985), the current diagnoses are:
   a. MHS: definite susceptibility to MH.
   b. MHN: non-susceptible subject from a proven MH pedigree.
   c. MHE: equivocal result; consider as MHS.
2. Failure to relax after suxamethonium. Severe muscle spasm after suxamethonium is an abnormal reaction (Ellis & Halsall 1984) and may be an early sign of MH, although other neurological conditions such as the myotonic dystrophies can be responsible. Susceptibility to MH was found in about half of a series of 77 patients who developed masseter rigidity (Rosenberg & Fletcher 1986). (See also Section 4, Masseter muscle rigidity.)
3. Increasing temperature tachycardia and ventricular ectopics beats.
4. Tachypnoea occurs in a spontaneously breathing patient, while in the paralysed patient there is an apparently increased requirement for muscle relaxants. Both states are initially due to stimulation of respiration by a rising alveolar CO_2. If a capnograph is being used, an increase in $ETCO_2$ may be the earliest sign of MH. In the later stages, cyanosis may be due to the combination of a massive increase in oxygen consumption, and ventilation perfusion defects.

5. A metabolic acidosis occurs. In early reports of fulminating cases, an arterial pH of less than 7.0 was not uncommon. Severe acidosis may have been responsible for the cases where sudden death occurred unexpectedly in the operating theatre.

6. Rigidity of certain, but not necessarily all, groups of muscles. Although a non-rigid group has been described, it is not yet known whether this is a different biochemical process, or an earlier stage of the same process. A contracture of the muscle actually takes place and if the process is not aborted, oedema, and subsequently ischaemia, of the muscle can develop.

7. Myoglobin and potassium may be released in large quantities. Myoglobinuria and renal failure may result. The serum CPK can be elevated to greatly exceed 100 000 iu/l.

8. Disseminated intravascular coagulation may occur in advanced cases.

9. Cerebral and pulmonary oedema can occur.

Management

1. Criteria for preoperative diagnosis. Following a strict protocol (Ellis et al 1984, European MH Group 1985), a quadriceps muscle biospy, which includes the motor point, is subjected to:

   a. A static caffeine test.

   b. A static halothane test.

   c. A dynamic halothane test.

The results should allow classification of patients into the three groups: MHS, MHN and MHE.

2. A patient who is known to be MHS, MHE, or possibly has a family history of MH, should be given a non-triggering anaesthetic.

   Known triggering agents include:

   a. All the inhalational agents.

   b. Suxamethonium.

   Agents not definitely implicated but avoidance suggested (Gronert 1980):

   a. Ketamine.

   b. Phenothiazines.

   c. Atropine.

   d. Lignocaine.

Discussion continues over the safety of giving calcium, which may be needed to treat severe hyperkalaemia. Its avoidance has been suggested, but there is clinical and experimental evidence against it acting as a trigger agent (Gronert et al 1986, Murakawa et al 1988).

   Agents thought to be safe, or for use if necessary, include:

   a. Thiopentone.

   b. Nitrous oxide.

   c. Opiates.

   d. Droperidol.

e. Pancuronium.

f. Benzodiazepines.

g. Bupivacaine.

The routine use of dantrolene preoperatively in MHS and MHE patients remains controversial. There is now no indication for the use of oral dantrolene, in view of its side-effects and the uncertainty of achieving therapeutic levels (Harrison 1988). Many believe that it is sufficient to give a non-triggering anaesthetic, provided that an entirely volatile agent-free anaesthetic machine is used, the monitoring of $ETCO_2$ is available, and intravenous dantrolene is readily to hand. Of 956 patients who had muscle biopsy without pretreatment with dantrolene, only four developed mild MH episodes, all of which responded to general measures (Cunliffe & Britt 1987).

Occasionally, treatment may be considered to be appropriate before prolonged surgery, in which case, dantrolene i.v. 2.4 mg/kg should be given, after induction of anaesthesia.

3. If an unexpected intraoperative diagnosis of MH is made, the treatment required will depend upon the severity of the reaction at the time of diagnosis. The patient's susceptibility, the promptness of the diagnosis and hence the dose of the triggering agent received, are all important factors.

A short exposure and rapid diagnosis may mean that the syndrome can be aborted at the initial stage of treatment. The fulminant MH syndrome may require the whole scheme to be executed rapidly.

Management of an episode of malignant hyperpyrexia:

a. Stop the use of all MH trigger agents. Terminate surgery if possible. Observe the ECG and capnograph.

b. Delegate one person to prepare dantrolene sodium 1 mg/kg.

c. Record core temperature, pulse rate and blood pressure every 5 minutes.

d. Estimate arterial pH and blood gases. Hypercarbia should be treated with vigorous hyperventilation, acidosis with sodium bicarbonate 2–4 mmol/kg. Oxygenation must be maintained.

e. Save one venous sample for CPK and send one for electrolytes and serum calcium estimations.

f. Give dantrolene sodium i.v. 1 mg/kg. Repeat at 10-minute intervals if necessary, up to a maximum of 10 mg/kg.

g. If the syndrome is severe, treat the symptoms. Cool the patient and treat hyperkalaemia if necessary.

h. Keep the first urine sample for myoglobin estimation. Measure urine output. If obvious myoglobinuria occurs, give intravenous fluids, and mannitol or frusemide to promote urine flow.

i. The use of steroids is controversial, but may be indicated for cerebral oedema in the severe case.

j. Repeat the CPK estimation at 24 hours.

k. Treat DIC if necessary.

1. Dantrolene may need to be repeated for up to 24 hours as further retriggering may occur. Its half-life is only 5 hours.

4. The social implications for a family, particularly in certain cultures, may be devastating (Fletcher 1987, Ellis 1988).

BIBLIOGRAPHY

Cunliffe M, Lerman J, Britt B A 1987 Is prophylactic dantrolene indicated for MHS patients undergoing elective surgery? Anesthesia and Analgesia 66: S35
Ellis F R 1988 The diagnosis of MH: its social implications. British Journal of Anaesthesia 60; 251–252
Ellis F R, Halsall P J 1984 Suxamethonium spasm. British Journal of Anaesthesia 56: 381–384
Ellis F R, Heffron J J A 1985 Clinical and biochemical aspects of malignant hyperpyrexia. In: Recent advances in anaesthesia and analgesia 15. Churchill Livingstone, Edinburgh
Ellis F R, Fletcher R, Halsall P J 1984 A protocol for the investigation of malignant hyperpyrexia by the European Malignant Hyperpyrexia Group. British Journal of Anaesthesia 56: 1267–1269
Ellis F R, Halsall P J, Harriman D G F 1986 The work of the Leeds Malignant Hyperpyrexia Unit, 1971–1984. Anaesthesia 41: 809–815
Ellis F R, Halsall P J, Harriman D G F 1988 Malignant hyperpyrexia and sudden infant death syndrome. British Journal of Anaesthesia 60: 28–30
European MH Group 1985 Laboratory diagnosis of malignant hyperpyrexia susceptibility (MHS). British Journal of Anaesthesia 57: 1038
Fletcher R 1987 4th International Hyperpyrexia Workshop. Report of a meeting. Anaesthesia 42: 206
Gronert G A 1980 Malignant hyperthermia. Anesthesiology 53: 395–423
Gronert G A, Ahern C P, Milde J, White R D 1986 Effect of CO_2, calcium, digoxin and potassium on cardiac and skeletal muscle in malignant hyperthermia susceptible swine. Anesthesiology 64: 24–28
Gronert G A, Mott J, Lee J 1988 Aetiology of malignant hyperthermia. British Journal of Anaesthesia 60: 253–267
Harrison G G 1988 Dantrolene – dynamics and kinetics. British Journal of Anaesthesia 60: 279–286
Krivosic-Horber R, Adnet P, Guevart E, Theunyck D, Lestavel P 1987 Neuroleptic malignant syndrome and malignant hyperthermia. British Journal of Anaesthesia 59: 1554–1556
Murakawa M, Hatano Y, Magaribuchi T, Mori K 1988 Should calcium administration be avoided in treatment of hyperkalaemia in malignant hyperthermia? Anesthesia and Analgesia 67: 604–605
Rosenberg H, Fletcher J E 1986 Masseter muscle rigidity and malignant hyperthermia susceptibility. Anesthesia and Analgesia 65: 161–164

MARCUS GUNN JAW WINKING PHENOMENON

A rare congenital abnormality in which there appears to be abnormal connections between the external pterygoid and ocular muscles. This results in ptosis, which can be partly corrected by the patient either opening the jaw or moving it to the contralateral side. A number of other abnormal reflexes may occur.

Preoperative abnormalities

1. Ptosis is present, but lid retraction is associated with jaw opening.
2. Abnormal pupillary reflexes may occur.

Anaesthetic problems

Unusual oculocardiac reflexes were reported during three separate operations on the eyelid in a young man with Marcus–Gunn syndrome (Kwik 1980). Arrhythmias, which appeared on manipulation of the eyelid and also occurred in the recovery room, included premature atrial contractions, wandering pacemaker, and bradycardia.

Management

1. It has been suggested that the use of IPPV and a retrobulbar block may decrease the incidence of arrhythmias (Kwik 1980).
2. ECG monitoring should begin in the anaesthetic room and be continued in the recovery room.

BIBLIOGRAPHY

Kwik R S H 1980 Marcus–Gunn syndrome associated with an unusual oculo-cardiac reflex. Anaesthesia 35: 46–49

MARFAN'S SYNDROME

An autosomal dominant inherited condition involving a connective tissue deficit. The tensile strength of collagen is reduced, while its elasticity is increased. Skeletal, cardiovascular and ocular features occur. Surgery may be required for the correction of any of these. The diagnosis is made on clinical grounds and there are variable manifestations of the condition. At least two of these four criteria should be present: a family history of the condition, the ocular, cardiovascular or skeletal features (Pyeritz & McKusick 1979).

Premature death is common and typically occurs between 23 and 34 years.

Preoperative abnormalities

1. Skeletal abnormalities include arachnodactyly, a high arched palate, increased length of tubular bones, scoliosis (40–70%), pectus excavatus and ligamentous laxity.
2. Ectopia lentis occurs in up to 80% of cases. Patients are prone to myopia and retinal detachment.
3. Cardiovascular complications are the commonest cause of death. Structural changes in the heart and great vessels may be present and can result in mitral or aortic incompetence, dissecting aortic aneurysm, aortic or pulmonary artery dilatation and coronary artery disease. Mitral valve prolapse can also occur. Pathological changes in arteries include cystic

degeneration of the media and replacement of elastic fibres by mucoid material.

Anaesthetic problems

1. A number of deaths have been reported in association with surgery but there has been no consistent cause of death. In a study of 13 patients, two of four who died had been assessed as having no cardiovascular involvement (Verghese 1984). Neither had, however, undergone echocardiography. In a report of general life-expectancy, cardiovascular complications accounted for 95% of deaths in those cases where a definite diagnosis was confirmed.
2. Hypotonia and ligamentous laxity may predispose the patient to accidental injury during anaesthesia. Joints, including the temporomandibular, are prone to dislocation.
3. Skeletal changes such as scoliosis, hypotonia, a high incidence of emphysema, lung cysts, spontaneous pneumothoraces and honeycomb lungs all increase the risk of intra- and postoperative pulmonary complications. Midtracheal obstruction and respiratory distress occurred after Harrington rod placement in a patient with scoliosis (Mesrobian & Epps 1986). This was attributed to a combination of structural weakness of cartilage and skeletal abnormalities.
4. If ascending aortic dilatation already exists, especially if it is greater than 6 cm in an adult, the risk of rupture is high and hypertensive peaks may predispose to aortic dissection (Pyeritz & McKusick 1979).

Management

1. Detailed examination of the cardiovascular system is essential and should include assessment of aortic size, and a search for evidence of aortic or mitral incompetence, coronary artery disease and heart failure. Echocardiography has been suggested as being mandatory in all patients requiring surgery (Wells & Podolakin 1984).
2. High pulsatile pressures must be avoided to reduce the risks of aortic dissection. Beta blocker therapy has decreased the risk of sudden death in animal models (Wells & Podolakin 1984).
3. Direct arterial monitoring may assist in the process of controlling sudden increases in blood pressure, but may carry a higher than normal risk of damage to the artery.

BIBLIOGRAPHY

Mesrobian R B, Epps J L 1986 Midtracheal obstruction after Harrington rod placement in a patient with Marfan's syndrome. Anesthesia and Analgesia 65: 411–413
Pyeritz R E, McKusick V A 1979 The Marfan syndrome: diagnosis and management. New England Journal of Medicine 300: 772–777
Verghese C 1984 Anaesthesia in Marfan's syndrome. Anaesthesia 39: 917–922
Wells D G, Podolakin W 1987 Anaesthesia and Marfan's syndrome: case report. Canadian Journal of Anaesthesia 34: 311–314

MASTOCYTOSIS

A rare group of diseases in which there are abnormal aggregations of mast cells within the skin, and in other organs. The organs most commonly affected are bone, liver, spleen and lymph nodes. When there is involvement of the skin alone without other viscera, the condition is known as urticaria pigmentosa. This mostly occurs in infants and children, may be associated with mastocytomas, and is relatively benign (Coleman et al 1980). The various forms of systemic mastocytosis occurring in adult life may be associated with intermittent symptoms varying from a mild disturbance, to the occasional fatal attack. These episodes are due to mast cell disruption and the resultant release of one or more of a number of biochemical substances from granules within the cells. Histamine and heparin were thought to be the most important of these. However, prostaglandin D2 has also been implicated as being a cause of symptoms in certain patients who failed to respond to histamine antagonists (Roberts et al 1980). Other substances which may be released in small amounts include serotonin and hyaluronic acid. Among the precipitating factors are trauma, extremes of temperature, toxins, alcohol, and a variety of drugs.

Preoperative abnormalities

1. Symptoms are variable, and can include episodic attacks of itching, urticaria, dermographia, headache, flushing, syncope, palpitations, diarrhoea and vomiting. The flush is bright red and lasts for about 20 minutes, in contrast to that associated with carcinoid syndrome, which is more cyanotic and lasts for less than 10 minutes.
2. Skin lesions vary in type and colour, but small, reddish brown maculopapular lesions are common. A positive Darier's sign may be demonstrated. Light stroking of the affected skin with a blunt, but pointed, object produces dermographia (due to localized urticaria) and a flare.
3. Skin biopsy shows an increased number of mast cells (>5 per high power field).
4. Increased blood and urinary levels of histamine, and urinary prostaglandin D2 metabolite levels, may be demonstrated.
5. Coagulation studies are occasionally abnormal.

Anaesthetic problems

1. Disruption of mast cells may produce severe cardiovascular effects. Drugs reported to have precipitated symptoms in individual patients include salicylates, opiates, polymyxin, thiopentone, lignocaine, gallamine and d-tubocurarine.

1

2. Both regional and general anaesthesia can produce life-threatening complications. In one series, complications occurred in six out of 42 cases (Parris et al 1986). Hypotension and bronchospasm were the most frequently encountered.

3. Although heparin may also be released, it has rarely been reported as producing clinically significant problems.

4. If systemic mastocytosis is present and an anaphylactoid reaction occurs, the reaction is likely to be more severe than in a normal patient. It has been suggested this particularly applies to blood transfusion reactions (Scott et al 1983).

5. The presence of cutaneous lesions alone does not guarantee freedom from anaesthetic problems. Profound hypotension and flushing were reported during surgery in a patient with asymptomatic urticaria pigmentosa (Hosking & Warner 1987).

Management

1. Symptoms should be controlled preoperatively by the use of H1 and H2 receptor antagonists, and prostaglandin inhibitors such as indomethacin or salicylates. Sodium cromoglycate, a mast cell stabilizer, improves preoperative symptoms. Plasma histamine levels did not rise during a portacaval shunt in a patient who was treated with histamine antagonists and cromoglycate (Smith et al 1987).

2. Preoperative intradermal skin testing, with drugs likely to be used during anaesthesia, is recommended (Parris et al 1986). Positive skin tests occurred in 15 out of a series of 42 patients. Drugs likely to produce reactions should be avoided.

3. Sedation with a benzodiazepine helps to reduce anxiety.

4. It is recommended that adrenaline, both as a 1 in 1000 bolus and as an infusion of 1 mg in 25 ml saline, should be available for immediate use to treat severe hypotension (Parris et al 1986).

5. There have been no reports of inhalational agents causing degranulation of mast cells. It has been suggested that ether-linked anaesthetics, such as isoflurane, may actually inhibit degranulation.

6. Care should be taken to avoid precipitating factors such as trauma, hypothermia and hyperthermia (Parris et al 1981).

7. Dextrans are probably better avoided (Scott et al 1983).

BIBLIOGRAPHY

Coleman M A, Liberthson R R, Crone R K, Levine F H 1980 General anesthesia in a child with urticaria pigmentosa. Anesthesia and Analgesia 59: 704–706
Hosking M P, Warner M A 1987 Sudden intraoperative hypotension in a patient with asymptomatic urticaria pigmentosa. Anesthesia and Analgesia 66: 344–346
Parris W C V, Sandidge P C, Petrinely G 1981 Anesthetic management of mastocytosis. Anesthesiology Review 8: 32–35
Parris W C V, Scott H W, Smith B E 1986 Anesthetic management of systemic mastocytosis: experience with 42 cases. Anesthesia and Analgesia 65: S117

Roberts L J, Sweetman B J, Lewis R A, Austen K F, Oates J A 1980 Increased production of prostaglandin D2 in patients with systemic mastocytosis. New England Journal of Medicine 303: 1400–1404
Rosenbaum K J, Strobel G E 1973 Anesthetic considerations in mastocytosis. Anesthesiology 38: 398–401
Scott H W, Parris W C V, Sandidge P C, Oates J A, Roberts L J 1983 Hazards in operative management of patients with systemic mastocytosis. Annals of Surgery 197: 507–514
Smith G B, Gusberg R J, Jordan R H, Kim B 1987 Histamine levels and cardiovascular responses during splenectomy and splenorenal shunt formation in a patient with systemic mastocytosis. Anaesthesia 42: 861–867

McARDLE'S SYNDROME

A type V glycogen storage disease, which appears as an autosomal recessive myopathy. It results from the single enzyme defect of muscle phosphorylase. Failure of conversion of glycogen into lactate results in increased muscle glycogen. Skeletal muscle is mainly involved, although reports of cardiac muscle and ECG abnormalities have appeared. Males are more commonly affected.

Preoperative abnormalities

1. Symptoms of cramp, stiffness, muscle pains and fatiguability may appear in childhood. Muscle contractions are relieved by rest. A family history may be elicited.
2. Occasional episodes of myoglobinuria can occur after exercise.
3. Progressive atrophy of muscle may occur in the fifth decade.
4. The diagnosis can be made with neurohistochemical techniques, or by demonstrating decreased venous lactate and pyruvate concentrations with ischaemic exercise. EMG shows a decrease in evoked muscle response, after supramaximal stimuli.

Anaesthetic problems

1. Suxamethonium may cause myoglobinuria, with the risk of renal failure.
2. The use of a limb tourniquet may result in muscle atrophy.
3. Shivering can produce muscle damage.

Management

1. Suxamethonium should not be given. Atracurium has been used in a child, without producing myoglobinuria or CPK elevation (Rajah & Bell 1986). A Caesarean section using alcuronium has also been reported (Coleman 1984). A peripheral nerve stimulator must be used.
2. A tourniquet should only be applied if absolutely essential.
3. Core temperature should be monitored. The operating theatre must

be warm. A water blanket and blood warmer are required for long operations, to avoid shivering and heat loss. Patients are intolerant of a hypermetabolic state (Ellis 1980).

4. A usable energy source such as dextrose, fructose or lactate should be given during the procedure and continued until oral intake is resumed.

5. If myoglobinuria occurs, i.v. fluids and mannitol should be given to reduce the possibility of renal failure.

BIBLIOGRAPHY

Coleman P 1984 McArdle's disease. Problems of anaesthetic management for Caesarean section. Anaesthesia 39: 784–787
Ellis F R 1980 Inherited muscle disease. British Journal of Anaesthesia 52: 153–164
Rajah A, Bell C F 1986 Atracurium and McArdle's disease. Anaesthesia 41: 93

MEDIASTINAL MASSES

Can occur in the posterior, middle or anterior mediastinum. The age of the patient indicates the most likely cause. In babies they can be bronchial cysts, teratomas or due to oesophageal duplication. In infants and children the commonest masses are neurogenic in origin, and are in the posterior mediastinum. In adults, middle mediastinal masses are usually carcinoma or lymphoma. Anterior masses usually involve the thymus or thyroid.

Patients with mediastinal masses may present for diagnostic procedures or thoracotomy. Bronchoscopy, lymph node biopsy, mediastinoscopy and staging laparotomy are the commonest operations.

Anaesthesia in patients with large mediastinal masses is extremely hazardous, in the presence of either superior vena caval (SVC) obstruction, or compression of the trachea or a main bronchus. The literature continues to report fatalities in these cases (Mackie 1987).

Preoperative abnormalities

1. SVC obstruction
Is diagnosed on clinical examination. It is four times more likely to occur with right-sided lesions than it is with those on the left, and will be more severe when the obstruction is below the azygos vein. At post-mortem examination, actual venous thrombosis has been found to be present in over a third of cases of SVC obstruction (Lokich & Goodman 1975). Initially there is dilatation of the veins in the neck and upper thorax, but this may progress to oedema of the face, arms and breasts. In these latter cases, signs of cerebral oedema may develop, and increasing respiratory difficulty due to laryngeal oedema may indicate the need for urgent radiotherapy.

2. Signs of airway obstruction or invasion

A careful history, and in particular, questioning about positional respiratory difficulty, stridor, dyspnoea and non-productive cough. Lesions may progress rapidly, therefore a recent CXR is essential. A normal PA X-ray does not exclude obstruction. Anterior-posterior compression of the trachea may only be demonstrated on a penetrated lateral view. In difficult cases, a CT scan of the airway can be invaluable.

3. Myocardial or pericardial involvement

Arrhythmias can occur, or the patient may have signs of a pericardial effusion. In cases of cardiac tamponade, there is respiratory distress and pulsus paradoxicus. There may be cyanosis and syncope on straining (Keon 1981).

4. Obstruction of the pulmonary artery

Due to compression.

5. Spinal cord involvement

Can occur in posterior mediastinal tumours.

6. Recurrent laryngeal nerve problems

Primarily occur with left-sided lesions.

7. Systemic non metastatic effects of tumours such as hormone secretion, neuropathies and myasthenia gravis.

Anaesthetic problems

1. In the presence of SVC obstruction, if a venous wall is breached anywhere in the area which drains into the SVC, severe haemorrhage will occur. Drugs given via venous access in the arm will have a markedly delayed action.

2. In cases of severe obstruction, cerebral and glottic oedema may occur.

3. There can be tracheal compression or invasion. Sudden respiratory obstruction, which may happen at any stage of the anaesthetic, has been described. It most commonly occurs after administration of a muscle relaxant and endotracheal intubation (Bray & Fernandes 1982, O'Leary 1983), but problems have also been encountered in the recovery room (Bittar 1975) and during inhalation induction (Mackie & Watson 1985). Deaths continue to be reported (Neuman et al 1984, Levin et al 1985, Northrip et al 1986).

Difficulty in inflation after intubation might be a result of external pressure, producing distortion or obstruction of the tube. However, it is more probably due to the change in lung mechanics which occurs after administration of a muscle relaxant. During spontaneous respiration there is a subatmospheric intrapleural pressure and a widening of airways on inspiration. Administration of a muscle relaxant will alter the support of the bronchial tree, such that in the presence of external pressure, collapse of the airway can occur and cause complete obstruction. Softening of the tracheal wall may contribute to this. In most of the cases described, partial relief of the obstruction coincided with the return of spontaneous respiration or recovery of consciousness.

4. Pulmonary artery involvement will decrease pulmonary perfusion and cardiac output.

5. Myocardial or pericardial involvement results in arrhythmias, and occasionally cardiac tamponade. Death on induction of anaesthesia occurred in a 9-year-old boy who was about to have a cervical node biopsy (Keon 1981). Autopsy showed an extensive lymphoma, enveloping the heart and infiltrating the pericardium and pulmonary artery.
6. Spinal cord involvement occurs most commonly in children with neurogenic tumours.

Management

1. If there are obvious signs of SVC obstruction, then this is an indication for urgent radiotherapy or chemotherapy prior to surgical intervention. The size of the tumour is reduced, as well as the degree of venous obstruction, provided that actual venous thrombosis has not occurred. Some authors have advocated the use of fibrinolytic agents or anticoagulants if thrombosis is suspected (Lokich & Goodman 1975).
2. If there is any suggestion of tracheal obstruction, the procedure should be performed under local anaesthetic. Should this not be possible, an inhalational induction should be administered and no muscle relaxants given. In cases where the patient is symptomatic, radiotherapy must be undertaken before surgery. Five life-threatening complications were associated with intubation anaesthesia in 74 cases of untreated mediastinal or hilar Hodgkin's disease (Piro et al 1976). By contrast, no complications were seen in 24 cases with mediastinal involvement when anaesthesia took place after initial radiotherapy, or in 78 anaesthetics where there was no mediastinal disease. Planned extracorporeal oxygenation may be indicated under certain circumstances (Hall & Friedman 1975).

BIBLIOGRAPHY

Bittar D 1975 Respiratory obstruction associated with induction of general anesthesia in a patient with mediastinal Hodgkin's disease. Anesthesia and Analgesia 54: 399–403
Bray R J, Fernandes F J 1982 Mediastinal tumour causing airway obstruction in anaesthetised children. Anaesthesia 37: 571–575
Hall K D, Friedman M 1975 Extracorporeal oxygenation for induction of anesthesia in a patient with an intrathoracic tumor. Anesthesiology 42: 493–495
Keon T P 1981 Death on induction of anesthesia for cervical node biopsy. Anesthesiology 55: 471–472
Levin H, Bursztein S, Heifetz M 1985 Cardiac arrest in a child with an anterior mediastinal mass. Anesthesia and Analgesia 64: 1129–1130
Lokich J J, Goodman R 1975 Superior vena cava syndrome. Journal of the American Medical Association 231: 58–61
Mackie A 1987 Anesthetic management of mediastinal masses – again. Anesthesia and Analgesia 66: 696
Mackie A M, Watson C B 1984 Anaesthesia and mediastinal masses. Anaesthesia 39: 899–903
Neuman G G, Weingarten A E, Abramowitz R M, Kushins L G, Abramson A L, Ladner W 1984 The anesthetic management of the patient with an anterior mediastinal mass. Anesthesiology 60: 144–147
Northrip D R, Bowman B K, Tsueda K 1986 Total airway occlusion and superior vena cava syndrome in a child with an anterior mediastinal tumour. Anesthesia and Analgesia 65: 1079–1082

O'Leary H T, Tracey J A 1983 Mediastinal tumours causing airway obstruction. Anaesthesia 38: 66–67

Piro A J, Weiss D R, Hellman S 1976 Mediastinal Hodgkin's disease: a possible danger for intubation anesthesia. International Journal of Radiation, Oncology, Biology, Physics 1: 415–419

MENDELSON'S SYNDROME, PULMONARY ASPIRATION SYNDROME

A syndrome which follows aspiration of acid gastric contents. Gastric fluid, particularly that with a pH of 2.5 or less, causes chemical damage to the alveolar epithelium and the capillary endothelium. As a result of permeability changes, fluid leaks from the capillaries into the alveoli and interstitial spaces, causing pulmonary oedema and hypoxia. This leakage is enhanced by increases in pulmonary artery pressure. It is particularly, but not exclusively, associated with obstetric anaesthesia. In a computer-aided study, an incidence of aspiration during anesthesia of 0.046% was found. Eighty-three per cent of the patients had increased risk factors. Only 17% occurred in elective cases, and two-thirds of these were associated with airway difficulties (Olsson et al 1986).

Presentation

1. Regurgitation and aspiration may be obvious at induction, or it may be unnoticed, particularly if intubation problems are encountered. In the latter case, signs may be delayed for several hours. The syndrome has been reported with the inhalation of as little as 25 ml of acid.

2. Unexplained bronchospasm may occur during the anaesthetic. In the absence of a history of asthma, aspiration should be suspected.

3. Postoperative tachycardia, tachypnoea, cyanosis and respiratory difficulty may develop.

4. CXR, which may be initially normal, can progress from showing patchy pulmonary infiltration, most commonly in the basal or perihilar regions, to signs of gross pulmonary oedema.

5. If clinically significant aspiration has occurred, serial arterial blood gases will show a deterioration in oxygenation. A decreasing PaO_2 and a metabolic acidosis will occur.

Diagnosis

This is usually made on clinical grounds. Testing of the initial fluid aspirate with litmus may indicate its gastric origin. Mortality rates of 100% have been recorded where the pH was <1.75, but no mortality if it was >2.4.

Management

1. Prophylaxis is the best form of management. The use of H_2 receptor antagonists and 0.3 mol/l sodium citrate prior to surgery in cases considered to be at risk, will reduce the pH of the gastric contents, should aspiration take place.

2. The patient should be placed in a head-down position and the pharynx or endotracheal tube sucked out. There is little place for bronchoscopy unless solid food pieces have been inhaled.

3. If inhalation has occurred or is suspected, treatment should be aggressive. The endotracheal tube should be kept in situ and IPPV and PEEP instituted. A policy of waiting for deterioration may prove to be disastrous.

4. The advisability of using high-dose steroids remains controversial. One view is that there is little evidence to support their use, and that if infection occurs they may interfere with tissue immunity. High-dose steroids were of no benefit in treating a pneumonitis induced in rabbits (Wynne et al 1979). On the contrary, a clinical impression has been gained that in man, their use for a 72-hour period may limit the extent of damage (Zorab 1984).

5. If the inhaled material is obviously contaminated, then antibiotics can be given. Otherwise they should be reserved for the presence of proven infection, using the appropriate antibiotic to which the organism is sensitive.

6. Bronchodilators can be given for bronchospasm. Aminophylline 5 mg/kg over 10–15 minutes can be followed by an infusion of 0.5 mg/kg/h.

7. Occasionally dopamine 5–20 μg/kg/min may be required for inotropic support.

BIBLIOGRAPHY

Coombs D W 1983 Editorial. Aspiration pneumonia prophylaxis. Anesthesia and Analgesia 62: 1055–1058
Olsson G L, Hallen B, Hambraeus-Jonzon K 1986 Aspiration during anaesthesia: a computer-aided study of 185 358 anaesthetics. Acta Anaesthesiologica Scandinavica 30: 84–92
Wynne J W, Reynolds J C, Hood I, Auerbach D, Ondrasick J 1979 Steroid therapy for pneumonitis in rabbits by aspiration of foodstuffs. Anesthesiology 51: 11–19
Zorab J S M 1984 Pulmonary aspiration. British Medical Journal 288: 1631–1632

METHAEMOGLOBINAEMIA

Methaemoglobin is produced when the iron in the haem group of the haemoglobin molecule is oxidized from the ferrous to the ferric form. Methaemoglobin is continuously formed during red cell metabolism, but it is then converted back to reduced Hb. Under normal circumstances, its concentration never exceeds 1%. Methaemoglobinaemia is a clinical condition in which more than 1% of the blood has been oxidized to the ferric form. It can arise from:

1. Congenital methaemoglobinaemia due to NADH-diaphorase deficiency. The inheritance is autosomal recessive.
2. Toxic methaemoglobinaemia, which occurs when various drugs or toxic substances oxidize haemoglobin, e.g. aniline and nitrobenzene.
3. Haemoglobin M disease, a form of haemoglobinopathy.

Cyanosis is seen when the level of methaemoglobin exceeds 1.5 g/dl. In congenital methaemoglobinaemia, the level of methaemoglobin varies between 8 and 40%. In general 20% of methaemoglobin is required before symptoms occur. Higher levels can be tolerated without symptoms in the congenital condition, as compared with the acute toxic form.

Presentation

1. The patient looks cyanosed, his actual appearance often being described as a 'slatey grey'. Arterial blood takes on an unusual chocolate brown colour. 1.5 g/dl of methaemoglobin causes cyanosis, compared with the 5 g/dl required for reduced Hb. The diagnosis may also be suspected when unexpectedly low oxygen saturation readings are recorded using a pulse oximeter, in the presence of a normal PaO_2 on a blood gas sample. Carboxyhaemoglobin, and dyes such as methylene blue, have also caused spurious oximeter readings (Eisenkraft 1988).
2. Methaemoglobinaemia, in normal subjects, has been reported to have been caused by a variety of substances:
   a. Ingestion of aniline or nitrobenzene compounds (Harrison 1977).
   b. Prilocaine in doses exceeding 600–900 mg (or 8 mg/kg), due to a metabolite, orthotoluidine (Duncan & Kobrinsky 1983).
   c. Benzocaine in toxic doses (O'Donohue et al 1980).
   d. Methylene blue, in doses of >7 mg/kg, due to oxidation of haemoglobin.
   e. Treatment with antimalarials.
   f. Antileprosy drugs (Mayo et al 1987).
   g. A combination of 'EMLA' cream (prilocaine and lignocaine) and a sulphonamide in a baby (Jakobsen & Nilsson 1985).

Anaesthetic or resuscitative problems

1. The oxygen-carrying capacity is reduced, and the oxygen dissociation curve is shifted to the left.
   a. 20% methaemoglobin is required before symptoms occur
   b. 20–50% produces tachycardia, dizziness, headache and dyspnoea
   c. 60–70% or more may be associated with vascular collapse, coma and death.

2. Unexplained cyanosis may occur. Cyanosis during appendicectomy in a child was subsequently found to be due to dapsone 200 mg, administered to him by his father (Mayo et al 1987).

While methylene blue 1–2 mg/kg is used in the treatment of methaemoglobinaemia, higher doses may oxidize haemoglobin to methaemoglobin. Thus, a rapid infusion of methylene blue can itself produce transient cyanosis. An infusion of methylene blue 5 mg/kg is frequently used to assist identification of the parathyroid glands during parathyroid surgery. Studies of the resulting methaemoglobin levels have shown a peak of 7.1% (Whitwam et al 1979) in one, and a range from 4.5 to 17.4% (Lamont et al 1986) in another. The first authors thought that such levels might be dangerous in a patient with haemoglobin M disease, or where there was an abnormality of the hexose monophosphate pathway. The second paper concluded that with normal doses, problems were unlikely.

Management

1. Ascorbic acid 300–600 mg daily can be used for chronic methaemoglobinaemia.
2. If acute symptomatic methaemoglobinaemia occurs, methylene blue 1–2 mg/kg should be given. This stimulates the relevant reducing enzymes. Excess methylene blue (>7 mg/kg) can itself cause methaemoglobinaemia.
3. In cases of severe poisoning, exchange transfusion may be required (Harrison 1977).

BIBLIOGRAPHY

Duncan P, Kobrinsky N 1983 Prilocaine-induced methemoglobinemia in a newborn infant. Anesthesiology 59: 75–76
Eisenkraft J B 1988 Pulse oximeter desaturation due to methaemoglobinaemia. Anesthesiology 68: 279–280
Harrison M R 1977 Toxic methaemoglobinaemia. Anaesthesia 32: 270–272
Jakobson B, Nilsson A 1985 Methemoglobinaemia associated with a prilocaine-lidocaine cream and trimethoprim-sulphamethoxazole. Acta Anaesthesiologica Scandinavica 29: 453–455
Lamont A S M, Roberts M S, Holdsworth D G, Atherton A, Shepherd J J 1986 Relationship between methaemoglobin production and methylene blue plasma concentrations under general anaesthesia. Anaesthesia and Intensive Care 14: 360–364
Mayo W, Leighton K, Robertson B, Ruedy J 1987 Intraoperative cyanosis: a case of dapsone-induced methaemoglobinaemia. Canadian Journal of Anaesthesia 34: 79–82
O'Donohue W J, Mos L M, Angelillo V A 1980 Acute methemoglobinemia induced by topical benzocaine and lidocaine. Archives of Internal Medicine 140: 1508–1509
Whitwam J G, Taylor A R, White J M 1979 Potential hazard of methylene blue. Anaesthesia 34: 181–182

MILLER'S SYNDROME

A recently described syndrome of postaxial acrofacial dysostosis.

Preoperative abnormalities

1. Craniofacial abnormalities similar to those found in Treacher Collin's syndrome, including micrognathia and cleft palate.
2. Limb and cardiac defects, including ASD, VSD and PDA also occur.
3. The patient is usually of normal intelligence.
4. Multiple anaesthetics may be required for plastic surgery.

Anaesthetic problems

1. Only one case so far has been reported in the anaesthetic literature (Richards 1987). The potential anaesthetic problems described were:
   a. Intubation difficulties due to micrognathia.
   b. Postoperative respiratory obstruction.
   c. Limb shortening causing venous access problems.
   d. Difficulties with positioning of the patient.

Management

1. The following were recommended (Richards 1987):
   a. Identification of cardiac problems, if present.
   b. An inhalation induction to anticipate intubation difficulties.
   c. Support for the limbs is required to prevent stress on joints, nerves and blood vessels.

BIBLIOGRAPHY

Richards M 1987 Miller's syndrome. Anaesthetic management of postaxial acrofacial dysostosis. Anaesthesia 42: 871–874

MITRAL VALVE DISEASE

Two main problems confront the anaesthetist when dealing with a patient with cardiac valvular disease. The first is that of the preoperative assessment of the severity of the lesion, and the degree of myocardial dysfunction resulting from it. The second, and crucial to the conduct of anaesthesia, is an understanding of the compensatory mechanisms which may have taken place. These will depend on whether the valvular disease is acute or longstanding.

The pathophysiology and compensatory mechanisms of an acute valve lesion following endocarditis or myocardial infarction, are very different from those of chronic valve disease, where gradual compensatory cardiac hypertrophy or dilatation has taken place. In either case, the aim is to give an anaesthetic which will cause as little disturbance as possible to these compensatory mechanisms.

The serious effects of decompensation range from pulmonary oedema and hypoxia, to a severe drop in left ventricular output resulting in myocardial ischaemia, infarction or arrhythmias. Whilst in mild disease there may be few problems, severe valvular disease requires close cardiovascular monitoring, a careful choice of anaesthetic technique, and anticipation and cautious correction of the factors causing decompensation.

MITRAL STENOSIS

Normal left ventricular filling is restricted by the decreased area across the stenosed valve. The normal area of the valve is 4 cm². Symptoms appear when this is reduced to about 2.5 cm². Below 1 cm² the symptoms are severe.

Compensation is normally achieved by increasing the pressure gradient across the mitral valve, and is dependent upon atrial contraction and the duration of diastole. Decompensation often begins with the onset of atrial fibrillation with a fast ventricular rate.

Preoperative abnormalities

1. The pulse may be irregular due to atrial fibrillation. Palpation of the precordium may reveal a palpable first sound ('tapping apex beat'). On auscultation there may be an opening snap (the closer to the second sound, the more severe the stenosis), followed by a mid diastolic murmur, with presystolic accentuation if the patient remains in sinus rhythm. The loudness of the murmur is no guide to severity, and may be inaudible if the cardiac output is low, in neglected disease. Atrial fibrillation causes decompensation by decreasing the left ventricular filling time and by reducing cardiac output. This is manifest clinically by cool, possibly cyanosed peripheries, and a low volume pulse. A malar flush is common.
2. Left atrial pressure (LAP) is increased, while dilatation and hypertrophy of left atrium occurs. When LAP rises, so does pulmonary capillary pressure, and when this exceeds colloid osmotic pressure (25–30 mmHg), pulmonary oedema develops. A sudden increase in LAP may be precipitated by tachycardia due to exercise, emotion, fever, pregnancy or by an arrhythmia. A proportion of the patients will develop irreversible pulmonary hypertension, right ventricular hypertrophy, pulmonary and tricuspid incompetence, and occasionally right heart failure.
3. CXR shows left atrial enlargement, with a prominent left atrial appendage and double contour of the right heart border. Kerley B lines may be present. ECG may show P mitrale. Definitive diagnosis is by echocardiography which allows precise measurement of left atrial dimensions and demonstration of the abnormal movement of the thickened or calcified valve cusps. If combined with Doppler techniques, valve area can be estimated.
4. In the presence of AF, systemic thromboembolism may occur.

5. The patient is usually taking digoxin, and sometimes beta blockers and anticoagulants.

6. Symptomatic history is a good guide to severity. Dyspnoea on mild exertion, with episodes of paroxysmal nocturnal dyspnoea, indicate a LAP of 15–20 mmHg. Occasionally angina occurs.

Anaesthetic problems

1. Tachycardia or fast atrial fibrillation reduces diastolic filling time and may precipitate pulmonary oedema.

2. Large decreases in systemic vascular resistance may result in severe hypotension, as there is limited capacity to increase cardiac output in compensation.

3. Volume overload may produce pulmonary oedema; conversely; hypovolaemia, accentuated by diuretics, may reduce cardiac output.

4. Myocardial depressant drugs can cause severe hypotension.

5. The Trendelenburg position may result in hypoxia and pulmonary oedema.

6. Hypoxia and acidosis can cause pulmonary vasoconstriction.

7. Nitrous oxide may be unsafe if pulmonary vascular resistance is raised (Schulte-Sasse et al 1982).

8. Bacteraemia during surgery or instrumentation carries the risk of bacterial endocarditis.

Management

1. Prophylactic antibiotics are required for any surgery which carries a risk of producing a bacteraemia. This includes dental, genitourinary and bowel operations, and childbirth. (See Subacute bacterial endocarditis.)

2. AF must be controlled prior to surgery.

3. While digoxin is the mainstay of treatment, care should be taken to prevent tachycardia. Atropine should be avoided. A sedative premedication reduces anxiety. An adequate depth of anaesthesia and good analgesia are essential.

4. Inotropic agents, particularly a dilating inotrope such as dobutamine, may be required to treat hypotension, although they can worsen pulmonary vasoconstriction.

5. Myocardial depressants should be avoided if possible.

6. Prevention of peripheral vasoconstriction due to cold, pain and hypovolaemia, is essential. CVP monitoring will assist the assessment of volume requirement for optimum right ventricular function. In severe mitral stenosis and before corrective surgery, it may be necessary to use dilating agents such as nitroprusside or nitrates. IPPV may be life saving.

7. The degree of monitoring used depends upon the severity of the lesion and the magnitude of the surgery. In the absence of pulmonary hypertension the changes in CVP will mirror those in the left atrium. However, if it is present, the PAWP does not correlate very well with the LAP.

8. If there is right ventricular dysfunction, nitrous oxide should be avoided.

9. In obstetrics, epidural anaesthesia may be appropriate for delivery or Caesarean section. The use of PAP monitoring to demonstrate the beneficial effects of epidural anaesthesia in a patient during delivery, has been reported (Hemmings et al 1987). The technique of bedside measurement of pulmonary artery and pulmonary capillary wedge pressures has been well described (George & Banks 1983).

MITRAL REGURGITATION

Causes include rheumatic endocarditis, frequently as a mixed lesion, mitral valve prolapse, papillary muscle dysfunction or rupture of chordae tendinae. The latter conditions usually follow myocardial infarction.

Preoperative abnormalities

1. An apical pansystolic murmur radiating to the axilla.
2. During systole a part of the stroke volume enters the aorta, while the rest is regurgitated into the left atrium. The ratio between the two depends upon the degree of incompetence and the impedance of each pathway.
3. There is left ventricular hypertrophy due to increased work and in severe chronic cases, LVF may eventually occur. In acute mitral incompetence pulmonary oedema occurs early.
4. During diastole the left atrium has to eject the normal pulmonary venous flow as well as the regurgitated fraction. Left atrial dilatation therefore takes place.
5. AF usually only occurs in mixed lesions or in advanced cases.
6. CXR will show left atrial dilatation and left ventricular hypertrophy. Echocardiography provides precise information about chamber dimensions, wall thickness and movement, and will demonstrate a rheumatic or prolapsing valve.
7. In general, in a patient with rheumatic mitral incompetence, the progression of exercise intolerance is slow, unless complications such as heart failure or bacterial endocarditis occur. If however the incompetence follows myocardial infarction, there may be sudden onset of acute pulmonary oedema and death.

Anaesthetic problems

1. Even when the disease is mild, there is a greater risk of bacterial endocarditis than with any other valve lesion.
2. There is a risk of systemic embolism and the patient may be on anticoagulants.

3. An increase in systemic vascular resistance will increase the regurgitated volume and decrease the cardiac output.
4. Hypovolaemia will decrease the LAP and the stroke work.
5. A bradycardia can worsen the regurgitation, as distortion of the valve may be enhanced by an increased diameter of the ventricle during diastole.

Management

1. Prophylactic antibiotics will be required.
2. Situations of heat loss, untreated pain and hypovolaemia, which all produce peripheral vasoconstriction, should be avoided.
3. Left atrial filling pressure should be maintained to increase the forward output of the left ventricle. Hypovolaemia must therefore be avoided.
4. A mild tachycardia is advantageous to avoid excess diastolic filling of the ventricle and valve distortion.

MITRAL VALVE PROLAPSE

The recognition of this condition has increased with the advent of echocardiography, although there is argument about its diagnosis, significance and prognosis (Oakley 1984). It has been reported to occur in up to 5% of healthy patients. However, the diagnosis is non-specific, and would appear to cover a wide spectrum, with considerable variations in significance. A chance finding on echocardiography in thin, young patients who are asymptomatic, is probably not of importance. In older patients who are symptomatic, and have elongated or ruptured chordae tendinae or pathological valve changes, the prognosis may be less good. Each patient should be assessed in relation to the clinical symptoms and findings. Patients with previously undiagnosed MVP may occasionally present with arrhythmias during anaesthesia.

Preoperative abnormalities

1. Abnormalities vary from slight prolapse of the posterior mitral valve leaflet with no regurgitation, to gross prolapse associated with marked regurgitation as the ventricles contract. The first is probably an anatomical variation, the second can arise from pathological changes in the chordae tendinae or valve leaflets.
2. MVP has also been found in a number of genetic conditions in which there are connective tissue defects. These include Marfan's and Ehlers–Danlos syndromes and pseudoxanthoma elasticum.
3. The patient is frequently asymptomatic, but symptoms such as syncope, chest pain and palpitations may feature. There is an increased incidence of bacterial endocarditis and a small risk of cerebral embolism.

4. Clinical signs may include a mid systolic click and a late systolic murmur. If gross regurgitation occurs during systole, then left atrial dilatation and left ventricular hypertrophy may be present. Atrial and ventricular arrhythmias may occur and there are occasional reports of sudden death.

Anaesthetic problems

1. The degree of valve prolapse is increased by anything which reduces ventricular volume, thus resulting in redundancy of the mitral leaflet (Thiagarajah & Frost 1983). Conversely prolapse is reduced by increases in ventricular volume. The following situations may accentuate valve prolapse:

    a. Increased myocardial contractility.

    b. Decreased preload due to hypovolaemia or sympathetic nervous system blockade.

    c. Tachycardia, which reduces the time for ventricular filling.

    d. High airways pressure produced by straining.

2. Most case reports are of unexpected atrial or ventricular arrhythmias arising in the perioperative period, and in over half of the cases the diagnosis was made postoperatively on echocardiography (Krantz et al 1980, Thiagarajah & Frost 1983, Berry et al 1985). Occasionally ventricular fibrillation or profound bradycardia can occur.

Management

1. The anaesthetic technique in known cases of MVP should aim to minimize the effects of factors known to worsen the prolapse.

    a. Avoid sympathetic stimulation and increases in myocardial contractility. A good premedication relieves anxiety. Atropine, and agents producing arrhythmias, are avoided. Hypoxia, hypercarbia and acidosis are prevented. Avoid light anaesthesia. If tachycardia occurs in spite of these manoeuvres, propranolol can be used.

    b. Prevent hypovolaemia. Circulating blood volume is maintained by expansion of the intravascular volume.

    c. Minimize decreases in systemic vascular resistance. Sympathetic blockade produced by regional anaesthesia may worsen the prolapse. However, sometimes there may be no choice. Epidural anaesthesia was required for Caesarean section in a patient with MVP, asthma and pneumonia (Alcantara & Marx 1987). The importance of adequately preloading the patient, and fractionating the doses of local anaesthetic, were stressed. Hypotension due to sympathetic blockade should be treated with a dilute phenylephrine solution, rather than ephedrine. Induced hypotension may also worsen the prolapse and should preferably not be used (Thiagarajah & Frost 1983).

2. High airway pressures should be avoided.

3. Prophylactic antibiotics for bacterial endocarditis are required.

BIBLIOGRAPHY

Alcantara L G, Marx G F 1987 Cesarean section under epidural analgesia in a parturient with mitral valve prolapse. Anesthesia and Analgesia 66: 902–903

Berry F A, Lake C L, Johns R A, Rogers B M 1985 Mitral valve prolapse – another cause of intraoperative dysrhythmias in the pediatric patient. Anesthesiology 62: 662–664

George R J D, Banks R A 1983 Bedside measurement of pulmonary capillary wedge pressure. British Journal of Hospital Medicine 29: 286–291

Hemmings G T, Whalley D G, O'Connor P J, Benjamin A, Dunn C 1987 Invasive monitoring and anaesthetic management of a parturient with mitral stenosis. Canadian Journal of Anaesthesia 34: 182–185

Krantz J M, Viljoen J F, Schermer R, Canas M 1980 Mitral valve prolapse. Anesthesia and Analgesia 59: 379–383

Leonard J C 1979 Mitral valve disease. British Journal of Hospital Medicine 22: 204–212

Oakley C M Mitral valve prolapse: harbinger of death or variant of normal? British Medical Journal 288: 1853–1854

Schulte-Sasse U, Hess W, Tarnow J 1982 Pulmonary vascular responses to nitrous oxide in patients with normal and high pulmonary vascular resistance. Anesthesiology 57: 9–13

Thiagarajah S, Frost E A M 1983 Anaesthetic considerations in patients with mitral valve prolapse. Anaesthesia 38: 560–566

MORQUIO'S SYNDROME
(see also MUCOPOLYSACCHARIDOSES)

One of the mucopolysaccharidoses (type IV), this autosomal recessive connective tissue disorder results from the abnormal metabolism of certain polysaccharides (Baines & Kelly 1983, Kempthorne & Browne 1983). Excessive amounts of some metabolites of these substances are laid down in the body tissues and result in a variety of defects. Skeletal, cardiac, eye and hearing problems develop, but there is no mental retardation. Death frequently occurs before the age of 30.

Preoperative abnormalities

1. Skeletal abnormalities include dwarfism, kyphosis, genu valgum, hand deformity, joint mobility, pigeon chest, vertebral flattening with wide disc spaces, and neck instability due to hypoplasia of the odontoid peg. Spinal cord compression may develop in late childhood with slow-onset paraplegia. The face is flattened, and the teeth may be widely spaced, and have defective enamel.

2. Both the mitral and aortic valves can become infiltrated. Late-onset aortic incompetence may occur. Heart disease may also develop secondary to the progressive chest deformity.

3. Corneal opacities commonly develop.

4. Nerve deafness may occur.

5. Inguinal herniae are common and may require surgery.

6. Excess keratin sulphate is found in the urine.

Anaesthetic problems

1. Atlanto-axial subluxation may occur and result in spinal cord transection. Acute tetraplegia, and subsequent death due to pneumonia, was reported in an 8-year-old girl having a myelogram under general anaesthesia (Beighton & Craig 1973). Displacement of the atlas on the axis was found to have occurred. This was attributed to excess movement of the head during the anaesthetic.
2. Chest deformities impair respiration postoperatively. Respiratory failure, and subsequent death from pneumonia, occurred in a patient following radical cervical lymph node resection for melanoma of the scalp (Jones & Croley 1979).
3. Intubation difficulties have been described due to facial deformity and redundant pharyngeal mucosa (Jones & Croley).
4. Upper airway obstruction may be produced during head flexion (Pritzaker et al 1980).

Management

1. A careful assessment of respiratory function is required so as to detect those patients with seriously impaired reserve. In view of the increased risk of major postoperative problems, and the reduced life expectancy, a decision to embark on non-essential major surgery should not be made lightly.
2. Cervical spine X-rays should be examined for signs of C1/C2 instability, and pre-existing neurological defects documented. If hypoplasia of the dens or instability is suspected, some means of immobilizing the neck is required to prevent flexion damage to the spinal cord. The management of appendicectomy in a young boy, who already had paraplegia due to cord compression, was described (Birkinshaw 1975). The child lay prone with his head propped on his hands and a plaster cast was applied to his head, back and sides. When the plaster was dry the patient was carefully rolled into a supine position. After an inhalation induction with halothane, intubation was achieved with deep ether anaesthesia.
3. If intubation difficulties are suspected, either an inhalation induction or an awake intubation should be considered.

BIBLIOGRAPHY

Baines D, Keneally J 1983 Anaesthetic implications of the mucopolysaccharidoses: a fifteen year experience in a Children's Hospital. Anaesthesia and Intensive Care 11: 198–202
Beighton P, Craig J 1973 Atlanto-axial subluxation in the Morquio syndrome. Journal of Bone and Joint Surgery 55B: 478–481
Birkinshaw K J 1975 Anaesthesia in a patient with an unstable neck: Morquio's syndrome; Anaesthesia 30: 46–49
Jones A E P, Croley T F 1979 Morquio syndrome and anesthesia. Anesthesiology 51: 261–262
Kempthorne P M, Brown T C K 1983 Anaesthesia and the mucopolysaccharidoses: A survey of techniques and problems. Anaesthesia and Intensive Care 11: 203–207

Pritzaker M R, King R A, Kronenberg R S 1980 Upper airway obstruction during head flexion in Morquio's disease. American Journal of Medicine 69: 467–470

MOTOR NEURONE DISEASE
(AMYOTROPHIC LATERAL SCLEROSIS)

A degenerative disease of unknown aetiology. It involves both upper and lower motor neurones and presents in late middle age with muscle weakness and fasciculations. There may be bulbar involvement. The prognosis is poor.

Preoperative abnormalities

1. A combination of signs and symptoms of upper and lower motor neurone disease. Muscle cramps, weakness, wasting, fasciculations, spasticity, hyperreflexia and extensor plantar reflexes, may coexist with bulbar signs, such as impairment of speech, swallowing and laryngeal reflexes. The ocular muscles are spared. The disease is progressive.
2. EMG indicates muscle denervation and shows fibrillation potentials.
3. A form of the disease may occur in conjunction with a carcinoma, usually bronchial.

Anaesthetic problems

1. Administration of suxamethonium has been reported to have produced marked hyperkalaemia and cardiovascular collapse (Beach et al 1971).
2. Patients may be sensitive to the effects of non-depolarizing muscle relaxants (Rosenbaum et al 1971).
3. There is a risk of perioperative aspiration and airway obstruction in cases where bulbar signs are present.
4. Postoperative respiratory insufficiency may occur.

Management

1. In view of the report of cardiovascular collapse due to hyperkalaemia, the use of suxamethonium should be avoided.
2. Due to the possibility of sensitivity to non-depolarizing drugs, small doses are given initially and neuromuscular function monitored.
3. If bulbar muscle function is impaired, then precautions should be taken to prevent perioperative pulmonary aspiration.
4. In advanced cases of the disease, careful consideration should be given to the appropriateness of surgery. Severe problems may arise once a patient is committed to IPPV.

BIBLIOGRAPHY

Beach T P, Stone W A, Hamelberg W 1971 Circulatory collapse following succinylcholine: report of a patient with diffuse lower motor neurone disease. Anesthesia and Analgesia 50: 431–437
Rosenbaum K J, Neigh J L, Strobel G E 1971 Sensitivity to non depolarising muscle relaxants in amyotrophic lateral sclerosis. Anesthesiology 35: 638–641

MOYA-MOYA DISEASE

A rare abnormality of the cerebral circulation, first described in Japan, in which gradual occlusion or severe stenosis of the internal carotid arteries occurs. Cerebral angiography shows a fine hazy network of vessels (the moya-moya collaterals) around the base of the brain. Patients usually present with signs of cerebrovascular insufficiency, either in childhood, or as adults.

Preoperative abnormalities

1. The patient may present with a variety of features suggestive of inadequate cerebral blood flow. These may range from transient ischaemic attacks to fixed neurological deficits.
2. Cerebral angiography demonstrates the occluded arteries and the abnormal 'net-like' collateral circulation.
3. Normal cerebral blood flow may be reduced by as much as a half.
4. In adults there is an increased incidence of intracranial aneurysms.

Anaesthetic problems

1. Hyperventilation can produce a reduction in arterial PCO_2 which may compromise the already poor cerebral circulation. Cases have been described in which hypocapnoea during anaesthesia was associated with a deterioration in neurological status. No deterioration occurred in those patients in whom normocapnoea was maintained (Sumikawa & Nagai 1983, Bingham & Wilkinson 1985). Anaesthesia using pancuronium, fentanyl and 0.5–1% isoflurane, while maintaining normocapnoea, was used in eight procedures on seven patients (Brown & Lam 1987).
2. In one series, four out of seven patients were found to have abnormal ECGs. One 27-year-old developed a ventricular tachycardia during surgery (Brown & Lam 1987).
3. Postoperatively, subjects are prone to develop fits.

Management

1. Surgical treatment is directed towards increasing the cerebral blood flow. Various surgical manoeuvres have been tried, including anastomosis

1

of the superficial temporal to the middle cerebral artery and encephaloduroarteriosynangiosis.

2. The maintenance of an $ETCO_2$ between 5.5 kPa and 6 kPa has been advocated.

3. Normothermia should be maintained.

BIBLIOGRAPHY

Bingham R M, Wilkinson D J 1985 Anaesthetic management in Moya-moya disease. Anaesthesia 40: 1198–1202
Brown S C, Lam A 1987 Moya-moya disease. A review of clinical experience and anaesthetic management. Canadian Journal of Anaesthesia 34: 71–75
Sumikawa K, Nagai H 1983 Moya-moya disease and anesthesia. Anesthesiology 58: 204–205

MUCOPOLYSACCHARIDOSES
(MPS)

A group of inherited connective tissue syndromes which result from enzyme deficiencies. The mucopolysaccharides (or glycoaminoglycans) are constituents of connective tissue, and are made up of repeating disaccharide units connected to protein. They are normally broken down in the cell lysosomes to monosaccharides and amino acids. In the absence of certain enzymes, accumulation of intermediate products of the degradation process takes place. These substances increase cell size and cause impairment of function. The effects depend upon the enzyme defect, and the specific organs involved. The disease progresses with age, and life-expectancy is greatly reduced.

Surgery is required most frequently for inguinal and umbilical herniae, ENT, orthopaedic or neurosurgical operations. More recently there have been attempts to replace missing enzymes by regular implantation of tissue such as human amnion (King et al 1984). Although these syndromes are rare, the more commonly encountered ones provide a considerable anaesthetic challenge. The classification is shown below. Some are dealt with under their individual names. Abnormalities in the least common types are included here.

Type I

Type I H	Hurler's syndrome (gargoylism)	(see Hurler)
Type I S	Scheie's syndrome	(see Hurler)
Type I H/S	Hurler–Scheie syndrome	(see Hurler)

Type II   Hunter's syndrome   (see Hurler)

Type III   Sanfilippo's syndrome
Craniofacial: Mild coarsening of facial features.
Skeletal: None
Cardiac: None
Mental: Severe progressive retardation

Other organs: None
Anaesthetic: Difficult intubation has been reported (Kempthorne & Brown 1983).

Type IV   Morquio' syndrome   (see Morquio)

Type VI   Maroteaux–Lamy syndrome
Craniofacial: coarse features and macroglossia
Skeletal: kyphosis, flat vertebrae, genu valgum
Cardiac: none
Mental: normal
Other organs: none
Anaesthetic: four out of six patients had either a difficult airway or
   difficult intubation (Baines & Keneally 1983, Kempthorne & Brown
   1983). Atlanto axial instability has been reported

Type VII   β-glucuronidase

Type VIII   ? like Morquio and Sanfilippo

BIBLIOGRAPHY

Baines D, Keneally J 1983 Anaesthetic implications of the mucopolysaccharidoses.
   Anaesthesia and Intensive Care 11: 198–202
Herrick I A, Rhine E J 1988 The mucopolysaccharidoses and anaesthesia. Canadian Journal
   of Anaesthesia 35: 67–73
Kempthorne P M, Brown T C K 1983 Anaesthesia and the mucopolysaccharidoses.
   Anaesthesia and Intensive Care 11: 203–207
King D H, Jones R M, Barnett M B 1984 Anaesthetic considerations in the
   mucopolysaccharidoses. Anaesthesia 39: 126–131

MUSCULAR DYSTROPHY
(see also DUCHENNE MUSCULAR DYSTROPHY)

A group of inherited muscle disorders. The severe Duchenne type, which is the most common, also produces the most serious anaesthetic problems. This condition is described separately. Precise diagnosis is not always possible, but the other types are less severe (Ellis 1980). In general these other dystrophies do not affect the muscles of respiration or swallowing, and cardiac involvement is less common. However, marked sensitivity to curare was reported with ocular muscular dystrophy (Robertson 1984) and therefore neuromuscular monitoring is mandatory in these patients.

1. X-linked:
   a. Duchenne (severe).
   b. Becker   (mild).
2. Autosomal recessive:
   a. Severe.
   b. Mild limb girdle with facial involvement.
                     without facial involvement.

3. Autosomal dominant:
   a. Facio-scapulo-humeral.
   b. Distal.
   c. Ocular.
   d. Oculopharyngeal.

BIBLIOGRAPHY

Ellis F R 1980 Inherited muscle disease. British Journal of Anaesthesia 52: 153–164
Robertson J A 1984 Ocular muscular dystrophy. A cause of curare sensitivity. Anaesthesia
   39: 251–253

MYASTHENIA GRAVIS

An autoimmune disease of the neuromuscular junction involving the
postjunctional acetylcholine receptors. Specific autoantibodies have been
identified and microscopic changes in the membrane demonstrated. Not
only is there a reduction in the number of acetylcholine receptors at the
postjunctional membrane, but there also appears to be a variation in the
functional ability of the antibodies to block the receptors (Drachman
1978). The condition is characterized by muscle weakness and fatiguability
on repeated use of that muscle. Females are more commonly affected than
males, in a two to one ratio. There is an association with thymic
enlargement and thymomas, both benign and malignant.

Preoperative abnormalities

1. Symptoms are primarily those of increasing muscle weakness and
neuromuscular fatigue which improve after resting. Muscles of the eye
and face are affected early in the disease and result in ptosis and diplopia.
Bulbar palsy may produce swallowing and speech difficulties, and neck
muscles may be affected. Sometimes respiratory muscle involvement
occurs early. Variable progression or remission may occur. The
involvement of particular muscle groups is inconstant, but proximal
muscles of the upper limbs are affected more frequently than the lower
limbs.
2. Antibodies against acetylcholine receptors are found in 80–90% of
patients with myasthenia gravis.
3. Diagnosis may be confirmed by demonstrating an improvement
within 10–30 seconds of giving edrophonium i.v. 2–10 mg. This lasts for
about 5 minutes.
4. Current treatment includes:
   a. Immunological suppression to eliminate the antibody. Azathioprine
   or steroids are used and benefit 90% of cases. This has become the first
   line of treatment.
   b. Thymectomy, increasingly via the transcervical approach.

c. Symptomatic relief with anticholinesterase preparations which potentiate the effects of acetylcholine. Pyridostigmine and neostigmine are most commonly used. Concurrent use of atropine or propantheline may be required to block muscarinic effects, such as intestinal colic.

d. Plasma exchange, for short-term treatment, particularly in a crisis.

Anaesthetic problems

1. The operation

Anaesthesia may be required for thymectomy, or for other incidental surgery. Thymectomy is performed either via a median sternotomy or a transcervical approach. The former produces the greater anaesthetic difficulties.

2. The variables

The main problem revolves around the anaesthetist's ability to anticipate and manage three variables:

    a. The muscle weakness produced by the patient's disease.

    b. His preoperative anticholinesterase medication.

    c. The surgeon's requirement for muscle relaxation.

Adequate respiratory function must be maintained in the pre- and postoperative period, and yet adequate intraoperative muscle relaxation may be needed for surgical access.

3. Muscle relaxants

Myasthenics may or may not have an increased sensitivity to non depolarizing muscle relaxants. The blockade of the acetylcholine receptors by antibody resembles partial curarization, and therefore the amount of a drug required to produce effective paralysis is often reduced. There is, however, wide patient variation in response to relaxants. The actual amount of relaxant needed will depend upon factors such as the stage of the disease, the presence or absence of a remission, the actual muscles being tested and whether anticholinesterase medication has been given preoperatively.

4. Excess anticholinesterase

Excessive amounts of an anticholinesterase may itself cause increased muscle weakness. This can be confused with that due to the myasthenia. Experimentally, an excess of anticholinesterase has been shown to reduce the number of functioning receptors. Patients in a cholinergic crisis may require ventilation.

5. Respiratory dysfunction

Respiratory muscle or bulbar weakness may occur pre- or postoperatively and can predispose the patient to aspiration, chest infection or respiratory failure.

6. Immunosuppression may lead to neutropenia and serious infection.

Management

1. Management of muscle relaxation

The method of management depends on the severity of the myasthenia, the type of operation and the anaesthetist's personal preference. In a series of 100 cases of transcervical thymectomy (Girnar et al 1976), those patients with mild myasthenia were given half their normal dose of pyridostigmine, while those with severe disease received their full dose. Anaesthesia and intubation were achieved with thiopentone, nitrous oxide, oxygen and either halothane or ethrane. IPPV was maintained without a muscle relaxant and 92 patients were extubated successfully within 2 hours of operation.

Upper abdominal surgery requires a greater degree of muscle relaxation than can be produced by inhalation agents alone. With the advent of clinical neuromuscular monitors, good control can be achieved using only small doses of a relaxant. The satisfactory use of atracurium in incremental doses has been reported (MacDonald et al 1984, Ward & Wright 1984). While the final doses required to produce 90–95% blockade varied from 0.05 mg/kg to 0.33 mg/kg, it was agreed that with atracurium, a relatively rapid rate of spontaneous recovery took place when compared with other relaxants. Vecuronium 0.02–0.04 mg/kg has been used in six patients for thymectomy, without problems in reversal (Hunter et al 1985).

2. Muscle relaxant reversal and anticholinesterases

Either reversal of muscle relaxants, or restoration of respiration in the myasthenic, may be achieved by the routine use of neostigmine and atropine. However, care must be taken not to give a dose in excess of the patient's normal requirements, otherwise a cholinergic crisis may occur (Eisencraft & Papatestas 1988). Equivalent doses are:

Neostigmine i.v.   1 mg
Neostigmine oral   30 mg
Pyridostigmine i.v.   4 mg
Pyridostigmine oral   120 mg

The patient's usual anticholinesterases may have to be given i.v. until oral medication can be taken.

3. Postoperative care

All patients require postoperative high-dependency facilities. Some patients will need postoperative IPPV. The surgical approach to the thymus is still controversial, although the transcervical approach is being increasingly used, rather than the more traumatic trans-sternal route. The cervical approach is associated with a reduced requirement for prolonged postoperative IPPV.

4. Will scoring systems predict patients who will require prolonged postoperative IPPV?

The contradictory reports of the sensitivity of such scoring systems are probably in part due to the variation in the surgical approach to the thymus. A scoring system utilizing four factors and claiming a predictive sensitivity of 100% has been devised (Leventhal et al 1980).

The factors were:
  a. Length of disease greater than 6 years.
  b. Concomitant respiratory disease.
  c. Pyridostigmine requirement of >750 mg/day.
  d. Vital capacity of <2.9 litres.
All the patients had transthoracic thymectomy. In another paper, these predictors were utilized in 92 patients, and a sensitivity of only 37.5% was achieved (Eisencraft et al 1986). However, all of these patients had a transcervical thymectomy which involved a much lower (8.7%) requirement for postoperative IPPV. This was a significant improvement on previously reported series of trans-sternal procedures for which the IPPV rates varied from 33 to 50%. A further attempt to utilize the scoring system included both approaches to the thymus, as well as a variety of non-thymectomy operations (Grant & Jenkins 1982). In the thymectomy group, only three out of seven who required IPPV were predicted. In contrast, none of the 24 non-thymectomy patients needed ventilation, despite 11 having scores of >10.

5. Tracheostomy
Occasionally tracheostomy may be required, but only if ventilation is prolonged and excess secretions are a problem.

6. Respiratory failure in myasthenia
Respiratory failure in myasthenic patients may be secondary to either a myasthenic or a cholinergic crisis. IPPV should be instituted, anticholinesterase therapy stopped, and then only cautiously reintroduced after testing with i.v. edrophonium. An improvement suggests a myasthenic cause, and deterioration, a cholinergic crisis. Facilities should be available for the rapid institution of IPPV.

BIBLIOGRAPHY

Drachman D B 1978 Myasthenia gravis. New England Journal of Medicine 298: 186–193
Drachman D B 1987 Present and future treatment of myasthenia gravis. New England Journal of Medicine 316: 743–745
Eisencraft J B, Papatestas A E, Kahn C H, Mora C T, Fagerstrom R, Genkins G 1986 Predicting the need for postoperative mechanical ventilation in myasthenia gravis. Anesthesiology 65: 79–82
Eisencraft J B, Papatestas A E 1988 Anaesthesia for trans-sternal thymectomy in myasthenia gravis. Annals of the Royal College of Surgeons of England 70; 257–258
Girnar D S, Weinreich A I 1976 Anesthesia for transcervical thymectomy in myasthenia gravis. Anesthesia and Analgesia 55: 13–17
Grant R P, Jenkins L C 1982 Prediction of the need for postoperative mechanical ventilation in myasthenia gravis: thymectomy compared with other surgical procedures. Canadian Anaesthetists' Society Journal 29: 112–116
Hunter J M, Bell C F, Florence A M, Jones R S, Utting J E 1985 Vecuronium in the myasthenic patient. Anaesthesia 40: 848–853
Leventhal S R, Orkin F K, Hirsch R A 1980 Prediction of the need for postoperative mechanical ventilation in myasthenia gravis. Anesthesiology 53: 26–30
MacDonald A M, Keen R I, Pugh N D 1984 Myasthenia gravis and atracurium. British Journal of Anaesthesia 56: 651–654
Ward S, Wright D J 1984 Neuromuscular blockade in myasthenia gravis with atracurium besylate. Anaesthesia 39: 51–53

1

MYASTHENIC SYNDROME
(see EATON–LAMBERT SYNDROME)

MYELOMA, MULTIPLE

This plasma cell neoplasm is one of the paraproteinaemias, whose peak incidence is in the seventh decade. It erodes bone and infiltrates bone marrow.

Preoperative abnormalities

1. Myeloma may present with bone pain, pathological fractures, anaemia, renal disease or hypercalcaemia. Punched-out lytic lesions may occur anywhere in the skeleton, but are most frequent in the skull, vertebrae, ribs and long bones. Peripheral neuropathy may occur, or paraplegia may arise due to an epidural plasmacytoma or vertebral collapse. The patient may become confused as a result of hyperviscosity.
2. There is usually anaemia, a high ESR, excretion of Bence-Jones protein in the urine, and abnormal protein electrophoresis. Bone marrow is infiltrated with plasma cells.
3. Patients may be on steroids or a variety of cytotoxic agents.

Anaesthetic problems

1. Bone involvement may result in rib fracture or vertebral collapse either spontaneously or with relatively minor trauma.
2. Hypercalcaemia, due to widespread bone disease, is present in about 30% of cases and may be associated with severe dehydration.
3. Renal impairment occurs in almost half of the cases, and actual renal failure in 25% (McIntyre 1980).
4. There is an increased susceptibility to infection due to impairment of the normal production of IgG.
5. Thrombocytopenia or coagulation defects occasionally occur.
6. Hyperviscosity may produce vascular and CNS problems, which include headaches, visual disturbances and retinopathy (McIntyre 1980).

Management

1. Hb, WCC and platelets should be checked. A coagulation screen should be performed if there is any suggestion of abnormal bleeding.
2. Patients should be moved and positioned particularly carefully during anaesthesia to prevent pathological fractures.
3. Hypercalcaemia >3.2 mmol/l is dangerous and requires urgent treatment (see Hypercalcaemia).

4. Regional anaesthesia should be avoided if a neuropathy or a coagulation abnormality is suspected.
5. Steroid supplements may be required.
6. If the patient is receiving cytotoxic agents, see Section 2.

BIBLIOGRAPHY

McIntyre O R 1980 Current concepts in cancer: multiple myeloma. New England Journal of Medicine 301: 193–196

MYOGLOBINURIA
(see RHABDOMYOLYSIS)

MYXOEDEMA
(see HYPOTHYROIDISM)

NEUROFIBROMATOSIS

An autosomal dominant inherited condition characterized by multiple neurofibromas and flat, brown, pigmented skin patches. Neurofibromas may occur anywhere in the body and can cause a variety of symptoms. A wide spectrum of associated abnormalities has been described. The condition is progressive and the effects vary from mild to very severe. There is an increased incidence of malignancies. The exact aetiology of the condition is unknown, but the abnormalities may originate from neural crest defects.

Preoperative abnormalities

1. Skin and nerves
Cafe au lait spots are found in 99% of patients. For diagnostic purposes at least six, having one diameter of more than 1.5 cm, should be present (Riccardi 1981). Freckling often occurs, particularly in the skin folds. Neurofibromas may be cutaneous or subcutaneous. They can occur on deep nerves or roots, or be associated with the autonomic nerves on viscera and blood vessels.
2. Central nervous system
In one series, two-thirds of cases had some neurological involvement (Riccardi 1981). Neurofibromas may appear in the vertebral foramina and cause dumbell tumours. Cerebral tumours such as gliomas and meningiomas occur in 5–10% of cases. There is some intellectual impairment in 40% of cases and 2–5% of patients have frank mental retardation.
3. Pulmonary
An associated fibrosing alveolitis may occur in up to 20% of cases.

4. Skeletal
Kyphoscoliosis develops in 2% of patients. Bone sarcoma can occur.
5. Endocrine
Phaeochromocytomas are present in up to 1% of patients and medullary thyroid carcinomas have been described.
6. Renal
There may be renal artery stenosis and hypertension.
7. Airway
Oral and upper airway tumours have been reported.

Anaesthetic problems

1. Airway difficulties can occur due to neurofibromas in the upper respiratory tract. A laryngeal tumour caused these during laryngoscopy in a 13-year-old boy (Fisher 1975). Such tumours are very rare. Emergency cricothyroidotomy had to be performed in one patient, who could not be ventilated after induction of anaesthesia for stabilization of a mandibular fracture (Crozier 1987). Subsequently a large neurofibroma of the tongue was removed. Oral lesions are said to be present in 5% of cases (Baden et al 1955).
2. Difficulty in performing regional anaesthesia, thought to be due to the presence of a neurofibroma in the needle path, has been reported (Fisher 1975).
3. If kyphoscoliosis and pulmonary disease coexist, they may contribute to postoperative respiratory complications.
4. There is a higher incidence of phaeochromocytoma than in the normal population, so signs of this should be sought. Ventricular tachycardia occurred in one patient having surgery for renal artery stenosis, but no evidence of a phaeochromocytoma was found (Krishna 1975). Renin release, and sensitization of the heart to the effect of catecholamines due to halothane, were postulated as contributing factors.
5. A small number of patients have been reported to have a prolonged neuromuscular blockade in response to relaxants (Nagao et al 1983).

Management

1. Careful preoperative assessment is essential, with particular attention being paid to mouth and airway lesions, chest and neurological complications.
2. Urinary catecholamine estimation should be performed.
3. Neuromuscular monitoring is advisable.

BIBLIOGRAPHY

Baden E, Pierce H E, Jackson W F 1955 Multiple neurofibromatosis with oral lesions; review of the literature. Oral Surgery 8: 263–280
Crozier W C 1987 Upper airway obstruction in neurofibromatosis. Anaesthesia 42: 1209–1211

Fisher M McD 1975 Anaesthetic difficulties in neurofibromatosis. Anaesthesia 30: 648–650
Krishna G 1975 Neurofibromatosis, renal hypertension, and cardiac dysrhythmias.
    Anesthesia and Analgesia 54: 542–545
Nagao H, Yamashita M, Shinozaki Y, Oyama T 1983 Hypersensitivity to pancuronium in a
    patient with von Recklinghausen's disease. British Journal of Anaesthesia 55: 253
Riccardi V M 1981 Von Recklinghausen neurofibromatosis. New England Journal of Medicine
    305: 1617–1627

NEUROGENIC PULMONARY OEDEMA
(see PULMONARY OEDEMA)

NEUROLEPTIC MALIGNANT SYNDROME
(NMS)

A rare but serious complication of treatment with neuroleptic drugs, characterized by the development of catatonic, extrapyramidal and autonomic effects. Its aetiology is unknown, but appears to be related to the antidopaminergic activity of the precipitating drug. Clinical features include hyperthermia, muscle rigidity, sympathetic overactivity and a variable conscious level. A mortality of 20% has been reported (Caroff et al 1983). The concept that NMS is related to anaesthetic-induced MH is supported in some quarters (Caroff et al 1983, Denborough et al 1985), but others suggest that, despite the superficial clinical similarities, MH and NMS are two distinct and unrelated entities (Krivosic-Horber et al 1987). When the criteria of the European MH Group for muscle testing were applied to six NMS survivors, five were found to be normal and one was equivocal (Krivosic-Horber et al 1987).

Presentation

1. Haloperidol and fluphenazine are the drugs most frequently reported as being associated with NMS. Others include chlorpromazine, trifluoperazine, droperidol, thioridazine, thiapride and metoclopramide. In most cases these drugs have been given for a variety of psychiatric disorders. NMS has also occurred with tetrabenazine, and after stopping treatment with levodopa. The condition may occur within hours of starting the drug, or after some months of treatment. Lithium therapy may facilitate its development. A probable case has been described which was associated with anaesthesia, in a young man given normal doses of droperidol and metoclopramide (Patel & Bristow 1987).
2. Clinical features include catatonia, hyperthermia, sweating, stupor, tremor, muscle rigidity, akinesia, autonomic dysfunction, incontinence and renal failure.
3. Rhabdomyolysis may occur. The CPK is usually increased. Levels >10 000 iu/l have been reported. LFTs may be abnormal and leucocytosis often occurs.

Management

1. The relevant medication is discontinued.

2. The patient is cooled.

3. Dantrolene sodium, 50 mg q.d.s. for 5 days, and bromocriptine mesylate, 5 mg t.d.s. increasing to 10 mg t.d.s., have both been used, apparently successfully, to treat NMS (Mueller et al 1983).

4. In severe cases, IPPV, fluid replacement and intensive care facilities will be required.

5. Whether a survivor of NMS who requires an anaesthetic should be treated as MH susceptible is contentious. Two papers have reported positive MH testing in NMS survivors (Denborough et al 1985, Caroff et al 1987), whereas a third, using the European MH Group criteria, could not confirm an association between the two conditions (Krivosic-Horber et al 1987).

BIBLIOGRAPHY

Caroff S, Rosenberg H, Gerber J C 1983 Neuroleptic malignant syndrome and malignant hyperthermia. Lancet 1983; i: 244

Caroff S N, Rosenberg H, Fletcher J E, Heiman-Patterson T D, Mann S C 1987 Malignant hyperthermia susceptibility in neuroleptic malignant syndrome. Anesthesiology 67: 20–25

Denborough M A, Collins S P, Hopkinson K C 1985 Rhabdomyolysis and malignant hyperpyrexia. British Medical Journal 288: 1878–1879

Krivosic-Horber R, Adnet P, Guevart E, Theunynck D, Lestavel P 1987 Neuroleptic malignant syndrome and malignant hyperthermia. British Journal of Anaesthesia 59: 1554–1556

Mueller P S, Vester J W, Fermaglich J 1983 Neuroleptic malignant syndrome: successful treatment with bromocriptine. Journal of the American Medical Association 249: 386–388

Patel P, Bristow G 1987 Postoperative neuroleptic malignant syndrome. A case report. Canadian Journal of Anaesthesia 1987; 34: 515–518

Szabadi E 1984 Neuroleptic malignant syndrome. British Medical Journal 288: 1399–1400

OBESITY

Morbid obesity has been defined as occurring when a subject's weight is more than 70% greater than the ideal weight for his or her age and height. Insurance statistics show a greatly increased mortality rate for such patients, and surgery and anaesthesia carry a number of risks. In addition to incidental procedures, the obese patient may be subjected to weight-reducing intestinal bypass operations, particularly in North America. A number of studies have been undertaken to identify the problems and determine the best method of anaesthesia.

Preoperative abnormalities

1. Respiratory

FRC is reduced, mainly due to a decrease in expiratory reserve volume. Tidal ventilation occurs below the closing volume, particularly in the supine position. The PaO_2 may be reduced, and the work and oxygen cost of respiration are increased.

2. Cardiovascular
An increased incidence of hypertension and coronary artery disease.
3. Increased glucose intolerance and diabetes.
4. The Pickwickian syndrome, characterized by hypoventilation,
somnolence, cor pulmonale and hypoxia, is very rare.

Anaesthetic problems

1. Difficulties with venous access.
2. Mechanical problems due to the size and weight of the patient.
3. Difficulties in locating the epidural or subarachnoid space. Standard
length needles may be too short.
4. Intubation problems.
5. Cyanosis occurs rapidly, due to a reduced FRC.
6. Rapid dehydration and a poor response to hypovolaemia results from
a reduced blood volume per unit weight.
7. Reliable indirect blood pressure monitoring is difficult to achieve.
8. Difficulties in maintaining an airway during mask anaesthesia.
9. Problems with intraoperative oxygenation during abdominal surgery,
particularly when in the head-down position, or when intra-abdominal
packs are in place.
10. For the first 48 postoperative hours, the supine position is associated
with a significant fall in PaO_2 (Vaughan et al 1976a).
11. Increased incidence of postoperative respiratory problems.
12. Venous thrombosis and pulmonary embolism.
13. An increased risk of wound infection (8–28%).

Management

1. Detailed cardiovascular and respiratory assessment is required. If
there is pre-existing hypoxia or hypercarbia, then some weight loss is
advisable before elective surgery. Mandibular wiring has been
advocated to aid this, prior to abdominal weight-reducing surgery.
2. Thoracic epidural anaesthesia has been recommended as an adjunct
to general anaesthesia. The rationale is that as a consequence, only light
general anaesthesia is required, good postoperative pain relief is
provided, and early extubation and mobilization are permitted. Epidural
analgesia was given to 70 patients in a series of 110 undergoing weight-
reducing surgery (Fox et al 1981). There was an incidence of postoperative
lung collapse of 18.5% in these patients, compared with 27.5% for
those just receiving pethidine i.m.. However, there was a suggestion that
pulmonary emboli might be slightly more common in the epidural
group.

Others do not believe that there are significant advantages in epidural
analgesia. Thoracic epidurals are technically difficult to perform in the
very obese and there was a 20% failure rate in one series (Buckley et al
1983). Some improvement in cardiovascular function, as evidenced by a

decrease in left ventricular stroke volume and myocardial oxygen requirement, was reported in patients with a thoracic epidural block and general anaesthesia compared with opiates and general anaesthesia (Gelman et al 1980). However, it was found to be no better than intravenous morphine in terms of postoperative pain relief, vital capacity and gas exchange. A lesser number of pulmonary complications were experienced with epidural analgesia, but a greater incidence of intraoperative hypotension and bradycardia (Buckley et al 1983).

Care must be taken to avoid giving an excessive volume of local anaesthetic to the morbidly obese. The reduced dose of bupivacaine required for epidural anaesthesia in obese pregnant patients (Hodgkinson & Hussain 1980), has been confirmed by others (Buckley et al 1983). This is probably due to venous engorgement in the epidural space.

3. The use of antacids and H_2 receptor antagonists as a precaution against acid aspiration syndrome is recommended.

4. If intubation difficulties are anticipated, awake intubation may be advisable. The incidence of difficult intubation under general anaesthesia has been reported to be between 6 and 13%.

5. A comparison of adjuvants with IPPV were made in 67 patients for gastric stapling (Cork et al 1981). There was no difference between halothane, enflurane or fentanyl in terms of early postoperative recovery. However, the use of isoflurane, which is the least metabolized, would seem rational.

6. During abdominal surgery, frequent blood gas sampling is advisable and an increased inspired oxygen concentration is required when the head-down position is employed. The use of subdiaphragmatic intra-abdominal packs may produce severe hypoxia and should be avoided if possible. Oxygenation in otherwise healthy obese subjects having abdominal surgery was studied (Vaughan et al 1976b). Fourteen per cent of patients in the supine position, and 77% with a 15° head-down tilt, had a PaO_2 of <10.6 kPa on 40% oxygen. In 23% of those in the latter group, the PaO_2 fell to <8.0 kPa. Four patients in whom subdiaphragmatic packs were used all had a PaO_2 of <8.6 kPa.

BIBLIOGRAPHY

Buckley F P, Robinson N B, Simonowitz D A, Dellinger E P 1983 Anaesthesia in the morbidly obese. Anaesthesia 38: 840–851
Cork R C, Vaughan R W, Bentley J B 1981 General anesthesia for morbidly obese patients: an examination of postoperative outcomes. Anesthesiology 54: 310–313
Fisher A, Waterhouse T D, Adams A P 1975 Obesity: its relation to anaesthesia. Anaesthesia 30: 633–647
Fox G S, Whalley D G, Bevan D R 1981 Anaesthesia for the morbidly obese, experience with 110 patients. British Journal of Anaesthesia 53: 811–816
Gelman S, Laws H L, Potzick J, Strong S, Smith L, Erdemir M 1980 Thoracic epidural versus balanced anesthesia in morbid obesity. An intraoperative and postoperative hemodynamic study. Anesthesia and Analgesia 59: 902–908
Hodgkinson R, Hussain F J 1980 Obesity and the cephalad spread of analgesia following epidural administration of bupivacaine for Cesarean section. Anesthesia and Analgesia 59: 89–92

Vaughan R W, Bauer S, Wise L 1976a Effect of position (semirecumbent versus supine) on postoperative oxygenation in markedly obese subjects. Anesthesia and Analgesia 55: 37–41
Vaughan R W, Wise L 1976b Intraoperative arterial oxygenation in obese patients. Annals of Surgery 184: 35–42

OPIATE ADDICTION

Dependence on opiates is present when a physical withdrawal state occurs on abrupt cessation of the drug, and when tolerance to the drug develops. Psychological dependence can alsc occur. The anaesthetist may be involved, either because a dependent patient requires surgery, or for resuscitation when accidental or deliberate overdosage occurs. The problem may be admitted by the patient, or concealed. He may or may not be registered as an addict. Occasionally a cured addict may come for surgery. Opiates should be scrupulously avoided in these patients. Alternatives such as continuous epidural analgesia should be considered for postoperative pain.

In the absence of a history of drug abuse, bizarre behaviour, malnutrition, or social deterioration in a patient under 40, should prompt the search for injection marks.

Preoperative abnormalities

1. Malnutrition, skin infection, superficial venous thrombosis, anaemia or jaundice may be present.
2. There is a high incidence of liver disease. A 10% incidence of hepatitis has been reported. In one study of multiple attacks, 32% of cases were due to HAV, 42% to HBV and 25% to NANBV (Norkrans et al 1980). Malnutrition may contribute to liver disease. There is a significant risk of transmission of hepatitis and possibly AIDS.
3. An increased risk of bacterial or fungal endocarditis, most frequently due to *Staphylococcus aureus*, but sometimes to pseudomonas. Arterial emboli, sometimes septic, can result.
4. Pulmonary infection, infarction and atelectasis are common. Pulmonary hypertension or oedema can occur.
5. Tetanus may be seen, in part due to additives such as quinine which allow the growth of anaerobes (McGoldrick 1980).
6. Adrenocortical function is suppressed.

Anaesthetic problems

1. Venous access may be difficult.
2. Problems of management of HBV- or HIV-positive patients.
3. Physical dependence and withdrawal symptoms. These include tachycardia, tremor, acute anxiety, sweating, piloerection, mydriasis,

nausea, vomiting. There is evidence to suggest that brain catecholamines play some part in the aetiology of this syndrome (McGoldrick 1980).

The time-course of the individual abstinence syndromes has been described (McCammon 1986):

Pethidine: onset 3 hours, peak 8–12 hours, duration 4–5 days.
Morphine: onset 8–12 hours, peak 36–48 hours, duration 7–10 days.
Heroin: onset 8–12 hours, peak 36–48 hours, duration 7–10 days.
Methadone: onset 1–2 days, peak 3–6 days, duration 2–3 weeks.

4. Tolerance to all the effects of opiates occurs. Anaesthetic techniques relying on opioids are therefore unsuitable, as very high doses will be required to suppress sympathetic responses to surgical stimulation.
5. The administration of partial or pure narcotic antagonists may precipitate a withdrawal state.
6. Hypotension may occur.

Management

1. A careful history should be taken, and a thorough examination made. If the patient is registered, then the drug centre or his psychiatrist should be contacted to verify details. Expert advice on management may be necessary. If doubt exists, urine may be tested for the presence of drugs. Belongings should be checked for concealed drugs.
2. Patients should be presumed to be HBV- and HIV-positive unless proved otherwise.
3. Most authorities are agreed that the correct time to institute detoxification is not during the period of surgery. Opiates will therefore need to be given. This may be the preparation already being used, or the equivalent dose of methadone might be substituted.

Approximately equivalent dosages (DHSS 1984) are reported as:
a. Methadone: 10 mg (some authorities quote 5 mg).
b. Morphine: 10 mg.
c. Pethidine: 100 mg.
d. Dextromoramide: 5 mg.
e. Heroin: 10 mg.
f. Dipipanone: 20 mg.
g. Buprenorphine: 0.8 mg.
h. Pentazocine: 125 mg.

If genuine organic pain does exist then, as a result of tolerance, higher than normal doses of opiates will be required.
4. If there is venous thrombosis, internal jugular or subclavian venous cannulation, or a venous cutdown, may be required.
5. Partial opiate antagonists such as pentazocine, or pure antagonists such as naloxone, may produce severe withdrawal symptoms, and should not be used.

6. The use of other drugs with addictive potential, such as the benzodiazepines, should be avoided.
7. Hypotension has been described preoperatively in opiate addicts. When it occurs during surgery, responses to various forms of treatment including opiates, fluids, vasoconstrictors or hydrocortisone have been reported.

BIBLIOGRAPHY

Caldwell T 1981 Anesthesia for patients with behavioral and environmental disorders. In: Anesthesia and uncommon diseases. W B Saunders, Philadelphia
DHSS 1984 Guidelines of good clinical practice in the treatment of drug misuse. Report of the Medical Working Group on Drug Dependence. HMSO, London
McCammon R L 1986 Anesthesia for the chemically dependent patient. International Anesthesia Research Society Review Course Lectures 47–55
McGoldrick K E 1980 Anesthetic implications of drug abuse. Anesthesiology Review 7: 12–17
Norkrans G, Frosner G, Hermodsson S, Iwarson S 1980 Multiple hepatitis attacks in drug addicts. Journal of the American Medical Association 243: 1056–1058

OPITZ–FRIAS SYNDROME

A rare congenital disorder whose features include craniofacial and genital abnormalities, and functional swallowing and laryngeal problems. Males are more severely affected than females.

Preoperative abnormalities

1. Hypertelorism, prominent parietal and occipital areas, micrognathia and a high-arched palate.
2. Hypospadias and bifid scrotum.
3. Dysphagia, probably of neuromuscular origin, oesophageal achalasia, hiatus hernia, gastric aspiration and pulmonary problems. There may be wheezing and inspiratory stridor, with a hoarse cry.

Anaesthetic problems

1. Recurrent gastric aspiration may cause cyanotic episodes, apnoea and asystole.
2. Craniofacial abnormalities can lead to intubation problems.

Management

Anaesthetic management of a 9-month-old child for fundoplication and feeding jejunostomy has been reported (Bolsin & Gillbe 1985). Several episodes of cyanosis and CXR changes had occurred after birth. A scan of an isotopic milk feed demonstrated reflux, and the child was fed through a nasogastric tube. Prior to surgery two admissions for respiratory distress and inhalation had been required. Some intubation difficulty was reported due to an immature larynx.

BIBLIOGRAPHY

Bolsin S N, Gillbe C 1985 Opitz–Frias syndrome. A case with potentially hazardous anaesthetic implications. Anaesthesia 40: 1189–1193

OSTEOGENESIS IMPERFECTA

The general term given to a group of inherited disorders of collagen. Four distinct types have been identified (Smith 1984).

Type I is of autosomal dominant inheritance and present in 80% of cases. Extraskeletal tissues are mainly involved and the bone disease is mild. Fractures mainly occur in childhood but become less common after puberty. The joints are hypermobile and the tendons susceptible to rupture. Patients are almost normal in stature. The sclera are blue, there is early-onset deafness and some children have dental problems. The aortic valve is thin, and sometimes incompetent.

Type II have severe skeletal abnormalities and usually die in the perinatal period.

Type III have severe skeletal deformities which are progressive. Chest deformity, with kyphoscoliosis and prominent sternum, often results in respiratory problems. Long bones are narrow and bent. The skull is large and asymmetrical. Patients with this type have white sclera.

Type IV is similar to type I, but with more bone abnormalities and some dwarfing. Teeth may be involved. Sclera are white.

Recent work has indicated that the defect is in type I collagen.

Preoperative abnormalities

1. Individual features have been described. A number of other defects may occur in association.
2. There is some evidence of hypermetabolism. Half the patients have raised serum thyroxine levels.
3. Platelet dysfunction may occur and produce a mild bleeding tendency. The platelet count may be normal.
4. Congenital heart disease has been described.

Anaesthetic problems

1. Bones and teeth are easy to break. The mandible is prone to fracture, but the facial bones are less so.

2. In the severe form, forced extension of the head during intubation carries a risk of vertebral fracture.

3. Airway problems may occur if the head is large, if there is macroglossia, or if the skeletal deformities are severe.

4. Hyperthermia and excess sweating during anaesthesia has been reported. An MH-like syndrome, which was terminated with dantrolene, has been described in a young man who refused further investigation. His sister had died aged 14 after a prolonged mask anaesthetic for reduction of a fracture (Rampton et al 1984).

5. Multiple general anaesthetics may be required for orthopaedic procedures.

6. Violent suxamethonium fasciculations can produce fractures.

Management

1. Patients should be positioned on the operating table and handled with extreme care. Padding should be used. If the head is large, a pillow under the chest may assist intubation.

2. Surgery should be avoided in the pyrexial patient. Core temperature must be monitored throughout surgery. Hyperthermia is reported to have responded to cooling alone.

3. In the severe cases, concern has been expressed that a blood pressure cuff may damage the humerus. Direct arterial monitoring has been suggested (Libman 1981).

4. Suxamethonium should be avoided where risk of fractures is high.

5. The use of ketamine has been reported (Oliverio 1973, Robinson & Wright 1986). This offers a convenient method of avoiding mask and intubation anaesthesia.

6. Although skeletal deformity may make regional anaesthesia technically difficult, epidural anaesthesia has been used for the management of a Caesarean section (Cunningham et al 1984). In this patient platelet studies were normal. This is not a suitable technique if serious intubation difficulties are anticipated.

BIBLIOGRAPHY

Cunningham A J, Donnelly M, Comerford J 1984 Osteogenesis imperfecta: anesthetic management of a patient for Cesarean section. Anesthesiology 61: 91–93

Libman R H 1981 Anaesthetic considerations for the patient with osteogenesis imperfecta. Clinical Orthopaedics and Related Research 159: 123–125

Oliverio R O 1973 Anesthetic management of intramedullary nailing in osteogenesis imperfecta. Anesthesia and Analgesia 52: 232–236

Rampton A J, Kelly D A, Shanahan E C, Ingram G S 1984 Occurrence of malignant hyperpyrexia in a patient with osteogenesis imperfecta. British Journal of Anaesthesia 56: 1443–1446

Robinson C, Wright D J 1986 Anaesthesia for osteogenesis imperfecta. Today's Anaesthetist 1,2: 22–23

Smith R 1984 Osteogenesis imperfecta. British Medical Journal 289: 394–396

PACEMAKERS
(see HEART BLOCK)

PAGET'S DISEASE

A metabolic bone disease which may be either focal or diffuse. The aetiology is unknown, but epidemiological studies and the presence of inclusion bodies in osteoclasts suggest a viral origin. The primary process appears to be unusually active resorption of bone by abnormal osteoclasts, and although osteoblasts replace it, the architecture is disorganized and mineralization defective. There is fibrosis of the marrow, and both marrow and bone are very vascular. In the later, sclerotic stage, vascularity decreases and the bone becomes dense and hard.

Preoperative abnormalities

1. The patient may be asymptomatic, or have bone pain. Affected bones may be enlarged and deformed, and the overlying skin warm. The pelvis, femur, tibia, skull and spine are the most commonly involved.
2. The bone is more vulnerable to fractures than normal bone. About 1% of patients develop bone sarcoma.
3. Bone enlargement and deformity may cause a variety of neurological symptoms. Deafness, paraplegia, brainstem compression and hydrocephalus have been described.
4. If the disease is widespread, the vascular stage may be associated with a high cardiac output. Cardiac failure, due to the disease itself, occurs rarely.
5. Most patients require no treatment or mild analgesics only. Specific treatment is indicated in those with bone pain, complications of deformity, neurological symptoms or heart failure. Mithramycin has been used for the rapid relief of pain and in spinal cord compression. Calcitonin (i.m. or i.v.) reduces the vascularity of bone before orthopaedic procedures, and is used for bone pain and in osteolytic disease. Etidronate is increasingly used. It reduces bone turnover and may interfere with mineralization. Treatment is usually limited to 6 months, but the effect may be prolonged.

Anaesthetic problems

1. Bone fracture is a common complication of Paget's disease (Guyer 1980).
2. In view of the marked vascularity of the bone, there may be considerable blood loss during orthopaedic procedures.
3. Paget's disease may affect the atlas and axis (Brown et al 1971). Cervical spine disease can be associated with serious neurological complications. Bone hypertrophy and narrowing of the spinal canal may

1

cause cord compression, or interference with the blood supply. Vertebral displacement can occur due to fracture or subluxation. Invagination of the foramen magnum into the posterior fossa is present in one-third of patients with Paget's disease of the skull (Guyer 1980).
4. If the lumbar spine is involved, regional anaesthesia may be technically difficult.

Management

1. To avoid fractures, patients should be moved and positioned very gently under anaesthesia. Limbs should be supported and padded.
2. Treatment with calcitonin has been reported to decrease the bone vascularity. However, its effect is maximal in the early stages of treatment but may progressively diminish after the first 3 months.
3. Patients with cervical spine and skull disease should be treated with extreme care. Neurological symptoms and signs should be sought and documented in advance. Atlantoaxial subluxation must be excluded.
4. Cardiac failure, if present, should be treated.

BIBLIOGRAPHY

Brown H P, LaRocca H, Wickstrom J K 1971 Paget's disease of the atlas and axis. Journal of
    Bone and Joint Surgery 53B: 1441–1444
Guyer P B 1980 Radiology in Paget's disease. Hospital Update 6: 1079–1091

PAPILLOMATOSIS
(see LARYNGEAL PAPILLOMATOSIS)

PARKINSON'S DISEASE

A disorder of the extrapyramidal motor system of unknown aetiology. Onset is gradual, and usually occurs after the age of 50. Pathological changes include degeneration of cells and loss of pigmented neurones in the substantia nigra. Biochemical abnormalities in brain neurotransmitters, and in particular a deficiency of dopamine in the striatum and substantia nigra, have been demonstrated. Parkinsonism has also occurred following insults to the brain such as encephalitis lethargia, trauma, certain chemicals, major psychotropic drugs, cerebrovascular disease or hypoxia. Parkinsonian features may occur in other degenerative CNS diseases, which may exhibit additional signs such as autonomic failure (e.g. Shy–Drager).

The aim of drug treatment is to increase dopamine concentrations in the basal ganglia, or to decrease the effects of acetylcholine.
The introduction of levodopa, which increases the dopamine levels in the striatum, has produced a considerable improvement in the quality of

life for many patients. Symptomatic relief and side-effects have to be balanced to find the optimum dosage. Improvements in drug therapy have decreased the requirement for stereotactic surgery. The future of embryonic brain tissue transplants is at present unknown. In addition, significant ethical considerations are raised (Editorial 1988).

Preoperative abnormalities

1. The main features are progressive akinesia, increased muscle tone with 'cogwheel' rigidity, and a tremor which is increased with stress, decreased during action, and absent during sleep. Postural changes involve flexion of the head and body. Symptoms may be asymmetrical. The facies becomes expressionless, giving a false impression of disinterest or poor cerebral function. However, the subject is usually intellectually unimpaired, although dementia or depression may occur in the later stages of the disease.
2. Drug therapy depends on the symptoms and stage of the disease. In the early stages, anticholinergics may ameliorate tremor and rigidity. Levodopa is appropriate when postural changes and akinesia develop. As only 5% of the drug crosses the blood–brain barrier, and the rest is broken down by dopa decarboxylase, large doses have to be given. However, the dose, and hence the side-effects due to high peripheral levels of levodopa metabolites, can be reduced by as much as 75% when it is combined with an inhibitor of extracerebral dopa decarboxylase, such as carbidopa or benserazide.

Anaesthetic problems

1. Arrhythmias may occur in patients taking high doses of levodopa alone without a decarboxylase inhibitor, due to metabolism to dopamine. However, the half-life is only 4 hours. The concomitant use of carbidopa reduces dopaminergic side-effects.
2. Orthostatic hypotension may occur in patients on chronic levodopa therapy. This may be due to a combination of decreased intravascular volume, decreased noradrenaline production and reduction of noradrenaline stores.
3. If levodopa is stopped completely in the perioperative period, the patient will become rigid and immobile. Maintenance of adequate ventilation may be difficult. The risks of venous thrombosis and respiratory restriction are then increased.
4. Phenothiazines and butyrophenones antagonize levodopa and may cause a deterioration in the Parkinson's disease.
5. Levodopa can interact with direct-acting sympathomimetic amines and monoamine oxidase inhibitors to cause severe hypertension.
6. Autonomic dysfunction has been described in advanced disease.
7. Suxamethonium-induced hyperkalaemia (4.2–7.6 mmol/l) occurred in

a patient with poorly controlled Parkinsonism (Gravlee 1980). This occurred during induction of anaesthesia for CABG, when a number of drugs had been given. Levodopa had been stopped for 5 days.
8. The theoretical possibility that high dose opioid/nitrous oxide anaesthesia may be dangerous, on the grounds that opioid-induced rigidity resembles Parkinson's disease, has been suggested (Severn 1988). As yet, this has not been supported by clinical reports.

Management

1. The patient's current drug therapy must be known. If levodopa alone is being given, then it should be stopped 12–24 hours before surgery. If, as in most cases, it is being given in combination with a dopa decarboxylase inhibitor, then the drugs can be given up to the time of surgery.
2. Medication should be continued after surgery, by nasogastric tube if necessary.
3. Evidence of autonomic neuropathy should be sought.
4. Careful cardiovascular monitoring for arrhythmias, hypotension and hypertension. If intravascular volume is decreased, colloids may be required.
5. Regional anaesthesia may be inadvisable in certain patients, if they are on complex drug regimens, or if there is a suggestion of autonomic neuropathy.
6. The use of ketamine in one patient with severe disease taking levodopa was reported to have greatly improved tremor and rigidity for several hours (Hetherington & Rosenblatt 1980).

BIBLIOGRAPHY

Editorial 1984 Surgery and long-term medication: Parkinsonism. Drugs and Therapeutics Bulletin 22: 75
Editorial 1988 Embryos and Parkinson's disease. Lancet i: 1087
Gravlee G P 1980 Succinylcholine-induced hyperkalaemia in a patient with Parkinson's disease. Anesthesia and Analgesia 59: 444–446
Hetherington A, Rosenblatt R M 1980 Ketamine and paralysis agitans. Anesthesiology 52: 527
Severn A 1988 Parkinsonism and the anaesthetist. British Journal of Anaesthesia 61: 761–770

PERICARDIAL DISEASE
(see CARDIAC TAMPONADE)

PHAEOCHROMOCYTOMA
(see also Section 4)

A rare catecholamine-secreting tumour, which usually originates in the adrenal gland, but may arise from anywhere in the sympathetic chain.

Secretion of noradrenaline is more common than adrenaline. Diagnosis may be made preoperatively, in which case adrenergic blockade must be instituted before surgery, or as soon as the diagnosis is made. Rarely it may present unexpectedly during operation, or in labour as a life-threatening crisis (see Section 4). In these cases the presenting features include tachycardia, hypertension, pulmonary oedema and sudden death. Phaeochromocytomas may feature in a number of rare syndromes which include neurofibromatosis, von Hippel–Lindau syndrome and the multiple endocrine neoplasias.

Preoperative abnormalities

1. Episodes of headache, sweating and palpitations are the commonest presenting symptoms. The majority of patients have two or more of these complaints. If none of the three are present, or if flushing is a feature, then phaeochromocytoma is almost certainly not the cause (Bravo & Gifford 1984).
2. Persistent hypertension occurs in 50% of cases. In most of the remaining patients it is episodic.
3. Patients are frequently thin, appear anxious and may be peripherally vasoconstricted. Preoperative adrenergic blockade, with the accompanying expansion of the vascular volume, often causes the patient's face to fill out.
4. A number of cases have been reported in which cardiac failure has occurred in conjunction with a phaeochromocytoma. It has been suggested that a cardiomyopathy, secondary to the chronic high levels of catecholamines, occurs more frequently than has been recognized (Gilsanz et al 1983).
5. Biochemical diagnosis involves the initial screening of at least three 24-hour urine collections for catecholamine metabolites. Measurement of urinary HMMA (3-hydroxy 4-methoxy mandelic acid; sometimes called VMA or vanillylmandelic acid), or urinary metadrenalines can be done. The latter is more accurate.

Should the screening tests prove positive, then direct plasma adrenaline and noradrenaline estimations can be performed but special laboratory facilities may be required. If the levels are only slightly elevated in the presence of hypertension, then the diagnosis is unlikely. Patients with phaeochromocytomas become less sensitive than normal patients to catecholamines. Thus, in a patient with a phaeochromocytoma who has hypertension, plasma catecholamines are likely to be at least twice normal levels (Brown 1987).

A number of drugs, including l-dopa, methyl dopa and MAOIs, may interfere with the biochemical tests.

Several provocation and suppression tests have been described for cases in which the diagnosis is in doubt. However, the provocation tests are dangerous and should not be used. Suppression of plasma catecholamine levels with pentolinium and clonidine will occur with physiologically raised levels, but not where the catecholamines are tumour generated.

6. Ninety per cent of tumours are adrenal in origin and are bilateral in 10% of cases. If adrenaline constitutes at least 20% of the total plasma catecholamines, then the tumour is likely to be in the adrenal (Brown 1987). This is so because the synthesis of adrenaline from noradrenaline is dependent on the presence of high levels of glucocorticoids, which are carried to the medulla in blood from the cortex.

For accurate localization, a CT scan is now the first line of investigation. Provided that the tumours are more than 1 cm in diameter, over 90% of tumours will be identified.

Radioisotope meta-iodobenzylguanidine (mIBG) scanning has been reported to assist in both diagnosis and treatment of malignant tumours. mIBG is similar to noradrenaline in structure and is taken up and concentrated in the storage granules of chromaffin tissue. Imaging takes place at 24, 48 and 72 hours. Adrenergic tissue is thus located (Editorial 1984). In cases where the site is still in doubt, selective venous sampling from the inferior vena cava, or arteriography, may be necessary. Preoperative adrenergic blocking must be performed.

Anaesthetic problems

1. Problems during anaesthesia in the untreated patient
The undiagnosed, or the diagnosed but unblocked patient, is greatly at risk from hypertensive crises, particularly during arteriography, anaesthesia, surgery or delivery. In the past, prior to the introduction of preoperative adrenergic blocking, the mortality from surgery was 25–40%. The risks in the undiagnosed case having incidental surgery (Sutton et al 1981), or occurring in association with pregnancy (Mitchell et al 1987), remain high. Major problems are:

a. Severe hypertension and tachycardia, with the risk of cerebral haemorrhage, encephalopathy, pulmonary oedema, myocardial infarction, ventricular fibrillation and renal failure. This may occur at induction and intubation, during handling of the tumour, or in labour during uterine contractions. Hypertension can also be precipitated if a beta blocker is administered alone, before alpha blockade has been established. This is due to the removal of the beta vasodilator effects thus leaving the vasoconstrictor alpha effects totally unopposed.

b. Severe hypotension following removal of the tumour, due to hypovolaemia and the sudden decrease in circulating catecholamines. Before adrenergic blockade, this was usually treated with noradrenaline or adrenaline infusions, and the patient frequently died in a state of profound vasoconstriction and hypotension.

2. Formerly, a request for only partial preoperative blockade was often made by the surgeon, in order to assess, after initial tumour removal, whether or not a second was present. Improved methods of tumour location have now made this much less necessary. In practice, however, some hypertensive response to tumour handling often occurs.

Management

1. Diagnosis of the phaeochromocytoma and location of tumour.
2. Pharmacological treatment with adrenergic blocking agents.
This is the most crucial part of the patient's management. Preparation with oral drugs should be undertaken for at least 10–14 days to allow gradual re-expansion of vascular volume. The patient is saline depleted, commonly manifest by postural hypotension. Thus, during the period of vasodilatation, i.v. repletion may be necessary. Criteria for the adequacy of blockade have been specified (Roizen et al 1982). They require that there must be control of blood pressure without undue postural hypotension, control of major symptoms, and 2 weeks' freedom from ST- and T-wave changes on ECG. A number of regimens have been described. The choice will depend upon individual preference.

    a. Phenoxybenzamine oral 10 mg b.d. initially, increasing gradually until hypertension is controlled. Between 80 and 200 mg may be required. At least 10 days' treatment will be needed.

    b. If a tachycardia develops, then a beta blocker, propranolol 40–80 mg daily, increasing gradually if necessary, should be given.

If ischaemic heart disease is present, blocking should be instituted very cautiously to prevent sudden hypotension or tachycardia.

Occasionally, intravenous blocking may be required. This should take a minimum of 3 days. There should be close monitoring by medical staff throughout the procedure, particularly in patients with a degree of myocardial ischaemia.

> Day 1:
> Phenoxybenzamine 1 mg/kg in 500 ml 5% dextrose over 2 hours.
> Propranolol orally if pulse rate above 120/min.
> Day 2:
> Phenoxybenzamine 1–1.5 mg/kg over 2 hours.
> Propranolol to keep pulse rate below 100/min.
> Day 3:
> Phenoxybenzamine 1–2 mg/kg over 2 hours.
> Propranolol as necessary.
> Day of operation
> Phenoxybenzamine 50 mg.
> Propranolol as necessary.

At this stage the BP should be 110/70 and pulse rate <90/min.

Other suggested methods of preoperative adrenergic blocking:

a. Prazosin, an alpha$_1$ receptor antagonist

Recent work has shown that there is more than one alpha adrenergic receptor site. Alpha$_1$ receptors are postsynaptic whereas alpha$_2$ are presynaptic. It appears that stimulation of the alpha$_2$ receptors has an inhibiting effect on the release of noradrenaline from the nerve terminal. Blocking of these receptors therefore will enhance the release of noradrenaline (Hoffman & Lefkowitz 1980). Phentolamine and phenoxybenzamine block both types of receptor, and the resultant tachycardia from the use of these drugs is said to be due to cardiac beta receptor stimulation.

Prazosin is a selective alpha$_1$ blocker and does not usually produce a tachycardia. Its use for preoperative preparation has been reported in four patients (Nicholson et al 1983). An initial test dose of prazosin 1 mg only was given, as sudden hypotension has been described in some subjects (Wallace & Gill 1978). On the basis of the response to this, further doses were prescribed. Satisfactory preoperative stabilization was produced with between 6 and 16 mg prazosin. However, all four patients had marked hypertensive responses during surgery, which required phentolamine infusion, and in one case, surgery was abandoned to allow treatment with phenoxybenzamine for 2 weeks. Prazosin alone therefore may not provide the best protection from the effects of high catecholamine levels produced during surgery.

b. Labetalol, a combined alpha and beta blocker

Its beta effects are three to seven times those of its alpha effects and it is therefore potentially dangerous in patients with phaeochromocytomas. Paradoxical severe hypertension has been reported following its use (Navaratnarajah & White 1984).

c. Alpha methylparatyrosine has been used to achieve blockade by generation of a false transmitter.

3. Anaesthetic technique

A wide variety of techniques and drugs have been advocated. After a randomized trial of four anaesthetic methods, it was concluded that the choice of technique was not the crucial factor in patient outcome (Roizen et al 1982). Adequacy of preoperative adrenergic blockade was probably of more importance.

The aim is to provide conditions under which catecholamine release by the tumour, or the effect of any catecholamines released, is kept to a minimum. Intubation, handling of the tumour, and certain drugs are known stimuli. A sedative premedication and a quiet, unhurried induction of anaesthesia are essential.

Both morphine and pethidine release histamine, and atropine may produce a tachycardia. Droperidol has been advocated, but there have been reports of pressor responses, possibly due to inhibition of catecholamine uptake (Sumikawa & Amakata 1977). Suxamethonium is traditionally avoided, as fasciculations increase intra-abdominal pressure.

Although total epidural anaesthesia has been reported (Cousins & Rubin 1974), it may be disadvantageous to add a further uncontrollable factor to the already complicated pharmacophysiological situation. Patients with epidural blockade are often very sensitive to circulating catecholamines (Hull 1986).

Pancuronium has been used on many occasions in the past but hypertension has been reported (Jones & Hill 1981). Vecuronium is a more logical substitute as it avoids the hypertension and tachycardia produced by pancuronium.

Halothane sensitises the heart to the effect of catecholamines.

4. Monitoring

Direct arterial monitoring should begin in the anaesthetic room. Measurement of central venous pressure, $ETCO_2$, urine output and neuromuscular monitoring are required.

5. Treatment of intraoperative complications

a. Hypertension

Phentolamine, sodium nitroprusside and nitroglycerin have all been used. The choice again depends on individual preference. Phentolamine causes a tachycardia, whereas sodium nitroprusside may produce swings in blood pressure, with hypotension occurring when tumour stimulation stops. Magnesium sulphate has been used to control the blood pressure in a pregnant patient (James et al 1988). Magnesium inhibits the release of catecholamines from the adrenal medulla, decreases the sensitivity of alpha adrenergic receptors, and causes direct vasodilatation.

b. Tachycardia

This usually responds to beta blockers, propranolol i.v. 1–2 mg being the most frequently used. The author has observed bronchospasm in one non-asthmatic patient, occurring 2 hours after operation. In asthmatic patients, a cardioselective blocker, such as practolol or atenolol, may be more appropriate.

If there is heart failure, beta blockers may not be suitable. Amiodarone has been used to treat a tachycardia in a patient with phaeochromocytoma and a cardiomyopathy (Solares et al 1986).

c. Hypotension

May occur after ligation of the main veins from the tumour. Sudden reduction in catecholamine output by the tumour is in part responsible, but hypovolaemia may contribute. Patients with adrenergic blockade are very sensitive to changes in blood volume. Rapid infusion and CVP monitoring will usually correct the hypotension. If this fails, the use of phenylephrine or dopamine has been suggested (Roizen et al 1982).

BIBLIOGRAPHY

Bravo E L, Gifford R W 1984 Pheochromocytoma: diagnosis, localisation and management. New England Journal of Medicine 311: 1298–1303

Brown M J 1987 The measurement of autonomic function in clinical practice. Journal of the Royal College of Physicians 21: 206–209

Cousins M J, Rubin R B 1974 The intraoperative management of phaeochromocytoma with total epidural sympathetic blockade. British Journal of Anaesthesia 46: 78–81

Editorial 1984 Iodobenzylguanidine for location and treatment of phaeochromocytoma. Lancet ii: 905–907

Gilsanz F J, Luengo C, Conejero P, Peral P, Avello F 1983 Cardiomyopathy and phaeochromocytoma. Anaesthesia 38: 888–891

Hoffman B B, Lefkowitz R J 1980 Alpha-adrenergic receptor subtypes. New England Journal of Medicine 302; 1390–1396

Hull C J 1986 Phaeochromocytoma. Diagnosis, preoperative preparation and management. British Journal of Anaesthesia 58: 1453–1468

James M F M, Huddle K R L, Owen A D, van der Veen B W 1988 Use of magnesium sulphate in the anaesthetic management of phaeochromocytoma in pregnancy. Canadian Journal of Anaesthesia 35: 178–182

Jones R M, Hill A B 1981 Severe hypertension associated with pancuronium in a patient with phaeochromocytoma. Canadian Anaesthetists' Society Journal 28: 394–396

Mitchell S Z, Freilich J D, Brant D, Flynn M 1987 Anesthetic management of pheochromocytoma resection during pregnancy. Anesthesia and Analgesia 66: 478–480

Navaratnarajah M, White D C 1984 Labetolol and phaeochromocytoma. British Journal of Anaesthesia 56: 1179

Nicholson J P, Vaughn E D, Pickering T G et al 1983 Pheochromocytoma and prazosin. Annals of Internal Medicine 99: 477–479

Roizen M F, Horrigan R W, Koike M et al 1982 A prospective randomised trial of four anesthetic techniques for resection of pheochromocytoma. Anesthesiology 57: A43

Solares G, Ramos F, Martin-Duran R, San-Jose J M, Buitrago M 1986 Amiodarone, phaeochromocytoma and cardiomyopathy. Anaesthesia 41: 186–190

Sumikawa K, Amakata Y 1977 The pressor effect of droperidol on a patient with phaeochromocytoma. Anesthesiology 46: 359–361

Sutton M St J, Sheps S G, Lie J T 1981 Prevalence of clinically unsuspected phaeochromocytoma. Mayo Clinic Proceedings 56: 354–360

Wallace J M, Gill D P 1978 Prazosin in diagnosis and treatment of pheochromocytoma. Journal of the American Medical Association 240: 2752–2753

PIERRE ROBIN SYNDROME

A rare syndrome in which the combination of severe micrognathia and posterior prolapse of the tongue, results in respiratory obstruction in infancy. Other congenital abnormalities such as cleft palate and oesophageal atresia may occur.

Preoperative abnormalities

1. In early life, micrognathia and glossoptosis cause breathing and feeding difficulties, with episodes of cyanosis when the child is in the supine position. A number of manoeuvres have been tried in an attempt to minimize respiratory obstruction and permit safe feeding. Nursing in the prone position is required, and suturing of the tongue to the lower gum may be needed. Feeding may be undertaken via a nasogastric tube or a gastrostomy. Occasionally tracheostomy is required.

As the child grows, the obstruction tends to improve. It has been suggested that obstruction is primarily due to the tongue being drawn backwards by the negative pressure created during inspiration, rather than passively falling back (Mallory & Paradise 1979). The improvement with age may result not so much from growth of the mandible, but from the increase in voluntary control of tongue muscles.

2. Cleft palate occurs in 60%, and eye problems in 40% of patients.

3. Chronic upper airway obstruction can result in cor pulmonale (Mallory & Paradise 1979). A raised pulmonary artery pressure may produce right to left shunting through a patent foramen ovale or a persistent ductus arteriosus. Anaesthesia for cardiac catheterization in an infant with cor pulmonale, and subsequent management of the airway obstruction for a month by means of a nasopharyngeal tube, has been described (Freeman & Manners 1980).

4. Obstructive sleep apnoea has been reported (Brouillette et al 1982).

Anaesthetic problems

1. Even in the unanaesthetized infant, during the first few months of life, respiratory obstruction occurs in the supine position.

2. The unusual facial configuration, due to the receding lower jaw, makes it difficult to maintain an airtight fit with the anaesthetic mask.

3. Difficulties in endotracheal intubation result from a combination of micrognathia, and prolapse or inward sucking of the posteriorly attached, and often enlarged, tongue.

Management

1. Methods to overcome the problem of difficult intubation have been proposed:

a. An understanding of the precise problems posed by mandibular hypoplasia according to Handler & Keon (1983). This well-illustrated account corrects the impression created on laryngoscopy, and given in some texts, that the larynx is anteriorly placed. In fact this is not so. It is the posterior placement of the tongue, due to its attachment to the hypoplastic mandible which is the prime cause of the problems. In the supine position, aided by the effects of gravity, the tongue drops back and completely obscures the larynx. A technique for intubation was described, for the anaesthetized spontaneously breathing patient, in which a Jackson anterior commissure laryngoscope is used.

The head is elevated above the shoulders, with flexion of the lower cervical vertebrae and extension at the atlanto-occipital joint. The larynogoscope is introduced into the right side of the mouth. Only the tip is directed towards the midline, the proximal end remaining laterally, so that a further 30° of anterior angulation can be obtained. The narrow closed blade prevents the tongue from falling in and obscuring the view of the larynx. When visualized, the epiglottis is elevated, and the larynx entered. Intubation is then achieved by passing a lubricated tube, without its adaptor, down the laryngoscope. It is then held in place with alligator forceps while the laryngoscope is withdrawn.

1

b. The realization of the problems caused by gravity acting on the tongue and mandible in the supine position led to the description of a successful blind nasal intubation with the patient prone (Populaire et al 1985). This position allows the tongue and mandible to fall forward under the effect of gravity and leave the larynx exposed.

c. A fibreoptic bronchoscopic technique has been described (Howardy-Hansen & Berthelsen 1988). In small infants, the 'tube over bronchoscope' technique is not possible because of the smallness of the tube, therefore a Seldinger type approach is necessary. After the administration of atropine, ketamine i.m. and topical lignocaine, a fibreoptic bronchoscope (OD 3.6 mm, L 60 cm and suction channel 1.2 mm) was passed through one nostril. The tongue was held forward with Magill forceps until the vocal cords were seen, but not entered, because of the risk of total obstruction. Under direct vision, a Teflon-coated guide wire with a flexible tip was passed via the suction channel into the trachea. The bronchoscope was carefully removed leaving the wire in place, and a 3 mm nasotracheal tube then passed over it into the trachea.

BIBLIOGRAPHY

Brouillette R T, Fernbach S K, Hunt C E 1982 Obstructive sleep apnea in infants and children. Journal of Pediatrics 100: 31–40
Freeman M K, Manners J M 1980 Cor pulmonale and the Pierre Robin anomaly. Anaesthesia 35: 282–286
Handler S D, Keon T P 1983 Difficult laryngoscopy/intubation: the child with mandibular hypoplasia. Annals of Otology, Rhinology and Laryngology 92: 401–404
Howardy-Hansen P, Berthelsen P 1988 Fibreoptic bronchoscopic nasotracheal intubation of a neonate with Pierre Robin syndrome. Anaesthesia 43: 121–122
Mallory S B, Paradise J L 1979 Glossoptosis revisited: on the development and resolution of airway obstruction in the Pierre-Robin syndrome. Pediatrics 64: 946–948
Populaire C, Lundi J N, Pinaud M, Souron R 1985 Elective tracheal intubation in the prone position for a neonate with Pierre-Robin syndrome. Anesthesiology 62: 214–215

PLASMA CHOLINESTERASE ABNORMALITIES
(see also Section 4)

Plasma cholinesterase (ChE) is present in plasma and most other tissues, apart from erythrocytes, and is an enzyme capable of hydrolysing many esters. It must be distinguished from acetylcholinesterase (AChE), which is found in erythrocytes and at the neuromuscular junction. ChE is a protein manufactured in the liver and its half-life is thought to be approximately 8–12 days. No physiological role for the enzyme has as yet been unequivocally demonstrated.

Its anaesthetic significance lies in the fact that it hydrolyses the depolarizing muscle relaxant suxamethonium, thus terminating its action after 1–5 minutes. In the presence of normal ChE activity, a two-stage hydrolysis of suxamethonium occurs.

succinyl dicholine + water → succinyl monocholine + choline
$$\downarrow$$
succinic acid + choline

If there is a low level of normal plasma cholinesterase, or if the cholinesterase is abnormal, prolonged apnoea may occur. In either case, following suxamethonium administration, the duration of muscle paralysis can vary from about 10 minutes to 2 hours. Decreased ChE activity may be due to genetic variants of the enzyme, pre-existing disease, or iatrogenic causes.

Genetic variants

Plasma cholinesterase synthesis is controlled by two allelic genes, the normal genotype being designated $E_1^u E_1^u$. There are several genetic defects which result in an individual having a diminished ability to metabolize suxamethonium (Whittaker et al 1980).

Differentiation between the normal and an atypical cholinesterase was first demonstrated by comparing the rates at which each hydrolysed benzoylcholine, in the presence of varying concentrations of an inhibitor, dibucaine. The percentage inhibition by a 10^{-5} molar concentration of dibucaine is known as the dibucaine number. Homozygous individuals for the atypical (or dibucaine-resistant) genotype ($E_1^a E_1^a$) have a dibucaine number about 20, heterozygotes ($E_1^u E_1^a$) about 60, and those with normal enzyme, about 80. Further genetic variants have subsequently been found. These include a 'silent' gene, E_1^s, which has little or no enzymic activity, and a fluoride-resistant gene, E_1^f. The fluoride number is determined in a similar way to the dibucaine number, but sodium fluoride is used as the inhibitor.

The distribution of the genotypes in suxamethonium-sensitive individuals has been studied by Whittaker and Britten (1987). So far, more than 12 genotypes have been recognized. As ChE is a large molecule of four polypeptide chains, it is likely that further variants will be described.

The main categories of subjects sensitive to suxamethonium have the genotypes $E_1^a E_1^a$ and $E_1^a E_1^s$, and their frequency is about 1 in 1800.

Disease states

Low levels of normal enzyme have been reported in association with a number of pathological conditions. These include severe liver disease, malnutrition, renal failure, malignant disease, tetanus, Huntington's chorea and collagen disorders.

Pregnancy

In late pregnancy, there may also be decreased ChE activity, although not necessarily to such a degree as to produce clinical problems. However, two circumstances have been reported in which problems may arise.

a. The use of plasmapheresis in the treatment of rhesus isoimmunization is associated with marked reduction in maternal ChE activity (Whittaker et al 1988). A patient with a normal phenotype was reported to have been apnoeic for 50 minutes following suxamethonium 75 mg. This was given during a Caesarean section undertaken 2 days after the seventh plasmapheresis, and was associated with very low ChE activity (Evans et al 1980).
b. The heterozygous patient. Pregnancy can also cause clinically detectable apnoea in a heterozygous patient, which would not normally be manifested in the non-pregnant patient, and especially if a suxamethonium infusion is used (Whittaker et al 1988).

Iatrogenic causes

Reported iatrogenic associations include radiotherapy, renal dialysis, plasmapheresis, cardiac bypass, cytotoxic drugs, ecothiopate eye drops, oral contraceptives, propanidid, neostigmine, chlorpromazine, pancuronium and exposure to organophosphorus compounds.

Anaesthetic problems

1. In individuals with suxamethonium sensitivity, varying lengths of apnoea can follow the administration of suxamethonium. By the use of a peripheral nerve stimulator, apnoea from this cause may be distinguished from that due to other causes.
2. If suxamethonium sensitivity is confirmed, subsequent investigation of the patient, and if possible his close relatives, is required.

Management

1. When spontaneous respiration fails to return after the administration of suxamethonium, IPPV should be continued. Light anaesthesia must be maintained to prevent the patient becoming distressed. The presence of a neuromuscular blockade should be confirmed with a peripheral nerve stimulator. This is most important as about 30% of patients referred to the Cholinesterase Research Unit have a normal phenotype. The routine use of a nerve stimulator might influence this figure. IPPV should be continued until adequate respiration can be maintained.
2. When the patient has recovered, detailed anaesthetic, family and drug histories should be taken. A simple explanation of the need for further investigation should be given.
3. Plasma cholinesterase activity, dibucaine and fluoride numbers should be investigated. While this may be done in a local laboratory, there are advantages of using the service provided by the Cholinesterase Research Unit.

A rapid service can be obtained, by sending 10 ml heparinized or whole blood, or separated plasma or serum, by first class post, to Dr J. Britten, Cholinesterase Research Unit, Royal Postgraduate Medical School, Hammersmith Hospital, London (Whittaker & Britten 1987).

BIBLIOGRAPHY

Evans R T, MacDonald R, Robinson A 1980 Suxamethonium apnoea associated with plasmapheresis. Anaesthesia 35: 198–201
Whittaker M 1980 Plasma cholinesterase variants and the anaesthetist. Anaesthesia 35: 174–197
Whittaker M, Britten J J 1987 Phenotyping of individuals sensitive to suxamethonium. British Journal of Anaesthesia 59: 1052–1055
Whittaker M, Crawford J S, Lewis M 1988 Some observations of levels of plasma cholinesterase activity within an obstetric population. Anaesthesia 43: 42–45

POLYCYTHAEMIA VERA

Polycythaemia is a general term for an increased haemoglobin, red cell count or packed cell volume. It can be relative, due to a reduction in plasma volume, or absolute due to increased red cell mass. Absolute polycythaemia can be primary or secondary. Causes of secondary polycythaemia include pulmonary disease, cyanotic heart disease and inappropriate production of erythropoietin. The primary disease, polycythaemia vera, is a neoplastic condition and is one of the chronic myeloproliferative diseases. Surgery in an untreated polycythaemic carries a high risk of either thrombotic or bleeding complications.

Preoperative abnormalities

1. Occurs most commonly in men, usually over 50 years of age. Patients can present with a range of symptoms due to hyperviscosity, a thrombotic or a bleeding episode or a high haemoglobin found on routine testing.
2. Splenomegaly, hepatomegaly and hypertension are common.
3. Haematological abnormalities include a high haemoglobin, an increased red cell mass and packed cell volume (50–70%), and often a leucocytosis and thrombocythaemia. A venous haematocrit of >0.50 in males and >0.47 in females is suggested as being sufficient to warrant further investigation (Pearson 1980). A high incidence of vascular occlusion is found when the platelet count is >400 × 10^9/l (Pearson 1980). The diagnosis should also be considered in patients with a normal haemoglobin but a microcytosis. This may be due to slow blood loss from the gastrointestinal tract, resulting in severe iron deficiency.
4. Platelet function may be abnormal.
5. Hyperuricaemia and secondary gout is common.
6. The method of treatment is controversial. It may involve venesection to keep the PCV below 50%, radioactive phosphorus, busulphan or hydroxyurea.

Anaesthetic problems

1. Patients may present for emergency surgery. In a study involving 200 patients, nearly 50% presented with vascular complications (Barabas 1980). Seventy-eight arterial complications occurred in 68 patients, 66 venous complications in 57 patients, and there were 27 patients who had both. Distal arterial disease is more common than that involving major vessels.

2. Despite being primarily a thrombotic condition, bleeding can also occur due to abnormal platelet function. A history of recurrent nose bleeds is common and gastrointestinal haemorrhage may occur. One patient presented with a spontaneous retropharyngeal haematoma and emergency intubation for airway obstruction was required (Mackenzie & Jellicoe 1986). Patients with polycythaemia may occasionally be anaemic secondary to bleeding, in which case the diagnosis may not be immediately obvious.

3. Increases in total blood volume and the presence of a high blood viscosity increase both the cardiac output, and the work of the heart. Cerebral blood flow is low, and this contributes to the high incidence of cerebrovascular occlusion.

4. Cyanosis occurs readily.

5. If a patient presents for surgery with a high haemoglobin and a raised haematocrit, problems may arise in deciding rapidly whether the polycythaemia is primary, or secondary to respiratory disease. In the first case cerebral blood flow will be low, and venesection is appropriate, while in the second, it is not.

Management

1. If a high haemoglobin and a raised haematocrit is found, arterial blood gases can be done. The presence of hypoxia or hypercarbia may suggest a respiratory cause. Other causes of secondary polycythaemia should be sought. If polycythaemia vera is likely, elective surgery should be postponed until there is medical control of the condition. It has been suggested that the peripheral blood picture and the blood volume should be normal for at least 4 months preoperatively (Barabas 1980).

2. If emergency surgery is required, venesection should be performed, and the volume replaced with the same volume of PPF or colloid. The decreased cerebral blood flow is increased as the venous haematocrit is reduced (Pearson 1980).

3. Prevention of venous stasis.

4. Extremes of hypotension and hypertension should be avoided.

5. Anticoagulants are inadvisable, as bleeding may occur.

BIBLIOGRAPHY

Barabas A P 1980 Surgical problems associated with polycythaemia. British Journal of Hospital Medicine 23: 289–294

Mackenzie J W, Jellicoe J A 1986 Acute upper airway obstruction. Spontaneous retropharyngeal haematoma in a patient with polycythaemia rubra vera. Anaesthesia 41: 57–59

Pearson T C 1980 Who should you treat for polycythaemia? British Journal of Hospital Medicine 24: 66–73

POMPE'S DISEASE

A glycogen storage disease, type IIa, in which there is a deficiency of alpha-1,4-glucosidase (acid maltase). This enzyme is present in lysosomes and involved in glycogen breakdown. Glycogen deposits are found in cardiac, skeletal and smooth muscle, kidney, liver, spleen, brain, spinal cord and tongue. Three different modes of presentation are now recognized (Howell & Williams 1983). The most severely affected patients present with cardiac failure in the first 3 months of life, and usually die in the first year. There is a less severe form appearing in infancy, with death before adulthood. A third form presents as a myopathy in the 20–40 year age group. Anaesthesia may be required for diagnostic muscle biopsy, cardiac catheterization or bronchoscopy.

Preoperative abnormalities

1. There is generalized hypotonia and muscle weakness, although muscle mass is normal.
2. The heart is greatly enlarged due to a hypertrophic cardiomyopathy. Outflow obstruction due to enlargement of the interventricular septum occurs in 50% of patients. Murmurs are usually absent. Cardiac failure rapidly supervenes.
3. CXR shows massive biventricular hypertrophy. Lobar collapse is common due to bronchial obstruction.
4. ECG shows a short PR interval (<0.09 seconds) and massive, wide QRS complexes.
5. Glucose, lactate and lipid levels are normal. Muscle enzymes are moderately raised.
6. Cardiorespiratory failure, pulmonary aspiration and pneumonia all contribute towards death in the most severe form of the disease.

Anaesthetic problems

1. Problems associated with cardiomyopathies and cardiac failure. Inhalational induction with halothane resulted in bradycardia and ventricular fibrillation in a 5-month-old baby (McFarlane & Soni 1986) and cardiac arrest occurred in a child having a muscle biopsy (Ellis 1980). In the latter case, the diagnosis of Pompe's disease was only made at post-mortem examination. Outflow tract obstruction often occurs, and the diseased muscle of the ventricles cannot compensate by hypertrophy and

increased contractility. Massive cardiomegaly may produce lobar collapse by bronchial compression.

2. Muscle weakness can predispose to respiratory failure.

3. Macroglossia may occur and can cause upper airway obstruction and difficult intubation. It has also been suggested that protrusion of the tongue secondary to respiratory distress gives a false impression of macroglossia (McFarlane & Soni 1986).

4. Impaired neurological function depresses cough and swallowing reflexes and predisposes to aspiration, atelectasis and pneumonia. All these factors may contribute to hypoxia.

5. Patients are sensitive to respiratory depressants.

Management

1. The importance of monitoring and the avoidance of hypoxia has been stressed (McFarlane & Soni 1986). Two anaesthetics were given to the same patient a week apart. The first, a halothane induction, began without monitoring and ended with ventricular fibrillation and the abandonment of the procedure. In the second, direct arterial monitoring and subsequent induction were established with ketamine, and the patient then ventilated using vecuronium.

Ketamine, halothane and suxamethonium were used successfully on different occasions in two patients (Kaplan 1980). However, on the evidence of a limited number of case reports, induction with halothane in these patients may be hazardous. Whether this is due to the effect of halothane on the myocardium, or to hypoxia secondary to airway obstruction, is impossible to judge. Undoubtedly, if intubation and control of respiration are rapidly achieved, this will reduce the potential for hypoxia and the need for high concentrations of inhalation agents.

2. Doubts have been cast on the wisdom of using suxamethonium in a patient with any myopathy, in view of the risk of hyperkalaemia or rhabdomyolysis.

3. It has been suggested that muscle relaxants may not be required, as muscle hypotonia facilitates ventilation.

4. Local anaesthesia should be considered. Diagnostic muscle biopsy has been described using a modified femoral nerve block and a peripheral nerve stimulator. Ketamine was used for sedation (Rosen & Broadman 1986). Caudal anaesthesia has also been suggested as a suitable technique (Kaplan 1980).

5. If macroglossia is present, and the possibility of difficult intubation exists, awake intubation may be advisable.

BIBLIOGRAPHY

Ellis F R 1980 Inherited muscle disease. British Journal of Anaesthesia 52: 153–164
Howell R R, Williams J C 1983 The glycogen storage diseases. In: The Metabolic basis of inherited disease. McGraw Hill, New York

Kaplan R 1980 Pompe's disease presenting for anesthesia. Anesthesiology Review 7: 21–28
McFarlane H J, Soni N 1986 Pompe's disease and anaesthesia. Anaesthesia 41: 1219–1224
Rosen K R, Broadman L M 1986 Anaesthesia for diagnostic muscle biopsy in an infant with
   Pompe's disease. Canadian Anaesthetists' Society Journal 33: 790–794

PORPHYRIA

A group of disorders of porphyrin metabolism due to defects in certain
enzymes involved in the synthesis of haem. They may be inherited or
acquired. While porphyria is very rare in the UK, one type, variegate
porphyria, is common in certain regions of South Africa. As a result, much
of the clinical and experimental work on the subject originates from that
country.

Haem, which is synthesized in the liver, bone marrow and erythrocytes, is
required for the manufacture of haemoglobin, myoglobin and a number of
other respiratory pigments, such as the cytochrome enzymes.

In the hepatic porphyrias, only the liver is involved in the abnormality of
haem synthesis. It is this group of porphyrias which is of particular
concern to the anaesthetist, and only they are discussed. In each of these,
there is a different relative deficiency of one of the enzymes involved in
the hepatic synthesis of haem. The majority of haem manufactured by the
liver is used in the biosynthesis of the cytochrome P-450 enzyme system.
This system is important for drug metabolism.

The administration of certain drugs to patients with porphyria, can, on
occasions, result in serious neurological defects. Most of the drugs which
are potentially dangerous in porphyria can increase delta-
aminolaevulinic acid (ALA) synthase activity. This is the first enzyme
required to initiate the sequence which results in the manufacture of
haem. These drugs are usually lipid soluble, and to assist their excretion
by the kidneys, they require transformation into water-soluble compounds
by the cytochrome P-450 enzyme system. The presence of any of these
drugs can therefore increase the activity of this system. In other words,
they share the common property of being enzyme inducers of the
cytochrome P-450 system. A demand for haem secondary to this induction
of cytochrome P-450 results in a feedback mechanism stimulating
further production of ALA synthase. The hepatic haem metabolic pathway
is thus stimulated, but because the underlying enzyme deficiencies
cannot fully cope with this extra activity, there is an accumulation of
certain porphyrins or precursors at specific levels in the metabolic chain.
These levels will vary according to the particular relative enzyme
deficiency.

The exact relationship between the biochemistry, and the clinical
features of the porphyric crises and neurological deficits, is not known.

However, there are characteristic pathological lesions in the central nervous system, the spinal cord and the autonomic ganglia. Axon degeneration and demyelination are particular features. It has been suggested that the signs and symptoms of porphyria can be entirely attributed to neurological damage (Laiwah et al 1987). However, porphyrin precursors do not seem to be the main cause of the neurotoxicity, as has been previously postulated. Existing evidence suggests that the nervous system lesions are primarily due to a deficiency of haem, while neurotoxicity due to increased levels of ALA may be an additional factor in their evolution.

Preoperative abnormalities

1. The clinical and biochemical features of the hepatic porphyrias rarely appear before puberty, and some patients remain permanently asymptomatic. Symptoms, which depend on the particular type of porphyria, may involve the gastrointestinal tract, the nervous system and the skin. Intermittent acute crises, which may result in severe neurological deficits and occasionally death, may be precipitated by a variety of drugs. Crises may also be associated with menstruation, acute infection and pregnancy.
2. Clinical features of the individual types of porphyria
    a. Acute intermittent porphyria (AIP) is an autosomal dominant condition in which there is a reduction in porphobilinogen deaminase. During an attack there are increased amounts of ALA and porphobilinogen produced and excreted. AIP often presents with episodes of acute abdominal pain, vomiting and pyrexia in adult life. Motor, sensory or autonomic deficits may occur. There may be severe neuropsychiatric manifestations.
    b. Hereditary coproporphyria (HC) is a rare condition which is similar to AIP. There is a deficiency of coproporphyrinogen oxidase, so that coproporphyrin levels may be elevated, in addition to those of ALA and porphobilinogen.
    c. Variegate porphyria (VP) results from a deficiency of protoporphyrinogen oxidase; the enzymic block is therefore one step further on. Cutaneous lesions are also present in this condition, commonly on the hands and face. Photosensitivity is due to the presence of certain porphyrins in the skin.
3. In the screening test for porphobilinogen, the patient's urine turns dark red on the addition of Ehrlich's aldehyde. Specific tests exist for different precursors and/or porphyrins to elicit the exact type of porphyria.
4. Acute crises can vary in length from hours to days. Tachycardia and hypertension may occur during an attack.
5. Haematin, which suppresses ALA synthase activity, has been used to relieve the symptoms of porphyria.

Anaesthetic problems

1. Drug porphyrinogenicity

A wide range of drugs possess a potential for increasing the production of porphyrins or their precursors, thus precipitating an acute attack. The use of any of these drugs may result in severe neurological deficits, including paraplegia or quadriplegia.

As the overall number of patients with porphyria presenting for anaesthesia is small, experience with any individual anaesthetic drug is limited. In addition, a patient's response to a particular drug will vary according to the state of their porphyria. A retrospective analysis of 78 anaesthetics given to 47 patients, suggested that if the patient was in a latent period, the risks of using thiopentone were small. In contrast, seven out of ten patients given thiopentone during an acute episode had a worsening of porphyric symptoms (Mustajoki & Heinonen 1980). However, with such potentially devastating complications, the scope for prospective human 'studies' is limited.

For this reason, experimental models are being used to assess the porphyrinogenicity of certain anaesthetic drugs. Rats primed with 3,5-dicarbethoxy-1,4-dihydrocolidine (DDC) provide a model for latent variegate porphyria. With this system, various drugs have been tested for their ability to increase hepatic ALA synthase activity and produce intermediate porphyrins (Blekkenhorst et al 1980, Harrison et al 1985). While animal studies cannot necessarily be extrapolated to man, additional testing with known safe and unsafe drugs have provided some measure of control (Blekkenhorst et al 1980).

A simple method of drug classification has been suggested as a clinical guide to therapy in porphyria (Disler et al 1982):

> Category A:
> Drugs reported in terms of clinical experience as dangerous or safe by three or more authorities.
> Category B:
> As Category A, but reported by only two or fewer authorities.

> These two categories are usually associated with corroborated experimental animal data:
> Category C:
> Drugs evaluated only in the experimental rat model.
> Category D:
> Drugs evaluated in chick embryo liver cell culture or 'in ovo'.
> Neither Categories C nor D have corroborative reports of human cases.
> For some drugs the data is conflicting.

For detailed information on general prescribing, reference to Disler's article is recommended.

Probably dangerous drugs include:

barbiturates, carbamazepine, carbromal, chloramphenicol, chloridiazepoxide, cimetidine, ergot alkaloids, erythromycin, flunitrazepam, frusemide, glutethimide, griseofulvin, hydantoins, imipramine, meprobamate, methyl dopa, metoclopramide, nalidixic acid, nikethimide, nitrazepam, pargyline, pentazocine, phenoxybenzamine, steroids, sulphonamides, sulphonylurea antidiabetic agents, theophylline and tranylcypromine.

Possibly dangerous drugs:
A number of drugs have often been used without complication, but a single case report or experimental data exists, implicating it as being porphyrogenic. This group includes corticosteroids, diazepam, enflurane*, etomidate*, fentanyl*, halothane*, hydralazine, ketamine*, lignocaine*, pancuronium*, pethidine*, paraldehyde, and the sex hormones.
(* Drugs on which further comment is made below.)

Although a single dose of etomidate produced equivocal results using the DDC-primed rat model, a continuous infusion of etomidate caused an increase in ALA synthase, coproporphyrin and protoporphyrin levels. The authors of this study believed it should be considered as category C, and thus potentially porphyrinogenic (Harrison et al 1985). In this same study, ketamine did not produce any change. While a single case report has implicated ketamine as porphyrinogenic, there is clinical and experimental evidence suggesting that it is safe (Rizk et al 1977, Blekkenhorst et al 1980, Capouet et al 1987).
   Halothane, lignocaine, fentanyl, pethidine and pancuronium have been implicated in single case reports only, and have been used on other occasions without complication (Disler et al 1982).
2. Acute abdominal crises can cause undiagnosed porphyrics to be subjected to surgery. There may be an accompanying tachycardia and hypertension.
3. A porphyric crisis may last for several days and result in dehydration, hyponatraemia and hypokalaemia.
4. Local and regional techniques are inadvisable for medicolegal reasons. Any subsequent neurological deterioration due to the disease might be attributed to the procedure itself.
5. Fasting prior to surgery induces cytochrome P-450 enzyme activity.

Management

1. All drugs known to precipitate acute crises should be avoided. Individual clinical judgements must be made about the controversial ones, taking into account the presence or absence of an acute attack (see above).
2. Drugs which are reported to be safe in porphyrics (Disler et al 1982, Magnus 1984) include:

adrenaline, aminoglycosides, aspirin, atropine, beta blockers, biguanides, bupivacaine, buprenorphine, cephalosporins, chlorpheniramine, chlorpromazine, codeine, coumarins, diazoxide, digitalis, droperidol, d-tubocurarine, erythromycin, ether, heparin, hyoscine, insulin, labetolol, lorazepam, morphine, neostigmine, nitroglycerin, nitrous oxide, paracetamol, penicillins, procaine, prochlorperazine, promazine, promethazine, propranolol, sodium nitroprusside, suxamethonium, thyroxine and trifluoperazine.

3. Clinical and experimental reports have suggested that propofol may be safe (Mitterschiffthaler et al 1988). The safety of alcuronium, atracurium and vecuronium is not yet known.

4. A careful history and examination must be made, to document existing neurological deficits.

5. A patient admitted in a porphyric crisis may require correction of fluid and electrolyte balance. Tachycardia and hypertension may be treated with beta blockers.

6. Glucose administration inhibits enzyme induction and fasting increases it. Administration of dextrose should therefore begin before a period of starvation.

7. Haematin has been reported to be effective in aborting clinical episodes of porphyria, by decreasing ALA synthase activity. A haematin infusion has been used to treat increased urinary porphobilinogen levels in a patient following cardiopulmonary bypass (Roby and Harrison 1982).

BIBLIOGRAPHY

Blekkenhorst G H, Harrison G G, Cook E S, Eales L 1980 Screening of certain anaesthetic agents for their ability to elicit acute porphyric phases in susceptible patients. British Journal of Anaesthesia 52: 759–762

Capouet V, Dernovoi B, Azagra J S 1987 Induction of anaesthesia with ketamine during an acute crisis of hereditary coproporphyria. Canadian Journal of Anaesthesia 34: 388–390

Disler P B, Blekkenhorst G H, Eales L, Moore M R, Straughan J 1982 Guidelines for drug prescription in patients with the acute porphyrias. South African Medical Journal 61: 656–660

Harrison G G, Moore M R, Meissner P N 1985 Porphyrinogenicity of etomidate and ketamine as continuous infusions. British Journal of Anaesthesia 57: 420–423

Laiwah A C Y, Moore M R, Goldberg A 1987 Pathogenesis of acute porphyria. Quarterly Journal of Medicine 63: 377–392

Magnus I A 1984 Drugs and porphyria. British Medical Journal 288: 1474–1475

Mitterschiffthaler G, Theiner A, Hetzel H, Fuith L C 1988 Safe use of propofol in a patient with acute intermittent porphyria. British Journal of Anaesthesia 60: 109–111

Mustajoki P, Heinonen J 1980 General anesthesia in 'inducible' porphyrias. Anesthesiology 53: 15–20

Rizk S K, Jacobsen J H, Silvay G 1977 Ketamine as an induction agent for acute intermittent porphyria. Anesthesiology 46: 305–306

Roby H P, Harrison G A 1982 Anaesthesia for coronary artery bypass in a patient with porphyria variegata. Anaesthesia and Intensive Care 10: 276–278

PRADER–WILLI SYNDROME

A syndrome of unknown aetiology, in which obesity is associated with disturbances of carbohydrate and fat metabolism. It usually presents in infancy with hypotonia, and feeding and respiratory difficulties. Despite the hypotonia, no histological, biochemical or neurophysiological abnormalities of the muscle have been demonstrated. Obesity develops by the age of 3, and a non-insulin-dependent diabetes around 10. Orchidopexy is commonly required for undescended testes. Dental and orthopaedic surgery may also be needed.

Preoperative abnormalities

1. Obesity and hyperphagia develop from about the age of 3. Children are of small stature. Mental retardation is usual.
2. Abnormal glucose tolerance curves are recorded and episodes of hypoglycaemia may occur. A mild non-insulin-dependent diabetes develops around the age of 10. This may be secondary to obesity.
3. Enamel defects and dental caries are common.
4. Skeletal abnormalities include, a straight ulnar border and hand and finger anomalies.

Anaesthetic problems

There have been at least 12 reports of anaesthetics given to these patients (Mayhew & Taylor 1983, Palmer & Atlee 1976, Yamashita et al 1983). Some have been uneventful, in others a variety of complications have been described.

1. The general problems of obesity.
2. Disturbances of thermoregulation may occur. Two cases had fever and acidosis during anaesthesia, and in six, fever occurred in the postoperative period (Yamashita et al). In one child, intubation difficulty was experienced after suxamethonium (Mayhew & Taylor). The anaesthetic was continued with halothane and curare, but was terminated due to a rise in temperature. However, the postoperative CPK only rose to 240 u/l. A subsequent anaesthetic, in which pancuronium, nitrous oxide and fentanyl were used, was uneventful. Although comparisons with MH patients have been made, as yet, there is nothing to suggest that the episodes of fever originate from abnormal muscle metabolism. A hypothalamic mechanism would seem more likely.
3. Cardiac arrhythmias were reported in four cases. A fifth, an 8-year-old child, was having a pacemaker implanted for sick sinus syndrome.
4. Difficulty in intubation was reported in two cases, but its origins were not stated.
5. Episodes of hypoglycaemia have been reported.

6. Micrognathia, high-arched palate and scoliosis are sometimes associated.

7. Convulsions have been recorded.

8. Hypotonia has been noted. The cause has not been elucidated, but it is said to improve with age.

Management

1. Blood glucose should be monitored carefully, and a glucose infusion given pre- and intraoperatively.

2. ECG, core temperature and $ETCO_2$ should be monitored from the beginning of the anaesthetic.

3. In view of the obesity, a technique using IPPV is advisable. No prolongation of response to muscle relaxants has been reported, despite depolarizing and non-depolarizing drugs having been used.

BIBLIOGRAPHY

Mayhew J F, Taylor B 1983 Anaesthetic considerations in the Prader–Willi syndrome. Canadian Anaesthetists' Society Journal 30: 565–566
Palmer S K, Atlee J L 1976 Anesthetic management of the Prader–Willi syndrome. Anesthesiology 44: 161–163
Yamashita M, Koishi K, Yamaya R, Tsubo T, Matsuki A, Oyama T 1983 Anaesthetic considerations in the Prader–Willi syndrome. Canadian Anaesthetists' Society Journal 30: 179–184

PROTEIN C DEFICIENCY

In the normal subject, protein C is an essential anticoagulant. It acts by selective inhibition of activated factors V and VIII, and by stimulation of fibrinolysis. Synthesis occurs in the liver and is vitamin K dependent.

Inherited and acquired deficiencies may occur. Since the first report in 1981 by Griffin et al, a number of families have been described in which relatively young members have had recurrent spontaneous venous thromboses in association with reduced levels (between 35 and 65% of normal) of protein C.

However, the situation has proved to be more complicated than was initially thought. When attempting to define the normal range of values of protein C, it was found that 1 in 60 of healthy adults had levels of 55–65%, and conversely, 1 in 200–300 patients with heterozygous protein C deficiency had no history of venous thrombosis (Miletich et al 1986). It is therefore possible that heterozygous subjects with venous thromboses have some additional predisposing abnormality, or conversely, heterozygous subjects without venous thrombosis have some compensating mechanism. A recently developed technique for functional assay has helped to detect patients who have reduced protein C activity, but normal levels of protein C as measured by immunological assay.

Severe congenital homozygous protein C deficiency (often with no detectable levels) has been described in infants of parents who both had heterozygous deficiency. These presented with widespread skin lesions and necrosis due to thrombosis of small veins.

Levels of protein C may also be reduced in liver disease, ARDS, and following surgery. They may be very low or undetectable in DIC states.

Preoperative abnormalities

1. When the condition presents in infancy, it is usually homozygous, and often fatal, as it is associated with purpura fulminans, cutaneous necrosis and extensive venous thrombosis.
2. Adults with the familial heterozygous deficiency may present for surgery. They will have a high risk of venous thrombosis.
3. Patients known to have the condition, and who have already had venous thromboses, will usually be on permanent coumarin therapy. Warfarin, despite one of its actions being to lower protein C levels, has been found to be beneficial in preventing recurrent venous thromboembolism in protein C deficiency (Broekmans et al 1983).
4. In a young patient who has had a previous spontaneous venous thrombosis, or who has a family history of thromboses, the possible presence of this condition should be considered. Other inherited thrombophilias include antithrombin III deficiency, dysfibrinogenaemia and plasminogen abnormalities (Schafer 1985).

Anaesthetic problems

1. Homozygous infant
   a. Skin necrosis over pressure points.
   b. There is a theoretical risk of tracheal damage during the period of endotracheal intubation.
2. Heterozygous adult
   a. The problems of the management of a patient for anaesthesia and surgery who is anticoagulated.
   b. The risk of venous thrombosis and pulmonary embolism.

Management

1. Homozygous infant
   a. The anaesthetic literature is very limited. Three consecutive anaesthetics were reported for partial omentectomy and insertion of Tenkhoff catheter, in a homozygous infant with renal failure (Wetzel et al 1986). Despite the theoretical risks, endotracheal intubation was

employed, using a small tube to reduce tracheal pressure. The trachea was examined with a flexible laryngoscope at the subsequent anaesthetics and no damage was found.

b. The advice of a haematologist should be sought for the correction of the protein C deficiency. Current treatment includes fresh frozen plasma and factor IX concentrate. As yet, no specific therapy is available.

2. Heterozygous Adult

a. If the patient is taking warfarin, heparin should be substituted to obtain more flexible control. Anticoagulants should be restarted as soon as the surgery allows.

b. If the patient is not anticoagulated, low-dose heparin should be started preoperatively.

BIBLIOGRAPHY

Broekmans A W, Veltkamp J J, Bertina R M 1983 Congenital protein C deficiency and venous thromboembolism. New England Journal of Medicine 309: 340–344
Griffin J H, Evatt B, Zimmerman T S, Kleiss A J, Wideman C 1981 Deficiency of protein C in congenital thrombotic disease. Journal of Clinical Investigation 68: 1370–1373
Miletich J, Sherman L, Broze G 1986 Absence of thrombosis in subjects with heterozygous protein C deficiency. New England Journal of Medicine 317: 991–996
Schafer A I 1985 The hypercoagulable states. Annals of Internal Medicine; 102: 814–828
Wetzel R C, Marsh B R, Yaster M, Casella J F 1986 Anesthetic implications of protein C deficiency. Anesthesia and Analgesia 65: 982–984

PULMONARY HYPERTENSION

Can be applied to any condition in which the pulmonary artery pressure is increased above 35/15 mmHg, or a mean of 15–18 mmHg (N = 15–30/ 5–12 mmHg). Can be primary or secondary. Secondary pulmonary hypertension may be due to pulmonary emboli, chronic lung disease, left to right shunts, sickle cell anaemia, raised left ventricular filling pressures, left atrial outflow obstruction and vasculitis.

Primary pulmonary hypertension (PPH) is a rare disease of the pulmonary vasculature and of unknown aetiology. After elimination of other causes, the diagnosis is one of exclusion. In PPH none of these is found. It is more common in women than in men and there may be a family history. There is a raised pulmonary artery pressure and pulmonary vascular resistance. The mortality in PPH is high and the average survival time is 2 years (Rich & Brundage 1984). Heart-lung transplantation has been successful.

Preoperative abnormalities

1. Increasing dyspnoea and intense fatigue occurs, initially on exertion, but later at rest. Chest pain and haemoptysis may feature. Cyanosis appears in advanced disease.

2. Signs of a low cardiac output, signs of the original disease, an elevated JVP, and a right ventricular heave. A loud pulmonary second sound, right ventricular gallop (loud third sound at the left sternal edge) and possibly an early diastolic murmur due to pulmonary incompetence. Right heart failure will develop, with hepatomegaly, and peripheral oedema. Tricuspid incompetence may occur.

3. ECG shows right axis deviation, right ventricular hypertrophy and right atrial hypertrophy (P pulmonale). Right bundle branch block is common.

4. CXR shows a prominent pulmonary artery and an increased cardiothoracic ratio at a later stage. There are oligaemic lung fields, except where the secondary disease is due to increased blood flow, when the lung fields are plethoric.

5. Certain conditions are more commonly associated with PPH. These include collagen vascular disease, Raynaud's disease, hepatic cirrhosis and sickle cell disease.

6. Patients may be on prophylactic anticoagulants.

7. Although vasodilators have been used for treatment, there is as yet no evidence that they improve long-term survival. Calcium antagonists are currently being used.

Anaesthetic problems

1. The pre-existing high pulmonary vascular resistance (PVR) may be further increased by hypoxia, acidosis, hypercarbia, cold, alpha adrenergic stimulation, nitrous oxide, anxiety and PEEP.

2. A further rise in PVR during anaesthesia can increase the degree of right ventricular failure or decrease venous return to the left heart, thus causing systemic hypotension.

3. There is a poor correlation between RAP and LAP, therefore PAP and PCWP measurement has been suggested for severe cases. However, there is an increased risk of pulmonary vessel perforation during PAWP measurement in patients with acute pulmonary hypertension (Kranz & Viljoen 1979).

4. The patient is often on anticoagulants, and there may be pressure to restart them soon after surgery. Death from haemorrhage occurred in a patient in whom heparin was restarted within hours of a Caesarean section performed using the classical approach (Roessler & Lambert 1986).

Management

1. The risks of surgery must be weighed against the benefits. There are relatively few case reports of anaesthesia in patients with PPH. In those reported, the perioperative mortality was high, especially in the pregnant patient (Nelson et al 1983).

2. An adequate preoperative assessment of the degree of cardiorespiratory impairment. Treatment is difficult. Although diuretics improve peripheral oedema, they produce a fall in right ventricular, and hence cardiac output. Pulmonary vasodilators are not very effective.

3. Pulmonary artery, pulmonary capillary wedge and systemic artery pressures need to be monitored with care to avoid pulmonary vessel perforation. Monitoring of pulmonary pressures allows rational treatment of perioperative pressure changes with appropriate vasodilators, or fluid replacement.

4. Avoidance of factors known to increase pulmonary vascular resistance. A sedative premedication relieves anxiety. Oxygenation should be maintained and hypercarbia and acidosis avoided. The theatre should be warm, and a heated water blanket and blood warmer used. Nitrous oxide has been shown to produce a significant elevation of PAP in patients with pre-existing high levels, but not in those with normal PAP (Schulte-Sasse et al 1982).

5. Pulmonary vasodilators may be required during anaesthesia. It has been suggested that patients should be admitted to the ITU prior to surgery to assess the effect of various forms of therapy on the above parameters (Roessler & Lambert 1986). A patient due for Caesarean section under epidural anaesthesia was tested for the haemodynamic effects of a fluid load, changes in inspired oxygen percentage, tolazoline, sodium nitroprusside, and glyceryl nitrate. In this patient, sodium nitroprusside reduced pulmonary artery pressure the most, but this was achieved at the expense of systemic hypotension. Epidural anaesthesia was also reported in a patient undergoing vascular surgery (Davies & Beavis 1984). Although hypotension responded to colloid and metaraminol, a simultaneous moderate increase in PAP occurred. Isoflurane has been reported to have a beneficial effect on pulmonary pressures. (Cheng & Edelist 1988). A young man with primary pulmonary hypertension, whose pre-induction PAP was equal to his systemic pressure, showed a marked decrease in PVR and PAP during oxygen/isoflurane anaesthesia.

BIBLIOGRAPHY

Cheng D C H, Edelist G 1988 Isoflurane and primary pulmonary hypertension. Anaesthesia 43: 22–24
Davies M J, Beavis R E 1984 Epidural anaesthesia for vascular surgery in a patient with primary pulmonary hypertension. Anaesthesia and Intensive Care 12: 165–167
Kranz E M, Viljoen J F 1979 Haemoptysis following insertion of a Swan-Ganz catheter. British Journal of Anaesthesia 51: 457–459
Nelson D M, Main E, Crafford W, Ahumada G G 1983 Peripartum heart failure due to primary pulmonary hypertension. Obstetrics and Gynaecology 62: 58S–62S
Rich S, Brundage B H 1984 Primary pulmonary hypertension. Journal of the American Medical Association 251: 2252 2254
Roessler P, Lambert T F 1986 Anaesthesia for Caesarean section in the presence of primary pulmonary hypertension. Anaesthesia and Intensive Care 14: 317–320
Schulte-Sasse U, Hess W, Tarnow J 1982 Pulmonary vascular responses to nitrous oxide in patients with normal and high pulmonary vascular resistance. Anesthesiology 57: 9–13

1

PULMONARY OEDEMA

Causes of acute pulmonary oedema occurring in the perioperative period can be broadly divided into two groups: those of cardiogenic, and those of non-cardiogenic, origin. There are some cases in which the aetiology may not be clearly defined, and in which a number of factors may contribute. Broadly, one of two basic abnormalities may develop to produce pulmonary oedema. The first is an increase in the gradient between hydrostatic and colloid osmotic pressure across the pulmonary capillary wall and the second is an increase in capillary permeability.

1. Increased pulmonary hydrostatic pressure may be due to:
   a. Increase in right atrial pressure or preload due to fluid retention or fluid overload.
   b. Decreased myocardial contractility due to myocardial infarction or cardiomyopathy.
   c. Increase in left atrial pressure, e.g. in mitral stenosis.
   d. Increased afterload due to severe hypertension, peripheral vasoconstriction, anatomical or pathological obstruction.
2. Increased capillary permeability may be due to:
   a. Pulmonary aspiration of acid gastric contents.
   b. Air, gas or amniotic fluid embolism.
   c. Allergic reactions to drugs or blood products.
   d. Poisoning with higher oxides of nitrogen.
   e. Pneumonias and septicaemias.
   f. Shock lung or ARDS.

There are a number of specific types of non-cardiogenic pulmonary oedema whose mechanisms have not been completely elucidated, but which may present in the perioperative period. These include neurogenic pulmonary oedema, oedema associated with the relief of severe upper airway obstruction, the therapeutic use of beta 2 sympathomimetics for premature labour or naloxone for opiate antagonism, and gas or amniotic fluid embolism. As the treatment required may differ, these conditions will be considered separately.

Differentiation between cardiogenic and permeability pulmonary oedema.

1. History
In many cases the diagnosis will be obvious. There may be history of previous myocardial infarction, hypertension, valvular heart disease, or episodes of cardiac failure. The sudden onset of an arrhythmia, such as atrial fibrillation, may cause cardiac decompensation. If none of these is found, the presence of a known precipitating factor for non-cardiogenic oedema should be sought.

2. Clinical examination

In general the physical signs are similar. In both there will be tachycardia, cool peripheries, respiratory distress, frothy sputum, cyanosis and basal and parasternal crepitations. In primary cardiac disease there may be obvious cardiac enlargement, murmurs or an arrhythmia. An added third sound points to a cardiac cause.

3. CXR may show cardiac enlargement in addition to the pulmonary oedema.

4. ECG may show evidence of infarction, an arrhythmia or chamber hypertrophy.

5. In difficult cases, measurement of PAP and PCWP may be required.

6. Measurement of protein levels in pulmonary oedema fluid

This can only be done where there is copious, uncontaminated fluid for sampling.

A number of studies have shown that, depending on the cause, the protein content in oedema fluid varies. When due to an increased hydrostatic pressure, i.e. cardiogenic, there is a low protein content, whereas when due to permeability problems the protein content tends to be high.

A study of 21 patients showed that all patients with a PCWP of <20 mmHg had an oedema fluid to plasma protein ratio >0.6, whereas the mean ratio in four patients with cardiogenic oedema was 0.46 (Fein et al 1979). Where permeability problems exist, large protein molecules such as globulins will be present in oedema fluid and the protein content will approach that of blood. It has been suggested that the use of globulin ratios in conjunction with total protein ratios gives a more clearcut differentiation between cardiac and non-cardiac causes (Sprung et al 1981).

If oedema protein levels are high, and pulmonary artery catheterization is unavailable, it is reasonable to assume that the cause is likely to be a permeability problem.

BIBLIOGRAPHY

Fein I A, Grossman R F, Jones J G, Overland E, Pitts L, Murray J F, Staub N C 1979 The value of edema fluid protein measurement in patients with pulmonary edema. American Journal of Medicine 67: 32–38

Sprung C L, Rackow E C, Fein A, Jacob A I, Isikoff S K 1981 The spectrum of pulmonary edema. American Review of Respiratory Diseases 124: 718–722

CARDIOGENIC PULMONARY OEDEMA

This is secondary to an increase in pulmonary capillary pressure due to a high left atrial pressure, and results in an increase in lung water. This may be due to left atrial outflow obstruction (mitral valve disease, myxoma), left ventricular dysfunction (ischaemic or myopathic), left ventricular outflow obstruction or an increased afterload. Cardiogenic pulmonary oedema may be associated with a fluid overload, or with normovolaemia.

Presentation

In a patient with cardiac disease, pulmonary oedema may occur at any time during the perioperative period.

1. In the preoperative period it presents as a sudden onset of dyspnoea, tachycardia, a third heart sound (gallop rhythm), sweating and hypertension, with bilateral basal or parasternal crepitations on auscultation. It is most likely to occur in a patient with known ischaemic, hypertensive or rheumatic heart disease and may be associated with overenthusiastic fluid therapy prior to emergency surgery.
2. Pulmonary oedema is relatively rare during surgery, as IPPV and the decreased peripheral vascular resistance during anaesthesia tend to oppose the hydrostatic forces and reduce the afterload. Early signs are tachycardia, decreased compliance and reduced oxygen saturation (Mason 1987). The patient may try to breathe against the ventilator. In severe cases, pulmonary oedema fluid may emerge from the endotracheal tube.
3. In the postoperative period a combination of factors may tip a patient from borderline into florid pulmonary oedema, usually within the first half hour of the recovery period. The main factor is the redistribution of fluid from the peripheral into the pulmonary circulation. Peripheral vasoconstriction may be due to pain or cold, coinciding with the effects of the anaesthetic wearing off. In addition, intravenous fluids administered during the operation may compound the problem. In obstetrics, the use of ergometrine has in the past been associated with pulmonary oedema in patients with cardiac lesions.

Differential diagnosis

1. Inhalation of gastric contents.
2. Post upper airway obstruction.
3. Neurogenic pulmonary oedema.
4. Pulmonary oedema associated with naloxone administration.

Management

1. If the patient is conscious, he should be placed in an upright position and oxygen administered. If not, IPPV should be continued or started.
2. Morphine i.v. should be given in 2 mg increments at 2-minute intervals to a total of 10 mg. This reduces preload by venodilatation and relieves agitation.
3. Frusemide i.v. or i.m. 20–50 mg, especially if there is fluid overload. Acute venodilatation and subsequent diuresis results.
4. A vasodilator, such as isosorbide dinitrate, nitroglycerin, or nitroprusside may be used. An isosorbide dinitrate infusion (diluted) can be given at a rate of 2–10 mg/h.
5. If the patient is in fast AF, control of the heart rate with verapamil or

digoxin is required. With ECG control, verapamil 5–10 mg i.v. is given slowly.

n.b. Verapamil i.v. is contraindicated if the patient is taking beta blockers.

6. In severe myocardial dysfunction, a dilating inotrope such as dobutamine may be required.

BIBLIOGRAPHY

Mason R A 1987 The pulse oximeter: an early warning device? Anaesthesia 42: 784–785

NEUROGENIC PULMONARY OEDEMA (NPO)

A rare complication associated with intracranial damage, which may be due to head injury, tumour or vascular accident. It is postulated that the primary brain insult produces raised intracranial pressure and a secondary disturbance in hypothalamic function. A massive sympthetic discharge results in pronounced systemic vasoconstriction, shifting blood from the systemic to the pulmonary circulation (Theodore & Robin 1975). Pulmonary oedema results from the sequential rise in left heart pressures, due to the left ventricle attempting to eject against a greatly increased systemic vascular resistance (i.e. increased LVEDP, LAP and pulmonary venous pressures), together with an increased pulmonary blood volume. Both will result in increased pulmonary capillary pressure. There is some evidence that altered pulmonary capillary permeability resulting from capillary damage may subsequently contribute to the oedema. Cases of NPO have been reported in which pulmonary oedema persisted after pulmonary pressures returned to normal, and in which the oedema protein content was similar to that of plasma (Harari et al 1976). There is a suggestion that the onset of NPO may be precipitated by noxious stimuli such as endotracheal intubation, when it is performed in the lightly unconscious patient. In the past NPO has been associated with a high mortality (Casey 1983). However, with the better understanding of the pathophysiology of the condition, and the general improvement in intensive care facilities, this may change.

Presentation

1. The patient (often a young adult or child who is unconscious after a head injury), develops sudden dyspnoea, cyanosis, marked tachycardia or bradycardia, and hypertension.

2. Clinical signs of intense peripheral vasoconstriction occur, with pallor, sweating and cold extremities.

3. If the patient is intubated, profuse frothy pink pulmonary secretions will pour out of the endotracheal tube. If the patient is ventilated, there will be a sudden decrease in lung compliance, and, unless fully paralysed, the patient will attempt to breathe against the ventilator. Oxygen saturation decreases rapidly.

Differential diagnosis

1. Inhalation of gastric contents.
2. Fluid overload during resuscitation.

Management

1. Maintenance of oxygenation
If not already instituted, IPPV with a high inspired oxygen is required.
PEEP may be needed.
2. Manoeuvres to reduce intracranial pressure (if raised)
   a. $PaCO_2$ should be kept around 3–4 kPa. A $PaCO_2$ of 3.4 kPa reduces cerebral blood flow by 33%.
   b. An infusion of thiopentone.
   c. Surgical decompression, if necessary.
   d. High-dose steroids. Dexamethasone is often used, but its value is doubtful.
3. Reduction of peripheral vasoconstriction
   a. Diuretics will assist in reducing the overall blood volume, especially if large quantities of crystalloid solution have been used in resuscitation. Frusemide 2 mg/kg may be used. Mannitol is usually only indicated immediately prior to surgical decompression, as it causes a subsequent rebound increase in intracranial pressure.
   b. Alpha adrenergic blockers such as phenoxybenzamine 0.5–2 mg/kg in 300 ml 5% dextrose as an infusion have been advocated on the grounds that the syndrome is thought to be due to massive sympathetic discharge. Experimentally, neurogenic pulmonary oedema can be produced in certain animals by the inflation of a balloon in the epidural space to produce a sudden rise in intracranial pressure. Pretreatment with alpha adrenergic blockers can prevent this occurrence of pulmonary oedema. Large doses of chlorpromazine were used successfully in a 17-month-old child with NPO following a head injury (Wauchob et al 1984). Other drugs which have been used are droperidol i.v. 200–300 μg/kg or a phentolamine infusion 30 μg/kg/min.
   c. Vasodilators, such as sodium nitroprusside, 1–8 μg/kg/min as a short term infusion, have also been advocated to reduce peripheral vascular resistance. Direct arterial monitoring is essential. The haemodynamic responses of a patient with intractable neurogenic pulmonary oedema were assessed, using sodium nitroprusside and isoprenaline in turn (Loughnan et al 1980). Both drugs transiently reduced PCWP and LVEDP, although the PaO_2 was not improved. However, when phenoxybenzamine was given (see b), the PaO_2 improved and the pulmonary oedema resolved rapidly.
4. Inotropic support may occasionally be required. Isoprenaline and dobutamine are both suitable, as neither has alpha adrenergic receptor stimulating properties.
5. Control of fits with benzodiazepines or thiopentone.

BIBLIOGRAPHY

Casey W F 1983 Neurogenic pulmonary oedema. Anaesthesia 38: 985–988
Harari A, Rapin M, Regnier B, Comoy J, Caron J P 1976 Normal pulmonary capillary
    pressures in the late phase of neurogenic pulmonary oedema. Lancet i: 494
Loughnan P M, Brown T C K, Edis B, Klug G L 1980 Neurogenic pulmonary oedema in man:
    aetiology and management with vasodilators based upon haemodynamic studies.
    Anaesthesia and Intensive Care 8: 65–71
Theodore J, Robin E D 1975 Pathogenesis of neurogenic pulmonary oedema. Lancet ii:
    749–751
Wauchob T D, Brooks R J, Harrison K M 1984 Neurogenic pulmonary oedema. Anaesthesia
    39: 529–534

PULMONARY OEDEMA ASSOCIATED WITH SEVERE UPPER AIRWAY OBSTRUCTION

A well-recognized complication of acute upper airway obstruction, and in over 50% of reported cases, the onset of clinical pulmonary oedema followed relief of the obstruction (Barin et al 1986). The exact mechanism is not known, but it has been suggested that the marked negative pressures produced by attempted inspiration against a closed glottis may permit either transudation of fluid into the alveoli, or increase capillary permeability (Weissman et al 1984). Other factors such as gastric inhalation and hypoxic pulmonary vasoconstriction may contribute. Although potentially dangerous because of the hypoxia produced, this type of pulmonary oedema is usually relatively shortlived.

Presentation

1. The onset pulmonary oedema is preceded by an episode of severe upper respiratory tract obstruction. Recognized causes include laryngeal spasm or oedema (Barin et al 1986), epiglottitis (Galvis et al 1980), malignancy and attempted strangulation.
2. Relief of the obstruction is usually accompanied by the outpouring of large amounts of pink, frothy oedema fluid. There is cyanosis and respiratory distress.

Diagnosis

1. Bilateral basal crepitations are heard on auscultation.
2. CXR shows diffuse pulmonary oedema. The heart size is usually normal.
3. Blood gases show a large arterial/alveolar PO_2 difference.

Management

1. Oxygenation, either via a mask or endotracheal intubation. A review of cases showed that more than 50% of patients had a PaO_2 of <8 kPa at the time of intubation or soon after (Barin et al 1986).

1

2. IPPV or PEEP may be required to improve oxygenation. A pneumothorax may occur as a complication of this.

3. The use of diuretics has been suggested. However, in cases where intracardiac pressures have been measured, these have not in general been found to be elevated (Weissman et al 1984).

BIBLIOGRAPHY

Barin E S, Stevenson I F, Donnelly G L 1986 Pulmonary oedema following acute upper airway obstruction. Anaesthesia and Intensive Care 14: 54–57
Galvis A G, Stool S E, Bluestone C D 1980 Pulmonary edema following relief of acute upper airway obstruction. Annals of Otology, Rhinology and Laryngology 89: 124–128
Weissman C, Damask M C, Yang J 1984 Non-cardiogenic pulmonary edema following laryngeal obstruction. Anesthesiology 60: 163–165

PULMONARY OEDEMA ASSOCIATED WITH BETA 2 SYMPATHOMIMETICS FOR PREMATURE LABOUR

Seventy-three case reports of pulmonary oedema associated with the use of beta 2 sympathomimetic agents to suppress premature labour have been reviewed (Hawker 1984a). There were seven deaths. The fetal and maternal benefits of their use have therefore been questioned.

The aetiology is unknown, although a number of mechanisms have been considered as possibly contributing. The few haemodynamic studies reported in patients with pulmonary oedema following tocolytics, are consistent with the oedema being primarily of a non-cardiogenic, permeability type (Hawker 1984a,b, Brown & Mullis 1985). However, there is evidence to suggest that fluid overload and persistent adrenergic stimulation are potent contributing factors (Hawker 1984a).

Predisposing factors

1. Drugs thought to be linked with this type of pulmonary oedema include terbutaline, ritodrine, isoxuprine, salbutamol and fenoterol. Tachycardia is a prominent feature.

It is known that the $beta_2$ agonists do have inotropic effects on the heart via $beta_1$ receptors. Indeed, tachycardia can be a very common and troublesome side-effect of the tocolytics. A further contributing feature may be a 'downgrading' of the beta receptors during continued stimulation. After chronic exposure to catecholamines, cardiac beta receptors may become 'downregulated', resulting in a decreased adrenergic support for the heart. This has been suggested to occur in severe heart failure, and is supported by the discovery of a decreased beta adrenergic receptor population in failing hearts (Bristow et al 1982). Myocardial changes have been found to occur with chronic administration of catecholamines both experimentally and clinically. Patients with phaeochromocytoma can develop a cardiomyopathy, which is usually reversible after removal of the tumour.

2. Pulmonary oedema has been reported with oral, subcutaneous and intravenous routes of administration. The duration of treatment prior to its onset varied from 6 to 96 hours (Hawker 1984a). The rates of infusion were similarly variable. Of those cases in which information was adequate, pulmonary oedema occurred in 29 before delivery, and in 17, within a further 11 hours. In one patient it developed at 5 days and she died at home on day 60. Late development may point to a cardiomyopathy. Thirty-three per cent of cases involved twin pregnancy and in 63% of patients, steroids were given in addition. In the four cases which had haemodynamic monitoring, three had a normal or low PAWP.
3. In 21 cases where fluid balance was recorded, 15 had a positive balance of at least 1 litre. Fluid overload can easily occur. In normal pregnancy, blood volume is already increased by 45%. Tocolytics, which are often given in large volumes of diluent, can increase ADH secretion. Fluid retention is a feature of treatment with steroids and indomethacin, both of which may be prescribed in premature labour.
4. Acute redistribution of vascular volumes can sometimes be the precipitating factor in the development of pulmonary oedema, when volume overload is present. The administration of ergometrine has been known to cause pulmonary oedema secondary to vasoconstrictor effects. During recovery from anaesthesia, vasoconstriction due to cold or pain can also cause movement of fluid from the peripheral into the central circulation.

Presentation

1. A history of a sudden onset of dyspnoea, cyanosis and expectoration of pink frothy sputum, during or after suppression of premature labour with beta$_2$ tocolytics. There is usually a pre-existing tachycardia and the patient is often in positive fluid balance.
2. On auscultation, bilateral basal crepitations are heard. CXR shows pulmonary oedema, and blood gases will indicate hypoxia.

Management

1. The justification for the use of tocolytics should be considered before instituting such treatment. The patient will require careful observation for the detection of a positive fluid balance. A persistent tachycardia during therapy may be a warning sign of impending pulmonary oedema.
2. If evidence of early pulmonary oedema occurs, the infusion should be stopped.
3. Oxygen should be administered and, if necessary, IPPV established.
4. Diuretics are required.

BIBLIOGRAPHY

Bristow M R, Ginsberg R, Minobe W et al 1982 Decreased catcholamine sensitivity and beta adrenergic receptor density in failing human hearts. New England Journal of Medicine 307: 205–211

Brown M, Mullis S 1985 Pulmonary oedema associated with tocolytic therapy. Anaesthesia and Intensive Care 13: 102–103

Hawker F 1984a Pulmonary oedema associated with beta 2 sympathomimetic treatment of premature labour. Anaesthesia and Intensive Care 12: 143–151

Hawker F 1984b Five cases of pulmonary oedema associated with beta 2 sympathomimetic treatment of premature labour. Anaesthesia and Intensive Care 12: 159–171

PULMONARY OEDEMA ASSOCIATED WITH NALOXONE REVERSAL OF OPIATES

Naloxone was originally thought to be a pure opiate antagonist, with no agonist action, and no side effects. This does not appear to be correct. A few cases have occurred in which opiate reversal with naloxone has been associated with a state of acute central adrenergic stimulation, resulting in cardiovascular complications. Pulmonary oedema is one of these, and appears to most closely resemble neurogenic pulmonary oedema.

In view of suggestions that opiates may in some way modulate the release of catecholamines, the report that a large dose (10 mg) of naloxone caused catecholamine release in a patient with a proven phaeochromocytoma is of interest (Mannelli et al 1983).

Presentation

The onset of pulmonary oedema has been reported in close association with the administration of naloxone to reverse the effect of opiates in the recovery period. It was first described in a 70-year-old man after cardiac surgery in which high-dose morphine was used (Flacke et al 1977). In view of the patient's pre-existing cardiac disease, this might not be considered to be remarkable. However, pulmonary oedema has also been reported after small doses of naloxone in four healthy patients having elective surgery (Andree 1980, Taff 1983, Prough et al 1984). One patient died.

Management

Oxygenation, and IPPV if necessary.

BIBLIOGRAPHY

Andree R A 1980 Sudden death following naloxone administration. Anesthesia and Analgesia 59: 782–784

Flacke J W, Flacke W E, Williams S G D 1977 Acute pulmonary edema following naloxone reversal of high dose morphine anesthesia. Anesthesiology 47: 376–378

Mannelli M, Maggi M, DeFeo M L, Cuomo S, Forti G, Moroni F, Guisti G 1983 Naloxone administration releases catecholamines. New England Journal of Medicine 308: 654–655

Prough D S, Roy R, Bumgarner J, Shannon G 1984 Acute pulmonary edema in healthy teenagers following conservative doses of i.v. naloxone. Anesthesiology 60: 485–486

Taff R H 1983 Pulmonary edema following naloxone administration in a patient without heart disease. Anesthesiology 59: 576–577

Q-T INTERVAL SYNDROME, PROLONGED
(ROMANO–WARD, JERVELL AND LANGE-NIELSEN SYNDROMES, FAMILIAL VENTRICULAR TACHYCARDIA)

The Q–T interval on the ECG represents depolarization and repolarization of the ventricle; that is, one complete ventricular contraction. There are two rare inherited conditions in which this is prolonged, and a third in which it is normal at rest, but prolonged on exercise. The first, described by Jervell and Lange-Nielsen, is recessive and associated with nerve deafness, but the second, the Romano–Ward syndrome, a dominant condition, is not. The third, familial ventricular tachycardia, is also autosomal dominant. The cause of the long Q–T interval is thought to be an imbalance between the sympathetic supply to the right and left sides of the heart.

In any of the conditions, emotion or exercise can provoke syncopal attacks, associated with either VT or VF, which can result in death. There is often a family history of sudden deaths.

The effects of long-term therapy on mortality in the long Q–T syndrome were studied in 203 patients (Schwartz et al 1975). Untreated patients had a mortality of 73%, while in those treated with beta blockers it was only 6%. A third group, who were treated, but not with beta blockers, had a mortality of 64%. In some patients left cervical sympathectomy has shortened the Q–T interval and reduced the incidence of syncopal attacks (Yanagida et al 1976). Other drugs which have been used for treatment include phenytoin, verapamil, bretylium and primidone.

The condition, and its treatment, has considerable anaesthetic significance. There have been a number of case reports in which VT, VF or cardiac arrest have occurred during anaesthesia in otherwise fit young patients. Most patients have been of the age where preoperative ECGs are unlikely to have been performed, or even if they have, the condition may not have been recognized. A history of recurrent syncope (which may be diagnosed as epilepsy), or a family history of sudden deaths, should alert the anaesthetist to the possibility of this condition. Although it is rare, its mere existence illustrates the importance of initiating ECG monitoring from the start of the anaesthetic, whatever the age of the patient.

Preoperative abnormalities

1. There may be a known family history of the condition, or of sudden and unexpected deaths in the family, at a young age.
2. The patient may give a history of syncopal attacks, or, as sometimes happens, may be diagnosed as being epileptic (Ponte & Lund 1981).
3. ECG abnormalities. The Q–T interval is measured from the beginning of the QRS complex to the end of the T wave. It varies with heart rate,

shortening as heart rate rises, and therefore must be corrected for rate (see below). In general, the normal Q–T interval should be less than 0.42 seconds, while in the prolonged Q–T interval syndrome it may be as long as 0.6 seconds. T waves are also usually abnormal, being broad and diphasic or altering in polarity. There is often a bradycardia, a feature which is unusual in normal children.

Approximate relationship between heart rate and Q–T interval in a normal subject:

50 b.p.m.	0.38–0.42 seconds
60 b.p.m.	0.35–0.41 seconds
70 b.p.m.	0.33–0.39 seconds
80 b.p.m.	0.29–0.37 seconds
90 b.p.m.	0.28–0.36 seconds
100 b.p.m.	0.26–0.34 seconds

4. Some patients with long Q–T syndrome have a prolapsed mitral valve (Forbes & Morton 1979).

Preoperative problems

1. VT, VF or cardiac arrest can occur during anaesthesia. Ten anaesthetic papers describe a total of 14 anaesthetics given to patients with congenital long Q–T interval syndrome. In eight anaesthetics the patients were treated with propranolol (Owitz et al 1979, O'Callaghan et al 1982, Medak & Benumof 1983, Carlock et al 1984, Galloway & Glass 1985), while one patient had a left cervical sympathetic block (Callaghan et al 1977). None of these had complications. In the five anaesthetics where no beta blocker was given, there were two episodes of VF, two of VT and one of asystole. (Forbes & Morton 1979, Wig et al 1979, Ponte & Lund 1981, Brown et al 1981, Medak & Benumof 1983). One patient died, the others were resuscitated.
2. The risk of transient attacks of VT or VF is increased by sympathetic stimulation, emotion or exercise.
3. Some drugs, including halothane and thiopentone (Martineau & Nadeau 1987), and large doses of opiates, may also prolong the Q–T interval.

Management

1. The patient should be fully beta blocked prior to anaesthesia, usually with propranolol. It has been suggested that pindolol and oxprenolol should be avoided, in view of their intrinsic sympathetic activity. (Galloway & Glass 1985).
2. ECG monitoring should be continued through the perioperative period and a defibrillator available.
3. A good premedication should help to relieve anxiety.

4. Left stellate ganglion block may shorten the Q–T interval and raise the threshold for ventricular fibrillation.

5. Intubation and extubation cause sympathetic stimulation, and they should not be performed during very light anaesthesia.

6. Any drug known to produce a tachycardia, or to prolong the Q–T interval, should be avoided. Drugs in these categories include pancuronium, atropine, thiopentone, halothane and high-dose opiates.

7. Isoflurane has been suggested as a suitable inhalation agent (Carlock et al 1984).

BIBLIOGRAPHY

Brown M, Liberthson R R, Ali H A, Lowenstein E 1981 Perioperative anesthetic management of a patient with long Q–T syndrome. Anesthesiology 55: 586–589

Callaghan M L, Nicholls A B, Sweet R B 1977 Anesthetic management of prolonged Q–T interval syndrome. Anesthesiology 47: 67–69

Carlock F J, Brown M, Brown E M 1984 Isoflurane anaesthesia for a patient with long Q–T syndrome. Canadian Anaesthetists' Society Journal 31: 83–85

Forbes R B, Morton G H 1979 Ventricular fibrillation in a patient with unsuspected mitral valve prolapse and prolonged Q–T interval. Canadian Anaesthetists' Society Journal 26: 424–427

Galloway P A, Glass P S A 1985 Anesthetic implications of prolonged Q–T interval syndrome. Anesthesia and Analgesia 64: 612–620

Martineau R J, Nadeau S G 1987 Q–Tc interval changes during induction of anaesthesia. Canadian Journal of Anaesthesia 34: S61–62

Medak R, Benumof J L 1983 Perioperative management of the prolonged Q–T interval syndrome. British Journal of Anaesthesia 55: 361–364

O'Callaghan A C, Normandale J P, Morgan M 1982 The prolonged Q–T syndrome. A review with anaesthetic implications and the report of two cases. Anaesthesia and Intensive Care 10: 50–55

Owitz S, Pratilas V, Pratila M G, Dimich I 1979 Anaesthetic considerations in the prolonged Q–T interval (LQTS). Canadian Anaesthetists' Society Journal 26: 50–54

Ponte J, Lund J 1981 Prolongation of the Q–T interval (Romano Ward syndrome): anaesthetic management. British Journal of Anaesthesia 53: 1347–1350

Schwartz P J, Periti M, Malliani A 1975 The long Q–T syndrome. American Heart Journal 89: 378–390

Wig J, Bali I M, Singh R G, Kataria R N, Khattri H N 1979 Prolonged Q–T interval syndrome. Sudden cardiac arrest during anaesthesia. Anaesthesia 34: 37–40

Yanagida H, Kemi C, Suwa K 1976 The effects of stellate ganglion block on the idiopathic prolongation of the Q–T interval with cardiac arrhythmia. (The Romano-Ward syndrome.) Anesthesia and Analgesia 55: 782–787

RABIES

An infectious acute neurological disease caused by a rhabdovirus, transmitted through saliva from the bite of a rabid animal. The virus accumulates locally and then ascends via the peripheral nerves to the central nervous system where it replicates in the neural cells. Peripheral dissemination then occurs via the nerves, to a number of different organ sites (Morrison & Wenzel 1985). Recovery is rare. Animals reported to transmit rabies include dogs, foxes, badgers, bats, skunks and racoons. Rabies is not yet endemic in Britain, although its relentless spread through Europe is such that its appearance is inevitable. Prophylaxis is crucial, and the new human diploid cell strain vaccines are very effective. No case of rabies has been reported in anyone given the vaccine correctly, with the hyperimmune serum, on the day of contact with the rabid animal (Editorial 1988).

Presentation

1. A patient who develops an acute neurological condition, and who has a history of an animal bite sustained in an endemic area, is suspect. Sensory changes may occur at the site of the bite.
2. Presentation may include acute hydrophobic spasms, opisthotonos, flaccid paralysis and coma. When the subject tries to drink water, there are painful inspiratory, pharyngeal and laryngeal muscle spasms (hydrophobia). Asphyxia may occur during a spasm. Autonomic involvement and haematemesis may occur. Those surviving this stage of 'furious rabies' may progress to a paralytic phase.
3. Recovery from the disease is extremely rare.

Anaesthetic problems

1. Although the outlook is poor in the established disease, intensive care provides the only hope for the patient (Cundy 1980). The three sole survivors of clinical rabies required intensive care facilities and prolonged hospitalization (Morrison & Wenzel 1985).
2. Management of the airway in hydrophobic spasms or respiratory support if paralysis occurs, may be required.
3. Serious cardiac arrhythmias may occur with autonomic involvement.
4. Other complications include cardiac and renal failure, raised intracranial pressure, hyperpyrexia, and inappropriate ADH secretion.

Management

The admission of rabid patients to British hospitals is rare, but the occasional case appears. The isolation and management of such a case for 12 days on a British ITU has been described (Cundy 1980). Consultation with microbiological and clinical experts is essential. An outline of management is given but the references offer more detailed advice.

1. A microbiologist must be consulted. Rabies prophylaxis requires local wound care and both passive and active rabies immunization. Animal studies have shown the importance of scrubbing the wound with soap, iodine or alcohol. Tetanus prophylaxis should also be given.
2. Barrier nursing, by a limited special staff who may be offered vaccination. Airborne transmission of rabies has been reported, so mask, gown and gloves should always be worn (Morrison & Wenzel 1985).

3. IPPV, sedation and treatment to control spasms.
4. Monitoring of cerebral and cardiovascular function.
5. The standard support required by a ventilated ITU patient.

BIBLIOGRAPHY

Cundy J M 1980 Rabies encephalitis: management in a district general hospital ICU.
   Anaesthesia 35: 35–41
Editorial 1988 Rabies vaccine failures. Lancet i: 917–918
Morrison A J, Wenzel R P 1985 Rabies: a review and current approach for the clinician.
   Southern Medical Journal 78: 1211–1218

RENAL FAILURE, CHRONIC

This term is intended to encompass a progressive reduction of
glomerular filtration rate, from decreased renal reserve, to renal
insufficiency, and finally to end-stage renal failure. In all cases an acute
reduction in function can be superimposed on the chronic disease. The
anaesthetist must ensure that neither omissions nor commissions
worsen renal function, cause drug-induced nephrotoxicity, or seriously
interfere with the patient's compensatory mechanisms for his disease.
The hyperbolic relationship between serum creatinine or urea, and GFR,
means that more than 50% of excretory function may be lost without
change in the serum chemistry outside the normal range. Many of the
patients will be on some form of dialysis. Dialysis provides the means
by which the most serious abnormalities of hyperkalaemia, circulatory
overload and acidosis can be corrected in the 12–24 hours prior to
surgery. Renal failure has a profound effect on all systems of the body.
Some of the abnormalities seen will be due to the renal disease itself,
others are associated with long-term dialysis.

Anaesthesia may be required for renal transplantation, insertion of
Tenckhoff catheters, CAPD, creation of arteriovenous fistulae, or for
parathyroid or incidental surgery.

Preoperative abnormalities

1. In contrast to acute renal failure where the causes are principally pre-
renal, the causes of chronic renal failure are primarily due to intrinsic
renal disease. These include glomerulonephritis, hypertension, diabetes,
chronic pyelonephritis, hereditary renal disease including polycystic
disease and Alport's disease, the systemic vasculitides including SLE, PAN
and Wegener's granulomatosis, the paraproteinaemias and amyloid.
Postrenal (obstructive) causes must also be considered, and include
prostatic hypertrophy, bladder and other pelvic tumours, calculus
disease, retroperitoneal fibrosis and tumours.

1

2. Renal failure has widespread systemic effects:
   a. Cardiovascular
   Hypertension is common, either due to retention of water and sodium, or secondary to increased renin secretion by the kidney. Left ventricular failure may be due to this, to the high cardiac output secondary to anaemia, or to uraemic cardiomyopathy. Occasionally, high blood flow through the arteriovenous fistula may contribute. Pericardial effusions can be associated with either terminal uraemia or with dialysis. Tamponade occasionally occurs. Cardiovascular lesions are numerically by far the most important causes of death in the dialysis population, with an increased incidence of atheroma, coronary artery disease and cerebrovascular accidents. Conduction defects may be associated with hyperkalaemia. Cardiovascular instability can occur during or after dialysis, or may be secondary to autonomic neuropathy.
   b. Pulmonary
   Pulmonary venous congestion or frank pulmonary oedema may occur. On CXR there is a typical symmetrical bat-wing appearance radiating from the lung hila. There is an increased susceptibility to lung infection. A low $PaCO_2$ is due to respiratory compensation for the metabolic acidosis.
   c. Nervous system
   There may be peripheral or autonomic neuropathies. Loss of nerve fibres and demyelination occur. Neuropathies are usually reversed after successful renal transplantation. Mental changes may be associated with chronic dialysis. Uraemic encephalopathy may reflect underdialysis, or be associated with disequilibrium (with probable elevated ICP) related to dialysis. A characteristic encephalopathy (associated with bone disease and anaemia) has been attributed to aluminium intoxication. Aluminium is excreted by the normal body, but accumulates during maintenance therapy, being derived from the softened waters (in certain geographical areas) used to make dialysate, or by ingestion of aluminium compounds used to chelate and inhibit gastrointestinal absorption of dietary phosphate. There are now stringent EEC recommendations limiting the concentration of aluminium in dialysate fluids. Some success in its removal has been achieved by desferrioxamine.
   d. Gastrointestinal
   Delayed gastric emptying and increased acid secretion occurs. There is a high incidence of gastrointestinal inflammation and bleeding. Liver function may be abnormal. An increased carrier rate for HBsAg occurs.
   e. Bone disease
   Renal bone disease may include elements of osteomalacia, osteitis fibrocystica and osteosclerosis. Failure of phosphate excretion is associated with raised serum phosphate levels, and hypocalcaemia. The latter induces secondary hyperparathyroidism and PTH secretion may then become autonomous.

3. Biochemical abnormalities

Nephron loss is associated with failure of hydrogen ion excretion and a metabolic acidosis ensues. Serum bicarbonate is further reduced by compensatory respiratory alkalosis.

4. Haematological abnormalities

A normochromic, normocytic, hypoproliferative anaemia occurs, in part due to inadequate production of erythropoietin. Anaemia starts as the creatinine level increases above 250 μmol/l, and a haemoglobin between 3 and 9 g/dl results. Repeated blood transfusion carries the danger of iron overload and may require therapy with desferrioxamine. Erythropoietin can now be manufactured by a recombinant DNA technique. The anaemia of renal failure can thus be corrected although the definitive place of this treatment is still being assessed (Cotes 1988). In untreated anaemia, compensation occurs by increase in cardiac output and a shift of the oxygen dissociation curve. Uraemia causes a prolonged bleeding time due to platelet dysfunction, but this improves on dialysis.

5. Treatment for end-stage renal failure may involve regular haemodialysis, continuous ambulatory peritoneal dialysis or renal transplantation.

6. The patient may have a permanent A-V fistula for vascular access.

Anaesthetic problems

1. A delayed gastric emptying time occurs, which is further prolonged by haemodialysis. Gastric acidity is increased.

2. The incidence of hepatitis in patients on dialysis was high (up to 25%), and a percentage of patients became chronic HBsAg carriers. With the advent of regular screening this has been greatly reduced. There is an increased risk to staff. Impaired liver function is common, due to hepatic venous congestion.

3. Hypertension and cardiovascular instability may be a problem.There is a decreased tolerance to variations in fluid balance. Both fluid overload and dehydration readily occur.

4. Drug excretion

While gallamine is the only anaesthetic drug which is entirely excreted by the kidney, the excretion of many drugs will be delayed. Cumulation of either the parent drug, or its metabolites may occur, especially if repeated doses are given (Drayer 1977).

   a. Benzodiazepines

The majority of benzodiazepines are relatively long acting and many have active metabolites. Lorazepam, oxazepam and diazepam all have increased half-lives in renal failure. This is not so with the shorter acting ones such as triazolam, temazepam and midazolam (Vinik et al 1983).

   b. Opiates

      i. There is increased sensitivity to morphine, which is in part due to decreased binding by plasma proteins, especially in the presence of an acidosis.

ii. Pethidine has CNS-depressant effects and has a short half-life, but one of its metabolites, norpethidine, has excitatory effects and a long half-life. With chronic administration or multiple doses of pethidine, norpethidine accumulates. Two cases were reported in which twitching and irritability were associated with high ratios of norpethidine to pethidine (Szeto et al 1977). One of these patients had impaired renal function.

c. Neuromuscular blocking agents

i. In renal failure a single dose of suxamethonium will normally only produce an increase in serum potassium of 0.5–0.7 mmol/l. However, a rise of 2.8 mmol/l occurred following a second dose of suxamethonium in a patient with uraemic neuropathy (Walton & Farman 1973).

ii. Early reports suggested that dialysis was associated with low plasma cholinesterase levels. A later study of 81 patients having renal transplants did not confirm this (Ryan 1977). Improvements in dialysis membranes may explain these discrepancies.

iii. d-Tubocurarine, alcuronium, and in particular pancuronium, have all been shown to produce prolonged neuromuscular blockade (McCleod et al 1976). The half-life of neostigmine is also prolonged (Cronnelly et al 1979). The half-life of vecuronium is only slightly longer than normal (Meistelman et al 1983).

d. Inhalation agents
Isoflurane, halothane and enflurane have all been used in renal failure. Although there have been a small number of reports of deterioration of renal function following enflurane, the levels of inorganic fluoride produced are usually well below those associated with renal toxicity. When halothane and enflurane were given to patients with mild to moderate renal failure, all showed a slight improvement in renal function (Mazze et al 1984).

5. Regional anaesthesia
A reduction in duration of brachial plexus block has been reported and attributed to an increased cardiac output (Bromage and Gertel 1972). However, this finding has been disputed (Martin et al, 1988). The presence of acidosis may increase CNS toxicity.

6. A-V fistula patency
There are risks of occluding the A-V fistula during surgery. Mechanical pressure, hypotension, cold and hypercoagulability, will predispose to this.

8. Hypercarbia and acidosis increase serum potassium levels. Both hypercarbia and hypocarbia reduce renal blood flow.

Management

1. Correction of fluid overload and electrolyte (particularly potassium) abnormalities. Dialysis should take place within 12–36 hours of surgery.

1

2. A coagulation screen, LFTs and HBsAg should be reviewed.

3. Prophylactic treatment for acid aspiration syndrome should be given, with antacid and H_2 receptor antagonists. The half-life of cimetidine is increased to 3–4 hours, so doses should be reduced.

4. Only short-acting benzodiazepines such as temazepam, triazolam or midazolam should be used. Triazolam has been recommended as the oral benzodiazepine of choice (Graybar & Tarpey 1987).

5. The hypertensive response to intubation may be reduced by treatment with propranolol, lignocaine or fentanyl.

6. Monitoring

The fistula arm should not be used for the blood pressure cuff, nor for i.v. infusions. Direct arterial monitoring should be avoided, so as to preserve arteries for subsequent vascular access. If monitoring of vascular volume is required, a CVP is preferred to a pulmonary artery catheter, which carries an increased risk of infection. Normocarbia is maintained by use of a capnograph. Serious increases in serum potassium can be detected by ECG monitoring of T-wave changes. Neuromuscular monitoring is essential. Pulse oximetry is a useful adjunct.

7. Venous access

Arteries and veins must be conserved, and the AV fistula protected from potentially occlusive insults. A bruit over the fistula must be heard both before and after surgery. The fistula arm should not be used and hypotension and cooling avoided. Occlusion of the fistula, if it occurs, is an indication for immediate thrombectomy. Wide-bore subclavian catheters are commonly employed as temporary access for haemodialysis and should not be used for routine intravenous purposes.

8. General Anaesthesia

a. Thiopentone is a suitable induction agent, although etomidate may be indicated if there is significant cardiac disease. A study of 15 patients given midazolam 0.2 mg/kg showed that the elimination half-life was identical to that in normal patients (Vinik et al 1983). Bradycardia frequently occurs in renal failure, so the use of an anti-cholinergic is indicated.

b. Suxamethonium should be avoided if the serum potassium is >5.5 mmol/l, or if there is a uraemic neuropathy. If suxamethonium is used, a second dose may produce a variety of arrhythmias. The pharmacokinetics and pharmacodynamics of atracurium, which is spontaneously broken into inactive components (Hofmann elimination), are unaltered by renal failure (Fahey et al 1984, de Bros et al 1985). Animal experiments suggest that laudanosine is unlikely to reach high enough levels to produce adverse EEG effects (Ingram et al 1985). Only small increases in the half-life of vecuronium have been found (Meistelman et al 1983). The half-life of neostigmine is prolonged, but the changes are similar to that occurring with d-tubocurarine and pancuronium.

c. Fentanyl is probably the most suitable analgesic. However, caution should be used with repeated doses, as rises in plasma fentanyl, probably due to drug redistribution, have been reported 2–5 hours after injection (Gulden et al 1984).

9. Regional anaesthesia

In the absence of bleeding problems, the use of regional anaesthesia reduces the need for giving cumulative doses of drugs. Brachial plexus block has been used for vascular access, and local anaesthesia for insertion of Tenckhoff catheters for CAPD. High spinal anaesthesia has been reported to produce satisfactory conditions for renal transplantation (Linke & Merin 1976). A reduction in local anaesthetic dosage by 25% has been recommended (Weir & Chung 1984). Severe hypertension, or uraemic neuropathy are contraindications to regional techniques.

10. Maintenance of cardiac output and blood pressure are essential.

BIBLIOGRAPHY

Bromage P R, Gertel M 1972 Brachial plexus anesthesia in chronic renal failure. Anesthesiology 36: 488–493
Cotes P M 1988 Erythropoietin: the developing story. British Medical Journal 296: 805–806
Cronnelly R, Stanski D R, Miller R D, Sheiner L B, Sohn Y J 1979 Renal function and the pharmacokinetics of neostigmine in anesthetised man. Anesthesiology 51: 222–226
de Bros F M, Lai A, Scott R et al 1985 Pharmacokinetics and pharmacodynamics of atracurium under isoflurane anesthesia in normal and anephric patients. Anesthesia and Analgesia 64: 207
Drayer D E 1977 Active drug metabolites and renal failure. American Journal of Medicine 62: 486–489
Fahey M R, Rupp S M, Fisher D M et al 1984 The pharmacokinetics and pharmacodynamics of atracurium in patients with and without renal failure. Anesthesiology 61: 699–702
Graybar G B, Tarpey M 1987 Kidney transplantation. In: Anesthesia and organ transplantation. W B Saunders, Philadelphia
Gulden D, Koehntop D, Rodman J, Brundage D, Hegland M 1984 Fentanyl pharmacokinetics during renal transplantation. Anesthesiology 61: A243
Ingram M D, Sclabassi R J, Stiller R L, Cook D R, Bennett M H 1985 Cardiovascular and electroencephalographic effects of laudanosine in 'nephrectomised' cats. Anesthesia and Analgesia 64: 232
Linke C L, Merin R G 1976 A regional anesthetic approach for renal transplantation. Anesthesia and Analgesia 55: 69–73
McCleod K, Watson M J, Rawlins M D 1976 Pharmacokinetics of pancuronium in patients with normal and impaired renal function. British Journal of Anaesthesia 48: 341–345
Maddern P J 1983 Anaesthesia for the patient with impaired renal function. Anaesthesia and Intensive Care 11: 321–328
Mazze R I, Sievenpiper T S, Stevenson J 1984 Renal effects of halothane and enflurane in patients with abnormal renal function. Anesthesiology 60: 161–163
Martin R, Beauregard L, Tetrault J P 1988 Brachial plexus block and chronic renal failure. Anaesthesiology 69: 405–406
Meistelman C, Leinhart A, Leveque C, Bitker M O, Pigot B, Viars P 1983 Pharmacology of vecuronium in patients in end stage renal failure. Anesthesiology 59: A293
Ryan D W 1977 Preoperative serum cholinesterase concentration in chronic renal failure. British Journal of Anaesthesia 49: 945–949
Szeto H H, Inturrisi C E, Houde R, Saal S, Cheigh J, Reidenberg M M 1977 Accumulation of normeperidine, an active metabolite of meperidine in patients with renal failure or cancer. Annals of Internal Medicine 86: 738–741

Vinik H R, Revers J G, Greenblatt D J, Abernethy D R, Smith L R 1983 The pharmacokinetics of midazolam in chronic renal failure patients. Anesthesiology 59: 390–394
Walton J D, Farman J V 1973 Suxamethonium hyperkalaemia in uraemic neuropathy. Anaesthesia 28: 666–668

Weir P H C, Chung F F 1984 Anaesthesia for patients with chronic renal disease. Canadian Anaesthetists' Society Journal 31: 468–480

RETROLENTAL FIBROPLASIA
(RLF)

A condition occurring in premature infants, or those with a birth weight <1500 g, in which an acute vascular retinopathy may progress to retinal scarring, detachment and possible blindness. Although originally attributed to exposure to high oxygen tensions in the neonatal period, it is now thought that there are many factors involved in the development of the severe form of the disease. Prematurity seems to be the most important of these, as approximately 45% of neonates weighing less than 1000 g develop acute retinal changes at birth. Out of this group however, only 10–20% will progress to cicatricial changes, retinal detachment and impairment of vision. Oxygen is probably only one of the factors which determines this unpredictable progression. The increase in incidence of RLF, despite care to limit oxygen tensions, probably reflects in part the increasing ability of neonatal units to salvage the lower birth weight infants.

Anaesthetic problems

1. The extent of risk to premature infants during major surgery is of concern. A twin (1140 g) who had surgery for duodenal atresia, and who had an increased inspired oxygen concentration for 4.5 hours, with the PaO_2 varying from 8.5–43 kPa, developed the cicatricial form of RLF, whereas the other normal twin (1440 g) did not. No retinal examination had been made prior to surgery (Betts et al 1977).

2. The multifactorial elements of this disorder have been stressed in a description of the clinical course of a 1445 g infant who developed severe RLF (Merritt et al 1981). No oxygen was given at delivery, but on day 7 abdominal surgery was required. The FIO_2 varied between 25% and 30% for the 45-minute procedure, apart from three separate 5-minute periods when it was 50%. Air only was given in the recovery room. Bicarbonate was required for a persistent metabolic acidosis over an 11-day period, and packed red cells were given for anaemia on day 12. A patent ductus arteriosus was also present, but asymptomatic. At 16 months the child was found to have severe RLF. It was suggested that the acidosis and the blood transfusion might have increased the oxygen delivery to the retinal tissues and hence the susceptibility of the immature vessels to damage.

3. The lack of data linking the development of RLF with concentrations of oxygen <50% has merited editorial comment (Flynn 1984). The view that a multiplicity of factors, including continual exposure to artificial

light, might render the immature retinal vessels more susceptible to oxygen damage than normal, was accepted. In an analysis of 134 cases of RLF in 639 infants, it was concluded that those who had major surgery in the course of their care were at no greater risk of developing permanent retinal damage than those who did not have surgery.

Management

1. All premature infants are at risk of developing RLF, presumbly until the retinal vessels are mature. If surgery is required in this period it has been suggested that ophthalmological assessment of vascular maturity should be made. There are practical difficulties in this (Merritt et al 1981).
2. An attempt should be made to maintain a PaO_2 of not greater than 10.6–12 kPa. In the presence of a patent ductus arteriosus, the most significant measurement is that of preductal PaO_2, as this will most accurately reflect retinal exposure. Inspired concentration and trancutaneous PO_2 give indirect information.

BIBLIOGRAPHY

Betts E K, Downes J J, Schaffer D B, Johns R 1977 Retrolental fibroplasia and oxygen administration during general anaesthesia. Anesthesiology 47: 518–520
Flynn J T 1984 Oxygen and retrolental fibroplasia. Anesthesiology 60: 397–399
Merritt J C, Sprague D H, Merritt W E, Ellis R A 1981 Retrolental fibroplasia: a multifactorial disease. Anesthesia and Analgesia 60: 109–111

RHABDOMYOLYSIS

Injury to skeletal muscle producing myoglobinaemia and myoglobinuria, and associated with a rise, sometimes massive, of the CPK. Free myoglobin appears in the blood soon after exposure to the cause. It may be detected in blood and urine almost immediately, and its transient appearance means it is frequently missed, whereas the CPK takes several hours to rise. Renal damage may occur, but the exact mechanism is unclear. Rhabdomyolysis of varying degrees of severity can be precipitated by a wide range of conditions, including the administration of certain anaesthetic drugs.

Preoperative abnormalities

1. Predisposing factors not associated with anaesthesia include crush and burns injury, ischaemia, viral infections, polymyositis, heat stroke, marathon running, McArdle's syndrome, Taurius' syndrome and neuroleptic malignant syndrome.
2. Conditions in which rhabdomyolysis may occur during anaesthesia include malignant hyperpyrexia myopathy, Duchenne muscular

dystrophy, Guillain–Barré syndrome, polyneuropathy, burns and a prolonged tourniquet time.

3. The passage of dark brown urine, positive for blood on reagent strip, but with no RBCs on microscopy, is suggestive of the diagnosis.

Anaesthetic problems

1. Rhabdomyolysis occurring in association with anaesthesia is most frequently precipitated by suxamethonium. It may occasionally occur after suxamethonium in an otherwise normal patient. Children are more susceptible to muscle injury after suxamethonium than adults, particularly if halothane has been used first (McKishnie et al 1983). However, those who have a significant degree of muscle destruction are often subsequently found to have some underlying muscle disease.

2. Rhabdomyolysis is one feature of the MH syndrome.

3. Masseter muscle rigidity (MMR) is a term applied to severe spasm of the muscles of mastication lasting for 2–3 minutes after suxamethonium. This is always accompanied by varying degrees of rhabdomyolysis.
About 50% of patients with severe MMR are reported to be susceptible to MH (Rosenberg & Fletcher 1986). (See also Section 4, Masseter muscle rigidity.)

4. The first sign of muscle destruction may be the occurrence of a serious cardiac arrhythmia, due to acute hyperkalaemia. Early cardiac arrest has been reported in Guillain–Barré syndrome (Hawker et al 1985), Duchenne muscular dystrophy (Seay et al 1978, Linter et al 1982), or non-specific myopathy (Schaer et al 1977).

5. Myoglobinuria may present unexpectedly in the postoperative period (Hool et al 1984, Rubiano et al 1987), and if severe or untreated, may progress to renal failure. Postoperative myoglobinuria and renal failure after suxamethonium and halothane was reported in a 3-year-old with a strong family history of DMD (McKishnie et al 1983).

6. Postoperative muscle weakness or stiffness may occur.

Management

1. Anticipation of the problem. Suxamethonium is best avoided in patients with myopathic or neuropathic types of disease. It should certainly not be given in DMD, Guillain–Barré syndrome, McArdle's Syndrome, MH myopathy, or after thermal injury.

2. Should sudden cardiac arrest occur after suxamethonium, myoglobinaemia and myoglobinuria should be anticipated.

3. If myoglobinuria occurs, intravenous fluid therapy and an osmotic diuretic should be given to maintain an adequate urine flow. Urine output, CPK, urea, creatinine and electrolytes should be checked regularly in the acute phase.

4. If renal failure ensues, dialysis should be instituted until renal function recovers (Hool et al 1984, Hawker et al 1985).

BIBLIOGRAPHY

Hawker F, Pearson I Y, Soni N, Woods P 1985 Rhabdomyolytic renal failure and suxamethonium. Anaesthesia and Intensive Care 13: 208–209

Hool G J, Lawrence P J, Sivaneswaran N 1984 Acute rhabdomyolytic renal failure due to suxamethonium. Anaesthesia and Intensive Care 12: 360–364

Linter S P K, Thomas P R, Withington P S, Hall M G 1982 Suxamethonium associated hypertonicity and cardiac arrest in unsuspected pseudohypertrophic muscular dystrophy. British Journal of Anaesthesia 54: 1331–1332

McKishnie J D, Muir J M, Girvan D P 1983 Anaesthesia induced rhabdomyolysis. Canadian Anaesthetists' Society Journal 30: 295–298

Rosenberg H, Fletcher J E 1986 Masseter muscle rigidity and malignant hyperthermia susceptibility. Anesthesia and Analgesia 65: 161–164

Rubiano R, Chang J-L, Carroll J, Sonbolian N, Larson C E 1987 Acute rhabdomyolysis following halothane anesthesia without succinylcholine. Anesthesiology 67: 856–857

Schaer H, Steinmann B, Jerusalem S, Maier C 1977 Rhabdomyolysis induced by anaesthesia with intraoperative cardiac arrest. British Journal of Anaesthesia 49: 495–499

Seay A R, Ziter F A, Thompson J A 1978 Cardiac arrest during induction of anesthesia in Duchenne muscular dystrophy. Journal of Pediatrics 93: 88–90

RHEUMATOID ARTHRITIS

A common autoimmune connective tissue disease, primarily involving the joints, but with widespread systemic effects. There is hypergammaglobulinaemia, and rheumatoid factors, which are autoantibodies of IgE, IgA and IgM classes, are present.

Preoperative abnormalities

1. The joint disease involves inflammation, the formation of granulation tissue, fibrosis, joint destruction and deformity. Any joint may be affected. Those of particular concern to the anaesthetist are the cervical, the temporomandibular and the cricoarytenoid joints.
2. Extra-articular problems occur in over 50% of patients.
   a. Lungs
   May be affected by effusions, nodular lesions, diffuse interstitial fibrosis or Caplan's syndrome. This is a form of massive pulmonary fibrosis seen in coalminers with rheumatoid arthritis or positive rheumatoid factor, and probably represents an abnormal tissue response to inorganic dust. There may be a restrictive lung defect, with a contribution from reduced chest wall compliance.
   b. Kidney
   Twenty-five percent of patients eventually die from renal failure. Renal damage may be related to the disease process itself, from secondary amyloid disease, or from drug treatment.
   c. Heart
   Is involved in 35% of cases. There may be endocarditis, pericarditis or left ventricular failure.
   d. Blood vessels
   A widespread vasculitis can occur. Small arteries and arterioles are

often involved, frequently in the presence of relatively disease-free main trunk vessels. Significant ischaemia may result, the actual effects depending on the tissue or organ supplied.

e. Peripheral neuropathy

Anaesthetic problems

1. Involvement of cervical vertebrae
Cervical instability is reported to occur in 25% of patients with rheumatoid arthritis. Of these, one-quarter will have no neurological symptoms (Norton & Ghanma 1982). This problem is not confined to those with longstanding disease. The commonest complication is atlanto-axial subluxation, although subaxial subluxations may occur in addition. Destruction of bone and weakening of the ligaments allow the odontoid peg to move backwards, thus compressing the spinal cord against the posterior arch of the atlas. The presenting symptoms of 31 patients with cervical myelopathy were analysed (Marks & Sharp 1981). Sensory disturbances occurred in 74% and were often dismissed as being due to peripheral neuropathy. Weakness occurred in 19%, flexor spasms in 16% and incontinence in 6%. By the time the diagnosis was made, 77% had spastic paraparesis or quadriparesis.

The dangers of anaesthesia and endoscopy have been emphasized. Flexion of the head and muscle relaxation may result in cervical cord damage (McConkey 1982, Norton & Ghanma 1982).

2. Laryngeal problems
A constant pattern of laryngeal and tracheal deviation is reported to occur in some patients, particularly those with proximal migration of the odontoid peg (Keenan et al 1983). The larynx is tilted forwards, displaced anteriorly and laterally to the left and the vocal cords rotated clockwise, with a forward tilt of the larynx. In addition, cricoarytenoid joint involvement may rarely produce upper respiratory tract obstruction.

3. Limitation of mouth opening may occur due to arthritis of the temporomandibular joints. This is a particular problem in juvenile rheumatoid arthritis (Hodgkinson 1981).

4. Lung disease may cause reduced pulmonary reserve and hypoxia.

5. There may be an increased sensitivity to anaesthetic agents.

Management

1. Assessment of neck and jaw mobility. The Sharp and Purser test gives a clinical indication of cervical instability (Norton & Ghanma 1982). The patient should be upright, relaxed and with the neck flexed. With a finger on the spinous process of the axis, the forehead should be pressed backwards with the other hand. Normally there is minimal movement. If subluxation is present, the head moves backwards as reduction occurs.

2. A lateral view of the cervical spine in flexion and extension will show the distance between the odontoid peg and the posterior border of the anterior arch of the atlas. If subluxation is present, this distance is greater than 3 mm.

3. Instability may be an indication for awake intubation and application of a collar or Crutchfield tongs, to maintain rigidity during surgery.

4. Deviation of the larynx may make fibreoptic laryngoscopy more difficult in some patients (Keenan et al 1983).

5. Assessment of pulmonary function and reserve.

6. Examination for other significant complications such as cricoarytenoid arthritis, valvular disease or pericardial effusion.

7. The use of epidural or caudal anaesthesia may be unwise in cases where intubation difficulties are anticipated.

BIBLIOGRAPHY

Hodgkinson R 1981 Anesthetic management of a parturient with severe juvenile rheumatoid arthritis. Anesthesia and Analgesia 60: 611–612
Keenan M A, Stiles C M, Kaufman R L 1983 Acquired laryngeal deviation associated with cervical spine disease in erosive polyarticular arthritis. Anesthesiology 58: 411–449
Marks J S, Sharp J 1981 Rheumatoid cervical myelopathy. Quarterly Journal of Medicine 50: 307–319
McConkey B (Editorial) 1982 Rheumatoid cervical myelopathy. British Medical Journal 284: 1731–1732
Norton M L, Ghanma M A 1982 Atlanto-axial instability revisited; an alert for endoscopists. Annals of Otology, Rhinology and Laryngology 91: 567–570

SARCOIDOSIS

A multisystem granulomatous disorder, most frequently presenting in young adults with bilateral hilar lymphadenopathy, pulmonary infiltration, cutaneous and ocular lesions.

Preoperative abnormalities

1. The patient may be asymptomatic, and about one-third of cases present because of an abnormality found on CXR. With more advanced disease there may be variable degrees of respiratory impairment. CXR usually shows bilateral hilar lymphadenopathy with increased reticular shadowing in the lung fields. Lung function tests may be impaired. Restrictive, gas transfer and obstructive defects may all occur at different stages of the disease. In advanced disease, pulmonary hypertension may develop.

2. Other more commonly involved organs are the skin, eyes, liver, spleen, and the bones of the hands and feet. Hypercalcaemia may occur.

3. Cardiac disease, although rare, is more common than was previously thought (Fleming 1986). Its diagnosis is of anaesthetic importance.

The pathological lesions can be diffuse or focal. Localized granulomata and fibrous scarring most commonly occur in the basal portion of the ventricular septum and left ventricular wall (Valantine et al 1987). These lesions will be asymptomatic unless they happen to involve the conducting system, in which case arrhythmias or conduction defects occur. Less commonly, the distribution of granulomata may be widespread, and they may coalesce to produce diffuse interstitial fibrosis. The resulting hypokinesia and subsequent heart failure will be clinically indistinguishable from other cardiomyopathies (Fleming 1986).

At autopsy on 84 patients with sarcoidosis, 27% were found to have myocardial granulomata, one-third of which had been unsuspected (Silverman et al 1978). In those patients diagnosed as having cardiac involvement, the signs in order of frequency of presentation were complete heart block, ventricular ectopics or ventricular tachycardia, myocardial disease causing heart failure, sudden death and first-degree heart block or bundle branch block. A further analysis of 57 patients with complete heart block and sarcoid revealed that in 72%, the heart block was the first sign of the disease (Pehrsson & Tornling 1985). Sudden death had occurred in two-thirds of patients in an autopsy study of cardiac sarcoid (Roberts et al 1977). In approximately 18% of these, death was the initial manifestation of cardiac involvement and in the vast majority of these, death occurred during a period of exercise.

4. Laryngeal sarcoidosis may occur. The commonest lesion reported is an oedematous, pale, diffuse enlargement of the supraglottic structures (Neel & McDonald 1982).

5. The diagnosis can be made on biopsy of a skin lesion, or lung and bronchial biospsy via a fibreoptic bronchoscope. The Kveim test has a high positivity in the active stages, but is lower in the chronic disease. Angiotensin-converting enzyme and 24-hour urinary calcium levels may be raised in active sarcoid.

Anaesthetic problems

1. In advanced disease, respiratory function may be markedly impaired.

2. Although rare, cardiac disease may be unexpected, and can occur in young, previously asymptomatic patients. The sudden onset of complete heart block during anaesthesia in an athletic young man with sarcoid was described (Thomas & Mason 1988). Permanent pacing was required after surgery. Difficulties with pacemaker management can be a feature of cardiac sarcoidosis (Lie et al 1974).

3. A case of upper airway obstruction due to sarcoid has been described (Wills & Harris 1987).

Management

1. If there is widespread pulmonary involvement and the patient is symptomatic, lung function tests, including blood gases, should be performed.

2. A preoperative ECG is essential, even in young patients. If there is evidence of a conduction defect, a temporary pacemaker should be inserted prior to anaesthesia.

3. Assessment and management of laryngeal sarcoid.

BIBLIOGRAPHY

Fleming H A 1986 Sarcoid heart disease. British Medical Journal 292: 1095–1096
Lie J T, Hunt D, Valentine P A 1974 Sudden death from cardiac sarcoidosis with involvement of the conduction system. American Journal of the Medical Sciences 267: 123–128
Neel H B, McDonald T J 1982 Laryngeal sarcoidosis: report of 13 patients. Annals of Otology, Rhinology and Laryngology 91: 359–362
Pehrsson S K, Tornling G 1985 Sarcoidosis associated with complete heart block. Sarcoidosis 2: 135–141
Roberts W C, McAllister H A, Ferrans V J 1977 Sarcoidosis of the heart. American Journal of Medicine 63: 86–108
Silverman K J, Hutchins G M, Bulkley B H 1978 Cardiac sarcoid: a clinicopathologic study of 84 unselected patients with systemic sarcoidosis. Circulation 58: 1204–1211
Thomas D W, Mason R A 1988 Complete heart block during anaesthesia in a patient with sarcoidosis. Anaesthesia 43: 578–580
Valantine H, McKenna W J, Nihoyannopoulos P, Mitchell A, Foale R A, Davies M J, Oakley C M 1987 Sarcoidosis: a pattern of clinical and morphological presentation. British Heart Journal 57: 256–263
Wills M H, Harris M M 1987 An unusual airway complication with sarcoidosis. Anesthesiology 66: 554–555

SCLERODERMA

A spectrum of diseases involving abnormal collagen deposition and vascular changes in the skin and other organs. Various forms have been described, including a localized cutaneous form (morphoea), systemic sclerosis, and the CREST syndrome (Calcinosis, Raynaud's, (o)Esophageal problems, Sclerodactyly and Telangiectasia). Scleroderma occurs more commonly in women, often in the 30–50 years age group. Pregnancy may worsen the disease, and there is a high incidence of fetal loss.

Preoperative abnormalities

1. The skin becomes taut, shiny and waxy looking. Skin folds are lost and there is a non-pitting oedema. Raynaud's of the hands and feet is the presenting feature in 90% of cases. Contractures of the joints and the mouth may develop. Multiple telangiectasia may occur. Sweating is reduced.

2. Oesophageal involvement has been reported in up to 80% of patients and may produce dysphagia, reflux oesophagitis and strictures. It has been suggested that the basis of the dysphagia lies in disturbances of motility, rather than structural changes in the oesophagus (Weisman & Calcaterra 1978).

3. Cardiac lesions may occur in 50–90% of cases of the systemic disease. A study of 46 patients with systemic sclerosis showed that 56% had arrhythmias or conduction defects, and 28% had a pericardial effusion demonstrated by echocardiography (Clements et al 1981).
4. Pulmonary fibrosis, mainly affecting the lower lobes, may progress to produce pulmonary hypertension. Weakness of the respiratory muscles and diaphragm may occur (Iliffe & Pettigrew 1983).
5. Gut involvement may cause malabsorption, and occasionally vitamin C deficiency. Intestinal obstruction can occur.
6. Renal disease and systemic hypertension are common in systemic disease. Clinical and pathological features of an accelerated phase occur, and the loss of renal function may be abrupt.
7. Antinuclear factor is positive in about 60% of cases.
8. Patients may be receiving steroids or immunosuppressants.

Anaesthetic problems

1. Skin changes may result in difficulties with venous access. The contractures of the mouth are susceptible to damage, and may result in poor access to the oral cavity. Problems occurred in a case during dental extraction. Injection into a peripheral cannula produced local complications in the patient's hand, and insertion of the mouth prop caused a tear of the angle of the mouth (Davidson-Lamb & Finlayson 1977).
2. Oesophageal involvement may make the patient more prone to acid reflux and regurgitation. Abnormalities of oesophageal function can occur even in asymptomatic patients, and there is an inability of the oesophagus to empty without the aid of gravity.
3. Complications have been described in association with local anaesthetic techniques. Prolonged sensory loss, which may be due to reduced blood flow, has been reported (Eisele & Reitan 1971, Lewis 1974). Injection of a large volume of solution can produce a degree of tension in the skin sufficient to interfere with local blood supply. Sclerotic skin may conceal landmarks.
4. Intubation may be more difficult than usual if there are mouth and neck contractures. Telangiectasia in the mouth or nose may bleed.
5. Problems occur associated with systemic or pulmonary hypertension. Left ventricular failure, arrhythmias or pericardial effusions may arise. A maternal death was reported associated with the development of pulmonary oedema and pulmonary hypertension following Caesarean section (Younker & Harrison 1985). Thus author has seen a maternal death due to severe hypertension and pulmonary oedema in the 32nd week of pregnancy.
6. The combination of pulmonary abnormalities and contraction of the skin of the chest wall, may contribute to postoperative respiratory inadequacy.

Management

1. Assessment of respiratory function, including lung function tests and blood gases, if there is pulmonary involvement.
2. Adequate venous access may require the use of a central vein or a venous cutdown. Vasoconstriction can be reduced by keeping the theatre temperature high and by warming intravenous fluids.
3. Precautions should be taken against acid aspiration.
4. Potential difficulties posed by intubation should be assessed preoperatively. Under certain circumstances, the possibility of an awake intubation or tracheostomy under local anaesthesia will need consideration.
5. Problems in measuring the blood pressure may be overcome by the use of an ultrasonic blood pressure device. If direct monitoring is necessary, then a large artery should be chosen.
6. For Caesarean section, the choice between a general or regional technique may be difficult. Successful epidural anaesthesia was reported in a patient with advanced systemic sclerosis and the CREST syndrome (Thompson & Conklin 1983). A coagulation screen should be performed, and care taken with the dose of local anaesthetic used.

BIBLIOGRAPHY

Clements P J, Furst D E, Cabeen W, Tashkin D, Paulus H E, Roberts N 1981 The relationship of arrhythmias and conduction disturbances to other manifestations of cardiopulmonary disease in progressive systemic sclerosis. American Journal of Medicine 71: 38–46
Davidson-Lamb R W, Finlayson M C K 1977 Scleroderma: complications encountered during dental anaesthesia. Anaesthesia 32: 893–895
Eisele J H, Reitan J A 1971 Scleroderma, Raynaud's phenomenon, and local anesthesics. Anesthesiology 34: 386–387
Iliffe G D, Pettigrew N M 1983 Hypoventilatory respiratory failure in generalised scleroderma. British Medical Journal 286: 337–338
Lewis G B 1974 Prolonged regional analgesia in scleroderma. Canadian Anaesthetists' Society Journal 21: 495–497
Thompson J, Conklin K A 1983 Anesthetic management of a pregnant patient wth scleroderma. Anesthesiology 59: 69–71
Weisman R A, Calcaterra J C 1978 Head and neck manifestations of scleroderma. Annals of Otology, Rhinology and Laryngology 87: 332–339
Younker D, Harrison B 1985 Scleroderma and pregnancy. Anaesthetic considerations. British Journal of Anaesthesia 57: 1136–1139

SCOLIOSIS

A lateral curvature of the spine occurring in association with actual rotation of the vertebral body and spine, in the direction of the concavity of the curve. There is wedging of the vertebral body and discs. The resulting prominence of the posterior part of the ribs on the side of the convexity may give a false impression of kyphosis.

Scoliosis can be broadly divided into three categories, the commonest of which is the idiopathic form. Otherwise, scoliosis may be congenital, or may develop as a secondary feature of a variety of neuromuscular or connective tissue disorders. Causes of secondary scoliosis include poliomyelitis, syringomyelia, Friedreich's ataxia, muscular dystrophy, neurofibromatosis, Marfan's syndrome and rheumatoid arthritis.

Scoliosis is described in terms of its angle. The greater the angle, the more severe the respiratory and subsequent cardiovascular impairment.

Preoperative abnormalities

1. Respiratory changes
Scoliosis causes respiratory impairment due to a number of factors. These include abnormalities in the development of the rib cage, the muscles of respiration, and in the distribution of the pulmonary vascular bed in relation to the alveoli. Respiratory impairment is usually restrictive, the vital capacity, total lung capacity and functional residual capacity being between 60% and 80% of that predicted. As the severity of the scoliosis increases, airway closure encroaches on the functional residual capacity. The greater the angle of scoliosis, the greater the abnormalities in lung function. Gas exchange is impaired due to ventilation blood flow inequalities, and it has been suggested that the greater maldistribution is on the side of the concavity. PaO_2 reduction occurs initially, and may worsen with increasing age. The respiratory response to CO_2 is abnormal and pulmonary vascular resistance may be elevated. Subsequently hypercapnoea may develop. Initially, the abnormalities may occur only during sleep, and studies have shown a decreased vital capacity, hypoxia and respiratory failure in some patients at night.

2. Cardiovascular changes
In the more severe cases, pulmonary vascular resistance increases due to a combination of structural changes in the pulmonary vascular bed and the effects of hypoxia. A raised pulmonary vascular pressure results. In the later stages there will be ECG changes of right atrial dilatation (P wave >2.5 mm in height) and right ventricular hypertrophy (R>S in leads V1 and V2). Right ventricular failure secondary to pulmonary disease may finally ensue.

3. Associated problems
  a. Neuropathic
  Poliomyelitis, Friedreich's ataxia, syringomyelia.
  b. Myopathic
  Muscular dystrophy.
  c. Miscellaneous
  Neurofibromatosis, Marfan's syndrome, rheumatoid arthritis.

Anaesthetic problems

Surgery may be incidental, or directed towards correction of the scoliosis. In general, the prognosis for patients with secondary scoliosis is less good than for the idiopathic form. Death due to cardiac failure occurred in the seventh hour of a scoliosis correction in a 13-year-old patient with DMD (Sethna et al 1988). One death was reported in a retrospective review of nine cases of DMD and one of Becker's muscle dystrophy, undergoing spinal fusion. The particular patient had a VC of only 12% of that predicted and could not be weaned off the ventilator (Milne & Rosales 1982).

Surgery in general

1. Problems attributable to the underlying cause, if the scoliosis is not idiopathic.
2. Respiratory problems depend upon the degree of existing impairment. An already decreased respiratory response to CO_2 may be made worse by the anaesthetic. While mild hypoxia is common, the onset of hypercarbia, unless precipitated by an acute infection, is of bad prognostic significance.
3. As a result of the anatomical changes, the respiratory muscles work at a mechanical disadvantage, so that postoperative respiratory inadequacy and retention of secretions may occur.
4. In advanced cases, there may be the problems of pulmonary hypertension and right ventricular failure. Cardiac abnormalities, including hypertrophic cardiomyopathy and conduction defects, occur in 90% of patients with Friedreich's ataxia.
   In DMD there may be hypertrophic cardiomyopathy and diastolic failure. Mitral valve prolapse may occur in some patients. Marfan's syndrome can be associated with mitral or aortic incompetence, dissecting aortic aneurysm, aortic or pulmonary dilatation or coronary artery disease.
5. A higher than expected incidence of MH, or an MH-like syndrome has been reported (Britt & Kalow 1970). Out of a total of 89 cases of MH studied, six had idiopathic scoliosis.
6. Hyperkalaemia following the use of suxamethonium has been reported in patients with neuromuscular problems, particularly in cases where there is a motor deficit.
7. Rhabdomyolysis and myoglobinuria may occur following the use of suxamethonium and halothane in patients with myopathies (including McArdle's syndrome).
8. Serious arrhythmias and cardiac arrest have been described following the use of halothane and suxamethonium in Duchenne muscular dystrophy (see also Duchenne muscular dystrophy).

Surgery for scoliosis

1. Inadequate preoperative respiratory reserve has resulted in postoperative deaths in patients subjected to surgery for scoliosis.

2. Evaluation of spinal cord function may be required after spinal distraction with Harrington rods. It may be necessary to waken the patient during the procedure, so that motor deficits can be detected and the spinal distraction decreased. The use of evoked cortical responses has also been suggested, although these have not always been reliable.

3. Blood loss may be substantial. Losses of up to 92% of the patient's blood volume have been recorded (Abott & Bentley 1980).

4. Deliberate hypotensive techniques have been associated with a decrease in blood supply to the spinal cord and subsequent paraplegia.

5. The problems of surgery performed in the prone position.

6. Hypothermia may occur in prolonged procedures and where extensive blood loss has been replaced.

7. Haemopneumothorax.

Management

Surgery in general

1. Respiratory assessment should include the VC measured in both seated and supine positions, FEV with and without bronchodilators, and blood gases (Kafer 1980).

2. Cardiovascular assessment. If the PVR and PAP are raised, and there are ECG changes and signs of RVH, then the prognosis is poor. Right ventricular failure must be treated.

3. In severe cases, a decision must be made as to whether or not elective surgery should be undertaken.

4. If possible, regional or local anaesthesia should be utilized.

5. Monitoring should include ECG, core temperature, $ETCO_2$, and blood pressure, directly or indirectly. Where indicated, urine output, CVP, blood gases, and occasionally PAP monitoring may be required.

Surgery for scoliosis

1. A VC of at least 20 ml/kg or 30% of predicted, and an inspiratory capacity of 15 ml/kg, have been suggested as being essential for scoliosis surgery (Milne & Rosales 1982).

2. The endotracheal tube must be firmly fastened.

3. A wake-up test should be performed, provided the patient is a suitable subject and the matter has been discussed in advance. Techniques described for this include N_2O/O_2/relaxants with morphine (Sudhir et al 1976, Abott & Bentley 1980), with fentanyl (MacEwen et al 1975) and with alfentanil (Chamberlain & Bradshaw 1985). The use of hypnosis (Crawford et al 1976) has also been reported. Reversal at the appropriate time is achieved with neostigmine and atropine, and by the use of a narcotic antagonist if necessary.

4. Sensory evoked potentials have been used both alone, and in conjunction with the wake-up test, to detect neurological damage.

(Grundy et al 1982). The reliability of sensory evoked potentials alone, in predicting cord damage, has not yet been established.

5. Theatre temperature should be maintained at a higher than usual level and a warming blanket and blood warmer used.

6. The use of deliberate hypotension should be carefully considered (Grundy et al 1982).

7. If the anterior approach through the diaphragm is used, postoperative IPPV may be required.

BIBLIOGRAPHY

Abott T R, Bentley G 1980 Intra-operative awakening during scoliosis surgery. Anaesthesia 35: 298–302
Britt B A, Kalow W 1970 Malignant hyperthermia: a statistical review. Canadian Anaesthetists's Society Journal 17: 293–315
Chamberlain M E, Bradshaw E G 1985 The 'wake-up test'. Anaesthesia 40: 780–782
Crawford A H, Jones C W, Perisho J A, Herring J A 1976 Hypnosis for monitoring intraoperative spinal cord function. Anesthesia and Analgesia 55: 42–44
Grundy B L, Nash C L, Brown R H 1982 Deliberate hypotension for spinal fusion: prospective randomised study with evoked potential monitoring. Canadian Anaesthetists' Society Journal 29: 452–461
Kafer E R 1980 Respiratory and cardiovascular functions in scoliosis and the principles of anesthetic management. Anesthesiology 52: 339–351
MacEwen G D, Bunnell W P, Sriram K 1975 Acute neurological complications in the treatment of scoliosis. Journal of Bone and Joint Surgery 57A: 404–408
Milne B, Rosales J K 1982 Anaesthetic considerations in patients with muscular dystrophy undergoing spinal fusion and Harrington rod insertion. Canadian Anaesthetists' Society Journal 29: 250–254
Sethna N F, Rockoff M A, Worthen M, Rosnow J M 1988 Anesthesia-related complications in children with Duchenne muscular dystrophy. Anesthesiology 68: 462–465
Sudhir K G, Smith R M, Hall J E, Hansen D D 1976 Intraoperative awakening for early recognition of possible neurological sequelae during Harrington rod spinal fusion. Anesthesia and Analgesia 55: 526–528

SHY-DRAGER SYNDROME
(see also AUTONOMIC DYSFUNCTION)

A condition presenting in late life, in which autonomic failure or dysfunction is associated with, or precedes, the onset of widespread central neuronal degeneration. In particular there is loss of cells in the intermediolateral nuclei of the lateral horn in the spinal cord which are the preganglionic sympathetic neurones.

Preoperative abnormalities

1. Postural hypotension and an inability, in response to stress, to produce the normal pressor response which depends on reflex vasoconstriction and tachycardia. There is reversal of the usual diurnal pattern of blood pressure and that normally produced by postural changes.

2. Anhidrosis, incontinence and impotence can occur.

3. Fluid and electrolyte homeostasis is disturbed, resulting in a failure to concentrate urine at night, and producing a nocturnal diuresis and sodium loss.

4. There may be a disordered respiratory pattern and sleep apnoea.

5. Denervation hypersensitivity has been reported.

6. Osteoporosis and aseptic necrosis of bone are thought to be a result of impaired periosteal vascular control. Orthopaedic surgery may therefore be required.

Anaesthetic problems

1. The inability of the cardiovascular system to respond to stress by vasoconstriction and tachycardia results in marked cardiovascular instability. The heart rate may be relatively fixed. An inability to release catecholamines has been suggested (Bannister 1979). A lack of pressor reponse to painful stimuli under light anaesthesia has been noted (Sweeney et al 1985).

2. Decreased sensitivity of the respiratory system to increased carbon dioxide levels under anaesthesia may make techniques using spontaneous respiration difficult to achieve (Sweeney et al 1985). Pulmonary respiratory reflexes are impaired.

3. Defective lacrimation, decreased sweating and sluggish pupillary reflexes may be present. The unreliability of these reflexes may cause difficulties in assessing the depth of anaesthesia.

4. A denervation hypersensitivity type of response to the infusion of catecholamines (Malan & Crago 1979) and a lack of response to indirectly acting amines such as ephedrine, methylamphetamine and tyramine have been reported. However, it has been suggested that these features should only be seen in conditions where there is peripheral, not central, autonomic dysfunction (Stirt et al 1982).

5. Sensitivity to the effects of intravenous and volatile anaesthetics (Sweeney et al 1987).

Management

1. Anaesthestic agents with minimal cardiovascular depression should be chosen.

2. Hypovolaemia should be corrected promptly (Bevan 1979).

3. Techniques using spontaneous respiration should probably be avoided.

4. Careful monitoring of blood pressure is essential for the correction of hypotension.

5. Postoperative observation to detect respiratory insufficiency.

6. Treatment with fludrocortisone may increase extracellular fluid volume (Watson 1987).

BIBLIOGRAPHY

Bannister R 1979 Chronic autonomic failure with postural hypotension. Lancet ii: 404–406
Bevan D R 1979 Shy–Drager Syndrome. Anaesthesia 34: 866–873
Malan M D, Crago R R 1979 Anaesthetic considerations in idiopathic orthostatic hypotension and the Shy–Drager syndrome. Canadian Anaesthetists' Society Journal 26: 322–327
Stirt J A, Frantz R A, Gunz E F, Conolly M E 1982 Anesthesia, catecholamines and hemodynamics in autonomic dysfunction. Anesthesia and Analgesia 61: 701–704
Sweeney B P, Jones S, Langford R M 1985 Anaesthesia in dysautonomia: further complications. Anaesthesia 40: 783–786
Watson R D S 1987 Treating postural hypotension. British Medical Journal 294: 390–391

SICK SINUS SYNDROME

A general term for various disorders of sino-atrial node function which usually present in the elderly, but can sometimes occur in young people. Patients may have a sinus bradycardia and periods of sinus arrest with escape rhythms, and sometimes intermittent episodes of tachyarrhythmias (the bradycardia/tachycardia syndrome). The sino-atrial node is under autonomic control and is a small area of specialized muscle situated at the junction of the superior vena cava and the base of the right atrial appendage. Its arterial supply is variable, arising from the right coronary artery in 65% and the left circumflex artery in 35% of cases. Dysfunction of the node is most commonly due to its replacement by fibrous tissue. Other causes include coronary artery disease, drugs and postcardiac surgery.

Preoperative abnormalities

1. A typical patient is commonly older than 60, and may complain of episodes of syncope, dizziness or palpitations. A 24-hour ambulatory ECG may show episodes of brady- or tachyarrhythmias which may be asymptomatic, but may coincide with the symptoms. Occasionally young people are affected, and this form may be familial. A group of nine people below the age of 25 with sino-atrial disease has been studied (Mackintosh 1981). They were all male, taller than average, and ambulatory monitoring of close relatives revealed an increased incidence of conducting system disorders.
2. Episodes of arrhythmia may cause fatigue, or precipitate angina or cardiac failure.
3. There is an inappropriate heart rate in response to stress or drugs. Often there is a sinus bradycardia of <60 b.p.m. during the awake state.
4. ECG may show alternate brady- and tachyarrhythmias. In sino-atrial block, P waves are dropped intermittently and the R–R intervals are multiples of cycle length.

1

Anaesthetic problems

1. The occurrence of brady- or tachyarrhythmias during anaesthesia may reduce cardiac output and compromise cerebral or coronary artery circulation. A number of such episodes have been reported. A sinus bradycardia of 40 b.p.m., which was unresponsive to atropine, occurred in a patient given ethrane with IPPV (Pratila & Pratilas 1976). Recurrent episodes of sinus arrest with nodal escape were described in a patient breathing spontaneously on halothane (Burt 1982). Asystole, which responded to cardiopulmonary resuscitation and atropine, occurred 10 minutes after administration of a spinal anaesthetic for prostatectomy in a patient with sinus bradycardia and RBBB (Cohen 1988). Several periods of asystole were reported in a 46-year-old lady, some hours after spinal anaesthesia for varicose vein surgery (Underwood & Glynn 1988). Sick sinus syndrome was diagnosed and a pacemaker inserted. Subsequent questioning revealed that the patient had a history of blackouts, usually related to vomiting.
2. A high incidence (15.3%) of systemic embolism has been reported in this syndrome. For this reason, the patient may already be taking anticoagulants.

Management

1. Twenty-four-hour ambulatory monitoring may be required to confirm the diagnosis. If there is inadequate time, and the diagnosis is in doubt, then the response of the patient to atropine may be tested. In a normal subject, atropine i.v. 0.02 mg/kg should increase the heart rate by more than 14 b.p.m.
2. If sick sinus syndrome is diagnosed, a temporary pacemaker should be inserted prior to anaesthesia. Halothane and enflurane may prolong conduction, and impair the ability of the myocardium to maintain cardiac output by increasing stroke volume. Under these circumstances there is no guarantee that cerebral or coronary perfusion will be adequate. Patients who are symptomatic are usually given a permanent pacemaker. Although this abolishes symptoms and improves the quality of life, studies have suggested that cardiac pacing does not affect long-term survival in the condition (Shaw et al 1980).
3. Anticoagulation may be required after surgery.

BIBLIOGRAPHY

Burt D E R 1982 The sick sinus syndrome. A complication during anaesthesia. Anaesthesia 37: 1108–1111
Cohen L I 1988 Asystole during spinal anesthesia in a patient with sick sinus syndrome. Anesthesiology 68: 787–788
Mackintosh A F 1981 Sinoatrial disease in young people. British Heart Journal 45: 62–66
Pratila M G, Pratilas V 1976 Sick-sinus syndrome manifest during anesthesia. Anesthesiology 44: 433–436
Shaw D B, Holman R R, Gowers J I 1980 Survival in sinoatrial disorders (sick-sinus syndrome). British Medical Journal 280: 139–141

Underwood S M, Glynn C J 1988 Sick sinus syndrome manifest after spinal anaesthesia. Anaesthesia 43: 307–309

SIPPLE'S SYNDROME
(MEN type IIa)

An autosomal dominant condition in which medullary carcinoma of the thyroid is frequently associated with phaeochromocytoma and, less commonly, with a parathyroid adenoma. Sipple's syndrome is one of a group of three familial diseases, and is otherwise known as multiple endocrine neoplasia (MEN) type IIa (Bouloux 1987).

Preoperative abnormalities

1. A thyroid mass may be associated with symptoms of hoarseness, dysphagia, cough and cervical lymphadenopathy.
2. The tumour may secrete a number of hormones including calcitonin, serotonin, prostaglandins and ACTH/MSH or insulin. Symptoms depend upon the hormone secreted.
3. Fifty per cent of cases have a phaeochromocytoma. Seventy per cent of the phaeochromocytomas are bilateral.
4. A parathyroid adenoma is present in 10% of cases.
5. Metastasis may occur to the liver, lungs and bone.

Anaesthetic problems

1. Those of a phaeochromocytoma, if present.
2. Cardiovascular complications, if hormones such as serotonin or prostaglandins are secreted.

Management

Exclude a phaeochromocytoma. If present, preoperative preparation will be required (see Phaeochromocytoma).

BIBLIOGRAPHY

Bouloux P-M 1987 Multiple endocrine neoplasia. Surgery 50: 1180–1185

SJÖGREN'S SYNDROME

A chronic inflammatory autoimmune disease which results in drying of secretions, and involves a number of exocrine organs, in particular the lacrimal and salivary glands (Isenberg & Crisp 1985). Sjögren's may be primary or secondary. About 75% of cases are secondary to a connective tissue disorder, of which the commonest is rheumatoid arthritis. In secondary Sjögren's, the glandular element is relatively mild. In the primary disease, infiltration of the salivary and lacrimal glands is predominant and there may be considerable swelling, accompanied by marked dryness of the eyes and mouth. Occasionally, in association with lymphadenopathy, this type may proceed to malignant lymphoma.

Preoperative abnormalities

1. Symptoms of the sicca syndrome include dryness of the eyes, mouth, vagina and skin.
2. Conditions associated with the secondary form include rheumatoid arthritis, systemic lupus, scleroderma, the polymyositis/dermatomyositis complex, polyarteritis nodosa, chronic active hepatitis and Graves' disease.
3. Swelling of the salivary and lacrimal glands may be prominent.
4. Other major organ involvement includes lung, kidney, liver, pancreas and lymphoid tissue. Either a sensory or motor neuropathy may occur and central nervous system lesions have been described.
5. The patient may be on corticosteroids or occasionally immunosuppressive agents.

Anaesthetic problems

1. Swelling of the salivary glands may make mask anaesthesia difficult (Eisele 1981).
2. Those of the primary disease (see under individual names).
3. The dry eyes are susceptible to damage during anaesthesia.

Management

1. If the Sjögren's is secondary to another disorder, there should be careful assessment of the primary disease.
2. Drying agents should be avoided if possible.
3. The eyes should be protected with pads.
4. Anaesthetic gases should be humidified.
5. Steroid supplements may be required.

BIBLIOGRAPHY

Eisele J H 1981 Connective tissue diseases. In: Anesthesia and uncommon diseases. W B Saunders, Philadelphia
Isenberg D, Crisp A 1985 Sjögren's syndrome. Hospital Update 11: 273–283

SNAKE BITES

The only poisonous snake in Britain is the adder (*Vipera berus*). The majority of adder bites are uncomplicated, and treatment is by immobilization of the affected part. It has been suggested that hospital admission for 12 hours is advisable, for observation and early treatment of complications, should they occur (Reid 1980). Deaths, although rare, have occurred between 6 and 60 hours after the bite. The venom causes local swelling, probably due to changes in vascular permeability. Occasionally, systemic absorption may cause activation of the complement and kinin systems, producing a severe anaphylactoid response with hypotension, ECG changes, raised CPK levels, and pulmonary oedema.

Presentation

1. Pain at the site of the bite.
2. Local swelling usually starts within 10 minutes, but may occur after an hour, and can last for 48–72 hours.
3. Regional lymph nodes draining the affected limb are enlarged.
4. Gastrointestinal symptoms. Vomiting can start within 5 minutes or up to several hours after the bite. Sweating, abdominal pain and diarrhoea may occur. The continuance of symptoms suggests a serious reaction.
5. Rarely there may be cardiovascular collapse, hypotension or peripheral vasoconstriction.
6. Angioneurotic oedema of the lips, face and tongue may develop at any time up to 48 hours after the event.
7. Bleeding is rare, although local bruising is common. Oozing from mucosal surfaces, such as the tooth sockets, is the first sign of generalized problems.

Management

1. The limb is immobilized and the patient reassured.
2. Monitor:
    a. Hourly pulse rate, blood pressure and respiratory rate.
    b. Any persistent symptoms. Continued vomiting, diarrhoea and abdominal pain, or the onset of spontaneous bleeding, is suggestive of a serious reaction.
    c. Local swelling. The circumference should be measured at an identified level on the affected limb.
    d. WCC, CPK, serum bicarbonate and ECG should be measured 12-hourly.
3. Zagreb antivenom should be given to reduce morbidity (Reid 1976) only if:
    a. Hypotension and peripheral vasoconstriction persists.

b. There is a leucocytosis of $>20 \times 10^9/l$.

c. An adult has swelling which extends up the forearm or the leg, within 2 hours of a bite.

Antivenom regimen

Zagreb antivenom 2 ampoules diluted with saline 0.9% 100 ml and given i.v., and repeated in 1–2 hours if no clinical improvement occurs.

n.b. Adrenaline 1 in 1000, 0.5 ml diluted to 10 ml, must be immediately available at the patient's side.

A known allergic history is an absolute contraindication to the use of antivenom.

Antivenoms for foreign venomous snakes

Contact either:

a. Pharmacy Department, Walton Hospital, Liverpool, UK (telephone 051-525-3611), or

b. Poisons Unit, Guy's Hospital, London, UK (telephone 01-955-5000).

BIBLIOGRAPHY

Reid H A 1976 Adder bites in Britain. British Medical Journal 2: 153–156
Reid H A 1980 Poisoning caused by snake bite. Hospital Update 6: 675–682

SOLVENT ABUSE

The incidence of solvent abuse is increasing in Britain. An epidemiological study reported 282 deaths in the period 1971–83 and 80 deaths in 1983 (Anderson et al 1985). The latter represented 2% of all deaths in males between the ages of 10 and 19 years. Fifty-one per cent of the deaths were attributed to direct toxic effects, 21% to plastic bag asphyxia, 18% to inhaled gastric contents and 11% to trauma.

Sudden death during 'sniffing' is thought to be due to arrhythmias associated with the sensitization of the heart to the effect of endogenous catecholamines, by the inhaled volatile hydrocarbon (Cunningham et al 1987). Death occurs therefore more commonly during periods of intense cardiac stimulation such as exercise. Animal studies with inhaled hydrocarbons would seem to confirm this. Serious ventricular arrhythmias can be provoked by both exogenous and endogenous catecholamines.

Volatile hydrocarbons also have chronic effects on the liver, kidney and brain. Chronic cardiotoxicity may also occur (Boon 1987).

It has been suggested that interactions may occur with halothane, whose chemical structure closely resembles that of 1,1,1-trichloroethane (McLeod et al 1987).

Typical products inhaled include glues, dry cleaning agents, nail polish, paint thinners, antifreeze and degreasing agents.

Preoperative abnormalities

1. Agents most frequently encountered:
   a. Toluene ($C_6H_5CH_3$)
   A solvent in cements and glues. Cardiac arrhythmias are common during inhalation, and the most frequent cause of death is cardiac arrest precipitated by exercise.
   b. 1,1,1-Trichloroethane
   An industrial cleaning solvent and paint remover. Is present in Tippex fluid thinner, audiovisual equipment cleaners, glues, adhesive plaster removers, and degreasing agents used in steel welding. Sudden deaths can occur either with solvent abuse or following industrial accidents. Cardiac arrhythmias can occur at the time of abuse, but may also persist for up to 2 weeks after the exposure. More recently, there has been a suggestion this agent may cause chronic cardiac damage, and that there may be provocation of symptoms of cardiac toxicity when re-exposure to the agent, or to chemically similar substances, occurs.
2. The abuser is most likely to be a teenager, 13–15 years being the peak age. There is a high incidence from social class V, and from the armed forces (Anderson et al 1985). Erythematous spots around the mouth and nose may indicate the use of a plastic bag.
3. Cardiac arrhythmias may be noticed preoperatively.

Anaesthetic problems

1. Cardiac arrhythmias
Cardiac problems in two patients chronically exposed to 1,1,1-trichloroethane were attributed to an interaction with halothane during anaesthesia (McLeod et al 1987). The first, a 14-year-old boy, developed multiple ventricular extrasystoles and ventricular tachycardia during tonsillectomy. The arrhythmias persisted postoperatively and needed treatment with a number of antiarrhythmic drugs. At one stage a pacemaker was required. Evidence of 1,1,1-trichloroethane abuse was subsequently found. The second was a 55-year-old man who had previously developed AF and cardiac failure. This was diagnosed as being due to industrial exposure to 1,1,1-trichloroethane in the steel industry. He was removed from exposure and his condition did not worsen. Two years later, and following an anaesthetic (halothane, but no details), he became symptomatic. Echocardiography and myocardial biopsy indicated a deterioration in cardiac function of recent onset. As halothane is very similar in structure to 1,1,1-trichloroethane, it was

postulated that this was reponsible for the cardiac problems encountered in both cases.

2. A cardiomyopathy developed in a 15-year-old boy, who had a 2-year history of solvent abuse with toluene-containing substances. He subsequently required cardiac transplantation (Wiseman & Banim 1987).

Management

1. The occurrence of unexpected arrhythmias in a teenager, particularly in the presence of spots around the mouth and nose, should alert the anaesthetist to the possibility of solvent abuse.

2. Continuous ECG monitoring. This underlines the importance of ECG monitoring from the start of the anaesthetic, even in apparently fit young patients.

BIBLIOGRAPHY

Anderson H R, Macnair R S, Ramsey J D 1985 Deaths from abuse of volatile substances: a national epidemiological study. British Medical Journal 290: 304–307

Boon N A 1987 Solvent abuse and the heart. British Medical Journal 294: 722

Cunningham S R, Dalzell G W N, McGirr P, Khan M M 1987 Myocardial infarction and primary ventricular fibrillation after glue sniffing. British Medical Journal 294: 739–740

McLeod A A, Marjot R, Monaghan M J, Hugh-Jones P, Jackson G 1987 Chronic cardiac toxicity after inhalation of 1,1,1-trichloroethane. British Medical Journal 294: 727–729

Wiseman M N, Banim S 1987 'Glue sniffer's' heart. British Medical Journal 294: 739

STURGE–WEBER SYNDROME

A congenital syndrome of unknown aetiology, in which a cavernous haemangioma of one side of the face is associated with an intracranial angioma. General anaesthesia may be required for the management of glaucoma.

Preoperative abnormalities

1. A naevus (port wine stain) of one side of the face, which may involve one or more divisions of the trigeminal nerve. It is often associated with progressive mental retardation.

2. Epilepsy, and a hemiparesis involving the contralateral side may occur. Fits may be difficult to control. Gum hypertrophy may occur secondary to phenytoin therapy.

3. There are variations in the full clinical picture. One side of the vault and the hemiparetic half of the body may be smaller than the other. There may be unilateral glaucoma, increased scalp vascularity and unilateral hypertrophy of the carotid artery.

4. A venous haemangioma usually involves the meninges of the occipitoparietal surface of the brain. The adjacent cortex is gradually destroyed, possibly due to pressure. Deeper arteriovenous malformations, which occur only rarely, may be fed by large arteries and increasingly large veins. If this happens, a considerable arteriovenous shunt may result in cardiac hypertrophy and failure.

5. Skull X-ray shows linear calcification of the underlying brain tissue.
6. Arteriography or DVI will demonstrate the extent of the lesion.

Anaesthetic problems

1. The patient is usually an epileptic.
2. Gross vascular hypertrophy of the lips, buccal mucosa, gums and tongue, caused airway obstruction during a difficult inhalational induction (Aldridge 1987).
3. The cerebral lesion is usually too large for operative surgery. However, should neurosurgery be required, it may be associated with massive bleeding.

Management

1. Assessment of the degree of significance of the arteriovenous shunt.
2. Extreme hyperventilation should be avoided.
3. Assessment of possible airway difficulties.
4. A hypotensive technique may be required for neurosurgical procedures.

BIBLIOGRAPHY

Aldridge L M 1987 An unusual cause of upper airway obstruction. Anaesthesia 42: 1239–1240

SUBACUTE BACTERIAL ENDOCARDITIS, PROPHYLAXIS DURING SURGERY

A serious infection of the endocardium, most frequently affecting the heart valves, and caused by circulating microorganisms. The uniformly fatal disease of the pre-antibiotic era has been reduced to one with a mortality of about 30% (Morris 1985). However its incidence has not declined, and there has been a noticeable change in the pattern of the disease.

In 1981/2 a joint study between the Royal College of Physicians and the British Cardiac Society of 544 cases of infective endocarditis has formed the basis of an interesting series of papers on various aspects of the disease (Bayliss et al 1983a,b, 1984). There is an increased risk for patients with pre-existing cardiac lesions when operations or venous procedures are undertaken. This has implications for the anaesthetist. The patients affected tend to be older than in the past, and with the decline in rheumatic heart disease, the aortic valve is now more often affected than the mitral. A proportion of patients had normal hearts, or previously undiagnosed abnormalities. Streptococcus is still the predominant organism. In some cases, the portal of entry was obvious. Nineteen per cent were probably dental in origin, 16% were from the gut, genitourinary, respiratory tract or skin, and 5% were from procedures involving access to the bloodstream. In 60% of cases, however, the source was unknown. While 13.7% of cases of endocarditis had had a dental procedure within the preceding 3 months, over half of these cases had pre-existing cardiac abnormalities, for which antibiotic prophylaxis had not been prescribed.

Any child with congenital heart disease is at risk, and endocarditis may present with fever, anaemia and leucocytosis. If the condition occurs in a child who has undergone open heart surgery, it carries a high mortality (Karl et al 1987).

Recommendations on the antibiotic prophylaxis of infective endocarditis were published by a Working Party of the British Society for Antimicrobial Chemotherapy in 1982:

1. Factors predisposing to the development of endocarditis
   a. High-risk patients:
      i. Prosthetic heart valves.
      ii. A previous attack of endocarditis.
   b. Standard-risk patients:
      i. Congenital heart disease, especially VSD and PDA, rarely ASD.
      ii. Rheumatic heart disease.
      iii. Other cardiac abnormalities, such as mitral valve prolapse and degenerative aortic valve disease.
      iv. Previous rheumatic fever.
      v. There is also an increased incidence in intravenous drug users, alcoholism, diabetes, renal failure, malignant disease and immunosuppression.
2. Bacteria involved in endocarditis
The organisms most commonly involved are *Streptococcus viridans*, *Streptococcus faecalis*, *Staphylococcus aureus* and Gram-negative organisms. In the 544 episodes studied in 1981/2, 63% were due to streptococci, 19% to staphylococci and 14% to bowel organisms (Bayliss et al 1983b). Infection with a staphyloccus carried the highest mortality (30%).
3. Types of surgery for which prophylaxis is recommended
   a. Necessary in both standard- and high-risk groups:
      i. Dental treatment including extractions, scaling, and surgery involving gingival tissues (Cawson 1982).
      ii. Genitourinary procedures, involving instrumentation.
      iii. Gastrointestinal surgery.
      iv. Respiratory tract operations.
   b. Not necessary in the standard- but necessary in the high-risk groups:

    i. Minor obstetric and gynaecological procedures.

    ii. GI endoscopic procedures.

    iii. Barium enema.

4. Recommended antibiotic prophylaxis

  a. Dental treatment without general anaesthesia

    i. Standard risk, not penicillin allergic:

Adult: amoxycillin oral, 3 g, 1 hour pre. op.

Child (5–10 yr): half adult dose.

Child (<5 yr): quarter adult dose.

    ii. Standard risk, penicillin allergic:

Adult: erythromycin oral 1.5 g, 90 minutes pre. op. and 500 mg 6
hours later

Child (5–10 yr): half adult dose.

Child (<5 yr): quarter adult dose.

    iii. High risk:

Amoxycillin i.m. 1 g and gentamicin i.m. 120 mg 15 minutes pre. op.
and amoxycillin oral 500 g 6 hours later.

  b. Dental treatment and upper respiratory tract surgery under general
anaesthesia

    i. Standard risk, not penicillin allergic:

Adult: amoxycillin i.m. 1 g in lignocaine 1% 2.5 ml before induction
and 500 mg oral 6 hours later.

Child (<10 yr): half adult dose.

    ii. Standard risk, penicillin allergic:

Adult: vancomycin infusion 1 g over 20–30 minutes, followed by
gentamicin i.v. 120 mg before induction.

    iii. High risk or those having been given penicillin in the preceding
month:

Vancomycin and gentamicin as above

In ii or iii, children (<10 yr) require vancomycin 20 mg/kg and
gentamicin 2 mg/kg.

  c. Genitourinary, gastrointestinal tract investigations or surgery

    i. Standard risk, not penicillin allergic:

Adult: amoxycillin i.m. 1 g in lignocaine 1% 2.5 ml and gentamicin
i.m. 120 mg immediately before induction, amoxycillin
500 mg 6 hours later.

Child (<10 yr): amoxycillin half adult dose and gentamicin 2 mg/kg.

    ii. Standard risk, penicillin allergic and high risk:

Adult: vancomycin infusion 1 g over 20–30 minutes, followed by
gentamicin i.v. 120 mg before induction.

Child (<10 yr): vancomycin 20 mg/kg and gentamicin 2 mg/kg by
i.v. infusion

BIBLIOGRAPHY

Bayliss R, Clarke C, Oakley C, Somerville W, Whitfield A G W 1983a The teeth and infective
endocarditis. British Heart Journal 50: 506–512

Bayliss R, Clarke C, Oakley C M, Somerville W, Whitfield A G W, Young S E J 1983b The microbiology and pathogenesis of infective endocarditis. British Heart Journal 50: 513–519
Bayliss R, Clarke C, Oakley C M, Somerville W, Whitfield A G W, Young S E J 1984 The bowel, the genitourinary tract, and infective endocarditis. British Heart Journal 51: 339–345
Cawson R A 1983 The antibiotic prophylaxis of infective endocarditis. British Dental Journal 154: 183–184
Karl T, Wensley D, Stark J, de Laval M, Rees P, Taylor J F N 1987 Infective endocarditis in children with congenital heart disease: comparison of selected features in patients with surgical correction or palliation and those without. British Heart Journal 58: 57–65
Morris G K 1985 Infective endocarditis: a preventable disease? British Medical Journal 290: 1532–1533
Report of a Working Party of the British Society for Antimicrobial Chemotherapy 1982 The antibiotic prophylaxis of infective endocarditis. Lancet ii: 1323–1326

SYSTEMIC LUPUS ERYTHEMATOSIS

An autoimmune connective tissue disorder predominantly occurring in females between the ages of 20 and 50.

Preoperative abnormalities

1. Arthritis and cutaneous lesions are the commonest presenting features, and occur in 86–100% of patients (Bellamy et al 1984). Skin lesions include the well-known, but often transient, butterfly facial rash, vasculitis, alopecia and a photosensitivity dermatitis. Other common features are nephritis (75% patients), CNS lesions (60%), myocarditis and pericarditis (20–30%). Pulmonary atelectasis is common and may be associated with lupus pneumonitis and occasionally fibrosing alveolitis. Pulmonary function tests may show a restrictive defect. The diaphragm may be elevated, and a diaphragmatic myopathy has been suggested as a cause of the 'vanishing lung' syndrome.
2. There may be anaemia, leucopenia and occasionally thrombocytopenia. Laboratory tests show a variety of antibodies to nuclear and cytoplasmic components (Bellamy et al 1984).
3. There can be exacerbations and remissions. The condition may be worsened by stress, drugs, infection and pregnancy. A significant proportion of the patients develop atherosclerotic disease in late life (Rubin et al 1985).
4. Medication may include corticosteroids, antimalarials, and occasionally cytotoxics.
5. Circulating lupus anticoagulant occurs in up to 37% of patients with SLE (Malinow et al 1987). Paradoxically, this is an autoantibody associated with systemic vascular thromboses, which actually causes prolongation of some coagulation tests. Pregnancies in the presence of this antibody usually result in fetal loss. The incidence of this may be reduced by antiplatelet therapy.

Anaesthetic problems

1. Pulmonary involvement may result in a restrictive lung defect.
2. Thrombotic problems. Up to 28% of patients with lupus anticoagulant may have arterial or venous thrombotic episodes.
3. Coagulation tests in patients with lupus anticoagulant may show a prolonged PT, APTT or KCCT, or platelet dysfunction.

Management

1. Assessment of pulmonary and cardiac function.
2. Coagulation studies should be performed.
3. The problems posed by the presence of lupus anticoagulant in the pregnant patient who is on aspirin therapy have been discussed (Malinow et al 1987). It is suggested that the benefits of epidural anaesthesia must be weighed against the possibility of an epidural haematoma developing.

BIBLIOGRAPHY

Bellamy N, Kean W F, Buchanan W W 1984. Connective tissue diseases: systemic lupus erythematosis. Hospital Update 10: 65–76
Malinow A M, Rickford W J K, Mokriski B L K, Saller D N, McGuinn W J 1987 Lupus anticoagulant. Implication for obstetric anaesthetists. Anaesthesia 42: 1291–1293
Rubin L A, Urowitz M B, Gladman D D 1985 Mortality in systemic lupus erythematosus: the bimodal pattern revisited. Quarterly Journal of Medicine 55: 87–98

TAKAYASU's ARTERITIS

A non-specific chronic panarteritis, usually occurring in young women, and originally described in the Far East. In the early stages there is an inflammatory process in the large arteries which progresses to chronic arterial occlusion (Hall et al 1985). It is also known as 'pulseless disease' as there are usually reduced or absent pulses in the affected arteries.

Type 1   involves the aortic arch and its branches.
Type 2   involves the descending thoracic and abdominal aorta, without arch involvement.
Type 3   is a mixed picture of I and II.
Type 4   can consist of any of the above features in association with pulmonary artery involvement.

Preoperative abnormalities

1. There may be pulse deficits, depending upon the stage of the disease and the arteries involved in the condition. Bruits may be heard over stenosed arteries. There are also ectatic lesions of the aorta with aneurysm formation.

2. Possible cerebrovascular or retinal insufficiency.
3. Renal involvement occurs in 63% of patients.
4. Hypertension.
5. In type IV (45%) there may be moderate pulmonary hypertension.
6. Heart failure can occur as a consequence of either systemic or pulmonary hypertension.
7. The ESR is related to the stage of the disease and is high in 78% of cases, notably in early inflammatory disease. There are ECG abnormalities in 40% and hypergammaglobulinaemia in 37%.
8. The patient may be on corticosteroids.

Anaesthetic problems

1. There may be difficulties in haemodynamic monitoring due to absent pulses (Ramanathan et al 1979, Warner et al 1983).
2. Pressure recording from one vessel does not necessarily reflect the pressure in another vessel.
3. Hypertension or pulmonary hypertension may be present, with or without heart failure.
4. The myocardium may be sensitive to drugs with negative inotropic effects (Thorburn & James 1986).
5. In the presence of pulmonary hypertension, high lung inflation pressures may be required.
6. Hyperextension of the neck during larygoscopy and intubation may reduce carotid artery blood flow.

Management

1. The nature and degree of organ involvement must be assessed. Particular evidence of cardiac, respiratory, cerebral and renal insufficiency should be sought.
2. Hypertension or heart failure should be treated, if present.
3. For the purposes of blood pressure monitoring, the arteries involved in the disease process must be fully assessed.
4. The degree of monitoring depends upon the state of the patient, the accessibility of the arteries and the magnitude of the surgery.

   a. Care must be taken to monitor an artery representative of true arterial pressure (Thorburn & James 1986).
   b. The use of a Doppler ultrasonic probe and a sphygmomanometer cuff, which permitted blood pressure recording despite an impalpable pulse, has been suggested (Warner et al 1983). The flow from a Doppler flow probe can also be displayed on an oscilloscope and recorded on a multichannel recorder (Ramanathan et al 1979).
   c. A cutdown onto the dorsalis pedis or superficial temporal arteries may be required for direct arterial monitoring. The appropriateness of these techniques will depend on the degree and distribution of the

underlying ischaemia and the nature of the surgery being performed. On occasions the surgeon can be requested to place a cannula in the aorta during surgery.

d. If pulmonary hypertension is present, a pulmonary artery catheter may be needed to measure PAP (Ramanathan et al 1979, Warner et al 1983). However, it must be remembered that PAWP may be unreliable.

e. Measurement of cardiac stroke volume using an impedance cardiograph has been described (Ramanathan et al 1979).

f. Urine output may need careful monitoring.

5. In a patient with pulmonary hypertension, invasive haemodynamic monitoring demonstrated that epidural anaesthesia had a more beneficial effect on blood pressure and afterload control than vasodilators (Thorburn & James 1986).

6. Before anaesthesia is induced, the head should be fixed in a position which does not produce symptoms of cerebral blood flow impairment.

BIBLIOGRAPHY

Hall S, Barr W, Lie J T, Stanson A W, Kazmier F J, Hunder G G 1985 Takayasu arteritis. Medicine 64: 89–99
Ramanathan S, Gupta U, Chalon J, Turndorf H 1979 Anesthetic considerations in Takayasu arteritis. Anesthesia and Analgesia 58: 247–249
Thorburn J R, James M F M 1986 Anaesthetic management of Takayasu's arteritis. Anaesthesia 41: 734–738
Warner M A, Hughes D R, Messick J M 1983 Anesthetic management of a patient with pulseless disease. Anesthesia and Analgesia 62: 532–535

TETANUS

An infection due to *Clostridium tetani*, an anaerobic bacillus present in soil and gut. It is able to survive for long periods outside the body. Under anaerobic conditions it multiplies and produces a potent neurotoxin which can travel up nerves into the spinal cord and medulla. The primary effect is on the spinal cord, with a lesser effect on the peripheral nerves. Tetanus neurotoxin is a high molecular weight protein, so its long half-life allows time for neural penetration (Flowers 1988). The incubation period of the disease is 3–21 days. In about 60–65% of cases there is a history of a wound, but it is often trivial. Cases may be classified (Edmondson & Flowers 1979) as:

Grade 1   Mild
Grade 2   Moderate
Grade 3a   Severe
Grade 3b   Very severe

In their report of 100 cases treated in Leeds, the mortality was 10%.

There is an increased risk of tetanus in heroin addicts, in part due to additives such as quinine, which provide anaerobic conditions for multiplication of the bacillus.

Presentation

1. General muscle hypertonicity.
2. Muscle spasm resulting in trismus (lockjaw), rigidity of the facial muscles (risus sardonicus), neck stiffness, dysphagia or opisthotonos. Intermittent muscle spasms are superimposed on hypertonicity. Breathing difficulties can occur due to spasm of the laryngeal or intercostal muscles, and respiratory failure may ensue.
3. Occasionally wounds in the head and neck may produce cephalic tetanus, which can result in a variety of cranial nerve palsies.
4. A small number of patients have localized tetanus only.
5. Sympathetic disturbances occur in 23–60% of severe cases. These consist of episodes of hypertension, tachycardia, arrhythmias, peripheral vasoconstriction, sweating, salivation and pyrexia. They are probably due to increased circulating catecholamine levels, associated with the presence of toxin within the sympathetic nerves (Domenighetti et al 1984).
6. Episodes of hypotension and bradycardia have been reported, particularly after tracheal suction. These may be due to autonomic dysfunction.

Diagnosis

1. Is generally made on clinical grounds.
2. Tetanus is not an immunizing disease, therefore it is possible to contract it on more than one occasion. This is probably due to the fact that toxin travels up the nerves and thus may not come into contact with gamma globulin. The blood level of tetanus antibody cannot be used as a diagnostic test for the disease (Stoddart 1979a).
3. Differentiation must be made from other causes which mimic tetanus. These include hysteria, and treatment with drugs, such as the phenothiazines and butyrophenones, which can produce dyskinetic symptoms (Stoddart 1979b).

Anaesthetic (or intensive care) problems

1. Any strong external stimulus can precipitate severe muscle spasm. Death may occur, as ventilation impairment coincides with a greatly increased oxygen consumption by the muscles.
2. Cardiovascular instability, with episodes of hypertension and tachycardia, is often associated with increased circulating catecholamine levels (Domenighetti et al 1984).

1

3. Hypotension and bradycardia may occur, particularly after endotracheal suction (Edmondson & Flowers 1979). There are several reports which suggest that treatment with beta blockers may predispose to bradycardias, and in one case, cardiac arrest occurred (Buchanan et al 1978).

4. Reduced serum cholinesterase levels have been reported, the level often correlating with the severity of the disease. In one report, there was no enzymic activity for the first 3 days after admission (Porath et al 1977).

5. The use of suxamethonium in the later stages of the disease may cause cardiac arrest due to hyperkalaemia.

6. Hypovolaemia occurs readily, due to a combination of sweating, excess salivation, and gastrointestinal losses. Hyponatraemia may occur secondary to inappropriate ADH secretion.

7. Gastrointestinal stasis is a problem.

8. Pyrexia can be due to infection, or it sometimes occurs as a result of autonomic dysfunction.

9. In patients who require ventilation for long periods, there is an increased risk of deep venous thrombosis and pulmonary embolism. In the Leeds series of 100 cases, nine venous thromboses, three pulmonary emboli and one death occurred (Edmondson & Flowers 1979). Another embolic death has been reported, despite the use of low-dose heparin (Jenkins & Keep 1976).

Management

1. Initial management
  a. Antitetanus immunoglobulin 30 units/kg i.m.
  b. Antibiotic: benzylpenicillin 600 mg i.m. 6-hourly.
  c. Tetanus toxoid course is started.
  d. The wound should be excised and cleaned, and tissue sent for microscopy and bacterial culture. It has been suggested that this should be delayed for several hours after the immunoglobulin has been given, so that any neurotoxin released can be neutralized. Mutilating surgery is not justified (Flowers 1988).

2. Management of spasm and hypertonus

Grade 1	Usually diazepam only
Grade 2	Diazepam, tracheostomy and nasogastric tube
Grade 3a and 3b	IPPV, sedatives, neuromuscular blockers and analgesics

3. Fluid replacement is required for sweating, salivation and gastrointestinal losses. The latter depends on measured loss, but may amount to as much as 6–8 l/day. Nutrition is also needed, which may be parenteral if there is gastrointestinal failure.

4. Sympathetic overactivity has been treated with very heavy sedation or with beta adrenergic blockade. However, the use of beta blockers is controversial, as profound bradycardia may occur. Extremely high catecholamine levels, equivalent to those encountered in a phaeochromocytoma, were reported in one case (Domenighetti et al 1984). During convalescence, these levels returned to normal. In this case, labetalol was used to treat sympathetic overactivity. The use of labetalol in 15 cases was reported to produce great variability of response and poor control of blood pressure (Wesley et al 1983). This is not surprising, as the beta blockade produced by labetalol is at least three to seven times greater than the alpha blockade. In addition, five of the treated patients had episodes of cardiac standstill. The death of a 4-year-old child was associated with the use of propranolol (Buchanan et al). In the Leeds series (Edmondson & Flowers 1979), only two of the patients were treated with propanolol. Both had severe bradycardias and cardiac standstill after tracheal suction.

5. Patients should be preoxygenated prior to tracheal suction to avoid hypoxia.

6. Low-dose heparin should be administered to prevent venous thrombosis. A fatal embolism occurred in an obese lady despite low-dose heparin. The use of full anticoagulation has been suggested (Jenkins & Keep 1976).

BIBLIOGRAPHY

Buchanan N, Smit L, Cane R D, De Andrade M 1978 Sympathetic overactivity in tetanus: fatality associated with propanolol. British Medical Journal 2: 254–255
Domenighetti G M, Savary G, Stricker H 1984 Hyperadrenergic syndrome in severe tetanus; extreme rise in catecholamines responsive to labetolol. British Medical Journal 288: 1483–1484
Edmondson R S, Flowers M W 1979 Intensive care in tetanus: management, complications, and mortality in 100 cases. British Medical Journal 1: 1401–1404
Flowers M W 1988 Tetanus. Surgery 55: 1300–1303
Jenkins J, Keep P 1976 Fatal embolism despite low dose heparin. Lancet i: 541
Porath A, Acker M, Perel A 1977 Serum cholinesterase in tetanus. Anaesthesia 32: 1009–1011
Stoddart J C 1979a The immunology of tetanus. Anaesthesia 34: 863–865
Stoddart J C 1979b Pseudotetanus. Anaesthesia 34: 877–881
Wesley A G, Hariparsad D, Pather M, Rocke D A 1983 Labetolol in tetanus. Anaesthesia 38: 243–249

THALASSAEMIA

An abnormality of haemoglobin resulting from an imbalance of globin chain synthesis, affecting the population in a wide geographical band from the Mediterranean area, through the Middle East, and into India and China.

In beta thalassaemia major (homozygous state) there is an absence, or a reduced production of beta chains, and therefore an increased production of alpha chains. The alpha chains precipitate in the red cell precursors, leading to ineffective erythropoiesis and shortened red cell survival. The haemolytic anaemia leads to tissue hypoxia and excess erythropoietin production, with marrow expansion and extramedullary erythropoiesis. Iron overload due to increase iron absorption and recurrent transfusion is another major clinical problem. Thalassaemia is therefore a quantitative haemoglobinopathy, as opposed to sickle cell anaemia, in which the defect is qualitative.

In alpha thalassaemia there is absent or deficient alpha chain synthesis. Excess beta chains produce HbH, which has a high affinity for oxygen, but will not release it. Excess gamma chains in fetal haemoglobin produce HbBarts. Both HbH and HbBarts are physiologically useless.

The prognosis in thalassaemia major has improved since more aggressive treatment has been undertaken. Multiple blood transfusions to maintain the Hb at 10–12 g/dl, help to suppress erythropoiesis and reduce bone deformity. Simultaneous iron chelation with desferrioxamine decreases iron deposition in the body. The effects of starting treatment at an earlier age are being tried.

Patients with thalassaemia minor (heterozygous state) are normally symptom free, except when exposed to stresses such as pregnancy, when they may become anaemic, usually due to folic acid deficiency.

Preoperative abnormalities

Homozygous disease

1. Haemolysis leads to gross anaemia.
2. Bony changes occur due to marrow hyperplasia.
3. Iron deposition takes place, particularly in the liver and myocardium.
4. There is gross hepatosplenomegaly.
5. A hyperdynamic circulation with an increase in the circulating blood volume results.
6. Neutropenia, and occasionally thrombocytopenia, secondary to hypersplenism or folate deficiency, may be seen.

Heterozygous beta thalassaemia

1. The haemoglobin level is normal, or there is only a mild anaemia, except during pregnancy.
2. The red cells are hypochromic and microcytic, therefore there is a low mean corpuscular haemoglobin and a low mean cellular volume.
3. The HbA$_2$ may be elevated to 4–6%. Fifty per cent of subjects have HbF levels of 1–5%.

Anaesthetic problems of homozygous disease

There are few case reports of anaesthesia in thalassaemia major. The management of open heart surgery in patients with haemoglobinopathies was described (de Laval et al 1974). No complications were experienced in the three patients with thalassaemia.

1. Anaemia, associated with a hyperdynamic circulation.
2. Intubation difficulties have been reported. Frontal bossing and maxillary bone enlargement may occur secondary to bone marrow hyperplasia. Intubation problems in an 11-year-old child were due to massive forward protrusion of the maxilla (Orr 1967). Marrow hyperplasia is now reduced by starting transfusion therapy at an earlier age.

Management

1. Patients with homozygous disease will be having regular transfusions to maintain the Hb at 10–12 g/dl and desferrioxamine i.v. or s.c. to chelate iron.
2. Possible potential intubation difficulties should be sought.
3. Serum ferritin levels will indicate the iron status in patients with thalassaemia minor.

BIBLIOGRAPHY

de Leval M R, Taswell H F, Bowie E J W, Danielson G K 1974 Open heart surgery in patients with inherited hemoglobinopathies, red cell dyscrasias and coagulopathies. Archives of Surgery 109: 618–622
Orr D 1967 Difficult intubation: a hazard in thalassaemia. British Journal of Anaesthesia 39: 585–587

THYROTOXICOSIS
(see also Section 4 THYROTOXIC CRISIS)

A state of thyroid overactivity, which should be controlled before elective surgery, to avoid precipitating a thyroid crisis. If antithyroid drugs are used, preparation for thyroid surgery may take up to 2 months. With beta blockers and potassium iodide alone control can be achieved within 2 weeks, but not all are agreed on the suitability of this method. Occasionally a thyrotoxic patient requires urgent surgery. Alternatively, surgery may be unwittingly undertaken in a thyrotoxic patient, because the diagnosis is obscured by other pathology. The diagnosis is most frequently missed in elderly patients. A further problem is that beta blockers only block the peripheral effects of the hormones. They do not affect their synthesis or release, and may obscure a crisis (Eriksson et al 1977).

Preoperative abnormalities

1. A history of weight loss, heat intolerance, tremor, diarrhoea and anxiety.
2. Tachycardia, in particular a raised sleeping pulse rate, atrial fibrillation in the elderly, and occasionally heart failure.
3. There may be thyroid swelling, exophthalmos and lid lag.
4. Investigations include T3, T4 and TSH. The TRH test may be needed in difficult cases.
5. Clinically obvious myopathy is infrequent, but there is some degree of EMG abnormality in 90% of thyrotoxic patients.

Anaesthetic problems

1. Tachyarrhythmias are common during anaesthesia.
2. A hypermetabolic state may occur, which can resemble malignant hyperpyrexia (Peters et al 1981, Stevens 1983).
3. Pulmonary oedema may develop intraoperatively. This can present as cyanosis, tachycardia and respiratory distress. It is due to a combination of hypertension, tachycardia and increased blood volume. A case was reported in which an undiagnosed thyrotoxic patient with a fractured hip developed pulmonary oedema, pyrexia and tachycardia during surgery (Stevens 1983). Again, this hypermetabolic state was diagnosed and treated as malignant hyperpyrexia. The true diagnosis was only revealed during postoperative investigations.
4. A thyroid crisis, or storm, may rarely develop postoperatively and present with agitation, pyrexia, sweating, tachycardia, hypertension and cardiac failure (Jamison & Done 1979).
5. The crisis can be masked by beta blockers, which do not block the output of thyroid hormones (Jones & Solomon 1981).
6. Thyrotoxic myopathy occasionally results in delayed recovery from neuromuscular blocking agents. A case was described in which beta blockers masked the signs of thyrotoxicosis, but not the thyrotoxic myopathy (Uusitupa et al 1980).
7. Proptosis makes the eyes more susceptible to damage than normal.

Management

1. The patient should be rendered euthyroid prior to surgery.
   a. Antithyroid drugs inhibit thyroid hormone synthesis and block T3 and T4, but will take 6–8 weeks to become fully effective. The physical size of the thyroid gland may significantly increase during this therapy.
   b. Potassium iodide will reduce the concentration of circulating hormone to well within the normal range, but its action only lasts for 10 days.
   c. Beta blockers will block the peripheral effects of the hormones, but

will not block hormone release. Therefore there will still be hormone present and a catabolic state. For the small gland, beta blockers are effective in combination with potassium iodide. This is not so for the more toxic patients.

i. Propanolol

40–120 mg daily in divided doses for 2–3 weeks, with the addition of potassium iodide for the last 10 days. However, the systemic clearance of propranolol is increased by thyrotoxicosis, and in combination with the half-life of the already circulating thyroxine means that it needs to be continued for a week after operation. It may also produce hypoglycaemia in the perioperative period. If propranolol cannot be given orally, an infusion will be required. The dose required to maintain therapeutic blood levels has been suggested to be 1 mg/h (Prys-Roberts 1984) and 3 mg/h (Smulyan et al 1982).

ii. Nadolol

Is more slowly metabolised by the liver, more slowly eliminated, and its clearance is not altered by thyrotoxicosis. It can be given in a single daily dose of 160 mg, which gives prolonged beta blockade and more satisfactory blood levels than propranolol (Peden et al 1982). Preoperative potassium iodide is added in the usual manner. Bradycardias have been more frequently noticed than with propranolol, and atropine has been recommended instead of hyoscine as a premedication.

2. Atrial fibrillation, heart failure or hypertension should be treated preoperatively.

3. The eyes should be carefully protected.

4. Treatment of a thyrotoxic crisis (see Section 4)

BIBLIOGRAPHY

Eriksson M, Rubenfeld S, Garber A J, Kohler P O 1977 Propranolol does not prevent thyroid storm. New England Journal of Medicine 296: 263–264

Jamison M H, Done H J 1979 Postoperative thyrotoxic crisis in a patient prepared for thyroidectomy with propranolol. British Journal of Clinical Practice 33: 82–83

Jones D K, Solomon S 1981 Thyrotoxic crisis masked by treatment with beta blockers. British Medical Journal 283: 659

Peden N R, Gunn A, Browning M C K, Crooks S J, Forrest A L, Hamilton W F, Isles T E 1982 Nadolol and potassium iodide in combination in the surgical treatment of thyrotoxicosis. British Journal of Surgery 69: 638–640

Peters K R, Nance P, Wingard D W 1981 Malignant hyperthyroidism or malignant hyperthermia. Anesthesia and Analgesia 60: 613–615

Prys-Roberts C 1984 Kinetics and dynamics of beta adrenoceptor antagonists. In: Pharmacokinetics of anaesthesia. Blackwell Scientific, Oxford

Smulyan H, Weinberg S E, Howanitz P J 1982 Continuous propranolol infusion following abdominal surgery. Journal of the American Medical Association 247: 2539–2542

Stevens J J 1983 A case of thyrotoxic crisis that mimicked malignant hyperthermia. Anesthesiology 59: 263

Uusitupa M, Aro A, Korhonen T, Jukka E 1980 Beta blockade, myopathy and thyrotoxicosis. British Medical Journal 1: 183

1

TORSADE DE POINTES
(ATYPICAL VENTRICULAR TACHYCARDIA)

An atypical paroxysmal ventricular tachycardia associated with delayed repolarization of the ventricle. It is frequently drug induced, but may also occur with metabolic abnormalities.

Presentation

1. The patient may complain of episodes of palpitations, faintness or fatigue.
2. As an unusual type of ventricular tachycardia. Instead of a rapid succession of extrasystoles of identical configuration, the axis of the QRS complex appears to rotate around the baseline. Before the event there is a characteristic 'long-short' sequence (Raehl et al 1985) in which a premature ectopic beat is followed by a long pause, then another premature ectopic initiates the torsade de pointes.
3. The ventricular tachycardia is not resolved by conventional antiarrhythmic treatment.
4. Factors which predispose to the development of torsade de pointes include:
   a. Drug therapy:
      Prenylamine
      Disopyramide
      Quinidine
      Tricyclic antidepressants
   b. Conduction problems:
      Sick sinus syndrome
      Congenital prolonged Q–T interval
      Atrioventricular block
   c. Electrolyte Imbalance
      Hypokalaemia
      Hypomagnesaemia
   d. Right radical neck dissection (Otteni et al 1983).
   Prolongation of the Q–T interval occurred in association with right-sided neck surgery, but not with left, and persisted in over a third of 32 patients studied. Three patients had episodes of torsade de pointes in the postoperative period.

Diagnosis

1. Is best made on a 12-lead ECG. A ventricular tachycardia is shown with the QRS axis undulating over 5–6 beats and with a change in direction. The 'long-short' initiating sequence may be seen.
2. In between episodes of torsade de pointes the corrected Q–T interval (Q–Tc) may be prolonged.

Management

1. The underlying cause is corrected.
   a. Any potentially causative drug is stopped. A recurrent ventricular tachycardia appeared 6 hours after pleurectomy in a patient with severe lung disease (Alexander & Potgieter 1983). A further 20 hours of treatment with a number of drugs including lignocaine, disopyramide, digoxin, procainamide and propranolol, and DC shock was unsuccessful. A 12-lead ECG showed an undulating QRS axis and the Q–Tc in between episodes of tachycardia was 0.863 seconds. A diagnosis of atypical ventricular tachycardia was made. All drugs were stopped and the hypokalaemia, corrected. Review of earlier ECGs also showed prolonged Q–Tc.
   b. Metabolic causes such as hypokalaemia, hypocalcaemia or hypomagnesaemia (Ramee et al 1985) are corrected.
2. Avoid the use of class I antiarrhythmics, and those drugs already mentioned.
3. In cases where the tachycardia persists, atrial pacing may be required.
4. If VF occurs, defibrillation will be necessary.
5. Isoprenaline may increase the heart rate and therefore shorten the Q–T interval. A dose of 1–2 μg/min has been recommended (Raehl et al 1985). However, extreme caution is required. Contraindications include myocardial ischaemia and hypertensive heart disease.
6. Bretylium, lignocaine and magnesium sulphate (Ramee et al 1985) have on occasions been successful.

BIBLIOGRAPHY

Alexander M G, Potgieter P D 1983 Atypical ventricular tachycardia (torsade de pointes). Anaesthesia 38: 269–274
Martinez R 1987 Torsade de pointes: atypical rhythm, atypical treatment. Annals of Emergency Medicine 16: 878–884
Otteni J C, Pottecher R T, Bronner G, Flesch H, Diebolt J R 1983 Prolongation of the Q–T interval and sudden cardiac arrest following right radical neck dissection. Anesthesiology 59: 358–361
Raehl C L, Patel A K, LeRoy M 1985 Drug-induced torsade de pointes. Clinical Pharmacy 4: 675–690
Ramee S R, White C J, Svinarich J T, Watson T D, Fox R F 1985 Torsade de pointes and magnesium deficiency. American Heart Journal 109: 164–167

TREACHER COLLINS SYNDROME

A craniofacial defect associated with developmental anomalies of the first arch. Abnormalities vary from minimal, to the complete syndrome. Patients may require anaesthesia for manoeuvres to temporarily improve upper airway obstruction, or for correction of some of the congenital defects.

Preoperative abnormalities

1. Features may include mandibular and malar hypoplasia, antimongoloid palpebral fissure, a large mouth and irregular maloccluded teeth, microphthalmia, lower lid defects, cleft palate, macroglossia and auricular deformities.
2. Associated abnormalities include mental retardation, deafness, dwarfism, cardiac defects and skeletal deformities.
3. The predominant problem is that of chronic upper respiratory tract obstruction, which in its severest form leads to retarded growth and occasionally cor pulmonale. If the child is failing to compensate for his airway dysfunction, his growth will be well below the average percentile (Mallory & Paradise 1979).
4. Sleep apnoea has been described.

Anaesthetic problems

1. Airway obstruction
In the small baby this may require urgent temporary corrective manoeuvres, such as stitching the tongue to the lower lip.
2. Excess secretions may hamper induction of anaesthesia.
3. Inhalation induction may be difficult.
4. Difficult intubation
A number of papers have described difficult or failed intubation, (Sklar & King 1976, Miyabe et al 1985, Rasch et al 1986). One resulted in a near fatality (Ross 1963).
5. Obstructive sleep apnoea may occur postoperatively (Roa & Moss 1984).
6. Pulmonary oedema
Respiratory arrest and pulmonary oedema was reported in a 15-year-old boy 40 minutes after a N_2O/O_2/halothane anaesthetic (Roa & Moss 1984).

Management

1. The use of respiratory depressant agents in the premedication, and postoperatively, should be avoided.
2. Drying agents should always be used.
3. A muscle relaxant must never be given until the airway has been secured.
4. Awake intubation or awake direct laryngoscopy to visualize the vocal cords, should be considered. A successful direct laryngoscopy, performed with the patient in the sitting position, and using a 5 gauge feeding tube taped to the side of the laryngoscope to give oxygen, has been described (Rasch et al 1986). The use of the fibreoptic bronchoscope or tracheostomy under local anaesthetic has been recommended in order to avoid the hazards of inhalational induction and failed intubation. In older children, some of whom are retarded, this may not be possible.

5. If general anaesthesia is essential, a number of techniques have been described to assist intubation.

a. The use of an anterior commissure laryngoscope, which prevents the tongue from falling in on the laryngoscope, has been described (Handler & Keon 1983, see Pierre Robin syndrome for a full description).

b. A tactile nasal intubation technique was used in a 4-year-old boy (Sklar & King 1976). Induction was with halothane followed by ether, and the tongue was pulled downwards and forwards. The tube was initially used as a nasal airway, while the index and middle finger were used to palpate the epiglottis, through which the tube was then passed.

c. The use of an assistant to pull out the tongue with forceps, and at the same time to apply cricoid pressure, was found to assist laryngoscopy (Miyabe et al 1985).

d. A 14-year-old boy was anaesthetized with incremental ketamine. A gum elastic bougie was inserted into the larynx and the tube was threaded over the top (MacLennan & Roberts 1981).

6. It is recommended that the endotracheal tube remain in situ until the patient is fully awake. There have been a number of reports of obstruction occurring during recovery. These have necessitated reintubation and, in one case, a tracheostomy.

7. Patients should be nursed in an intensive care area postoperatively. The combination of sleep apnoea and depressant drugs may make them very susceptible to respiratory arrest. The use of an oximeter is advantageous.

BIBLIOGRAPHY

Handler S D, Keon T P 1983 Difficult laryngoscopy/intubation: the child with mandibular hypoplasia. Annals of Otology, Rhinology and Laryngology 92: 401–404
MacLennan F, Robertson G S 1981 Ketamine for induction and intubation in Treacher-Collins syndrome. Anaesthesia 36: 196–198
Mallory S B, Paradise J L 1979 Glossoptosis revisited: on the development and resolution of airway obstruction in the Pierre-Robin syndrome. Pediatrics 64: 946–948
Miyabe M, Dohi S, Homma E 1985 Tracheal intubation in an infant with Treacher Collins syndrome – pulling out the tongue by a forceps. Anesthesiology 62: 213–214
Rasch D J, Browder F, Barr M, Greer D 1986 Anaesthesia for Treacher-Collins and Pierre-Robin syndromes: a report of three cases. Canadian Anaesthetists' Society Journal 33: 364–370
Roa N L, Moss K S 1984 Treacher-Collins syndrome with sleep apnea: anesthetic considerations. Anesthesiology 60: 71–73
Ross E D 1963 Treacher-Collins syndrome. An anaesthetic hazard. Anaesthesia 18: 350–354
Sklar G S, King B D 1976 Endotracheal intubation and Treacher-Collins syndrome. Anesthesiology 44: 247–249

TURNER'S SYNDROME

A syndrome due to a sex chromosome abnormality, and includes gonadal dysgenesis, primary amenorrhoea, skeletal, renal and other anomalies.

Preoperative abnormalities

1. Skeletal abnormalities may include short stature, a short webbed neck with fusion of cervical vertebrae, a low hairline, cubitus valgus, a high-arched palate, micrognathia, a shield chest, and a short fourth metacarpal.
2. Associated anomalies such as renal dysgenesis, coarctation of the aorta, peripheral lymphoedema and ocular and aural defects.
3. There is an increased incidence of diabetes and autoimmune thyroid disease.

Anaesthetic problems

1. Intubation difficulties may occur due to the short neck and fused cervical vertebrae.
2. The distance between the vocal cords and carina may be short. A patient developed left lung collapse following accidental one lung ventilation during laparoscopy (Divekar et al 1983). Subsequent X-rays showed that the bifurcation of the trachea was in an abnormally high position, at the level of the sternoclavicular joint.
3. Problems of renal disease.

Management

1. Assessment of abnormalities, particularly those of the cardiovascular system.
2. Potential intubation difficulties must be anticipated and the risk of inadvertent one lung ventilation borne in mind.

BIBLIOGRAPHY

Divekar V M, Kothari M D, Kamdar B M 1983 Anaesthesia in Turner's syndrome. Canadian Anaesthetists' Society Journal 30: 417–418

VIPOMA

One of the APUDomas (Amine Precursor Uptake and Decarboxylation), which secretes vasoactive intestinal polypeptide (VIP), but may also produce other hormones. Tumours in adults are most commonly of pancreatic endocrine origin, whereas in children they are usually ganglioneuroblastomas arising from the sympathetic chain. VIP may also be one of a number of hormones which can be secreted by bronchial carcinomas and paragangliomas. Intravenous administration of VIP produces hypotension due to vasodilatation, hyperglycaemia, diarrhoea, inhibition of gastric acid output and respiratory stimulation.

Preoperative abnormalities

1. The syndrome as it was originally described consisted of Watery Diarrhoea, Hypokalaemia and Achlor- or hypochlorhydria (WDHA syndrome). There is accompanying weight loss and dehydration, and a history of abdominal colic and cutaneous flushing.
2. The picture may be complicated by the effects of additional hormones (see Apudomas).
3. Biochemical changes include hypokalaemia, acidosis, hypercalcaemia, raised blood urea, a diabetic glucose tolerance, raised plasma VIP and a raised plasma pancreatic polypeptide.

Anaesthetic problems

1. A major problem can be gross fluid and electrolyte imbalance. Losses of up to 8 l/day may occur (Bouloux 1987). One patient whose serum potassium was only 1.3 mmol/l, presented with a quadriparesis. This resolved completely after potassium infusion (Taylor et al 1977).
2. Secretion of VIP during handling of the tumour may produce profound hypotension. The patient mentioned above had an adrenal ganglioneuroblastoma which secreted both VIP and noradrenaline. Prior to removal of the tumour, these had mutually antagonistic effects. However, following its removal there was severe hypotension, probably due to the more prolonged action of VIP.

BIBLIOGRAPHY

Bouloux P–M 1987 Multiple endocrine neoplasia. Surgery 1: 1180–1185
Taylor A R, Chulajata D, Jones D H, Whitwam J G 1977 Adrenal tumour secreting vasoaction intestinal peptide and noradrenaline. Anaesthesia 32: 1012–1016

VON GIERKE'S DISEASE

An autosomal recessive inherited glycogen storage disease (Cori type I) in which there is an absence, or reduction in levels, of glucose-6-phosphatase. Glycogen is a polymer made up of straight and branching chains of glucose monomer units. Blood glucose is normally maintained by breakdown of glycogen.

Glucose-6-phosphatase is present in the liver, kidney, gut and platelets. It is the enzyme involved in the final step in the conversion of glycogen to free glucose. An absence, or a reduction in levels of the enzyme, results in hypoglycaemia. Some patients have been improved by a portacaval shunt (Casson 1975).

Preoperative abnormalities

1. There is gross hepatomegaly, presenting in infancy and due to accumulation of glycogen and fat in the liver. The kidneys are also enlarged.
2. Severe hypoglycaemia occurs, which does not respond to glucagon, fructose or adrenaline. It may lead to fits and failure to thrive. In spite of this, patients tend to be obese, due to deposition of subcutaneous fat.
3. A chronic lactic acidosis exists, due to free conversion of pyruvate to lactate, and increased pyruvate levels.
4. Hypertriglyceridaemia and high free fatty acids due to increased synthesis, and stimulation of their release from fat.
5. Platelet dysfunction, secondary to biochemical derangements, may produce coagulation problems. These are reversed when treatment is instituted.
6. Diagnosis can be confirmed by liver biopsy, and histocytochemistry.
7. Management includes measures such as continuous intragastric, nasogastric, or parenteral feeding and portacaval shunt, all of which improve metabolic control.

Anaesthetic problems

1. Starvation produces severe hypoglycaemia and lactic acidosis. In a review of 12 patients, one 17-year-old boy developed a pH of 7.08 during surgery after 7 hours of starvation (Cox 1968). Death occurred in one child, who had a cardiac arrest at the end of a tonsillectomy. No details were given.
2. The current successful continuous metabolic management of these children reduces the tolerance to low blood glucose levels which normally occurs in the untreated child.
3. There may be epistaxis, bruising and coagulation problems due to platelet dysfunction, although this is reversed with treatment.
4. Muscle development is poor and may result in postoperative respiratory insufficiency.

Management

1. To prevent an acidosis occurring at the beginning of surgery, a dextrose infusion should be given during the period of preoperative starvation. In one case, intragastric feeding was maintained until 3 hours preoperatively, and replaced by an infusion of glucose to give 0.4 g/kg/h (Bevan 1980).
2. If major surgery, such as a portacaval shunt, is contemplated, preoperative parenteral nutrition is advisable (Casson 1975). Liver size is decreased and platelet function improved.
3. Plasma glucose and acid base status should be monitored regularly

1

throughout the perioperative period (Bevan 1980). Acidaemia can occur without ketonuria, therefore monitoring of urinary ketones alone may be unreliable.

4. Lactate-containing solutions are absolutely contraindicated.

5. In view of platetet dysfunction, regional anaesthesia is probably inadvisable.

6. Neuromuscular monitoring.

7. Careful postoperative observation is required, to detect respiratory insufficiency.

BIBLIOGRAPHY

Bevan J C 1980 Anaesthesia in Von Gierke's disease. Current approach to management. Anaesthesia 35: 699–702

Casson H 1975 Anaesthesia for portacaval bypass in patients with metabolic diseases. British Journal of Anaesthesia 47: 969–975

Cox J M 1968 Anesthesia and glycogen storage disease. Anesthesiology 29: 1221–1225

VON HIPPEL–LINDAU DISEASE

A rare familial neuroectodermal disorder, usually presenting in young adults with one or more of a variety of manifestations. Amongst the most serious of these are cerebellar, medullary or spinal haemangioblastomas, retinal angiomatosis, renal cell carcinoma and phaeochromocytoma (Horton et al 1976).

Preoperative abnormalities

1. Features usually present separately, and unless there is a known family history, the diagnosis of von Hippel–Lindau may only be made in retrospect. Tumours may recur, or new tumours appear. The author has seen a phaeochromocytoma in a 14-year-old boy, who subsequently presented with a cerebral haemangioblastoma, retinal angiomatosis and a second phaeochromocytoma.

2. Other associated conditions include pancreatic cysts, angiomas of the liver and kidneys, renal cysts and polycythaemia.

Anaesthetic problems

1. Those of the management of a phaeochromocytoma, if present.

2. Spinal anaesthesia may be hazardous in the presence of an undiagnosed cerebral or spinal tumour.

3. The safe management of the pregnant patient with a previously resected cerebral tumour (Matthews & Halshaw 1986).

Management

1. Careful assessment should be made for lesions other than the one for which anaesthesia is required, and in particular for any symptoms and signs of cerebral or cerebellar tumours.

2. Twenty-four-hour urinary screening for catecholamines.

3. Preparation for phaeochromocytoma surgery (see Phaeochromocytoma).

BIBLIOGRAPHY

Horton W A, Wong V, Eldridge R 1976 von Hippel–Lindau disease. Archives of Internal Medicine 136: 769–777
Matthews A J, Halshaw J 1986 Epidural anaesthesia in von Hippel–Lindau disease. Anaesthesia 41: 853–855

VON RECKLINGHAUSEN'S DISEASE
(see NEUROFIBROMATOSIS)

VON WILLEBRAND'S DISEASE

A group of autosomal dominant inherited haemorrhagic diseases associated with reduced, abnormal or absent von Willebrand factor (vWF : Ag). In plasma, vWF : Ag forms a complex with factor VIII (VIII/vWF : Ag), although the two proteins are controlled by genes on different chromosomes. During coagulation the complexes are dissociated.

As the formation of a complex with vWF : Ag protects factor VIII from premature destruction, factor VIII clotting activity levels are also reduced in most cases of von Willebrand's disease (vWd). However, levels usually remain above 5% and on occasions may even be normal.

vWF : Ag has been demonstrated to be present in endothelial cells and platelets, and is involved in the link between platelets and damaged endothelium. von Willebrand's disease is therefore associated with defects in platelet adhesiveness and aggregation, and a prolonged bleeding time. Electrophoretic techniques have allowed laboratory classification of three different types, and further subtypes, of von Willebrand's disease.

The different types of the disease vary in their clinical severity, mode of inheritance, laboratory abnormality and in their response to different methods of therapy.

Preoperative abnormalities

1. Clinically, the bleeding in vWd differs from that seen in haemophilia. Bruising occurs easily, and bleeding tends to be mucosal in type, from the nose, mouth, gastrointestinal tract, lungs and uterus. Immediate bleeding tends to follow trauma and surgery in vWd, whereas it is usually delayed in haemophilia.

2. The bleeding time is usually prolonged, and platelet aggregation and adhesion reduced. Factor VIII clotting activity may be reduced or normal, and therefore the partial thromboplastin time may or may not be abnormal. There are a number of laboratory tests for vWF : Ag activity, which remain in the province of the haematologist. The Ristocetin cofactor activity is the most reliable in clinical terms.

Anaesthetic problems

1. Bleeding after trauma or surgery may occur, the degree being dependent upon the severity of the disease. Although bleeding is not usually as severe as in haemophilia, major anaesthetic problems may arise from time to time. The anaesthetic management of haemoptysis and haemothorax in vWd has been described (Bowes 1969).

2. Pregnancy and delivery may be complicated. Vaginal delivery may cause trauma and haemorrhage in infants of severely affected mothers, and in these patients Caesarean section is required. In such cases, blood loss at Caesarean section may be considerable. Two patients have been described in which the use of desmopressin in labour was associated with water retention. In one patient hyponatraemic fits occurred (Chediak et al 1986).

Management

1. Careful clinical and haematological assessment of the type and severity of the disease is required. Advice must be obtained from a haematologist as to the appropriate therapy to cover the proposed surgery. In the less severe form of the disease, a clinical and laboratory improvement is associated with both pregnancy and the administration of oestrogens or desmopressin.

2. Blood samples for coagulation studies should be taken with care. Stasis, or damage to blood by difficult aspiration, may produce unreliable results with some tests.

3. Salicylates may worsen the defect and their use should be avoided.

4. Where treatment is required, either desmopressin 0.3 μg/kg, or both desmopressin and cryoprecipitate may be used, depending on the severity and type of vWd (Mannucci et al 1981).

5. Regional anaesthesia should not be used unless the partial thromboplastin time and the bleeding time are close to normal.

6. The clinical course of six pregnancies in patients with vWd has been described (Chediak et al 1986). Caesarean section will be required unless the defect is mild, as the trauma of delivery may cause haemorrhage in a susceptible infant. If both desmopressin and oxytocin are required, only small volumes of saline 0.9% should be used as the diluent, and the plasma sodium should be estimated regularly during treatment.

BIBLIOGRAPHY

Bowes J B 1969 Anaesthetic management of haemothorax and haemoptysis due to von
   Willebrand's disease. British Journal of Anaesthesia 41: 894–897
Chediak J R, Alban G M, Maxey B 1986 von Willebrand's disease and pregnancy:
   management during delivery and outcome of offspring. American Journal of Obstetrics and
   Gynaecology 155: 618–624
Mannucci P M, Canciani M T, Rota L, Donovan B S 1981 Response of factor VIII/von
   Willebrand factor to DDAVP in healthy subjects and patients with haemophilia and von
   Willebrand's disease. British Journal of Haematology 47: 283–293

WEGENER'S GRANULOMATOSIS

A systemic granulomatous vasculitis in which granulomas of the upper
and lower respiratory tract are associated with a focal necrotizing
glomerulonephritis, and a widespread vasculitis involving other organs.
The clinical features overlap with microscopic polyarteritis, and the
antineutrophil cytoplasmic antibody is positive in both. A survey of 85
cases showed that all patients had either upper or lower respiratory tract
involvement, and 85% had documented renal disease (Fauci et al 1983).
Without treatment, the prognosis is poor, and up to 90% of deaths are
associated with renal failure. Treatment with cyclophosphamide and
corticosteroids has improved the prognosis. Patients may require
anaesthesia for ENT procedures, or for biopsy of airway lesions, before the
diagnosis has been made.

Preoperative abnormalities

1. Upper airway problems include nasal discharge, crusting, bleeding and
ulceration, sometimes progressing to septal perforation and nasal collapse.
Infection or ulceration may occur in the sinuses, palate and pharynx.
Granulomas, ulceration and stenosis, may involve the larynx.
2. Over 90% of patients have pulmonary involvement. Symptoms include
cough, haemoptysis, chest pain and breathlessness. CXR shows changing
pulmonary opacities, which are often multiple and bilateral. Some of these
cavitate and simulate lung carcinoma.
3. Renal disease may present with haematuria, proteinuria or red cell
casts. Untreated, patients progress to kidney failure.
4. Ophthalmic and aural complications were reported in 58% and 61% of
cases respectively.
5. Other systems which may be involved in a diffuse vasculitis include the
skin (45%), nervous (22%) and cardiovascular systems (12%). Cardiac
complications include pericarditis, myopathy, valvular and coronary
disease.
6. General symptoms include joint pains, malaise and fever.
7. Patients may be taking cyclophosphamide and steroids.
8. There may be anaemia, raised ESR, hypergammaglobulinaemia and

leucocytosis (unless cyclophosphamide has caused a leucopenia).
9. Plasmapheresis may have a place for those in renal failure.

Anaesthetic problems

1. Granulomas of the upper airway may cause bleeding, or result in obstruction (Cohen et al 1978, Lake 1978). Subglottic stenosis, tracheal granulomas and tracheo-oesophageal fistula have all been described. Subglottic stenosis is usually circumferential, most frequently affects females, and usually requires permanent tracheostomy (Arauz & Fonseca 1982, McDonald et al 1982).
2. Nasal intubation may dislodge tissue or cause bleeding.
3. Renal failure is common.
4. A peripheral arteritis may result in digital ischaemia. In such cases arterial cannulation is hazardous.
5. Pulmonary lesions may lead to hypoxia or bleeding.
6. Cardiac lesions can cause heart failure, conduction defects or coronary insufficiency, although this is rare.
7. Treatment for the disease may cause immunosuppression. Cyclophosphamide most commonly causes leucopenia, hair loss and haemorrhagic cystitis (Fauci et al 1983). Cholinesterase activity may be reduced.

Management

1. A careful assessment of the systems which may be affected by the disease must be undertaken. If there are signs that the airway is involved then indirect laryngoscopy and airway tomography may be indicated.
2. Necessary investigations may include Hb, WCC, platelet count, ESR, CXR, blood gases and tests of renal and liver function.
3. Corticosteroid supplements may be needed.
4. If airway obstruction is diagnosed, examination or intubation under local anaesthesia, or occasionally tracheostomy may be necessary. Otherwise, examination of the palate, pharynx and larynx for lesions should be carried out during laryngoscopy.
5. The management of renal failure (see Renal failure).
6. If the patient has both airway lesions and renal failure, then local anaesthesia should be considered. However, any neurological lesions secondary to the disease should be accurately documented prior to anaesthesia.

BIBLIOGRAPHY

Arauz J C, Fonseca R 1982 Wegener's granulomatosis appearing initially in the trachea. Annals of Otology, Rhinology and Laryngology 91: 593–594
Cohen S R, Landing B H, King K K, Isaacs H 1978 Wegener's granulomatosis causing laryngeal and tracheobronchial obstruction in an adolescent girl. Annals of Otology, Rhinology and Laryngology 87: S52; 15–19

Fauci A S, Haynes B F, Katz P, Wolff S M 1983 Wegener's granulomatosis: prospective
clinical and therapeutic experiences. Annals of Internal Medicine 98: 76–85
Lake C L 1978 Anesthesia and Wegener's granulomatosis: case report and review of the
literature. Anesthesia and Analgesia 57: 353–359
McDonald T J, Neel H B, DeRemee R A 1982 Wegener's granulomatosis of the subglottis and
the upper portion of the trachea. Annals of Otology, Rhinology and Laryngology 91:
588–592

WOLFF–PARKINSON–WHITE SYNDROME

A congenital pre-excitation syndrome in which an accessory pathway
occurs between the atrial and ventricular myocardium (the Bundle of
Kent). This permits the initiation of excitation and contraction of the
ventricles before the normal atrial impulse has crossed the AV node to the
bundle of His (Wellens et al 1987). The different excitation recovery times
of the two pathways allow repeated circulation of impulses between the
atria and ventricles. Subjects are thus prone to episodes of
supraventricular tachycardia, and sometimes rapid atrial fibrillation. The
myocardium is usually normal, but prolonged periods of tachycardia may
cause hypotension, and occasionally heart failure.

It may occur in up to 0.3% of the general population, and the incidence
can be even higher in close relatives of affected individuals.

In cases which are refractory to medical treatment, surgical division of the
relevant accessory pathway may be required (Bennett 1988).

Preoperative abnormalities

1. The P–R interval is short, usually less than 0.12 seconds. This is best
seen in lead V1.
2. The QRS interval is broader than normal (>0.12 seconds, best seen in
leads II, V5 and V6), and the initial QRS deflection is slow rising and
slurred, and known as the delta wave. Early depolarization occurs via
the accessory pathway, but further spread is slow, as it does not involve
specialized conducting tissue. It therefore merges into the normal QRS
complex. In some cases the ECG may be entirely normal.
3. There are two types of WPW. In type A, the ventricular complex is
predominantly positive in V1; in type B it is predominantly negative.
4. The clinical history is of episodes of 'palpitations' which are
precipitated by exercise, stress or excitement. During an attack the patient
may complain of faintness, chest pain, breathlessness or polyuria. If the
arrhythmia persists, cardiac failure may occur.
5. The ECG during attacks may show an AV re-entrant tachycardia
(120–140 b.p.m.), atrial fibrillation or atrial flutter. Ventricular tachycardia,
flutter or fibrillation have been reported. Death occasionally occurs
(Brechenmacher et al 1977). During the re-entrant tachycardia there will

be narrow, regular ventricular complexes. If the P wave can be seen, it will occur midway between ventricular complexes. Atrial fibrillation will in general be faster than normal, most of the impulses will show delta waves although some will not.

Anaesthetic problems

1. Tachyarrhythmias may be precipitated by anxiety, surgical stimulation, induction of anaesthesia, intubation or hypotension (van der Starre 1976, Jacobsen et al 1985).
2. During an attack, hypotension and a marked fall in cardiac output may occur. Recurrent episodes of SVT were reported in a patient in late pregnancy. Failure to respond to drug therapy on one occasion, and the occurrence of hypotension and fetal distress due to practolol on the second, necessitated the use of direct current cardioversion on both occasions (Klepper 1981).

Management

1. If the patient is already on drug treatment, this should be maintained.
2. Sympathetic stimulants, atropine and pancuronium should be avoided.
3. There is no agreement about the optimal agents for anaesthesia. However, on general principles, drugs producing tachycardia, or techniques of light anaesthesia resulting in sympathetic stimulation, should be avoided. Neurolept anaesthesia with droperidol and fentanyl has been recommended (van der Starre 1978). However, another report based on 13 cases, nine of which were for His or Kent bundle surgery, recommended inhalational anaesthesia (Sadowski & Moyers 1979). Three of these 13 patients developed tachycardias. Two of the three patients had morphine and pancuronium, and the third had halothane and d-tubocurarine. Of the ten who had no arrhythmias, all but one had inhalation agents, and most received curare rather than pancuronium. It is possible that the episodes of tachycardia were triggered by a combination of pancuronium and light anaesthesia.

Anaesthesia has been described in a premature neonate for pyloric stenosis, using thiopentone, vecuronium and isoflurane (Richmond & Conroy 1988).

Relatively little work has been done on the effect of anaesthetic drugs on the electrical pathways in patients with WPW. In one electrophysiological study on patients about to undergo surgical section of the accessory pathway, droperidol, in doses of 0.2–0.6 mg/kg, was found to increase the antegrade and retrograde effective refractory period of the action potential (Gomez-Arnau et al 1983).
4. If an attack occurs, vagal stimulation by carotid sinus massage, a Valsalva manoeuvre, or squatting, can be tried. To be effective, these need

to be instituted as soon as possible after the beginning of the tachycardia (Wellens et al 1987). If they fail, then drug or other methods of treatment will be needed. Individual patients may respond differently to different drugs. In addition, if atrial fibrillation is present, it can be worsened by verapamil and digoxin.

a. For AV re-entrant tachycardias (Wellens et al 1987)

i. Verapamil 5–10 mg over 1 minute (but should not be used if the patient is on beta blockers).

ii. Other drugs which prolong the refractory period of either the aberrant pathway, or the AV node, can be tried. These include disopyramide, diltiazem, procainamide, adenosine phosphate and amiodarone.

iii. Drugs producing reflex bradycardia may occasionally be successful. Phenylephrine 200 μg, and a subsequent phenylephrine infusion, finally terminated a refractory tachycardia in a patient having squint surgery, when other drugs had failed (Jacobsen et al 1985).

b. For atrial fibrillation

i. Disopyramide, amiodarone and flecainide impair conduction in the bundle of Kent.

c. Direct current cardioversion should be considered early in atrial fibrillation, particularly if there is haemodynamic compromise. It can also be used if tachycardias fail to respond to drug treatment. Recurrent attacks of SVT in a patient in late pregnancy which produced marked maternal hypotension required cardioversion (Klepper 1981).

d. Atrial pacing may be used as a last resort.

e. Surgical transection may be considered for patients with recurrent arrhythmias or intolerance to drug therapy (Bennett 1988).

BIBLIOGRAPHY

Bennett J G 1988 Surgery for cardiac arrhythmias. British Medical Journal 296: 1687–1688
Brechenmacher C, Coumel P H, Fauchier J-P, Cachera J-P, James T M 1977 Intractable paroxysmal tachycardia which proved fatal in type A Wolff–Parkinson–White syndrome. Circulation 55: 408–417
Gomez-Arnau J, Marquez-Montes J, Avello F 1983 Fentanyl and droperidol effects on the refractoriness of the accessory pathway in the Wolff–Parkinson–White syndrome. Anesthesiology 58: 307–313
Jacobson L, Turnquist K, Masley S 1985 Wolff–Parkinson–White syndrome. Anaesthesia 40: 657–660
Klepper I 1981 Cardioversion in late pregnancy. Anaesthesia 36: 611–616
Richmond M N, Conroy P T 1988 Anesthetic management of a neonate born prematurely with Wolff–Parkinson–White. Anesthesia and Analgesia 67: 477–478
Sadowski A R, Moyers J R 1979 Anesthetic management of the Wolff–Parkinson–White syndrome. Anesthesiology 51: 553–556
van der Starre P J A 1978 Wolff–Parkinson–White syndrome during anaesthesia. Anesthesiology 48: 369–372
Wellens H J J, Brugada P, Penn O C 1987 The management of the preexcitation syndromes. Journal of the American Medical Association 257: 2325–2333

2

Preoperative Drugs

A. PROPRIETARY NAMES

2

Non-proprietary name	Use/type of drug	Other information (page)

Abidec		multivitamin prepn	
Acepril	captopril	ACE inhibitor	
Acetoxyl	benzoyl peroxide	antibacterial	
Acezide	captopril + hydrochlorothiazide	ACE inhibitor + diuretic	
Achromycin	tetracycline	antibiotic	
Acnidazil	benzoyl, miconazole	antibacterial	
Actal	alexitol sodium	antacid	
Actidil	triprolidine HCl	antihistamine	
Actifed	triprolidine HCl pseudoephedrine dextromethorphan	antihistamine sympathomimetic antitussive	
Actinac	chloramphenicol	antibacterial, topical	
Actonorm	aluminium OH magnesium OH	antacid	
Acupan	nefopam HCl	analgesic	
Adalat	nifedipine	calcium antagonist	376
Addiphos		potassium supplement	
Adriamycin	doxorubicin	cytotoxic antibiotic	363
Aerolin	salbutamol	bronchodilator spray	
Aerosporin	polymyxin B	antibiotic	350
Afrazine	oxymetazoline	sympathomimetic spray	
Agarol	paraffin	laxative	
Alcopar	bephenium	antihelminth	
Aldactide	spironolactone + hydroflumethiazide	potassium-sparing thiazide	
Aldactone potassium-sparing	spironolactone	aldosterone inhibitor	
Aldomet	methyldopa	antihypertensive	
Alembicol D	triglycerides	for fat malabsorption	
Alevaire	tyloxapol	bronchial mucolytic	
Alexan	cytarabine	antimetabolite	363
Alexitol Na	aluminium OH	antacid	
Algicon	alginate + antacid	antacid, antireflux	
Alkeran	melphalan	alkylating cytotoxic	363
Allbee with C		multivitamin	
Allegron	nortriptyline	tricyclic antidepressant	386
Allpyral		hyposensitizing treatment	
Almazine	lorazepam	benzodiazepine	368
Almevax	rubella vaccine	immunization	
Almodan	amoxycillin	antibiotic	
Alophen		laxative, anticholinergic	
Aloral	xanthine oxidase inhibitor	gout prophylaxis	
Alrheumat	ketoprofen	NSAID	
Altacite Plus		antacid	
Alu-Cap	aluminium OH	antacid	
Aludrox	aluminium OH	antacid	
Aluhyde	aluminium OH + belladonna	antacid, anticholinergic	

Proprietary name	Non-proprietary name	Use/type of drug	Other information (page)
Aluline	allopurinol	xanthine oxidase inhibitor	
Alupent	orciprenaline	bronchodilator, B-agonist suppress premature labour	
Alupram	diazepam	benzodiazepine	368
Aluzine	frusemide	loop diuretic	
Ambaxin	bacampicillin	antibiotic	
Amfipen	ampicillin	antibiotic	
Amikin	amikacin	aminoglycoside	350
Amilco	amiloride + hydrochlorothiazide	K$^+$-sparing/thiazide	
Amoxidin	amoxycillin	antibiotic	
Amoxil	amoxycillin	antibiotic	
Ampiclox	ampicillin + cloxacillin	antibiotic	
Ampilar	ampicillin	antibiotic	
Amsidine	amsacrine	cytotoxic	363
Amytal	amylobarbitone	barbiturate	
Anafranil	clomipramine	tricyclic antidepressant	386
Ananase Forte	bromelains	proteolytic enzyme	
Anapolon	oxymetholone	anabolic steroid for hypoplastic anaemias	
Ancoloxin	meclozine + pyridoxine	antiemetic	
Androcur	cyproterone	anti-androgen	
Andursil		antacid	
Angilol	propranolol	beta blocker	371
Anquil	benperidol	butyrophenone	368
Antabuse	disulfiram	alcoholism	
Antepar	piperazine	antihelminth	
Antepsin	sucralfate	peptic ulcer	
Antoin	aspirin, codeine, caffeine	analgesic	
Anturan	sulphinpyrazone	uricosuric	
Anxon	ketazolam	benzodiazepine	368
Apistate	diethylpropion + vitamins	CNS stimulant, anti-obesity	
Apresoline	hydralazine HCl	vasodilator	
Aprinox	bendrofluazide	thiazide diuretic	
Aproten	nutrition	aminoacidurias etc.	
Apsifen	ibuprofen	NSAID	
Apsin VK	penicillin V	antibiotic	
Apsolol	propranolol	beta blocker	371
Arelix	piretanide	loop diuretic	
Arobon	ceratonia, starch	anti-diarrhoeal	
Arpicolin	procyclidine	anticholinergic	
Arpimycin	erythromycin	antibiotic	
Artane	benzhexol	anti-Parkinsonian	
Artracin	indomethacin	NSAID	
Asacol	mesalazine	salicylate	
Asilone		antacid	
Asmaven	salbutamol	asthma, beta$_2$ agonist	
Aspav	salicylate + papaveretum	analgesic	
Atarax	hydroxyzine HCl	antihistamine, anxiety	
Atensine	diazepam	benzodiazepine	368
Ativan	lorazepam	benzodiazepine	368
Atromid S	clofibrate	hyperlipidaemia	

2

Proprietary name	Non-proprietary name	Use/type of drug	Other information (page)
Atrovent	ipratropium	anticholinergic, bronchodilator	
Audax	choline salicylate	analgesic	
Augmentin	clavulanic acid + amoxycillin	antibiotic	
Aureomycin	chlortetracycline	antibiotic	
Aventyl	nortriptyline	tricyclic antidepressant	386
Avloclor	chloroquine	malaria, amoebicide	
Axid	nizatidine	H_2-receptor antagonist	
Azactam	aztreonam	antibiotic	
Azamune	azathioprine	immunosuppressant	363
Bactrim	trimethoprim + sulphamethoxazole	folic acid inhibitor + sulphonamide	
Banocide	diethylcarbamazine	amoebicide	
Baratol	indoramin	alpha blocker	
Baxan	cefadroxil	cephalosporin antibiotic	
Baycaron	mefruside	thiazide-like diuretic	
Baypen	mezlocillin	antibiotic	
BC 500	vitamins B and C	vitamin deficiency	
Becloforte	beclomethasone	aerosol steroid, asthma	
Becosym	vitamin B	vitamin deficiency	
Becotide	beclomethasone	aerosol steroid, asthma	
Bedranol	propranolol	beta blocker	371
Bellocarb	belladonna + Mg	antacid	
Bendogen	bethanidine	hypertension	
Benerva	vitamin B	vitamin deficiency	
Benoral	benorylate	salicylate/paracetamol	
Bentex	benzhexol	anticholinergic	
Benztrone	oestradiol	oestrogen replacement	
Berkamil	amiloride	K^+-sparing diuretic	
Berkaprine	azathioprine	immunosuppressant	363
Berkatens	verapamil	calcium antagonist	376
Berkmycen	oxytetracycline	antibiotic	
Berkolol	propranolol	beta blocker	371
Berkozide	bendrofluazide	thiazide diuretic	
Berotec	fenoterol	aerosol bronchodilator beta$_2$ agonist	
Beta-cardone	sotalol	beta blocker	371
Betaloc	metoprolol	beta blocker	371
Betim	timolol	beta blocker	371
Betnelan	betamethasone	corticosteroid	380
Betnesol	betamethasone	corticosteroid	380
Bextasol	betamethasone	steroid aerosol	380
Bezalip-mono	bezafibrate	for hyperlipidaemia	
Bicillin	penicillin G + procaine penicillin	antibiotic	
Bicnu	carmustine	alkylating cytotoxic	363
Binovum	oestrogen + progestogen	oral contraceptive	
Biogastrone	carbenoxolone	gastric ulcer	
Biophylline	theophylline	bronchodilator	
Biorphen	orphenadrine	anti-Parkinsonian, anticholinergic	
Bleomycin	bleomycin	cytotoxic antibiotic	363
Blocadren	timolol	beta blocker	371
Bolvidon	mianserin	tetracyclic antidepressant	
Bradilan	nicofuranose	nicotinic acid derivative	

2

Proprietary name	Non-proprietary name	Use/type of drug	Other information (page)
Bretylate	bretylium	class II antiarrhythmic	356
Brevinor	ethinyloestradiol norethisterone	oral contraceptive	
Bricanyl	terbutaline	beta$_2$ agonist	
Brinaldix K	clopamide + K$^+$	thiazide-like diuretic	
Britiazem	diltiazem	Class III Ca^{++} antagonist	376
Brocadopa	levodopa	dopamine precursor	367
Broflex	benzhexol	anticholinergic	
Bronchodil	reproterol	beta$_2$ agonist	
Brovon	adrenaline, atropine papaverine	aerosol bronchodilator	
Broxil	phenethicillin	antibiotic	
Brufen	ibuprofen	NSAID	
Buccastem	prochlorperazine	Meniere's, phenothiazine	
Burinex	bumetanide	loop diuretic	
Buscopan	hyoscine	anticholinergic	
Butacote	phenylbutazone	NSAID	
Butazolidin	phenylbutazone	NSAID	
Cafadol	paracetamol + caffeine	analgesic	
Cafergot	ergotamine	migraine	
Calabren	glibenclamide	oral hypoglycaemic	355
Calcicard	diltiazem	calcium antagonist	376
Calcimax		calcium supplement	
Calcisorb	Na cellulose phosphate	ion-exchange, hypercalciuria	
Calcitare	calcitonin	Paget's, hypercalcaemia	
Calpol	paracetamol	analgesic	
Calsynar	salcatonin	Paget's, hypercalcaemia	
Calthor	ciclacillin	broad-spectrum penicillin	
CAM	ephedrine + butethamate	sympathomimetic, anticholinergic	
Camcolit	lithium	manic depression	383
Camoquin	amodiaquine	acute malaria	
Cantil	mepenzolate	anticholinergic	
Capastat	capreomycin	antituberculous	
Caplenal	allopurinol	gout prophylaxis	
Capoten	captopril	ACE inhibitor	
Capozide	captopril + hydrochlorothiazide	ACE inhibitor, thiazide	
Caprin	salicylate	analgesic	
Carace	lisinopril	ACE inhibitor	
Carbellon	belladonna + Mg + charcoal	antacid anticholinergic	
Cardene	nicardipine	calcium antagonist	376
Cardiacap	pentaerythritol tetranitrate	nitrate, vasodilator	
Carisoma	carisprodol	carbamate, centrally acting muscle relaxant	
Catapres	clonidine	central alpha agonist	362
Caved-S	liquorice based	cytoprotectant, ulcers	
CCNU	lomustine	alkylating cytotoxic	363
Ce-Cobalin	vitamins B12 and C	vitamins	
Cedilanid	lanatoside C	cardiac glycoside	381
Cedocard	isosorbide dinitrate	vasodilator, angina, heart failure	

2

Proprietary name	Non-proprietary name	Use/type of drug	Other information (page)
Cefizox	ceftizoxime	cephalosporin antibiotic	
Celbenin	methicillin Na	penicillinase-resistant penicillin	
Celevac	methylcellulose	bulking agent	
Cellucon	methylcellulose	bulking agent	
Centrax	prazepam	benzodiazepine	368
Centyl	bendrofluazide	thiazide diuretic	
Ceporex	cephalexin	cephalosporin antibiotic	
Cervagem	gemeprost	prostaglandin	
Cesamet	nabilone	anti-emetic	
Chemotrim	sulphamethoxazole + trimethoprim	antibiotic	
Chendol	chenodeoxycholic acid	cholesterol gallstones	
Chenocedon	chenodeoxycholic acid	cholesterol gallstones	
Chenofalk	chenodeoxycholic acid	cholesterol gallstones	
Chloromycetin	chloramphenicol	antibiotic	
Choledyl	choline theophyllinate	xanthine bronchodilator	
Chymar	chymotrypsin	proteolytic enzyme	
Chymocyclar	tetracycline + pancreatic conc.	antibiotic	
Chymoral	trypsin + chymotrypsin	proteolytic enzyme	
Cinobac	cinoxacin	quinolone bacteriocide	
Ciproxin	ciprofloxacin	quinolone bacteriocide	
Claradin	salicylate	analgesic	
Clinium	lidoflazine	calcium antagonist	376
Clinoril	sulindac	NSAID	
Clobazam	clobazam	benzodiazepine	368
Clomid	clomiphene	antioestrogen	
Clopixol	zuclopenthixol	thioxanthene antipsychotic	
Cobalin-H	Vitamin B12	vitamin	
Co-Betaloc	metoprolol + hydrochlorothiazide	beta blocker, thiazide diuretic	371
Cobutolin	salbutamol	beta₂ agonist	
Co-Codamol	codeine + paracetamol	analgesic	
Co-Codaprin	aspirin + codeine	analgesic	
Codis	aspirin + codeine	analgesic	
Co-Dydramol	dihydrocodeine + paracetamol	analgesic	
Cogentin	benztropine mesylate	anticholinergic	
Colestid	colestipol	ion exchange resin	
Colofac	mebeverine	antispasmodic	
Cologel	methylcellulose	bulking agent	
Colomycin	colistin sulphomethate	polymyxin antibiotic	350
Colpermin	peppermint oil	antispasmodic	
Colven	mebeverine + ispaghula husk	antispasmodic + bulking agent	
Combantrin	pyrantel embonate	antihelminthic	
Comox	trimethoprim + sulphamethoxazole	folic acid inhibitor + sulphonamide	
Comploment	pyridoxine	vitamin B6 deficiency	
Continus			
Concavit	multivitamin	vitamin deficiency	
Concordin	protriptyline	tricyclic antidepressant	386
Conova	ethinyloestradiol ethynodiol	oral contraceptive	
Controvlar	ethinyloestradiol norethisterone	menstrual disorders	

Proprietary name	Non-proprietary name	Use/type of drug	Other information (page)
Coparvax	corynebacterium	immunostimulant	
Co-Proxamol	dextropropoxyphene paracetamol	analgesic	
Cordarone X	amiodarone	class III antiarrhythmic	356
Cordilox	verapamil	calcium antagonist	376
Corgard	nadolol	beta blocker	371
Corgaretic	nadolol + bendrofluazide	beta blocker + thiazide diuretic	371
Coro-Nitro	glyceryl trinitrate	angina aerosol	
Cortelan	cortisone acetate	gluco-mineralocorticoid	380
Cortistab	cortisone acetate	gluco-mineralocorticoid	380
Cortisyl	cortisone acetate	gluco-mineralocorticoid	380
Corwin	xamoterol	partial alpha₁ agonist	
Cosmogen lyovac	actinomycin D	cytotoxic antibiotic	363
Cosuric	allopurinol	gout prophylaxis	
Cotazym	pancreatic enzymes	pancreatic insufficiency	
Creon	pancreatic enzymes	pancreatic insufficiency	
Crystapen	penicillin G	antibiotic	
Cyclobral	cyclandelate	peripheral vascular disease	
Cyclo-Progynova	oestradiol + norgestrel	hormone replacement, menopause symptoms	
Cyclospasmol	cyclandelate	peripheral vascular disease	
Cyklokapron	tranexamic acid	antifibrinolytic	
Cyprostat	cyproterone	prostatic carcinoma	
Cytacon	cyanocobalamin	vitamin B12 deficiency	
Cytosar	cytarabine	antimetabolite	363
Daktarin	miconazole	antifungal imidazole	
Dalacin C	clindamycin	lincosamide antibiotic	350
Dalmane	flurazepam	benzodiazepine	368
Daneral SA	pheniramine	antihistamine	
Danol	danazol	inhibits gonadotrophin release	
Dantrium	dantrolene Na	muscle spasticity	
Daonil	glibenclamide	sulphonylurea, diabetes	355
Dapsone	dapsone	sulphone, for leprosy	
Daranide	dichlorphenamide	carbonic anhydrase inhibitor, glaucoma	
Daraprim	pyrimethamine	malaria prophylaxis	
DDAVP	desmopressin	vasopressin analogue	
Decadron	dexamethasone	glucocorticoid	380
DecaDurabolin	nandrolone	anabolic steroid	
Decaserpyl-Plus	methoserpidine + benzthiazide	rauwolfia alkaloid + diuretic	
Declinax	debrisoquine	adrenergic neurone blocker	
Decortisyl	prednisone	glucocorticoid	380
Defencin	isoxuprine	beta₂ agonist, for vascular disorders	
Deltacortril	prednisolone	glucocorticoid	380
De-Noltab	bismuthate	cytoprotectant, ulcers	
Depixol	flupenthixol	antipsychotic	368
Depocillin	procaine penicillin	antibiotic	
Deponit	glyceryl trinitrate	nitrate patches, angina	
Deseril	methysergide	serotonin antagonist	
Destolit	ursodeoxycholic acid	cholesterol gallstones	
Deteclo	tetracycline	antibiotic	
Dexedrine	dexamphetamine	sympathomimetic	
Dextropropoxyphene	dextropropoxyphene	analgesic	
DF 118	dihydrocodeine	analgesic, antitussive	

2

Proprietary name	Non-proprietary name	Use/type of drug	Other information (page)
DHC Continus	dihydrocodeine	analgesic	
Diabinese	chlorpropamide	sulphonylurea, diabetes	355
Diamicron	gliclazide	sulphonylurea, diabetes	355
Diamox	acetazolamide	carbonic anhydrase inhibitor	
Diane	cyproterone + ethinyloestradiol	anti-androgen + oestrogen	
Diarrest	dicyclomine, NaCl codeine, KCl	diverticulitis	
Diatensec	spironolactone	K$^+$-sparing diuretic	
Diazemuls	diazepam	benzodiazepine	368
Dibenyline	phenoxybenzamine	alpha blocker	
Diconal	dipipanone + cyclizine	opiate analgesic + antiemetic	
Dicynene	ethamsylate	haemostatic	
Didronel	etidronate Na	chelating agent, Paget's	
Dimelor	acetohexamide	sulphonylurea, diabetes	355
Dimotapp	bromopheniramine + phenylephrine	antihistamine + sympathomimetic	
Dindevan	phenindione	anticoagulant	352
Dirythmin SA	disopyramide	class I antiarrhythmic	356
Disalcid	salsalate	NSAID	
Disipal	orphenadrine	anticholinergic, Parkinson's	
Distaclor	cefaclor	cephalosporin antibiotic	
Distalgesic	dextropropoxyphene, paracetamol	analgesic	
Distamine	penicillamine base	rheumatoid arthritis	
Distaquaine-V-K	penicillin V-potassium	antibiotic	
Diumide-K Continus	frusemide + potassium	loop diuretic, K$^+$	
Diuresal	frusemide	loop diuretic	
Diurexan	xipamide	thiazide-like diuretic	
Dixarit	clonidine	central alpha agonist	362
Dolmatil	sulpiride	antipsychotic	
Dolobid	diflunisal	NSAID, salicylate	
Doloxene	dextropropoxyphene	analgesic	
Domical	amitriptyline	tricyclic antidepressant	386
Dopamet	methyldopa	central alpha agonist	
Dormonoct	loprazolam	benzodiazepine	368
Doxatet	doxycycline	tetracycline antibiotic	
Dozic	haloperidol	antipsychotic	368
Dramamine	dimenhydrinate	antihistamine	
Droleptan	droperidol	butyrophenone	368
Dromoran	levorphanol	analgesic	
Droxalin	alexitol + magnesium	antacid	
Dryptal	frusemide	loop diuretic	
DTIC-Dome	dacarbazine	cytotoxic	363
Dulcodos	docusate + bisacodyl	constipation	
Dulcolax	bisacodyl	constipation	
Duogastrone	carbenoxolone	Cytoprotectant, ulcers	
Duovent	fenoterol + ipratropium	beta$_2$ agonist + anticholinergic	
Duphalac	lactulose	osmotic bowel stimulant	
Duphaston	dydrogesterone	progestogen	
Durabolin	nandrolone	anabolic steroid	
Duromine	phentermine	antiobesity, CNS stimulant	

2

Proprietary name	Non-proprietary name	Use/type of drug	Other information (page)
Duvadilan	isoxuprine	beta$_2$ agonist	
Dyazide	triamterene + hydrochlorothiazide	K$^+$-sparing + thiazide diuretic	
Dyspamet	cimetidine	H$_2$-receptor antagonist	
Dytac	triamterene	K$^+$-sparing diuretic	
Dytide	triamterene + benzthiazide	K$^+$-sparing + thiazide diuretic	
Ebufac	ibuprofen	NSAID	
Edecrin	ethacrynic acid	loop diuretic	
Effercitrate	citric acid + potassium bicarb.	alkalinizing agent	
Efudix	fluorouracil	antimetabolite	363
Elantan	isosorbide mononitrate	nitrate vasodilator	
Elavil	amitriptyline	tricyclic antidepressant	386
Eldepryl	selegiline	monoamine oxidase B inhibitor	
Eldisine	vindesine	vinca alkaloid	363
Eltroxin	thyroxine sodium	thyroid hormone	
Emcor	bisoprolol	beta blocker	371
Emeside	ethosuximide	petit mal epilepsy	
Emtexate	methotrexate	folic acid antagonist	363
Endoxana	cyclophosphamide	alkylating cytotoxic	363
Enduron	methyclothiazide	thiazide diuretic	
Enteromide	Ca sulphaloxate	sulphonamide	
Epanutin	phenytoin	anticonvulsant	354
Ephynal	tocopheryl acetate	vitamin E deficiency	
Epilim	sodium valproate	anticonvulsant	354
Epodyl	ethoglucid	alkylating agent	363
Equagesic	ethoheptazine + meprobamate + salicylate	opiate + muscle relaxant + aspirin	
Equanil	meprobamate	carbamate tranquilizer	
Eradacin	acrosoxacin	acute gonorrhoea	
Erycen	erythromycin	antibiotic	
Erymax	erythromycin	antibiotic	
Erythrocin	erythromycin	antibiotic	
Erythromid	erythromycin	antibiotic	
Erythroped A	erythromycin	antibiotic	
Esbatal	bethanidine	adrenergic neurone blocker	
Esidrex	hydrochlorothiazide	thiazide diuretic	
Eskornade	phenylpropanolamine diphenylpyramine	sympathomimetic + antihistamine	
Estracyt	estramustine	alkylating agent	363
Eudemine	diazoxide	vasodilator, hyperglycaemic	
Euglucon	glibenclamide	hypoglycaemic	355
Eugynon	ethinyloestradiol levonorgestrel	oestrogen + progestogen	
Evacalm	diazepam	benzodiazepine	368
Evadyne	butriptyline	tricyclic antidepressant	386
Evoxin	domperidone	antidopaminergic	
Exirel	pirbuterol	beta$_2$ agonist, asthma	
Fabahistin	mebhydrolin	antihistamine	
Fabrol	acetylcysteine	mucolytic	
Fansidar	sulfadoxine + pyrimethamine	sulphonamide + antimalarial	
Farlutal	medroxyprogesterone	progestogen	
Fasigyn	tinidazole	anaerobic infections	

2

Proprietary name	Non-proprietary name	Use/type of drug	Other information (page)
Faverin	fluvoxamine	5HT reuptake inhibitor	
Fectrim	trimethoprim + sulphamethoxazole	folic acid inhibitor + sulphonamide	
Fefol	iron + folic acid	haematinic	
Fefol Vit	iron + vitamins	haematinic + vitamins	
Fefol Z	iron + zinc	haematinic + zinc	
Feldene	piroxicam	NSAID	
Femerital	ambucetamide + paracetamol	antispasmodic + analgesic	
Femodene	ethinyloestradiol gestodene	oestrogen + progestogen	
Femulen	ethynodiol	progestogen	
Fenbid	ibuprofen	NSAID	
Fenopron	fenoprofen	NSAID	
Fenostil	dimethindene	antihistamine	
Fentazin	perphenazine	phenothiazine	
Feospan	iron	iron deficiency	
Feospan Z	iron + zinc	haematinic + zinc	
Ferfolic SV	iron + folic acid	haematinic	
Fergon	iron	haematinic	
Ferrocap	iron	haematinic	
Ferrocontin	iron	haematinic	
Ferrograd	iron	haematinic	
Ferrograd C	iron, ascorbic acid	haematinic + vitamin C	
Ferrograd-folic	iron, folic acid	haematinic	
Ferromyn	iron	haematinic	
Fersaday	iron	haematinic	
Fersamal	iron	haematinic	
Fertiral	gonadorelin	gonadotrophin releasing	
Fesovit	iron + vitamins	haematinic + vitamins	
Fesovit Z	iron, zinc, vitamin	haematinic, zinc, vitamin	
Flagyl	metronidazole	anaerobic infection	
Flolan	epoprostenol	prostaglandin	
Florinef	fludrocortisone	mineralocorticoid	380
Floxapen	flucloxacillin	penicillin	
Fluanxol	flupenthixol	antipsychotic	368
Folex 350	iron + folic acid	haematinic	
Folicin	folic acid, iron, Cu, manganese	haematinic, minerals	
Forceval	vitamins, minerals	vitamin deficiencies	
Fortagesic	pentazocine + paracetamol	analgesic	
Fortral	pentazocine	analgesic, narcotic antagonist	
Fortum	ceftazidime	cephalosporin antibiotic	
Fortunan	haloperidol	antipsychotic	368
Franol	ephedrine + theophylline + phenobarbitone	sympathomimetic, xanthine barbiturate	
Frisium	clobazam	benzodiazepine	368
Froben	flurbiprofen	propionic acid NSAID	
Frumil	frusemide + amiloride	loop + K$^+$-sparing diuretic	
Frusene	frusemide + triamterene	loop + K$^+$-sparing diuretic	
Frusetic	frusemide	loop diuretic	
Frusid	frusemide	loop diuretic	
Fucidin	sodium fusidate	antibiotic	
Fulcin	griseofulvin	antidermatophyte	
Fungilin	amphotericin	anticandidal	

2

Proprietary name	Non-proprietary name	Use/type of drug	Other information (page)
Furadantin	nitrofurantoin	antibiotic	
Fybranta	bran	bulking agent	
Galfer	iron	haematinic	
Galfervit	iron + vitamins	haematinic + vitamins	
Galpseud	pseudoephedrine	sympathomimetic	
Gamanil	lofepramine	tricyclic antidepressant	386
Gastrocote	alginate + antacid	oesophagitis	
Gastromax	metoclopramide	anticholinergic	
Gastron	alginate + antacid	oesophagitis	
Gastrozepin	pirenzepine	anticholinergic	
Gaviscon	alginate + antacid	oesophagitis	
Gelusil	antacid	hyperacidity	
Genticin	gentamicin	aminoglycoside	350
Gestanin	allyloestrenol	progestogen	
Gevral	multivitamins + minerals	deficiencies	
Givitol	iron + vitamins	deficiencies	
Glibenese	glipizide	sulphonylurea, diabetes	355
Glucophage	metformin	biguanide, diabetes	355
Glucotard	guar gum	bulking agent, diabetes	
Glurenorm	gliquidone	sulphonylurea, diabetes	355
Grisovin	griseofulvin	antidermatophyte	
Guarem	guar gum	bulking agent, diabetes	
Guarina	guar gum	bulking agent, diabetes	
Gynovlar 21	ethinyloestradiol norethisterone	oestrogen, progestogen	
Halcion	triazolam	benzodiazepine	368
Haldol	haloperidol	antipsychotic	368
Hamarin	allopurinol	gout prophylaxis	
Harmogen	piperazine oestrone	oestrogen	
Haymine	antihistamine + sympathomimetic	chlorpheniramine + ephedrine	
Heminevrin	chlormethiazole	sedative	
Hexopal	inositol nicotinate	vasodilator	
Hiprex	hexamine hippurate	antibacterial	
Hismanal	astemizole	antihistamine	
Histryl	diphenylpyraline	antihistamine	
Honvan	tetrasodium fosfestrol	oestrogen for carcinoma of prostate	
Hormonin	oestriol, oestrone, oestradiol	oestrogen	
Human insulin	insulin	hypoglycaemic	355
Hydergine	codergocrine mesylate	cerebral activator, ergot alkaloid	
Hydrea	hydroxyurea	cytotoxic	363
Hydrenox	hydroflumethiazide	thiazide diuretic	
Hydrocortistab	hydrocortisone	gluco-, mineralocorticoid	380
Hydrocortone	hydrocortisone	gluco-, mineralocorticoid	380
Hydromet	methyldopa + hydrochlorothiazide	central alpha agonist + thiazide diuretic	
Hydrosaluric	hydrochlorothiazide	thiazide diuretic	
Hydrotalcite	hydrotalcite	antacid	
Hygroton	chlorthalidone	thiazide-like diuretic	
Hypertane	hydrochlorothiazide amiloride	thiazide + K^+-sparing diuretic	
Hypon	aspirin, caffeine, codeine	analgesic	
Hypovase	prazosin	selective alpha$_1$ blocker	

2

Proprietary name	Non-proprietary name	Use/type of drug	Other information (page)
Hytrin	terazosin	selective alpha$_1$ blocker	
Ibumetin	ibuprofen	NSAID	
Ilosone	erythromycin	macrolide antibiotic	
Ilotycin	erythromycin	macrolide antibiotic	
Imbrilon	indomethacin	NSAID	
Imdur	isosorbide mononitrate	angina	
Imodium	loperamide	antidiarrhoeal	
Imperacin	oxytetracycline	antibiotic	
Imunovir	inosine pranobex	antiviral	
Imuran	azathioprine	immunosuppressant	363
Inderal	propranolol	beta blocker	371
Inderetic	propranolol + bendrofluazide	beta blocker + thiazide diuretic	371
Inderex	propranolol + bendrofluazide	beta blocker + thiazide diuretic	371
Indocid	indomethacin	NSAID	
Indoflex	indomethacin	NSAID	
Indolar	indomethacin	NSAID	
Indomod	indomethacin	NSAID	
Innovace	enalapril	ACE inhibitor	
Intal	sodium cromoglycate	asthma prophylaxis	
Integrin	oxypertine	phenothiazine-like	
Ionamin	phentermine	antiobesity	
Ipral	trimethoprim	folic acid inhibitor	
Irofol C	iron, vitamin C	haematinic, vitamin C	
Ironorm	iron	haematinic	
Ismelin	guanethidine	adrenergic neurone blocker	
Ismo	isosorbide mononitrate	angina prophylaxis	
Iso-autohaler	isoprenaline	asthma aerosol	
Isogel	ispaghula husk	bulking agent	
Isoket	isosorbide dinitrate	angina prophylaxis	
Isordil	isosorbide dinitrate	angina prophylaxis	
Juvel	multivitamin	deficiencies	
Kalspare	chlorthalidone + triamterene	thiazide-like + K$^+$-sparing diuretic	
Kalten	atenolol, amiloride hydrochlorothiazide	beta blocker, K$^+$-sparing + thiazide diuretic	371
Kannasyn	kanamycin	aminoglycoside antibiotic	350
K-Contin	potassium chloride	potassium depletion	
Kefadol	cefamandole	cephalosporin	
Keflex	cephalexin	cephalosporin	
Keflin	cephalothin	cephalosporin	
Kefzol	cephazolin	cephalosporin	
Kelfizine W	sulfametopyrazine	sulphonamide	
Kemadrin	procyclidine	anticholinergic	
Kemicetine	chloramphenicol	antibiotic	
Kerlone	betaxolol	beta blocker	371
Kest	magnesium sulphate phenolphthalein	constipation	
Ketovite	multivitamin	deficiency	
Kiditard	quinidine	class I antidysrhythmic	356
Kinidin	quinidine	class I antidysrhythmic	356
Kloref	potassium	potassium depletion	
Laboprin	salicylate	analgesic	

Proprietary name	Non-proprietary name	Use/type of drug	Other information (page)
Labrocol	labetalol	alpha & beta blocker	371
Ladropen	flucloxacillin	antibiotic	
Lamprene	clofazimine	leprosy	
Lanoxin	digoxin	cardiac glycoside	381
Lanvis	thioguanine	antimetabolite	363
Laractone	spironolactone	K^+-sparing diuretic	
Laraflex	propionic acid	NSAID	
Larapam	piroxicam	NSAID	
Laratrim	trimethoprim + sulphamethoxazole	folic acid inhibitor + sulphonamide	
Largactil	chlorpromazine	phenothiazine	368
Larodopa	levodopa	dopamine precursor	367
Lasikal	frusemide + potassium chloride	loop diuretic + potassium supplement	
Lasilactone	frusemide + spironolactone	loop diuretic + K^+-sparing diuretic	
Lasipressin	penbutolol + frusemide	beta blocker + loop diuretic	371
Lasix	frusemide	loop diuretic	
Lasma	theophylline	xanthine bronchodilator	
Lasoride	frusemide + amiloride	loop diuretic + K^+-sparing diuretic	
Ledercort	triamcinolone	glucocorticoid	380
Lederfen	fenbufen	NSAID	
Ledermycin	demeclocycline	tetracycline	
Lederspan	triamcinolone	glucocorticoid	380
Lejguar	guar gum	bulking agent, diabetes	
Lentizol	amitriptyline	tricyclic antidepressant	386
Leo-K	potassium chloride	potassium supplement	
Leukeran	chlorambucil	alkylating cytotoxic	363
Lexotan	bromazepam	benzodiazepine	368
Libanil	glibenclamide	sulphonylurea	355
Libraxin	chlordiazepoxide + clinidium bromide	benzodiazepine + anticholinergic	368
Librium	chlordiazepoxide	benzodiazepine	368
Lidifen	ibuprofen	NSAID	
Limbitrol	amitriptyline + chlordiazepoxide	tricyclic antidepressant + benzodiazepine	368, 386
Lincocin	lincomycin	lincosamide antibiotic	350
Lingraine	ergotamine tartrate	migraine	
Lioresal	baclofen	for muscle spasticity, GABA-mimetic, spinal level	
Lipoflavonoid	multivitamins	vitamin B deficiency	
Lipotriad	multivitamins	vitamin B deficiency	
Liskonum	lithium carbonate	manic depression	383
Litarex	lithium citrate	manic depression	383
Lo-Asid	Al & Mg hydroxide + dimethicone	antacid + deflatulent	
Lobak	chlormezanone + paracetamol	muscle antispasmodic + analgesic	
Lodine	etodolac	NSAID	
Loestrin	ethinyloestradiol + norethisterone	oestrogen + progestogen	
Logynon	ethinyloestradiol + levonorgestrel	oestrogen + progestogen	
Lomotil	diphenoxylate + atropine	opiate + anticholinergic	

Proprietary name	Non-proprietary name	Use/type of drug	Other information (page)
Loniten	minoxidil	vasodilator, hypertension	
Lopid	gemfibrozil	for hyperlipidaemias	
Loprazolam	loprazolam	benzodiazepine	368
Lopresor	metoprolol	beta blocker	371
Lopressoretic	metoprolol + chlorthalidone	beta blocker + thiazide diuretic	371
Lorazepam	lorazepam	benzodiazepine	368
Lormetazepam	lormetazepam	benzodiazepine	368
Ludiomil	maprotiline	tetracyclic antidepressant	
Luminal	phenobarbitone	anticonvulsant	354
Lurselle	probucol	hyperlipoproteinaemias	
Macrodantin	nitrofurantoin	antibiotic	
Madopar	levodopa	dopamine precursor	367
Magnapen	ampicillin + flucloxacillin	antibiotic	
Malinal	almasilate	antacid	
Malix	glibenclamide	sulphonylurea, diabetes	355
Maloprim	dapsone + pyrimethamine	malaria prophylaxis	
Marevan	warfarin	coumarin anticoagulant	352
Marplan	isocarboxazid	MAOI	384
Marvelon	ethinyloestradiol desogestrel	oestrogen, progestogen	
Masteril	drostanolone	anabolic steroid	
Maxepa	eicosapentaenoic + docosahexaenoic acid	hypertriglyceridaemia	
Maxolon	metoclopramide	antidopaminergic	
Maxtrex	methotrexate	folic and antagonist	363
Medihaler-Duo	isoprenaline + phenylephrine	bronchodilator aerosol	
Medihaler-Epi	adrenaline	anaphylaxis, aerosol	
Medihaler-Ergotamine	ergotamine tartrate	migraine, aerosol	
Medihaler-Iso	isoprenaline	bronchodilator aerosol	
Medocodene	paracetamol + codeine	analgesic	
Medomet	methyldopa	central alpha agonist	
Medrone	methylprednisolone	glucocorticoid	380
Mefoxin	cefoxitin	cephalosporin antibiotic	
Megace	megestrol	progestogen, neoplasms	
Megaclor	clomocycline	antibiotic	
Melleril	thioridazine	phenothiazine group II	368
Menophase	mestranol + norethisterone	oestrogen, progestogen	
Meptid	meptazinol	opiate partial agonist	
Merbentyl	dicyclomine	anticholinergic	
Mestinon	pyridostigmine	anticholinesterase	
Metefer	iron	haematinic	
Metenix	metolazone	thiazide-like diuretic	
Meterfolic	iron + folic acid	haematinic	
Metopirone	metyrapone	aldosterone inhibitor	
Metox	metoclopramide	antidopaminergic	
Metramid	metoclopramide	antidopaminergic	
Metrolyl	metronidazole	antibiotic	
Mexitil	mexiletine	class I antiarrhythmic	356

2

Proprietary name	Non-proprietary name	Use/type of drug	Other information (page)
Micro K	potassium chloride	potassium supplement	
Microgynon	ethinyloestradiol + levonorgestrel	oestrogen, progestogen	
Micronor	norethisterone	progestogen	
Microval	levonorgestrel	progestogen	
Mictral	nalidixic acid + sodium citrate	bacteriocide	
Midamor	amiloride	K$^+$-sparing diuretic	
Midrid	isometheptine + dichloralphenazone + paracetamol	sympathomimetic + sedative + analgesic	
Migraleve	buclizine + codeine paracetamol	antihistamine + analgesic	
Migravess	metoclopramide aspirin	antiemetic + analgesic	
Migril	ergotamine + cyclizine, caffeine	migraine	
Minilyn	ethinyloestradiol + lynoestranol	oestrogen, progestogen	
Minocin	minocycline	tetracycline	
Minodiab	glipizide	sulphonylurea, diabetes	355
Minovlar	ethinyloestradiol + norethisterone	oestrogen, progestogen	
Mintec	peppermint oil	antispasmodic	
Mintezol	thiabendazole	antihelminthic	
Miraxid	pivampicillin + pivmecillinam	antibiotic	
Mithracin	plicamycin	cytotoxic antibiotic	363
Mitoxana	ifosfamide	alkylating cytotoxic	363
Mitomycin C	mitomycin	cytotoxic antibiotic	363
Modecate	fluphenazine	depot phenothiazine	368
Moditen	fluphenazine	phenothiazine	368
Modrenal	trilostane	adrenal inhibitor	
Moducren	hydrochlorothiazide amiloride timolol	thiazide diuretic + K$^+$-sparing diuretic beta blocker	371
Moduret 25	hydrochlorothiazide amiloride	thiazide diuretic + K$^+$-sparing	
Moduretic	hydrochlorothiazide amiloride	thiazide diuretic + K$^+$-sparing	
Mogadon	nitrazepam	benzodiazepine	368
Molipaxin	trazadone	tricyclic related	
Monaspor	cefsulodin	cephalosporin antibiotic	
Monit	isosorbide mono-nitrate	angina prophylaxis	
Mono-Cedocard	isosorbide mono-nitrate	angina prophylaxis	
Monocor	bisoprolol	beta blocker	371
Monotrim	trimethoprim	folic acid inhibitor	
Monovent	terbutaline	beta$_2$ agonist	
Motilium	domperidone	antidopaminergic	
Motipress	fluphenazine + nortriptyline	phenothiazine + tricyclic antidepressant	368, 386
Motival	fluphenazine + nortriptyline	phenothiazine + tricyclic antidepressant	368, 386
Motrin	ibuprofen	NSAID	

Proprietary name	Non-proprietary name	Use/type of drug	Other information (page)
Moxalactam	latamoxef disodium	cephalosporin antibiotic	
MST continus	morphine	opiate analgesic	
Mucodyne	carbocisteine	mucolytic	
Mucolex	carbocisteine	mucolytic	
Multivite	multivitamins	vitamin deficiency	
Muripsin	glutamic acid + pepsin	hypochlorhydria	
Mustine HCl	mustine HCl	alkylating agent	363
Myambutol	ethambutol	antituberculous drug	
Mycardol	pentaerythritrol tetranitrate	angina, nitrate	
Myelobromol	mitobronitol	alkylating agent	363
Myleran	busulphan	alkylating cytotoxic	363
Mynah	ethambutol + isoniazid	antituberculous drug	
Myocrisin	Na aurothiomalate	gold salt, arthritis	
Myotonine	bethanechol	cholinergic	
Mysoline	primidone	anticonvulsant	354
Mysteclin	tetracycline	antibiotic	
Nacton	poldine methylsulphate	anticholinergic	
Nalcrom	sodium cromoglycate	mast cell stabiliser, asthma	
Naprosyn	naproxan	NSAID	
Nardil	phenelzine	MAOI	384
Narphen	phenazocine	opiate analgesic	
Natrilix	indapamide	vasorelaxant, hypertension	
Natulan	procarbazine	cytostatic, mild MAOI	363
Navidrex	cyclopenthiazide	thiazide diuretic	
Navidrex K	cyclopenthiazide + potassium chloride	thiazide diuretic + potassium supplement	
Naxogin	nimorazole	antiprotozoal	
Nebcin	tobramycin	aminoglycoside antibiotic	350
Negram	nalidixic acid	bacteriocide	
Neocon	ethinyloestradiol + norethisterone	oestrogen, progestogen	
Neogest	norgestrel	progestogen	
NeoMercazole	carbimazole	antithyroid	
NeoNaclex	bendrofluazide	thiazide diuretic	
NeoNaclex K	bendrofluazide + potassium	thiazide diuretic + potassium	
Neoplatin	cisplatin	alkylating cytotoxic	363
Nephril	polythiazide	thiazide diuretic	
Netillin	netilmicin	aminoglycoside antibiotic	350
Neulactil	pericyazine	phenothiazine	
Nicorette	nicotine	nicotine replacement	
Niferex	iron	haematinic	
Nilstim	methylcellulose	bulking agent, obesity	
Nitoman	tetrabenazine	dopamine-depleting agent	
Nitrados	nitrazepam	benzodiazepine	368
Nitrazepam	nitrazepam	benzodiazepine	368
Nitrocine	glyceryl trinitrate	angina	
Nitrocontin Continus	glyceryl trinitrate	angina	
Nitrolingual	glyceryl trinitrate	angina, aerosol	
Nitronal	glyceryl trinitrate	angina	
Nivaquine	chloroquine	malaria prophylaxis	

2

Proprietary name	Non-proprietary name	Use/type of drug	Other information (page)
Nivemycin	neomycin	aminoglycoside antibiotic	350
Nizoral	ketoconazole	antifungal	
Nobrium	medazepam	benzodiazepine	368
Noctec	chloral hydrate	sedative	
Noctesed	nitrazepam	benzodiazepine	368
Noltam	tamoxifen	antioestrogen	
Noludar	methyprylone	sedative	
Nolvadex	tamoxifen	antioestrogen	
Noradran	guaiphenesin diphenhydramine diprophylline ephedrine	expectorant + antihistamine + bronchodilator + sympathomimetic	
Nordox	doxycycline	tetracycline	
Norflex	orphenadrine	central anticholinergic	
Norgesic	orphenadrine + paracetamol	central anticholinergic + analgesic	
Norgestron	levonorgestrel	progestogen	
Noriday	norethisterone	progestogen	
Norimin	ethinyloestradiol + norethisterone	osetrogen + progestogen	
Norinyl-1	mestranol + norethisterone	oestrogen + progestogen	
Normacol	sterculia	bulking agent	
Normax	danthron + docusate sodium	constipation	
Normetic	hydrochlorothiazide amiloride	thiazide diuretic + K^+-sparing diuretic	
Normison	temazepam	benzodiazepine	368
Norval	mianserin	tetracyclic antidepressant	
Novantrone	mitozantrone	DNA-reactive cytotoxic	363
Nozinan	methotrimeprazine	phenothiazine	
Nuelin SA	theophylline	asthma	
Nu-K	potassium chloride	potassium supplement	
Nulacin	antacid	dyspepsia	
Numotac	isoetharine	beta agonist, asthma	
Nu-Seals aspirin	salicylate	analgesic	
Nutrizym	pancreatic enzymes	pancreatic replacement	
Nystan	nystatin	anticandidal drug	
Octovit	multivitamin	vitamin deficiencies	
Olbetam	acipimox	hyperlipoproteinaemias	
Oncovin	vincristine	vinca alkaloid	363
One-Alpha	alfacalcidol	vitamin-D analogue	
Opilon	thymoxamine	$alpha_1$ blocker	
Opobyl	bile salts etc.	constipation, biliary insufficiency	
Optimax	1-tryptophan + pyridoxine + vitamin C	5-HT precursor + vitamins	
Optimine	azatadine	antihistamine, antiserotonin	
Orabet	metformin	biguanide, diabetes	355
Oradexon	dexamethasone	glucocorticoid	380
Orap	pimozide	antipsychotic	
Orbenin	cloxacillin	antibiotic, penicillin	
Orimeten	aminoglutethimide	steroid synthesis inhibitor	
Orovite	vitamins B & C	vitamin deficiencies	

2

Proprietary name	Non-proprietary name	Use/type of drug	Other information (page)
Orovite 7	multivitamin	vitamin deficiencies	
Orudis	ketoprofen	NSAID	
Oruvail	ketoprofen	NSAID	
Ortho-Novin	mestranol norethisterone	oestrogen, progestogen	
Ossopan	hydroxyapatite	calcium/phosphorus supplement	
Ovran	ethinyloestradiol levonorgestrel	oestrogen, progestogen	
Ovranette	ethinyloestradiol levonorgestrel	oestrogen, progestogen	
Ovysmen	ethinyloestradiol norethisterone	oestrogen, progestogen	
Oxanid	oxazepam	benzodiazepine	368
Oxazepam	oxazepam	benzodiazepine	368
Oxymycin	oxytetracycline	antibiotic	
Pacitron	l-tryptophan	5-HT precursor, depression	
Palaprin Forte	aloxiprin	salicylate analgesic	
Palfium	dextromoramide	opiate analgesic	
Paludrine	proguanil	malaria prophylaxis	
Pameton	paracetamol + methionine	analgesic + antidote	
Panadeine	paracetamol + codeine	analgesic	
Panadol	paracetamol	analgesic	
Panasorb	paracetamol	analgesic	
Pancrease	pancreatic enzymes	pancreatic replacement	
Pancrex-V	pancreatic enzymes	pancreatic replacement	
Paracetamol	paracetamol	analgesic	
Paracodol	paracetamol + codeine	analgesic	
Parahypon	paracetamol + codeine + caffeine	analgesic	
Parake	paracetamol + codeine	analgesic	
Paramax	paracetamol + metoclopramide	analgesic, antiemetic	
Paramol	paracetamol + dihydrocodeine	compound opiate analgesic	
Paraplatin	carboplatin	alkylating cytotoxic	363
Pardale	paracetamol + codeine + caffeine	compound analgesic	
Paritane	oxprenolol	beta blocker	371
Parlodel	bromocriptine	dopamine agonist	
Parmid	metoclopramide	antidopaminergic antiemetic	
Parnate	tranylcypromine	MAOI	384
Paroven	oxerutins	for leg ulcers	
Parstelin	tranylcypromine + trifluoperazine	MAOI + phenothiazine	368, 384
Paxalgesic	dextropropoxyphene paracetamol	opiate + compound opiate analgesic	
Paxophen	ibuprofen	NSAID	
Paynocil	aspirin + glycine	analgesic	
Penbritin	ampicillin	antibiotic	
Pendramine	penicillamine	arthritis, penicillin deriv.	

Proprietary name	Non-proprietary name	Use/type of drug	Other information (page)
Penidural	benzathine penicillin	antibiotic	
Pentazocine	pentazocine	narcotic antagonist	
Pepcid PM	famotidine	H_2 antagonist, ulcers	
Peptard	hyoscyamine	anticholinergic	
Percutol	glyceryl trinitrate	antianginal ointment	
Periactin	cyproheptadine	antiserotonin/antihistamine	
Pernivit	acetomenaphthone	for chilblains	
Persantin	dipyridamole	antiplatelet	
Pertofran	desipramine	tricyclic antidepressant	386
Phanodorm	cyclobarbitone	barbiturate	
Pharmidone	codeine + caffeine diphenhydramine + paracetamol	analgesic/antihistamine	
Pharmorubicin	epirubicin	cytotoxic antibiotic	363
Phasal	lithium	manic/depression	383
Phazyme	dimethicone	deflatulent	
Phenergan	promethazine	phenothiazine, antihistamine	
Phensedyl	promethazine + codeine, ephedrine	antihistamine + opiate + sympathomimetic	
Pholcomed	pholcodine + papaverine	opiate, bronchorelaxant	
Pholtex	pholcodine + phenyltoloxamine	opiate, antihistamine	
Phyllocontin Continus	aminophylline	long-acting bronchodilator	
Physeptone	methadone	opiate	
Piportil	pipothiazine	depot phenothiazine	
Pipril	piperacillin	penicillin	
Piptal	pipenzolate	anticholinergic	
Piptalin	pipenzolate + dimethicone	anticholinergic + deflatulent	
Piriton	chlorpheniramine	antihistamine	
Plaquenil	hydroxychloroquine	antimalarial, NSAID	
Platet	low-dose aspirin	reduce graft occlusion	
Platinex	cisplatin	alkylating cytotoxic	363
Platosin	cisplatin	alkylating cytotoxic	363
Plesmet	iron	haematinic	
Polyvite	multivitamin	vitamin deficiency	
Ponderax	fenfluramine	serotoninergic	382
Pondocillin	pivampicillin	penicillin	
Ponstan	mefenamic acid	NSAID	
Pramidex	tolbutamide	tolbutamide	355
Praxilene	naftidrofuryl	vascular disorders	
Precortisyl	prednisolone	steroid	380
Prednesol	prednisolone	steroid	380
Prefil	sterculia	obesity	
Pregaday	ferrous fumarate	haematinic	
Pregnavite	iron/vitamin	haematinic/multivitamin	
Premarin	oestrogen	hormonal replacement	
Prempak	oestrogen + progestogen	hormonal replacement	
Prempak-C	oestrogen + progestogen	hormonal replacement	
Prestim	timolol maleate + bendrofluazide	beta blocker thiazide diuretic	371

Proprietary name	Non-proprietary name	Use/type of drug	Other information (page)
Priadel	lithium	manic depression	383
Primalan	mequitazine	antihistamine phenothiazine	
Primolut N	norethisterone	progestogen	
Primperan	metoclopramide	antidopaminergic	
Pripsen	piperazine	antihelminthic	
Pro-Actidil	triprolidine	antihistamine	
Pro-banthine	propantheline	anticholinergic	
Procainamide	procainamide	class I antiarrhythmic	356
Proctofibe	grain fibre	bulking agent	
Prodexin	aluminium glycinate	antacid	
Progesic	fenoprofen	NSAID	
Progynova	oestradiol	oestrogen	
Prominal	methylphenobarbitone	barbiturate	
Prondol	iprindole	tricyclic antidepressant	386
Pronestyl	procainamide	class I antiarrhythmic	356
Propain	codeine + diphehydramine + paracetamol	analgesic + antihistamine	
Prostigmin	neostigmine	anticholinesterase	
Prothiaden	dothiepin	tricyclic antidepressant	386
Pro-vent	theophylline	bronchodilator	
Provera	medroxyprogesterone	progestogen	
Pro-viron	mesterolone	androgen	
Pulmadil	rimiterol	beta$_2$ agonist aerosol	
Pulmicort	budesonide	steroid aerosol	
Puri-Nethol	mercaptopurine	antimetabolite	363
Pyopen	carbenicillin	penicillin	
Pyrogastrone	carbenoxolone + antacids	cytoprotectant antacid	
Questran	cholestyramine	ion-exchange resin	
Rabro	liquorice + antacid	cytoprotectant + antacid	
Ramodar	etodolac	NSAID	
Rapitard	insulin	biphasic	355
Rastinon	tolbutamide	sulphonylurea	355
Razoxin	razoxane	cytotoxic	363
Redeptin	fluspirilene	antipsychotic	
Redoxon	ascorbic acid	vitamin C deficiency	
Refolinon	folinic acid	megaloblastic anaemia	
Regulan	ispaghula husk	bulking agent	
Rehibin	cyclofenil	antioestrogen	
Relifex	nabumetone	NSAID	
Remnos	flunitrazepam	benzodiazepine	368
Rescufolin	folinic acid	megaloblastic anaemia	
Resonium A	sodium polystyrene sulphonate	ion-exchange resin	
Restandol	testosterone	androgen	
Retcin	erythromycin	antibiotic	
Retrovir	zidovudine	antiviral	
Rheumox	azapropazone	NSAID	
Rhinocort	bedesonide	steroid aerosol	
Rhumalgan	diclofenac	NSAID	
Ridaura	auranofin	gold salt NSAID	
Rifadin	rifampicin	antituberculous drug	
Rifater	isoniazid + pyrazinamide + rifampicin	antituberculous drug	

Proprietary name	Non-proprietary name	Use/type of drug	Other information (page)
Rifinah	rifampicin + isoniazid	antituberculous drug	
Rimactane	rifampicin	antituberculous drug	
Rimactazid	rifampicin + isonicotinic acid	antituberculous drug	
Rivotril	clonazepam	anticonvulsant	368
Ro-A-vit	vitamin A	vitamin A deficiency	
Robaxin	methocarbamol	muscle spasm	
Robaxisal	methocarbamol + salicylate	muscle spasm	
Robinul	glycopyrronium	anticholinergic	
Rocaltrol	calcitrol	vitamin D analogue	
Roferon-A	interferon	cytotoxic	
Rohypnol	flunitrazepam	benzodiazepine	368
Ronicol	nicotinyl alcohol	vasospasm	
Roter	bismuth + antacid	peptic ulceration	
Rynacrom	sodium cromoglycate	mast cell stabilizer spray	
Rythmodan	disopyramide	class I antiarrhythmic	356
Sabidal SR	theophylline	bronchodilator	
Salazopyrin	sulphasalazine	NSAID, colitis	
Salbulin	salbutamol	beta$_2$ agonist	
Saluric	chlorothiazide	thiazide diuretic	
Salzone	paracetamol	analgesic	
Sandocal	calcium	calcium supplement	
Sando-K	potassium	potassium deficiency	
Sanomigran	pizotifen	serotonin antagonist	
Saventrine	isoprenaline	beta agonist	
Secadrex	acebutolol + hydrochlorothiazide	beta blocker + thiazide diuretic	371
Seconal	quinalbarbitone	barbiturate	
Sectral	acebutolol	beta blocker	371
Securon	verapamil	calcium antagonist	376
Securopen	azlocillin	penicillin	
Selexid	pivmecillinam	penicillin	
Selexidin	mecillinam	penicillin	
Selora	potassium chloride	salt substitute	
Semidaonil	glibenclamide	sulphonylurea	355
Semitard	insulin	intermediate acting	355
Senna	sennoside	laxative	
Senokot	sennoside	laxative	
Septrin	trimethoprim + sulphamethoxazole	folic acid inhibitor + sulphonamide	
Serc	betahistine	histamine analogue	
Serenace	haloperidol	butyrophenone	368
Serophene	clomiphene	antioestrogen	
Serpasil	reserpine	antihypertensive	
Serpasil-Esidrex	reserpine + hydrochlorothiazide	antihypertensive diuretic	
Siloxyl	alum, dimethicone	dyspepsia	
Simeco	alum, dimethicone	dyspepsia	
Sinemet	levodopa + carbidopa	dopamine precursor dopa decarboxylase inhibitor	367
Sinequan	doxepin	tricyclic antidepressant	386
Sinthrome	nicoumalone	anticoagulant	352
Sintisone	prednisolone	steroid	380
Slo-Phyllin	theophylline	bronchodilator	
Slow-Fe	iron	haematinic	
Slow-Fe Folic	iron, folic acid	haematinic	
Slow K	potassium	potassium deficiency	

2

Proprietary name	Non-proprietary name	Use/type of drug	Other information (page)
Slow-Pren	oxprenolol	beta blocker	371
Slow-Trasicor	oxprenolol	beta blocker	371
Sodium amytal	amylobarbitone	barbiturate	
Soframycin	framycetin	aminoglycoside	350
Solis	diazepam	benzodiazepine	368
Solpadeine	paracetamol + codeine + caffeine	analgesic	
Solprin	salicylate	analgesic	
Solvazinc	zinc	zinc deficiency	
Sominex	promethazine	antihistamine	
Somnite	nitrazepam	benzodiazepine	368
Soneryl	butobarbitone	barbiturate	
Soni-Slo	isosorbide dinitrate	angina	
Sorbichew	isosorbide dinitrate	angina	
Sorbid-SA	isosorbide dinitrate	angina	
Sorbitrate	isosorbide dinitrate	angina	
Sotacor	sotalol	beta blocker	371
Sotazide	sotalol + hydrochlorothiazide	beta blocker + thiazide diuretic	371
Sparine	promazine	phenothiazine	
Spasmonal	alverine	dysmenorrhoea	
Spiretic	spironolactone	K^+-sparing diuretic	
Spiroctan	spironolactone	K^+-sparing diuretic	
Spirolone	spironolactone	K^+-sparing diuretic	
Stabillin VK	penicillin V	antibiotic	
Stafoxil	flucloxacillin	antibiotic	
Staphlipen	flucloxacillin	antibiotic	
Stelazine	trifluoperazine	phenothiazine	368
Stemetil	proclorperazine	phenothiazine	
Stesolid	diazepam	benzodiazepine	368
Stromba	stanozolol	anabolic steroid	
Stugeron	cinnarizine	antihistamine	
Sudafed	pseudoephedrine	sympathomimetic	
Sulphamezathine	sulphadimidine	sulphonamide	
Sulpitil	sulpiride	antipsychotic	
Surbex T	vitamins B and C	vitamin deficiency	
Surem	nitrazepam	benzodiazepine	368
Surgam	tiaprofenic acid	NSAID	
Surmontil	trimipramine	tricyclic antidepressant	386
Suscard	glyceryl trinitrate	angina	
Sustac	glyceryl trinitrate	angina	
Sustamycin	tetracycline	antibiotic	
Sustanon	testosterone	androgen	
Symmetrel	amantadine	dopaminergic	
Synadrin	prenylamine	calcium antagonist	376
Syndol	paracetamol, codeine, doxylamine, caffeine	analgesic + antihistamine	
Synflex	naproxen	NSAID	
Synkavit	menadiol	vitamin K analogue	
Synphase	ethinyloestradiol, norethisterone	oestrogen progestogen	
Syraprim	trimethoprim	folic acid inhibitor	
Sytron	iron edetate	haematinic	
Tachyrol	dihydrotachysterol	vitamin D analogue	
Tagamet	cimetidine	H_2 blocker	
Talpen	talampicillin	penicillin	

Proprietary name	Non-proprietary name	Use/type of drug	Other information (page)
Tambocor	flecainide	class I antiarrhythmic	356
Tamofen	tamoxifen	antioestrogen	
Tavegil	clemastine	antihistamine	
Tedral	theophylline + ephedrine	bronchodilator + sympathomimetic	
Tegretol	carbamazepine	anticonvulsant, neuralgia	
Temazepam	temazepam	benzodiazepine	368
Temgesic	buprenorphine	analgesic	
Tenavoid	meprobamate + bendrofluazide	premenstrual syndrome	
Tenoret	atenolol + chlorthalidone	beta blocker thiazide diuretic	371
Tenoretic	atenolol + chlorthalidone	beta blocker thiazide diuretic	371
Tenormin	atenolol	beta blocker	371
Tensium	diazepam	benzodiazepine	368
Tenuate-Dospan	diethylpropion	CNS stimulant, for obesity	
Terolin	terolidine	anticholinergic	
Teronac	mazindol	CNS stimulant, for obesity	
Terramycin	oxytetracycline	antibiotic	
Tertroxin	liothyronine	thyroid hormone	
Tetrabid	tetracycline	antibiotic	
Tetrachel	tetracycline	antibiotic	
Tetralysal	lymecycline	tetracycline	
Tetrex	tetracycline	antibiotic	
Theodrox	aminophylline	bronchodilator	
Theo-Dur	theophylline	bronchodilator	
Thiotepa	thiotepa	alkylating agent	363
Ticar	ticarcillin	penicillin	
Tiempe	trimethoprim	folic acid inhibitor	
Tigason	etretinate	vitamin A derivative	
Tilade	nedocromil	bronchodilator aerosol	
Tildiem	diltiazem	class III Ca antagonist	376
Timentin	clavulanic acid + ticarcillin	antibiotic	
Tinset	oxatomide	antihistamine	
Titralac	calcium	calcium supplement	
Tofranil	imipramine	tricyclic antidepressant	386
Tolanase	tolazamide	sulphonylurea	
Tolectin	tolmetin	NSAID	
Tolerzide	sotalol + hydrochlorothiazide	beta blocker + thiazide diuretic	371
Tonivitan	multivitamin	vitamin deficiency	
Tonocard	tocainide	class I antiarrhythmic	356
Topal	aluminium hydroxide dimethicone	antacid deflatulent	
Torecan	thiethylperazine	phenothiazine	
Trancopal	chlormezanone	anxiolytic	
Trancoprin	aspirin + chlormezanone	muscle spasm	
Trandate	labetalol	beta + mild alpha blocker	371
Tranxene	chlorazepate	benzodiazepine	368
Trasicor	oxprenolol	beta blocker	371
Trasidrex	oxprenolol + cyclopenthiazide	beta blocker + thiazide diuretic	371
Tremonil	methixene	anticholinergic	

2

Proprietary name	Non-proprietary name	Use/type of drug	Other information (page)
Trental	oxpentifylline	peripheral vascular disease	
Treosulphan	treosulphan	alkylating agent	363
Triamco	hydrochlorothiazide triamterene	thiazide diuretic + K^+-sparing diuretic	
Triazolam	triazolam	benzodiazepine	368
Tridil	glyceryl trinitrate	angina	
Trisilate	salicylate	NSAID	
Triludan	terfenadine	antihistamine	
Trimogal	trimethoprim	antibiotic	
Trimopan	trimethoprim	antibiotic	
Trinordiol	ethinyloestradiol + norethisterone	oestrogen progestogen	
TriNovum	ethinyloestradiol + norethisterone	oestrogen + progestogen	
Triperidol	trifluperidol	butyrophenone	368
Triptafen	amitriptyline	tricyclic antidepressant	386
Trisequens	oestrogen + norethisterone	oestrogen + progestogens	
Trobicin	spectinomycin	aminoglycoside-like	
Tropium	chlordiazepoxide	benzodiazepine	368
Tryptizol	amitriptyline	tricyclic antidepressant	386
Tuinal	quinalbarbitone	barbiturate	
Tylex	paracetamol + codeine	analgesic	
Ubretid	distigmine	anticholinesterase	
Unigesic	paracetamol + caffeine	analgesic	
Unigest	antacid + dimethicone	antacid deflatulent	
Unimycin	oxytetracycline	antibiotic	
Uniphyllin Continus	theophylline	long acting bronchodilator	
Unisomnia	nitrazepam	benzodiazepine	368
Univer	verapamil	class I Ca antagonist	376
Uriben	nalidixic acid	antibacterial	
Urisal	sodium citrate	alkalinising agent	
Urispas	flavoxate	antispasmodic	
Uromide	sulphacarbamide + phenazopyridine	sulphonamide + anaesthetic	
Ursofalk	ursodeoxycholic acid	bile acid	
Uticillin	carfecillin	penicillin	
Utovlan	norethisterone	progestogen	
Valium	diazepam	benzodiazepine	368
Vallergan	trimeprazine	antihistamine	
Valoid	cyclizine	antihistamine	
Vancocin	vancomycin	antibiotic	350
Vascardin	isosorbide dinitrate	angina	
Vasoxine	methoxamine	alpha agonist	
V-Cil-K	penicillin	antibiotic	
Velbe	vinblastine	vinca alkaloid	363
Velosef	cephradine	antibiotic	
Velosulin	insulin	short-acting insulin	355
Ventide	salbutamol + beclomethasone	beta$_2$ agonist + steroid aerosol	
Ventodisks	salbutamol	beta$_2$ agonist	
Ventolin	salbutamol	beta$_2$ agonist	
Vepesid	etoposide	antineoplastic	363
Veractil	methotrimeprazine	phenothiazine	

Proprietary name	Non-proprietary name	Use/type of drug	Other information (page)
Vermox	mebendazole	antihelminthic	
Vertigon	prochlorperazine	phenothiazine	
Vibramycin	doxycycline	tetracycline	
Vi-Daylin	multivitamin	vitamin deficiency	
Vidopen	ampicillin	antibiotic	
Villescon	prolintane + vitamins	sympathomimetic + vitamins	
Visclair	methylcysteine	mucolytic	
Viskaldix	pindolol + clopamide	beta blocker + thiazide diuretic	371
Visken	pindolol	beta blocker	371
Vita-E gels	tocopheryl acetate	intermittent claudication	
Vitavel	multivitamin	vitamin deficiency	
Vivalan	viloxazine	antidepressant	
Volital	pemoline	hyperkinesia in children	
Volmax	salbutamol	beta$_2$ agonist	
Voltarol	diclofenac	NSAID	
Welldorm	dichloralphenazone	hypnotic	
Xanax	alprazolam	benzodiazepine	368
Yomesan	niclosamide	antihelminthic	
Zaditen	ketotifen	mast cell stabiliser	
Zadstat	metronidazole	amoebicide	
Zantac	ranitidine	H$_2$-receptor antagonist	
Zarontin	ethosuximide	petit mal epilepsy	
Zinacef	cefuroxime	antibiotic	
Zinamide	pyrazinamide	nicotinic acid derivative	
Zinnat	cefuroxime	antibiotic	
Zovirax	acyclovir	antiviral, herpes	
Z-Span	zinc spansule	zinc deficiency	
Zyloric	allopurinol	gout	

B. NON-PROPRIETARY NAMES

2

Non-proprietary name	Use/type of drug	Other information (page)
Acebutolol	beta adrenergic blocker	371
acetazolamide	carbonic anhydrase inhibitor	
Acetohexamide	sulphonylurea hypoglycaemic	355
acetomenaphthone	for chilblains	
acetylcysteine	mucolytic for cystic fibrosis	
acetylsalicylic acid	aspirin	
acipimox	hyperlipoproteinaemias	
acrosoxacin	treatment of gonorrhoea	
Actinomycin D	cytotoxic antibiotic	363
acyclovir	antiviral agent	
alexitol sodium	antacid	
alfacalcidol	vitamin D analogue	
alginic acid	antacid constituent	
allopurinol	gout	
allyloestrenol	progestogen	
almasilate	antacid	
aloxiprin	salicylate	
Alprazolam	benzodiazepine	368
alverine citrate	antispasmodic	
amantadine hydrochloride	dopaminergic	
ambucetamide	antispasmodic	
amiloride	K$^+$-sparing diuretic	
aminoglutethimide	steroid synthesis inhibitor	
aminophylline	bronchodilator	
Amiodarone	class III antiarrhythmic	356
Amitriptyline	tricyclic antidepressant	386
amodiaquine	antimalarial	
amoxycillin	broad-spectrum penicillin	
amsacrine	DNA-reactive cytotoxic	363
amylobarbitone	barbiturate	
ascorbic acid	vitamin C	
astemizole	antihistamine	
Atenolol	beta blocker	371
auranofin	gold salt	
azapropazone	NSAID	
azatadine	antihistamine, antiserotonin	
azathioprine	cytotoxic immunosuppressant	363
azlocillin	antipseudomonal penicillin	
aztreonam	monobactam antibiotic	
bacampicillin	broad-spectrum penicillin	
baclofen	for muscle spasticity	
beclomethasone	corticosteroid	380
bendrofluazide	thiazide diuretic	
benorylate	salicylate/paracetamol	
benperidol	butyrophenone	368
benserazide	levodopa + dopa decarboxylase inhibitor	367
benzhexol	anticholinergic	
benzthiazide	thiazide diuretic	
benztropine mesylate	anticholinergic	

2

Non-proprietary name	Use/type of drug	Other information (page)
bephenium	antihelminthic	
betahistine	antihistamine	
betamethasone	corticosteroid	380
bethanechol	cholinergic	
bethanidine	adrenergic neurone blocker	
bezafibrate	for hyperlipidaemias	
bisoprolol	beta adrenergic blocker	371
bretylium	class II antiarrhythmic	356
bromazepam	benzodiazepine	368
bromocriptine	dopamine agonist	
bromopheniramine	antihistamine	
buclizine	antihistamine	
bumetanide	loop diuretic	
·buprenorphine	opiate analgesic	
buspirone	anxiolytic	
busulphan	alkylating cytotoxic	363
butobarbitone	barbiturate	
butriptyline	tricyclic antidepressant	386
calcitonin	hormone	
calcitriol	vitamin D analogue	
captopril	angiotensin-converting enzyme inhibitor	
carbamazepine	anticonvulsant	
carbenicillin	antipseudomonal penicillin	
carbenoxolone	cytoprotectant, peptic ulcers	
carbidopa	dopa decarboxylase inhibitor	367
carbimazole	antithyroid	
carboplatin	alkylating cytotoxic	363
carfecillin	antipseudomonal penicillin	
carisoprodol	for muscle spasm	
carmustine	alkylating cytotoxic	363
ceflaclor	cephalosporin antibiotic	
cefadroxil	cephalosporin	
cefotaxime	cephalosporin	
cefoxitin	cephalosporin	
cefsulodin	cephalosporin	
ceftazidime	cephalosporin	
ceftizoxime	cephalosporin	
cefuroxime	cephalosporin	
cephalexin	cephalosporin	
cephalothin	cephalosporin	
cephazolin	cephalosporin	
cephradine	cephalosporin	
chloral hydrate	hypnotic	
chlorambucil	alkylating cytotoxic	363
chloramphenicol	antibiotic	
chlordiazepoxide	benzodiazepine	368
chlormethiazole	sedative, hypnotic	
chlormezanone	tranquillizer	
chloroquine	antimalarial	
chlorothiazide	thiazide diuretic	
chlorpheniramine	antihistamine	
chlorpromazine	phenothiazine	368
chlorpropamide	sulphonylurea, hypoglycaemic	355
chlortetracycline	antibiotic	
chlorthalidone	thiazide-like diuretic	

Non-proprietary name	Use/type of drug	Other information (page)
cholestyramine	ion-exchange resin	
chymotrypsin	proteolytic enzyme	
ciclacillin	broad spectrum penicillin	
cimetidine	H$_2$-receptor blocker	
cinnarizine	antihistamine	
cinoxacin	quinolone antibacterial	
ciprofloxacin	antibiotic	
cisplatin	alkylating cytotoxic	363
clemastine	antihistamine	
clindamycin	lincosamide antibiotic	350
clobazam	benzodiazepine	368
clofazimine	phenothiazine	
clofibrate	hypolipidaemia	
clomiphene	antioestrogen	
clomipramine	tricyclic antidepressant	386
clomocycline	tetracycline	
clonazepam	benzodiazepine (epilepsy)	368
clonidine	central alpha agonist	362
clopamide	thiazide diuretic	
clorazepate	benzodiazepine	368
cloxacillin	penicillin	
colestipol	ion-exchange resin	
colistin	polymyxin antibiotic	350
corticotrophin	ACTH	
cortisone	gluco/mineralocorticoid	380
co-trimoxazole	antibacterial	
cyanocobalamin	vitamin B12	
cyclandelate	Ca^{++} overload regulator	
cyclobarbitone	barbiturate	
cyclofenil	antioestrogen	
cyclopenthiazide	thiazide diuretic	
cyclophosphamide	alkylating cytotoxic	363
cyclosporin	immunosuppressant	363
cyproheptadine	antiserotonin, antihistamine	
cyproterone acetate	antiandrogen	
cytarabine	antimetabolite	363
dacarbazine	alkylating cytotoxic	363
danazol	gonadotrophin release inhibitor	
dantrolene sodium	for muscle spasticity	
dapsone	sulphone, malaria prophylaxis	
debrisoquine sulphate	adrenergic neurone blocker	
demeclocycline	tetracycline	
desferrioxamine	chelating agent	
desipramine	tricyclic antidepressant	386
desmopressin	vasopressin analogue	
dexamethasone	glucocorticoid	380
dexamphetamine	sympathomimetic	
dextromethorphan	antitussive	
dextromoramide	opiate	
dextropropoxyphene	opiate	
diazepam	benzodiazepine	368
diazoxide	vasodilator, hyperglycaemic	
dichloralphenazone	sedative/hypnotic	
dichlorphenamide	carbonic anhydrase inhibitor	
diclofenac	NSAID	
dicyclomine	anticholinergic	
diethylcarbamazine	antihelminthic	

Non-proprietary name	Use/type of drug	Other information (page)
diethylpropion hydrochloride	CNS stimulant	
diflunisal	salicylate	
digoxin	cardiac glycoside	381
dihydrocodeine	opiate	
dihydrotachysterol	vitamin D analogue	
diltiazem	class III Ca^{++} antagonist	376
dimenhydrinate	antihistamine	
dimethindene maleate	antihistamine	
dipipanone	opiate	
dipyridamole	antiplatelet	
disopyramide	class I antiarrhythmic	356
distigmine	anticholinesterase	
disulfiram	aldehyde dehydrogenase inhibitor	
dobutamine	$beta_1$ agonist	
domperidone	antidopaminergic	
disulfiram	aldehyde dehydrogenase inhibitor	
dobutamine	$beta_1$ agonist	
domperidone	antidopaminergic	
dopamine	inotropic agent	
dothiepin	tricyclic antidepressant	386
doxepin	tricyclic antidepressant	386
doxycycline	tetracycline	
droperidol	butyrophenone	368
drostanolone	anabolic steroid	
dydrogesterone	progestogen	
enalapril	angiotensin-converting enzyme inhibitor	
ephedrine	sympathomimetic	
epirubicin	cytotoxic antibiotic	363
ergotamine	ergot alkaloid, migraine	
erythromycin	macrolide antibiotic	
estramustine	oestrogenic alkylating agent	363
ethacrynic acid	loop diuretic	
ethambutol	antituberculous agent	
ethamsylate	haemostatic agent	
ethoglucid	alkylating cytotoxic	363
ethosuximide	succinimide anticonvulsant	354
etidronate disodium	diphosphanate, hypocalcaemic	
etodolac	NSAID	
etoposide	podophylotoxin, antimitotic	363
famotidine	H_2-receptor antagonist	
fenbufen	NSAID	
fenfluramine	serotoninergic, obesity	382
fenoprofen calcium	NSAID	
fenoterol	selective $beta_2$ agonist	
flavoxate	antispasmodic	
flecainide	class I antiarrhythmic	356
flucloxacillin	penicillin	
fludrocortisone	mineralocorticoid	380
flumazenil	benzodiazepine antagonist	368
flunitrazepam	benzodiazepine	368
flupenthixol	antipsychotic	368
fluphenazine	phenothiazine	368
flurazepam	benzodiazepine	368
flurbiprofen	NSAID	
fluspirilene	antipsychotic	
fluvoxamine	serotonin reuptake inhibitor	

2

Non-proprietary name	Use/type of drug	Other information (page)
fosfestrol	oestrogen	
frusemide	loop diuretic	
gemfibrozil	hypolipidaemic agent	
gentamicin	aminoglycoside antibiotic	350
glibenclamide	sulphonylurea hypoglycaemic	355
gliclazide	sulphonylurea hypoglycaemic	355
glipizide	sulphonylurea hypoglycaemic	355
gliquidone	sulphonylurea hypoglycaemic	355
glyceryl trinitrate	vasodilator, antianginal	
goserelin	gonadotrophin-releasing homone analogue	
griseofulvin	antifungal	
guanethidine	adrenergic neurone blocker	
haloperidol	butyrophenone	368
hydralazine	vasodilator	
hydrochlorothiazide	thiazide diuretic	
hydrocortisone	gluco/mineralocorticoid	380
hydroflumethiazide	thiazide diuretic	
hydrotalcite	antacid	
hydroxyapatite	calcium/phosphorus supplement	
hydroxychloroquine	NSAID, antimalarial	
hydroxyurea	DNA reactive cytotoxic	363
hydroxyzine	antihistamine	
hyoscine	anticholinergic	
hyoscyamine	anticholinergic	
ibuprofen	NSAID	
ifosfamide	alkylating cytotoxic	363
imipramine	tricyclic antidepressant	386
indapamide	vasodilator	
indomethacin	NSAID	
indoramin	selective alpha$_1$ blocker	
inosine pranobex	antiviral immunopotentiator	
inositol nicotinate	Raynaud's phenomenon	
insulin	hypoglycaemic	355
interferon	subtype recombinant	
ipratropium	anticholinergic	
iprindole	tricyclic antidepressant	386
isocarboxazid	monoamine oxidase inhibitor	384
isoetharine	non-selective beta agonist	
isoniazid	antituberculous agent	
isosorbide dinitrate	vasodilator	
isosorbide mononitrate	vasodilator	
isoxsuprine	beta$_2$ agonist	
kanamycin	aminoglycoside antibiotic	350
ketazolam	benzodiazepine	368
ketoprofen	NSAID	
ketotifen	mast cell stabiliser	
labetalol	alpha/beta blocker	371
lanatoside C	cardiac glycoside	381
latamoxef	cephalosporin	
levodopa	dopamine precursor	367
levonorgestrel	progestogen	
levorphanol tartrate	opiate	
lidoflazine	class IV Ca^{++} antagonist	376
lincomycin	lincosamide antibiotic	350

2

Non-proprietary name	Use/type of drug	Other information (page)
liothyronine sodium	thyroid hormone	
lithium	manic depression	383
lofepramine	tricyclic antidepressant	386
lomustine	alkylating cytotoxic	363
loperamide	opiate	
loprazolam	benzodiazepine	368
lorazepam	benzodiazepine	368
lymecycline	tetracycline	
lypressin	vasopressin analogue	
maprotiline	tetracyclic antidepressant	386
mazindol	CNS stimulant, obesity	
mebendazole	antihelminthic	
mebeverine	antispasmodic	
mebhydrolin	antihistamine	
mecillinam	amidino penicillin	
medazepam	benzodiazepine	368
mefenamic acid	NSAID	
mefruside	thiazide-like diuretic	
megestrol	progestogen	
melphalan	alkylating cytotoxic	363
mepenzolate bromide	anticholinergic	
meprobamate	anxiolytic	
meptazinol	opiate partial agonist	
mequitazine	antihistamine	
mercaptopurine	antimetabolite	363
mesalazine	salicylate	
mesterolone	androgen	
metformin	biguanide hypoglycaemic	355
methadone	opiate	
methicillin	penicillin	
methixene	anticholinergic	
methocarbamol	skeletal muscle spasm	
methoserpidine	rauwolfia alkaloid	
methotrexate	folic acid antagonist	363
methotrimeprazine	phenothiazine, antiserotonin	
methoxamine	alpha agonist	
methyclothiazide	thiazide diuretic	
methylcysteine	mucolytic	
methyldopa	central alpha agonist	
methylphenobarbitone	barbiturate	
methylprednisolone	glucocorticoid	380
methyprylone	sedative	
methysergide	serotonin antagonist	
metoclopramide	antidopaminergic	
metolazone	thiazide-like diuretic	
metoprolol	cardioselective beta blocker	371
metronidazole	antiprotozoal, antibacterial	
metyrapone	aldosterone inhibitor	
mexiletine	class I antiarrhythmic	356
mezlocillin	broad-spectrum penicillin	
mianserin hydrochloride	tetracyclic antidepressant	
miconazole	antifungal	
midazolam	benzodiazepine	368
minocycline	tetracycline	
minoxidil	vasodilator	
mitozantrone	DNA-reactive cytotoxic	363

2

Non-proprietary name	Use/type of drug	Other information (page)
morphine	opiate	
nabilone	cannabinoid, antiemetic	
nabumetone	NSAID	
nadolol	beta blocker	371
naftidrofuryl	cerebral activator	
nalbuphine	opiate	
nalidixic acid	antibiotic	
naloxone	narcotic antagonist	
nandrolone	anabolic steroid	
naproxen	NSAID	
natamycin	antifungal	
nefopam	analgesic	
neomycin	aminoglycoside	350
neostigmine	anticholinesterase	
netilmicin	aminoglycoside	350
nicardipine	class II Ca^{++} antagonist	376
niclosamide	antihelminthic	
nicofuranose	nicotinic acid derivative	
nicoumalone	coumarin anticoagulant	352
nifedipine	class II Ca^{++} antagonist	376
nimodipine	class II Ca^{++} antagonist	376
nimorazole	antiprotozoal	
nitrazepam	benzodiazepine	368
nitrofurantoin	nitrofuran antibiotic	
nizatidine	H_2-receptor blocker	
noradrenaline	sympathomimetic amine	
norethisterone	progestogen	
norgestrel	progestogen	
nortriptyline	tricyclic antidepressant	386
oestradiol	oestrogen	
oestriol	oestrogen	
orciprenaline	beta agonist	
orphenadrine	anticholinergic	
oxatomide	antihistamine, mast cell stabilizer	
oxazepam	benzodiazepine	368
oxpentifylline	peripheral vascular disease	
oxprenolol	beta blocker	371
oxymetholone	anabolic steroid	
oxypertine	anxiolytic	
oxytetracycline	tetracycline	
oxytocin	uterine stimulant	
pancreatin	pancreatic enzyme	
papaveretum	opiate	
paracetamol	analgesic	
pemoline	childhood hyperkinesia	
penbutolol	beta blocker	371
penicillamine	penicillin derivative, NSAID	
pentaerythritrol tetranitrate	nitrate vasodilator	
pentazocine	narcotic antagonist	
pericyazine	phenothiazine	
perphenazine	phenothiazine	
pethidine	opiate	
phenazocine	opiate	
phenelzine	monoamine oxidase inhibitor	384
phenethicillin	penicillin	

Non-proprietary name	Use/type of drug	Other information (page)
phenindamine	antihistamine	
phenindione	oral anticoagulant	352
pheniramine	antihistamine	
phenobarbitone	barbiturate	354
phenoxybenzamine	non-selective alpha blocker	
phenoxymethylpenicillin	penicillin	
phentermine	CNS stimulant, obesity	
phentolamine	alpha adrenergic blocker	
phenylbutazone	NSAID	
phenylephrine	sympathomimetic	
phenytoin	anticonvulsant	354
phytomenadione	vitamin K1 derivative	
pimozide	antipsychotic	
pindolol	beta blocker	371
pipenzolate bromide	anticholinergic	
piperacillin	broad-spectrum penicillin	
piperazine	antihelminthic	
pipothiazine palmitate	antipsychotic	
pirbuterol	selective beta$_2$ agonist	
pirenzepine	anticholinergic	
piretanide	loop diuretic	
piroxicam	NSAID	
pivampicillin	broad-spectrum penicillin	
pivmecillinam	amidino-penicillin	
pizotifen hydrogen maleate	serotonin antagonist	
poldine methylsulphate	anticholinergic	
polymyxin B	polymyxin antibiotic	350
polystyrene sulphonate	ion-exchange resin	
polythiazide	thiazide diuretic	
prazosin	selective alpha$_1$ blocker	
prednisolone	glucocorticoid	380
prednisone	glucocorticoid	380
prenylamine lactate	class V Ca^{++} antagonist	376
primidone	anticonvulsant	354
probenecid	uricosuric	
procainamide	class I antiarrhythmic	356
procaine penicillin	penicillin	
procarbazine	cytostatic agent	363
prochlorperazine	phenothiazine	
procyclidine	anticholinergic	
progesterone	progestogen	
proguanil	antimalarial	
promazine	phenothiazine	
promethazine	phenothiazine	
propantheline bromide	anticholinergic	
propranolol	beta blocker	371
protriptyline	tricyclic antidepressant	386
pyrantel embonate	antihelminthic	
pyrazinamide	antituberculous, in combination	
pyridostigmine	anticholinesterase	
pyridoxine	vitamin B6	
pyrimethamine	malarial prophylaxis	
quinalbarbitone sodium	barbiturate	
quinidine bisulphate	class I antiarrhythmic	356
ranitidine	H$_2$-receptor blocker	

2

Non-proprietary name	Use/type of drug	Other information (page)
razoxane	antineoplastic	363
reproterol	selective beta$_2$ agonist	
reserpine	rauwolfia alkaloid	
rifampicin	antituberculous	
rimiterol	selective beta$_2$ agonist	
ritodrine	beta agonist	
salbutamol	beta agonist	
salcatonin	salmon calcitonin	
salsalate	salicylate	
selegiline	monoamine oxidase B inhibitor	
sodium cromoglycate	mast cell stabiliser, non-selective beta agonist	
sodium fusidate	antibiotic	
sodium nitroprusside	vasodilator	
sodium picosulphate	bowel stimulant	
sodium valproate	anticonvulsant	354
somatrem	growth hormone	
sotalol	beta blocker	371
spectinomycin	antibiotic	
spironolactone	K$^+$-sparing diuretic	
stanozolol	anabolic steroid	
streptokinase	fibrinolytic	
sucralfate	cytoprotectant for peptic ulcer	
sulfametopyrazine	sulphonamide	
sulindac	NSAID	
sulphadimidine	sulphonamide	
sulphamethoxazole	sulphonamide	
sulphasalazine	salicylate/sulphonamide	
sulphinpyrazone	uricosuric	
sulpiride	antipsychotic	
talampicillin	broad-spectrum penicillin	
tamoxifen	antioestrogen	
temazepam	benzodiazepine	368
terazosin	selective alpha$_1$ blocker	
terbutaline	selective beta$_2$ agonist	
terfenadine	antihistamine	
terlipressin	vasopressin analogue	
terodiline	anticholinergic	
tetrabenazine	dopamine-depleting agent	368
tetracycline	antibiotic	
tetracosactrin	adrenal stimulating hormone	
theophylline	xanthine bronchodilator	
thiabendazole	antihelminthic	
thiethylperazine	phenothiazine	
thioguanine	antimetabolite	363
thioridazine	phenothiazine	368
thymoxamine	selective alpha$_1$ blocker	
l-thyroxine sodium	thyroid hormone	
tiaprofenic acid	NSAID	
ticarcillin	antipseudomonal penicillin	
timolol maleate	beta blocker	371
tinidazole	antibiotic	
tobramycin	aminoglycoside	350
tocainide	class I antiarrhythmic	356

Non-proprietary name	Use/type of drug	Other information (page)
tolazamide	sulphonylurea hypoglycaemic	355
tolbutamide	sulphonylurea hypoglycaemic	355
tolmetin	NSAID	
tranexamic acid	antifibrinolytic	
tranylcypromine sulphate	monoamine oxidase inhibitor	384
trazodone	antidepressant	
triamcinolone	glucocorticoid	380
triamterene	K^+-sparing diuretic	
triazolam	benzodiazepine	368
trifluoperazine	phenothiazine	368
trimeprazine	antihistamine	
trimetaphan	ganglion blocker	
trimethoprim	folic acid inhibitor	
trimipramine acid maleate	tricyclic antidepressant	386
tripotassium dicitratobismuthate	for peptic ulcer	
triprolidine	antihistamine	
trisodium edetate	chelating agent	
l-tryptophan	serotonin precursor	
urokinase	fibrinolytic	
ursodeoxycholic acid	bile acid	
vancomycin	glycopeptide antibiotic	350
verapamil	class I Ca^{++} antagonist	376
vidarabine	antiviral	
viloxacine	antidepressant	
vinblastine	vinca alkaloid	363
vincristine	vinca alkaloid	363
vindesine	vinca alkaloid	363
warfarin	coumarin anticoagulant	352
xipamide	thiazide-like diuretic	
zidovudine	antiviral	
zuclopenthixol	antipsychotic	

C. INFORMATION ON IMPORTANT GROUPS OF DRUGS

2

ANTIBIOTICS

For preoperative antibiotic cover as prophylaxis against endocarditis (see Section 1: Subacute bacterial endocarditis)

Potential anaesthetic problems

1. Neuromuscular effects
Muscle paralysis can be caused by four main classes of antibiotics: the aminoglycosides, the polymyxins, the tetracyclines and the lincosamides. Experimental studies seem to indicate that this results from a combination of pre- and postjunctional effects (Singh et al 1982). In addition, any antibiotic from these four groups, when given in combination with muscle relaxants, can potentially contribute to the production of a mixed type of neuromuscular block. Problems are more likely to occur in patients with pre-existing neuromuscular diseases, such as myasthenia or Duchenne muscular dystrophy (Sokoll & Gergis 1981).
2. Renal toxicity
May occur with high doses of aminoglycosides, especially in combination with frusemide, ethacrynic acid, tetracyclines or zidovudine, or with prolonged therapy.
3. Ototoxicity
Therapeutic doses of aminoglycosides should not cause problems in normal patients. However, ototoxicity may occur in renal insufficiency, with courses of long duration, in patients with pre-existing hearing problems, or when used with frusemide, ethacrynic acid, piretanide or vancomycin.
4. Infusion interactions
May occur with aminoacid, lipid or dextrose infusions, or with other antibiotics in solution.
5. Other interactions
  a. Oral antibiotics potentiate the effects of anticoagulants.
  b. Sulphonamides, isoniazid and PAS may precipitate phenytoin toxicity.
6. Hypersensitivity
Penicillin produces a high incidence of anaphylactic reactions, a proportion of which are fatal. IgE is frequently involved (Sogn 1984). Up to 8% of patients sensitive to penicillin will also react to cephalosporins.

Management

1. Neuromuscular blockade

Although the use of a combination of calcium and neostigmine to reverse a mixed block has been suggested, it is probably safer to ventilate the patient until full neuromuscular function has returned. Calcium is shortlived in its action, and may antagonize the effects of the antibiotic (Choi et al 1985).

2. Therapeutic blood levels should be monitored during courses of aminoglycosides.

a. Gentamicin: Peak serum concentration should not exceed 8 μg/ml 15 minutes after i.v. dose, or 10 μg/ml 1 hour after i.m. injection. Trough concentrations just before the next dose should be less than 2 μg/ml.

3. Combinations of aminoglycosides with other potentially nephrotoxic drugs should be avoided.

These include frusemide, ethancrynic acid, piretanide, tetracylines and vancomycin. If combinations are necessary, doses should be kept apart. Tetracyclines should not be given to patients with renal disease, especially in the elderly.

4. Antibiotic infusions

a. In general, antibiotics should not be added to aminoacid or lipid solutions.

b. Dextrose solutions may reduce the activity of penicillin and gentamicin.

c. Penicillin and tetracyclines should not be mixed.

d. Kanamycin and methicillin should not be mixed.

e. Gentamicin and carbenicillin should not be mixed.

5. It has been suggested that all intraoperative antibiotics should be given slowly, having been diluted to 50–250 ml (Levy 1986).

Requests to give them at induction of anaesthesia should be resisted. Should a reaction occur, there may be problems in identifying the drug responsible.

BIBLIOGRAPHY

Choi W W, Gergis S D, Sokoll M D 1985 Controversies in muscle relaxants. In: Muscle relaxants: basic and clinical aspects. Grune and Stratton, New York

Levy J H 1986 Antibiotics. In: Anaphylactic reactions in anesthesia and intensive care. Butterworth, Guildford

Singh Y N, Marshall I G, Harvey A L 1982 Pre- and postjunctional blocking effects of aminoglycoside, polymyxin, tetracycline and lincosamide antibiotics. British Journal of Anaesthesia 54: 1295–1306

Sogn D D 1984 Penicillin allergy. Journal of Allergy and Clinical Immunology 74: 589–593

Sokoll M D, Gergis S D 1981 Antibiotics and neuromuscular function. Anesthesiology 55: 148–159

ANTICOAGULANT THERAPY

HEPARIN

1. Mode of action
Heparin potentiates the formation of complexes between antithrombin III and activated serine proteases which are thrombin, factor XIIa, XIa, Xa and IXa.

2. Onset of action
Heparin acts immediately. A continuous i.v. infusion gives less major bleeding problems than 4 hourly boluses i.v.

3. Duration of action
Plasma half-life: 90 minutes (range 30–360 minutes).

4. Dosage regimen
s.c. heparin for prophylaxis of DVT: 5000 units preoperatively and 5000 units 8–12-hourly.
i.v. heparin for anticoagulation: loading dose of 12 500 units. 30–40 000 units/24 h by infusion, according to monitoring.

5. Method of monitoring therapy
The method of monitoring and the control depends upon the laboratory. The activated partial thromboplastin time (APTT) (or kaolin cephalin clotting time, KCCT) is commonly used. The therapeutic range is 2–2.5 times the control.

6. Reversal of heparin
Cessation of therapy is usually sufficient. If there is life-threatening haemorrhage, or during CPB where heparin has been given within the previous 15 minutes, then protamine can be used for reversal. Give protamine sulphate i.v., 1 mg/100 units heparin. Excess protamine can act as an anticoagulant.

7. Anaphylactoid reactions to protamine
Serious haemodynamic effects and type I hypersensitivity reactions have been reported with protamine. These include increased airway pressure, acute pulmonary hypertension and systemic hypotension (Colman 1987). Protamine should be given slowly. Inotropes and fluid loading may be required.

ORAL ANTICOAGULANT THERAPY

1. Mode of action
Interference with the hepatic synthesis of vitamin K dependent clotting factors.

2. Onset of action
This is delayed, because clotting factors already synthesized must be cleared from the body. The peak effect does not occur for 36–72 hours.

3. Duration of action

Half-life: Warfarin   44 hours
              Nicoumalone   24 hours
              Phenindione   5 hours

4. Method of monitoring therapy
Prothrombin time:
Citrated plasma is incubated with tissue thromboplastin. Calcium ions
are added, and the time to record a visible fibrin clot is taken.
Thromboplastin source is now animal, rather than human, and in view
of the variance of preparations, the thomboplastin must be calibrated
against an International Reference Preparation to gain an International
Sensitivity Index (Brownell et al 1986). The ISI varies from 1.1 to 2.5,
therefore results are now expressed as the International Normalized
Ratio (INR). INR = Prothrombin ratio $\times$ ISI.

5. Recommended therapeutic range (Poller 1985)
  a. INR 2.0–2.5   DVT prophylaxis, and for high-risk surgery
  b. INR 2.0–3.0   DVT treatment, TIAs, pulmonary embolism
  c. INR 3.0–4.0   Recurrent DVT and PE. Arterial grafts, cardiac grafts
  and prostheses, myocardial infarction, arterial disease

6. Reversal of vitamin K antagonists
Depends upon whether the patient is bleeding, the urgency of the
surgery, and whether the stopping of anticoagulants carries a risk in itself.
Action required may vary from the omission of one or more doses, to
partial reversal, or sometimes full reversal of anticoagulation.
  n.b. If vitamin K is given, it takes 3–12 hours to start acting and
reanticoagulation will be prevented for up to 2 weeks
  Recommendations of the British Society for Haematology:
  a. INR 4.5–7.0 without haemorrhage:
Stop warfarin for one or more days according to INR.
  b. INR >7.0 without haemorrhage:
Stop warfarin and consider phytomenadione 5–10 mg orally.
  c. INR <4.5 with haemorrhage:
Give FFP and investigate cause.
  d. INR >2.0 with life-threatening haemorrhage:
Phytomenadione 2.5–10 mg i.v. and FFP or factors II, IX and X.

7. Anaesthetic management of patients with coagulation tests outside
the normal levels.
  a. No i.m. or s.c. injections should be given.
  b. If a CVP is necessary, subclavian and internal jugular routes
should be avoided and the antecubital fossa used.
  c. Nasotracheal intubation and nasogastric tubes should be avoided.
Laryngoscopy and oral endotracheal intubation must be performed with
care.
  d. Regional anaesthesia
Remains controversial. Series of epidural and subarachnoid blocks
have been performed, without untoward effect, on patients who were
receiving or subsequently received anticoagulants. However, the

degree of anticoagulation present was not always specified. On those occasions when it was specified, the results were not always within the therapeutic range (Cunningham et al 1980, Rao & El-Etr 1981, Fuchs et al 1982, Odoom & Sih 1983). Most standard textbooks do not recommend epidural or spinal anaesthesia in the presence of systemic anticoagulation.

Problems with low-dose heparin therapy have not yet been reported, although a case in which full anticoagulation occurred has been documented (Brozovic 1974). If there is an indication for an epidural or spinal block, coagulation tests must be normal.

BIBLIOGRAPHY

Brownell A, Mackie I J, Machin S J 1986 The prothrombin time and monitoring oral anticoagulant therapy. British Journal of Hospital Medicine 36: 442–443
Brozovic M, Stirling Y, Klenerman L, Lowe L 1974 Subcutaneous heparin and postoperative thromboembolism. Lancet 1974; ii: 99–100
Colman R W 1987 Humoral mediators of catastrophic reactions associated with protamine neutralization. Anesthesiology 66: 595–596
Cunningham F O, Egan J M, Inahara T 1980 Continuous epidural anesthesia in abdominal vascular surgery. American Journal of Surgery 139: 624–627
Fuchs J C A, Fagraeus L, Lumb P D 1982 The emerging role of epidural anesthesia in arteriography and in vascular operations. Annals of Surgery 195: 781–785
Odoom J A, Sih I L 1983 Epidural analgesia and anticoagulant therapy. Experience with 1000 cases of continuous epidurals. Anaesthesia 38: 254–259
Poller L 1985 Therapeutic ranges in anticoagulant administration. British Medical Journal 290: 1683–1686
Rao T L K, El-Etr A A 1981 Anticoagulation following placement of epidural and subarachnoid catheters. Anesthesiology 55: 618–620
Stow P J, Burrows F A 1987 Anticoagulants in anaesthesia. Canadian Journal of Anaesthesia 34: 632–649

ANTICONVULSANT DRUGS

Preoperative problems associated with anticonvulsant drugs

1. Most anticonvulsants are enzyme inducers, and can interfere with the metabolism of other drugs. Folate deficiency and megaloblastic anaemia, which are sometimes seen in patients on long-term therapy with phenytoin, phenobarbitone or primidone, are probably due to enzyme induction.

2. Sodium valproate (Epilim) may interfere with haemostasis (Editorial 1984). Thrombocytopenia is the commonest defect. Its incidence is dose related and it is commoner in children than in adults. Platelet dysfunction, prolonged bleeding time and hypofibrinogenaemia have been reported. Caution is necessary if anticoagulants or antiplatelet drugs are given.

3. Pregnancy is associated with an increased risk of fits, and therapy with a twofold increase in congenital malformations. During pregnancy phenytoin, phenobarbitone and primidone may precipitate vitamin K deficiency (Dalessio 1985). Bleeding may occur at delivery, or in the neonate.

4. Phenytoin has a narrow therapeutic range. The concurrent use of sulphonamides, isoniazid, PAS or cimetidine may precipitate phenytoin toxicity, producing ataxia, nystagmus and respiratory depression.

2

Potential perioperative problems in epileptics

1. Sudden cessation of anticonvulsant therapy may precipitate severe rebound convulsions.

2. Conversely, anticonvulsant toxicity due to drug interactions has been reported in the perioperative period. A young man taking phenobarbitone and phenytoin had a delayed recovery from a 90-minute halothane anaesthetic, only to lapse into coma 12 hours later (Karlin & Kutt 1970). Blood levels of phenytoin were found to be 41 mg/l (therapeutic level 10–20 mg/l, ataxia 30 mg/l, mental changes 40 mg/l). This was attributed to temporary hepatic dysfunction.

3. Some anaesthetic agents such as ketamine, methohexitone and enflurane increase cerebral activity and produce epileptiform changes on the EEG.

Management

1. Prior to surgery or tooth extraction, haemoglobin, platelet count and coagulation screening should be performed in patients on sodium valproate. A platelet count above $100 \times 10^9/l$ is of no significance. At levels below $50 \times 10^9/l$ there is an increasing possibility of problems. Stopping the drug usually results in recovery of the platelet count within a week. Levels below $20 \times 10^9/l$ will require active treatment with platelet concentrates. Platelet dysfunction is indicated if the platelet count is normal but the bleeding time is prolonged (above 12 minutes).

2. Anticonvulsants should be continued in the perioperative period.

3. If ataxia, mental changes or delayed recovery from anaesthesia occurs, the possibility of anticonvulsant toxicity must be considered.

BIBLIOGRAPHY

Dalessio D J 1985 Current concepts: seizure disorders and pregnancy. New England Journal of Medicine 312: 559–563
Editorial 1984 Sodium valproate and haemostasis – what to do. Drugs and Therapeutics Bulletin 22: 23–24
Karlin J M, Kutt H 1970 Acute diphenylhydantoin intoxication following halothane anaesthesia. Journal of Pediatrics 76: 941–944

2

ANTIDIABETIC MEDICATION

Oral hypoglycaemics

Drug	Duration of action	Half-life
Acetohexamide	12–24	6
Chlorpropamide	24–60	33
Glibenclamide	10–15	5–8
Gliclazide	12–18	12
Glipizide	8	2–4
Gliquidone	2–4	1.5
Metformin	6	3
Tolazamide	15	7
Tolbutamide	6–12	5

Insulins

Insulin	Onset (h)	Peak (h)	Duration (h)
Human actraphane	2	2–12	20
Human actrapid	1/2	2–5	8
Human initard 50/50	1/2	4–8	20
Human insulatard	2	4–8	20
Human mixtard	1/2	4–8	20
Human monotard	1–3	7–15	22
Human protaphane	2	4–8	20
Human ultratard	3	8–24	30
Human velosulin	1/2	1–3	8
Humulin	1/2	1–3	7
Humulin lente	2.5	4–16	24
Humulin M1	1/2	1–9	18
Humulin M2	1/2	1–9	16
Humulin M3	1/2	1–8	15
Humulin M4	1/2	1–8	15
Humulin S	1/2	1–3	8
Humulin Zn	3	6–14	24
Hypurin isophane	2	4–13	20
Hypurin lente	2	6–15	28
Hypurin neutral	1/2	2–6	8
Hypurin protamine zinc	4	8–16	36
Hypurin soluble	1/2	2–6	8
Initard 50/50	1/2	4–8	20
Insulatard	2	4–12	20
Lentard MC	3	7–15	20
Mixtard 30/70	1/2	4–8	20
Rapitard MC	2	4–12	20
Semitard MC	2	5–10	16
Velosulin	1/2	1–3	8

ANTIARRHYTHMIC DRUGS

Vaughan-Williams classification of antiarrhythmics based on their electrophysiological effects:

Class I   Drugs which have a direct effect upon the membrane.

Class IA   Drugs producing membrane stabilization, with a prolonged action potential duration, in both atria and ventricles.
e.g. disopyramide, procainamide, quinidine.

Class IB   Drugs producing membrane stabilization with a shortened action potential duration, but only in the ventricles.
e.g. lignocaine, mexiletine, tocainide.

Class IC   Drugs producing membrane stabilization, with a varied action potential duration, in both atria and ventricles.
e.g. flecainide.

Class II   Anti-adrenergic drugs, including beta blockers.
e.g. propranolol, bretylium.

Class III   Drugs producing action potential prolongation and increases in the refractory period without altering the rate of depolarization.
e.g. amiodarone, bretylium, sotalol.

Class IV   Drugs which interfere with calcium transport. The term calcium channel blocker, or calcium antagonist encompasses a wide range of drugs, which are further subdivided. They include verapamil, nifedipine, nicardipine, diltiazem, lidoflazine and prenylamine. However, only verapamil and diltiazem have significant antiarrhythmic effects.

Antiarrythmics can also be classified according to the sites of predominant clinical effect:

1. AV node
Drugs which primarily act by slowing conduction at the AV node are used for supraventricular arrhythmias. These include digoxin, beta blockers, verapamil and diltiazem.

2. Ventricles
Those used mainly for ventricular arrhythmias are lignocaine, phenytoin, mexiletine and tocainide.

3. Atria and ventricles
Drugs which act on both the atria and the ventricles (and accessory pathways, such as the Bundle of Kent in WPW) can be used for either supraventricular or ventricular arrhythmias. They include quinidine, disopyramide, flecainide, amiodarone and procainamide.

AMIODARONE

1. Uses:
WPW syndrome, to prolong conduction in the accessory pathway, and as a second-line drug for atrial, junctional and ventricular arrhythmias. It has no negative inotropic effects and is therefore useful when left ventricular dysfunction is present.

2. Route:

Oral/i.v.

3. Half-life:

7–40 days

4. Side-effects:

Skin photosensitivity, neurological and thyroid disorders, corneal deposits and prolongation of the Q–T interval.

5. Interactions:

Digoxin, warfarin, diltiazem and verapamil.

6. Contraindications:

Bradycardia and AV block.

DILTIAZEM

1. Uses:

SVT, angina and hypertension. Produces less arterial vasodilatation than verapamil.

2. Route:

Oral.

3. Half-life:

4–6 hours.

4. Side-effects:

Slowing of conduction through the AV node, bradycardia and hypotension.

5. Interactions:

With digoxin. Reduces digoxin elimination and potentiates the effects of lithium.

6. Contraindications:

Bradycardia, sick sinus syndrome, AV block

DIGOXIN

1. Uses:

Supraventricular arrhythmias such as atrial fibrillation and atrial flutter. It blocks the AV node and thus controls ventricular rate.

2. Route:

Oral/i.v.

3. Half-life:

33–38 hours.

4. Side-effects:

Arrhythmias, AV block. (See Digoxin toxicity.)

5. Interactions:

Quinine, quinidine, verapamil and amiodarone.

6. Contraindications:

SVT caused by WPW syndrome

DISOPYRAMIDE

1. Uses:
Supraventricular and ventricular arrhythmias, but has negative inotropic effects.
2. Route:
Oral/i.v.
3. Half-life:
5–10 hours.
4. Side-effects:
Anticholinergic effects, hypotension, heart failure, torsade de pointes ventricular tachycardia, AV block.
5. Interactions:
Amiodarone, anticholinergics, beta blockers and other Class I antiarrhythmics.
6. Contraindications:
Second- and third-degree AV block, sinus node dysfunction, severe heart failure and glaucoma.

FLECAINIDE

1. Uses:
Ventricular arrhythmias and pre-excitation syndromes.
Causes widespread prolongation of conduction time.
Possesses negative inotropic effects.
2. Route:
Oral/i.v.
3. Half-life:
16 hours.
4. Side-effects:
Prolongation of Q–T interval. Occasionally may cause serious arrhythmias. Possesses negative inotropic effects. Can increase the endocardial pacing threshold in patients with pacemakers. May cause dizziness and visual disturbances.
5. Interactions:
Amiodarone, other Class I antiarrhythmics.
6. Contraindications: AV block, sinoatrial disease and heart failure.

LIGNOCAINE

1. Uses:
As a first- line drug in the short term treatment of ventricular arrhythmias.
2. Route:
i.v.
3. Half-life:

1–3 hours.
4. Side-effects:
Central nervous system toxicity.
Lightheadedness, circumoral tingling, numbness of the tongue, anxiety, twitching, convulsions and apnoea (see also Section 4 Local anaesthetic toxicity).
5. Interactions:
Beta blockers
6. Contraindications:
Sinoatrial disorders, AV block and severe myocardial depression.

MEXILETINE

1. Uses:
Treatment of ventricular arrhythmias due to ischaemia, or those induced by digitalis.
2. Route:
Oral/i.v.
3. Half-life:
9 hours.
4. Side-effects:
Bradycardia, hypotension, nausea and vomiting.
5. Interactions:
Should not be administered concurrently with i.v. lignocaine.
6. Contraindications:
Bradycardia and heart block are relative contraindications.

PROCAINAMIDE

1. Uses:
Ventricular and supraventricular arrhythmias and ventricular arrhythmias due to digitalis. Is little used for long-term oral administration because of side-effects.
2. Route:
Oral/i.v.
3. Half-life:
3–5 hours.
4. Side-effects:
Lupus erythematosus-like syndrome, heart failure, gastrointestinal symptoms and agranulocytosis.
5. Interactions:
Amiodarone.
6. Contraindications:
Hypotension, heart block and heart failure.

QUINIDINE

1. Uses:
Supraventricular and ventricular arrhythmias.
2. Route:
Oral. (i.v. is dangerous.)
3. Half-life:
6–7 hours.
4. Side-effects:
Torsade de pointes ventricular tachycardia. Can increase the ventricular rate in atrial flutter and atrial fibrillation. Prolongation of QT and QRS complex lengthening.
5. Interactions:
With digoxin. May potentiate muscle relaxants. Antagonizes anticholinesterases.
6. Contraindications:
Heart block and quinidine idiosyncrasy.

TOCAINIDE

1. Uses:
Ventricular arrhythmias. Similar to lignocaine.
2. Route:
Oral/i.v.
3. Half-life:
10–15 hours.
4. Side-effects:
CNS and gastrointestinal effects, an SLE-like syndrome and bone marrow depression
5. Interactions:
Drugs causing hypokalaemia.
6. Contraindications:
Sinoatrial disorders, AV block and severe myocardial depression.

VERAPAMIL

1. Uses:
Supraventricular arrhythmias, angina, hypertension. Will terminate arrhythmias in which the AV node is involved, or slow the ventricular response rate to impulses originating from the atria.
2. Route:
Oral/i.v.
3. Half-life:
5–10 hours.
4. Side-effects:

2

Gastrointestinal symptoms, bradycardia, AV block, negative inotropic effects and asystole.

5. Interactions:

With beta blockers, to produce bradycardias or asystole. Do not give verapamil i.v. to patients taking beta blockers. Verapamil may worsen AF in WPW syndrome.

6. Contraindicatons:

Bradycardia, sick sinus syndrome, AV block, and atrial fibrillation complicating WPW syndrome.

ANTIHYPERTENSIVE THERAPY

1. Diuretics

The thiazide type are used either alone or in combination with other hypotensive therapy for mild hypertension. As well as having a diuretic action, they reduce peripheral vascular resistance. The main anaesthetic problems are the hypokalaemia or hyponatraemia of long-term use.

Potassium-retaining diuretics include amiloride, triamterene and spironolactone. However, these are only weak hypotensive agents. Hyperkalaemia may occur if these are given with potassium supplements, captopril or NSAIDs.

Loop diuretics such as frusemide, bumetanide, ethacrynic acid and piretanide may be used to promote diuresis with ACE inhibitors, in malignant hypertension or in hypertension associated with chronic renal failure. Again hypokalaemia and hyponatraemia may occur.

2. Beta adrenergic blockers

Reduce blood pressure in a number of ways. Noradrenaline release from sympathetic nerve endings is reduced, cardiac rate and contractility is decreased, and renin secretion inhibited. Side-effects include hypotension, bradycardia, bronchospasm, cardiac failure and a syndrome of sudden withdrawal. (See Beta blockers.)

3. Calcium channel blockers

Act by reducing tone in vascular smooth muscle, hence decreasing peripheral resistance. Verapamil, nicardipine and nifedipine can be used for hypertension. (See Calcium antagonists.)

4. Angiotensin-converting enzyme (ACE) inhibitors

Inhibit the conversion of angiotensin I to angiotensin II. Angiotensin II is a potent vasoconstrictor, and inhibition of its formation results in vasodilatation. Hyperkalaemia may occur when ACE inhibitors are used with indomethacin, cyclosporin, potassium supplements and potassium-sparing diuretics.

5. Alpha adrenergic blockers

Prazosin:

A postsynaptic, alpha$_1$, adrenergic receptor blocker causing venous and arterial vasodilatation.

Terazosin:
A postsynaptic, alpha$_1$, adrenergic receptor blocker.
Indoramin:
An alpha$_1$ receptor blocker with Class I antiarrhythmic properties but a high incidence of side-effects which include first dose hypotension and fluid retention.
Labetalol:
Although marketed as a combined alpha$_1$ and beta blocker, the beta effects predominate, being from three to seven times more potent than the alpha effects.

6. Centrally acting
Clonidine:
Severe rebound hypertension can occur on withdrawal.
Methyldopa:
Side-effects include haemolytic anaemia and jaundice.

7. Peripheral vasodilators
Rarely used as oral therapy. They are potent drugs with a high incidence of side-effects. Diazoxide and hydralazine may be used i.v. for hypertensive crises. Minoxidil is reserved for resistant hypertension.
Minoxidil:
Causes tachycardia and fluid retention. A diuretic and beta blocker will therefore also be required. The growth of body hair is stimulated. (See Section 3: Vasodilators.)
Hydralazine:
Causes tachycardia, fluid retention, and may produce an SLE-like syndrome with prolonged therapy. (See Section 3: Vasodilators.)
Diazoxide:
Produces tachycardia, hyperglycaemia, hyperuricaemia and reduction in glomerular filtration. (See Section 3: Vasodilators.)

8. Adrenergic neurone blockers
Prevent the release of noradrenaline from postganglionic adrenergic neurones. They include bethanidine, debrisoquine and guanethidine. Guanethidine also depletes the nerve endings of noradrenaline. Blood pressure control is inadequate and they are now infrequently used, except in combination with other drugs.

ANTIMITOTIC THERAPY

Classification of anticancer drugs:

1. Alkylating agents
Cause alkylation of nucleic acids: e.g. busulphan, carmustine, chlorambucil, cyclophosphamide, estramustine, ethoglucid, ifosfamide, lomustine, melphalan, mitobronitol, mustine hydrochloride, thiotepa, treosulfan.

2. Antimetabolites

Antagonists of normal cell metabolites. Bind with enzymes and prevent normal cell division: e.g. cytarabine, 5-fluorouracil, mercaptopurine, methotrexate, thioguanine.

3. Cytotoxic antibiotics

Form complexes with DNA and inhibit nucleic acid synthesis: e.g. actinomycin D, bleomycin, doxorubicin hydrochloride (Adriamycin), epirubicin hydrochloride, mitomycin, plicamycin (Mithramycin).

4. Plant alkaloids

Bind with cellular proteins:

e.g. etoposide, vinblastine sulphate, vincristine sulphate, vindesine sulphate.

5. Miscellaneous agents

e.g. amasacrine, carboplatin, cisplatin, dacarbazine, hydroxyurea, mitozantrone, procarbazine, razoxane.

6. Immunotherapy

e.g. azathioprine, corticosteroids, *Corynebacterium parvum* vaccine, cyclosporin.

7. Hormone antagonists

e.g. aminoglutethimide, buserelin, cyproterone acetate, goserelin, tamoxifen.

8. Sex hormones
  a. Oestrogens
  e.g. ethinyloestradiol, fosfestrol tetrasodium, polyestradiol phosphate, stilboestrol.
  b. Progestogens
  e.g. gestronol, medroxyprogesterone acetate, megestrol acetate, norethisterone, norethisterone acetate.
  c. Androgens and anabolic steroids
  e.g. drostanolone, nandrolone.

Potential anaesthetic problems

a. Toxic effects of the drugs themselves may produce clinically significant organ damage (Chung 1982). These toxic effects may be difficult to differentiate from the effects of the original cancer or its metastases.

b. Potential interactions between the antimitotic drug and anaesthetic agents.

Organs potentially involved

1. Heart

Doxorubicin (Adriamycin), daunorubicin, cisplatin and cyclophosphamide have been associated with cardiac toxicity. Doxorubicin may cause two types of cardiac problem:

a. A dose-related cardiomyopathy which, if it occurs, has a high mortality. Doses above 600 mg/m^2 have been associated with a 30% incidence of chronic cardiotoxicity. Although some deaths have occurred in patients on doxorubicin following surgery, only one has been reported intraoperatively. Ventricular fibrillation occurred during deep halothane anaesthesia for central venous catheter insertion in a child on doxorubicin (McQuillan et al 1988). Although there was evidence of a cardiomyopathy and pulmonary oedema at post-mortem, the child was in a poor state initially, with a serum sodium of 114 mmol/l and a serum potassium of 2.7 mmol/l.

b. Non-specific arrhythmias or ECG changes, which usually cease when treatment stops, occur in 10–25% of patients on doxorubicin (Selvin 1981). It is not dose related.

2. Liver

Hepatic damage can occur with thioguanine, 6-mercaptopurine, streptozocin, plicamycin, cyclophosphamide, daunorubicin, doxorubicin, methotrexate, dacarbazine and chlorambucil.

3. Kidney

Renal damage can be caused by high doses of busulphan, cisplatin, methotrexate, 6-mercaptopurine, plicamycin, carboplatin and streptozocin. Cisplatin, mitomycin and plicamycin may also cause problems at ordinary dosages.

4. Lungs

Bleomycin causes some degree of pulmonary impairment in 5–10% of patients. The effect is dose related, and is more common in the elderly and in those receiving radiation therapy. The role of perioperative oxygen therapy has also been implicated, but this is controversial. Pulmonary damage may also be a rare complication of treatment with busulphan, clorambucil, cyclophosphamide, doxorubicin, melphalan, thiotepa, cytarabine, methotrexate, carmustine and plicamycin.

5. Nervous system

Cisplatin, dacarbazine, procarbazine, vinblastine and vincristine can all cause a peripheral neuropathy or other CNS effects.

6. Bone marrow

Bone marrow suppression occurs to a greater or lesser extent with most agents. Problems include anaemia, leucopenia, thrombocytopenia and sometimes haemolytic anaemia. Marked depression may be produced by busulphan, thiotepa, methotrexate, 5-fluorouracil, cytarabine, vinblastine, plicamycin, mitomycin, lomustine, hydroxyurea and procarbazine.

7. Coagulation problems

Hypercoagulability, and occasionally DIC, can both occur with carcinomas.

8. Inappropriate ADH secretion

Can be caused by cyclophosphamide, vinblastine and vincristine, but may also be a secondary effect of the tumour.

Potential interactions with anaesthetic agents

1. The suggestion that there is a link between bleomycin and oxygen toxicity is both controversial and complicated. Fatal postoperative respiratory complications were reported in five patients who had received bleomycin 6–12 months prior to surgery (Goldiner et al 1978). It was postulated that bleomycin had sensitized the lungs to oxygen toxicity. This theory was apparently supported in reports of a further 14 patients in whom the perioperative inspired oxygen concentrations were kept between 20% and 25% and in whom there was no mortality (Goldiner & Schweizer 1979, Allen et al 1980). In another report, surgery for oesophageal carcinoma following bleomycin and radiotherapy was associated with interstitial pneumonitis, postoperative respiratory failure and a 50% mortality, whereas 10 patients given the same treatment without surgery had no pulmonary complications. However, a further 16 who had no surgery, but who were given higher doses of bleomycin and radiotherapy, also had lung infiltration and a 25% mortality (Nygaard et al 1979). Others have failed to find an association between bleomycin, oxygen toxicity and pulmonary complications (Douglas & Coppin 1980, Klein & Wilds 1984, LaMantia et al 1984).
2. Reduction in plasma cholinesterase activity may prolong the effects of suxamethonium. This has been reported with some of the alkylating agents, including cyclophosphamide and thiotepa.
3. Procarbazine is a mild monoamine oxidase inhibitor. In theory, there may be interaction with sympathomimetics and pethidine.
4. The hepatic metabolism of anaesthetic drugs may be decreased.
5. Prolongation of action of non-depolarizing agents has occurred with the use of some alkylating agents (Bennett et al 1977).

Management

1. A detailed history and examination is required.
2. Investigations should be undertaken to identify hepatic, renal and cardiac toxicity, and evidence of any bone marrow suppression.
3. If renal damage is present, adequate fluid intake should be maintained. Other potentially nephrotoxic drugs should be avoided, and those drugs dependent on renal excretion should be given in reduced doses.
4. All drugs dependent on hepatic metabolism should be used with caution in the presence of suspected hepatic damage.
5. Cardiac damage. Signs of pericardial effusion should be sought. Arrhythmias or heart failure should be treated.
6. Pulmonary toxicity. The relative roles of oxygen therapy and radiotherapy in the aetiology of bleomycin-induced lung damage is still not resolved. However, while doubt exists, it would seem prudent to limit perioperative oxygen therapy to that essential for the maintenance of safe oxygenation. This requires the monitoring and documentation of

oxygenation. The use of colloid rather than crystalloid infusions may reduce the risk of lung problems.

7. Regional anaesthesia may be appropriate in certain circumstances. However, it should be avoided if there is a peripheral neuropathy.

BIBLIOGRAPHY

Allen S C, Riddell G S, Butchart E G 1981 Bleomycin therapy and anaesthesia. Anaesthesia 36: 60–63
Bennett E J, Schmidt G B, Patel K P, Grundy E M 1977 Muscle relaxants, myasthenia and mustards. Anesthesiology 46: 220–221
Chung F 1982 Cancer, chemotherapy and anaesthesia. Canadian Anaesthetists' Society Journal 29:364–371
Douglas M J, Coppin C M L 1980 Bleomycin and subsequent anaesthesia: A retrospective study at Vancouver General Hospital. Canadian Anaesthetists' Society Journal 27: 449–452
Goldiner P L, Carlon G C, Cvitkovic E, Schweizer O, Howland W S 1978 Factors influencing postoperative morbidity and mortality in patients treated with bleomycin. British Medical Journal 1: 1664–1667
Goldiner P L, Schweizer O 1979 The hazards of anesthesia and surgery in bleomycin-treated patients. Seminars in Oncology 6: 121–124
Klein D S, Wilds P R 1983 Pulmonary toxicity of antineoplastic agents: anaesthetic and postoperative implications. Canadian Anaesthetists' Society Journal 30: 399–405
Lamantia K R, Glick J H, Marshall B E 1984 Supplemental oxygen does not cause respiratory failure in bleomycin-treated surgical patients. Anesthesiology 60: 65–67
McQuillan P J, Morgan B A, Ramwell J 1988 Adriamycin cardiomyopathy. Anaesthesia 43: 301–304
Nygaard K, Smith-Erichsen N, Hatlevoll R, Refsum S B 1978 Pulmonary complications after bleomycin, irradiation and surgery for oesophageal cancer. Cancer 41: 17–22
Selvin B L 1981 Cancer chemotherapy: implications for the anesthesiologist. Anesthesia and Analgesia 60: 425–434

ANTIPARKINSONIAN DRUGS

Potential problems of therapy with levodopa

1. Levodopa is a dopamine precursor which crosses the blood–brain barrier, whereas dopamine itself does not. In Parkinsonism, CNS dopamine is deficient, and levodopa is taken up by dopaminergic neurones in the brain. Levodopa, given alone, may cause arrhythmias when administered in high doses because it is rapidly metabolized in the circulation to dopamine. Therefore, if levodopa is being used alone, it should be stopped 12–24 hours prior to surgery.

2. If, however, levodopa is combined with small doses of carbidopa, a dopa decarboxylase inhibitor, selective dopa decarboxylase inhibition will occur in the sympathetic nerves, but not in the brain. This allows lower doses of levodopa to be used, with a consequent lower incidence of peripheral side-effects due to levodopa.

3. Levodopa can interact with direct-acting sympathetic amines to produce hypertension.

4. There is also interaction with phenothiazines and butyrophenones to cause a deterioration in Parkinson's disease.

5. If levodopa is stopped completely in the postoperative period, the patient becomes rigid and immobile. Such a state predisposes him to venous thrombosis and respiratory restriction. Medication, if necessary by nasogastric tube, should be restarted as soon as possible after surgery.

ANTIPSYCHOTIC AGENTS

1. Neuroleptic malignant syndrome (NMS, see also Section 1.)
A rare but serious complication of drug therapy with certain antipsychotic and neuroleptic drugs. The aetiology of the condition is unknown, but appears to be related to the antidopaminergic activity of the precipitating drug. Clinical features include muscle rigidity, hyperthermia, akinesia, tremor, sympathetic overactivity and stupor. Rhabdomyolysis and a raised CPK usually occur.

Although some authors support the concept that NMS is related to anaesthetic-induced malignant hyperpyrexia (Caroff et al 1983, 1987), others suggest that, despite the clinical similarities, MH and NMS are two distinct and unrelated entities (Krivosic-Horber et al 1987).

Drugs most frequently reported to cause NMS are haloperidol and fluphenazine. Others are chlorpromazine, trifluoperazine, droperidol, thioridazine, and thiapride.

2. Syndrome of withdrawal of antipsychotic drugs
Although uncommon, this syndrome may occur within a few days of abrupt cessation of medication. Dyskinesias, or rarely, a syndrome of acute cholinergic overactivity, may result.

BIBLIOGRAPHY

Caroff S, Rosenberg H, Gerber J C 1983 Neuroleptic malignant syndrome and malignant hyperpyrexia. Lancet i: 244
Caroff S, Rosenberg H, Fletcher J E, Heiman-Patterson T D, Mann S C 1987 Malignant hyperthermia susceptibility in neuroleptic malignant syndrome. Anesthesiology 67: 20–25
Krivosic-Horber R, Adnet P, Guevart E, Theunynk D, Lestavel P 1987 Neuroleptic malignant syndrome and malignant hyperthermia. British Journal of Anaesthesia 59: 1554–1556

BENZODIAZEPINES AND BENZODIAZEPINE ANTAGONISTS

The benzodiazepines are a group of drugs used for their sedative, anxiolytic, hypnotic, anticonvulsant and amnesic properties. Specific benzodiazepine receptors were discovered in 1977. They are found throughout the CNS, spinal cord and other tissues. At present their function outside neuronal tissue is not known. The receptors are located in a complex with GABA receptors, arranged around a chloride channel. GABA is a major inhibitory neurotransmitter and the benzodiazepines

2

are thought to facilitate GABA-nergic synaptic neurotransmission. They appear to reduce affinity of recognition sites for GABA. The release of GABA enhances morphine analgesia.

Many of the benzodiazepines in clinical use are metabolized into biologically active metabolites, giving them a prolonged action and a tendency to accumulate.

1. Benzodiazepines in clinical use

Name	Half-life (h)	Duration of action	Metabolites	Half-life (h)
Alprazolam	12–15	long	yes	12–15
Bromazepam	10–20	intermediate	yes	10–20
Chlordiazepoxide	4–6	long	yes	≤ 65
Clobazam	9–30	long	yes	≤ 46
Clorazepate K	2	long	yes	≤ 65
Diazepam	20–70	long	yes	≤ 65
Flunitrazepam	9–13	long	yes	≤ 30
Flurazepam	1–2	long	yes	≤ 75
Ketazolam	2	long	yes	≤ 70
Loprazolam	3–15	intermediate	no	
Lorazepam	10–15	intermediate	no	
Lormetazepam	<10	intermediate	yes	≤ 10
Medazepam	2	long	yes	≤ 65
Midazolam	1–2.5	short	no	
Nitrazepam	18–31	long	no	
Oxazepam	8	intermediate	no	
Temazepam	4–8	intermediate	no	
Triazolam	4–4.5	short	no	

2. Interactions
The actions of benzodiazepines are potentiated by many drugs, including alcohol, antidepressants, antihistamines, cimetidine, opiates and phenothiazines.
3. Addiction potential
Tolerance to the effects of benzodiazepines occurs after as little as 3–15 days' therapy, and dependence after only a few weeks (Murphy et al 1984). Withdrawal may be difficult and the withdrawal syndrome, with symptoms of sympathetic overactivity and insomnia, may last for up to 10 days.
4. Benzodiazepine antagonists
Flumazenil is a competitive inhibitor of the specific binding of benzodiazepines at the receptor level. Although some studies have suggested that it may have partial agonist activity, in man this appears to be insignificant in clinical dosages (Brogden & Goa 1988). Its onset of action is 2–3 minutes, with an elimination half-life of about 50 minutes. It is therefore relatively short acting, and of much shorter duration of action than most of the benzodiazepines. Concern has been expressed that this point may be overlooked, and that problems arising from the

inappropriate or indiscriminate use of the antagonist, may be blamed on the drug itself (Editorial 1988).

This brevity of action may be of particular significance if it is to be used for outpatient cases, or for the treatment of benzodiazepine toxicity. Thus, its exact place in clinical practice has yet to be established.

5. Suggested uses for benzodiazepine antagonists

a. Benzodiazepine intoxication

When used in 31 patients with benzodiazepine intoxication, after an initial improvement, some central depression returned 1 hour after administration (Knudsen et al 1988). In cases of self-poisoning involving multiple drugs, an i.v. dose of flumazenil may enable the benzodiazepine component to be transiently unmasked.

b. Intensive care

The ability to reverse benzodiazepine sedation, for the assessment of ventilated patients in intensive care, may prove to be a useful facility (Bodenham et al 1988).

c. Recovery after minor procedures

Acceleration of recovery after minor surgery under midazolam, fentanyl and nitrous oxide anaesthesia (Wolff et al 1986), and gastroscopy using diazepam (Kirkegaard et al 1986), has been reported. For outpatient use, its short duration of action may be disastrous.

d. Benzodiazepine withdrawal

It was originally suggested that the use of an antagonist in patients on chronic benzodiazepine therapy might precipitate a withdrawal syndrome. Although information is still sparse, these fears are thought to be unfounded (Whitwam 1987). Indeed, there is evidence that flumazenil may prove to be useful in benzodiazepine withdrawal (Nutt & Costello 1987). Not only does it appear that flumazenil can reverse dependence, but the effect may persist long after the drug has been cleared from the body. Flumazenil may precipitate fits in epileptics on long-term benzodiazepines.

BIBLIOGRAPHY

Bodenham A, Brownlie G, Dixon J S, Park G R 1988 Reversal of sedation by prolonged infusion of flumazenil. Anaesthesia 43: 376–378

Brogden R N, Goa K L 1988 Flumazenil: a preliminary review of its benzodiazepine antagonist properties, intrinsic activity and therapeutic use. Drugs 35: 448–467

Editorial 1988 Midazolam – is antagonism justified? Lancet ii: 140–142

Kirkegaard L, Knudsen L, Jensen S, Kruse A 1986 Benzodiazepine antagonist Ro 15–1788. Anaesthesia 41: 1184–1188

Knudsen L, Lonka L, Sorensen B H, Kirkegaard L, Jensen O V, Jensen S 1988 Benzodiazepine intoxication treated with flumazenil. Anaesthesia 43: 274–276

Murphy S M, Owen R T, Tyrer P J 1984 Withdrawal symptoms after six weeks' treatment with diazepam. Lancet ii: 1389

Nutt D, Costello M 1987 Flumazenil and benzodiazepine withdrawal. Lancet ii: 463

Whitwam J G 1987 Benzodiazepines. Anaesthesia 42: 1255–1257

Wolff J, Carl P, Clausen T G, Mikkelsen B O 1986 Ro 15–1788 for postoperative recovery. Anaesthesia 41: 1001–1006

BETA ADRENERGIC BLOCKERS

Beta adrenergic receptor sites are widely distributed throughout the body and can be divided into $beta_1$ and $beta_2$ types. Beta adrenoreceptor antagonists compete for receptor sites and displace the agonists. The presence of large amounts of the agonist may overcome the antagonism. Long-term administration of beta blockers may increase the receptor population.

1. Clinically important properties of beta blockers
   a. Some drugs have more $beta_1$ than $beta_2$ effects, and are relatively cardioselective, with a lesser risk of producing bronchoconstriction, e.g. atenolol, metoprolol, acebutolol, practolol and bisoprolol. However, bronchospasm can be precipitated by any beta blocker.
   b. Some are partial agonists and have intrinsic sympathomimetic activity, e.g. acebutolol, practolol, oxprenolol and pindolol. This group produces less bradycardia and cardiac depression, but the drugs are also less effective as antihypertensive agents.
   c. Absorption depends upon the lipophilic or hydrophilic properties of the particular drug. Metoprolol, pindolol, propranolol and timolol are lipophilic and thus more completely absorbed from the gastrointestinal tract. Liver disease may prolong the effects of some of these lipophilic drugs. Atenolol and nadolol are more hydrophilic and therefore less well absorbed after oral administration.
   d. Atenolol, nadolol, pindolol and sotalol are predominantly excreted by the kidney. Their elimination half-lives are increased in patients with renal insufficiency.
   e. Although beta blockers are often classified in terms of their membrane-stabilizing activity, this is not clinically relevant, as it only occurs only when they are given in large doses.
   f. Some drugs have active metabolites which may contribute to their action, e.g. atenolol, propranolol and metoprolol.
2. Effects of stimulation at different adrenergic receptor subtypes
   a. Beta$_1$ receptor
   Stimulation increases myocardial contractility, cardiac conduction, excitability and automaticity, and produces coronary artery vasodilatation, renin release and relaxation of intestinal muscle.
   b. Beta$_2$ receptor
   Stimulation results in peripheral vasodilatation, bronchodilatation, glycogenolysis, uterine relaxation (of the pregnant uterus), insulin secretion, prejunctional release of noradrenaline, and tremor. Beta$_2$ receptors are also present in the heart.
   c. Alpha$_1$ receptor
   Stimulation produces vasoconstriction, platelet aggregation, bronchoconstriction, pupillary dilatation and insulin suppression.

2

d. Alpha$_2$ receptor

Stimulation produces presynaptic inhibition of adrenergic nerve transmission. However, recent work indicates that the distinction between the alpha receptor types is more complex than was previously thought (Langer & Hicks 1984).

3. Uses of beta adrenergic receptor blockers

Treatment of hypertension, angina, arrhythmias, obstructive cardiomyopathies, thyrotoxicosis, and suppression of the beta effects of phaeochromocytoma.

4. Commonly used beta blockers

	Half life (h)	Receptor block	Oral dose range	i.v. dose range
Acebutolol	3–4	beta$_1$	400 mg b.d.	
Atenolol	6–8	beta$_1$	50–100 mg	2.5–10 mg
Betaxolol	16–20	beta$_1$	20–40 mg	
Bisoprolol	10–11	beta$_1$	10–20 mg	
Labetalol*	3–4	beta$_1$, beta$_2$	50–200 mg b.d.	50–200 mg slowly
Metoprolol	3–4	beta$_1$	100–400 mg	1–5 mg
Nadolol	12–24	beta$_1$, beta$_2$	80–240 mg	
Oxprenolol	1.3–2.0	beta$_1$, beta$_2$	80–160 mg b.d.	
Penbutolol		beta$_1$, beta$_2$	40 mg i.d. or b.d.	
Pindolol	2–5	beta$_1$, beta$_2$	10–45 mg	
Practolol	5–10	beta$_1$	—	5–10 mg slowly
Propranolol	4–6	beta$_1$, beta$_2$	40–240 mg b.d.	1–10 mg
Sotalol	5–13	beta$_1$, beta$_2$	80–300 mg b.d.	20–60 mg slowly
Timolol	4–5	beta$_1$, beta$_2$	5–30 mg b.d.	

* Some weak alpha-blocking activity.

5. Advantages of beta blockade during anaesthesia

a. Chronic beta blocker therapy decreases heart rate and cardiac output, reduces myocardial oxygen consumption and decreases both the inotropic and chronotropic effects of sympathomimetic agents.

b. The use of i.v. beta blockers during surgery is particularly beneficial under certain circumstances. They may reduce arrhythmias due to catecholamine release, precipitated by procedures such as intubation, dentistry, phaeochromocytoma surgery and thyroidectomy. Tachycardia produced by induced hypotension, or arrhythmias resulting from the surgical infiltration of adrenaline, may be decreased. There is some attenuation of the hypertensive response to intubation. Propranolol is used in the treatment of hypertrophic cardiomyopathies, and it has been reported to relieve infundibular spasm during cardiac catheterization in the tetralogy of Fallot (Kam 1978).

6. Potential problems during anaesthesia

a. Airway obstruction

Beta$_2$ receptor blockade is undesirable if there is a history of asthma or obstructive airways disease. However, all beta blockers can aggravate airway obstruction, although the relatively cardioselective ones cause less problems than the non-selective ones. If large enough doses of

2

beta$_1$ blockers are given, beta$_2$ receptors will be blocked as well.

b. Myocardial function

Myocardial depression with halothane and enflurane is dose dependent. In clinical use, the addition of beta blockers does not seem to significantly increase this. Using propranolol, only small additional reductions in cardiac output occur with halothane and enflurane. This effect is less with the partial agonists, oxprenolol and practolol, than with propranolol. Experimentally, high doses of enflurane with propranolol produce significant myocardial depression (Horan et al 1977b). However, myocardial function was not significantly impaired when oxprenolol, a partial agonist, was used with enflurane (Cutfield et al 1981). No adverse interactions have occurred with isoflurane.

c. Haemodynamic responses

i. Hypovolaemia

Fears that patients would respond poorly to blood loss during anaesthesia seem, in general, to be unfounded. In dogs given propranolol, blood loss was tolerated well in the presence of halothane and isoflurane. However, in the presence of enflurane, the combination of propranolol and hypovolaemia were associated with significant depression of cardiac output (Horan et al 1977 a, b).

ii. Assessment of blood loss

Pulse rate will be an unreliable monitor of hypovolaemia. During beta blockade, assessment of blood loss can only be made on decreases in blood pressure, CVP or cardiac output.

iii. Hypoxia

The haemodynamic responses to hypoxia are not impaired by beta blockers.

iv. Atropine

Unless there is complete blockade, atropine will increase the pulse rate. In the presence of high doses of beta blockers (propranolol 1–2.4 g/day), the response to atropine is impaired. Care must be taken with the use of neostigmine (Prys-Roberts 1980, Seidl & Martin 1984).

d. Diabetes

Beta blockers lengthen the recovery time from hypoglycaemia, and mask the normal sympathetic nervous system-mediated signs and responses.

e. Cardiac failure is occasionally precipitated by beta blockers.

f. Calcium antagonists

Undesirable drugs interactions can occur with calcium antagonists, and in particular with verapamil. During anaesthesia, left ventricular dysfunction, hypotension, heart block and death have been reported (Hartwell & Mark 1986). Problems are most likely to occur when more than one calcium antagonist is being used, or if i.v. verapamil is given to patients on long-term beta blockers. Bradycardia and cardiac arrest have been reported in a patient on timolol eye-drops having verapamil

(Pringle & MacEwen 1987). Prolonged bradycardia has occurred after neostigmine in a patient on nadolol (Seidl & Martin 1984).

g. Thyroid surgery

In the preoperative preparation of patients with thyrotoxicosis, beta antagonists only block the peripheral effects of thyroid hormone, and postoperative thyroid crisis has been reported (Eriksson et al 1977). If a thyroid crisis should occur, its clinical signs can be masked by beta blockers (Jones & Solomon 1981).

h. Anaphylactoid reactions

Experimentally, beta blockers interfere with the anti-anaphylactic effects of catecholamines. If an anaphylactoid reaction occurs in a patient treated with beta blockers, hypotension does not respond readily to adrenaline, and high doses of isoprenaline and i.v. fluids may be needed to restore the blood pressure (Laxenaire et al 1985).

i. The individual effects of beta blockers at different receptors sites may be unequal. Certain beta blockers can vary in their ability to reduce the response to catecholamines, depending on whether the latter are from endogenous or exogenous sources. Apparently adequate control of tachycardia on exercise can be produced by both propranolol and metoprolol. However propranolol is a more powerful inhibitor of the responses to exogenous adrenaline, such as that used in surgical infiltration.

7. Should beta blockers be withdrawn prior to surgery?

a. General anaesthesia

Sudden cessation of beta blockers can produce ventricular arrhythmias, angina, myocardial infarction or even death (Miller et al 1975). Withdrawal of beta blockade prior to aortocoronary bypass was found to be hazardous in terms of increased ischaemic episodes and new ventricular arrhythmias (Slogoff et al 1978). In addition, hypersensitivity to adrenergic stimulation has been shown to occur 24–48 hours after propranolol withdrawal in normal subjects (Boudoulas et al 1977). Even gradual withdrawal before surgery was found to be associated with a high incidence of myocardial ischaemia and arrhythmias (Ponten et al 1982a). The time taken for regression of beta blockade after cessation of propranolol therapy was found to be dose dependent (Prys-Roberts 1984). With doses of less than 240 mg/day there was no residual blockade at 24 hours, whereas with doses in excess of 2 g, regression could take more than 48 hours.

b. Spinal anaesthesia

Withdrawal of beta blockers prior to prostatectomy under spinal anaesthesia was associated with similar complications (Ponten et al 1982b). No such problems were encountered when therapy was continued.

8. Parenteral administration of beta blockers in the perioperative period

a. Ideally, the patient's normal dose should be continued, as soon as oral fluids can be taken.

b. If this is not possible, then an intravenous infusion should be used. A variety of suggestions have been made for likely dosage requirements. Propranolol 3 mg/h (Smuylan et al 1982), a bolus of 0.2 mg/kg followed by a continuous infusion of 1 mg/kg/24 h (Villers et al 1984) and 1 mg/h (Prys-Roberts 1980) have all been advocated. With labetalol, adequate beta blockade without hypotension has been reported using 5–10 mg/h (Prys-Roberts 1980).

Management

1. In general, beta blockers should not be stopped suddenly prior to surgery. Postoperatively they should be started again as soon as possible, either i.v. or orally.
2. During surgery, care should be taken to monitor vascular volume, and to correct hypovolaemia or blood loss.
3. If inotropic support is required, higher doses than normal may be needed to give the desired effect.
4. Occasionally beta blockade may require reversal, perhaps in the case of an overdose or severe bradycardia. Atropine may be tried first, but is usually ineffective. Isoprenaline should then be used for non-selective, and dobutamine for selective, beta blockers (Foex 1984).

BIBLIOGRAPHY

Boudoulas H, Lewis R P, Kates R E, Dalmangas G 1977 Hypersensitivity to adrenergic stimulation after propranolol withdrawal. Annals of Internal Medicine 87: 433–436
Cutfield G R, Francis C M, Foex P, Ryder W A, Jones L A 1981 Effects of oxprenolol on myocardial function during enflurane anaesthesia. British Journal of Anaesthesia 53: 668P–669P
Erikkson M, Rubenfeld S, Garber A J, Kohler P O 1977 Propranolol does not prevent thyroid storm. New England Journal of Medicine 296: 263–264
Foex P 1984 Alpha- and beta-adrenoceptor antagonists. British Journal of Anaesthesia 56: 751–765
Hartwell B L, Mark J B 1986 Combination of beta blockers and calcium channel blockers: a cause of malignant perioperative conduction disturbances. Anesthesia and Analgesia 65: 905–907
Horan B F, Prys-Roberts C, Roberts J G, Bennett M J, Foex P 1977a Haemodynamic responses to isoflurane anaesthesia and hypovolaemia in the dog, and their modification by propranolol. British Journal of Anaesthesia 49: 1179–1187
Horan B F, Prys-Roberts C, Hamilton W K, Roberts J G 1977b Haemodynamic responses to enflurane anaesthesia and hypovolaemia in the dog, and their modification by propranolol. British Journal of Anaesthesia 49; 1189–1197
Jones D K, Solomon S 1981 Thyrotoxic crisis masked by treatment with beta blockers. British Medical Journal 283: 659
Kam C A 1978 Infundibular spasm in Fallot's tetralogy. Anaesthesia and Intensive Care 6: 138–140
Langer S Z, Hicks P E 1984 Physiology of the sympathetic nerve ending. British Journal of Anaesthesia 56: 689–700
Laxenaire M-C, Moneret-Vautrin D-A, Vervloet D 1985 The French experience of anaphylactoid reactions. International Anaesthesiology Clinics 23: 145–160
Miller R R, Olson H G, Amsterdam E A, Mason D T 1975 Propranolol-withdrawal rebound phenomenon. New England Journal of Medicine 293; 416–418
Ponten J, Biber B, Bjuro T, Henriksson B A, Hjalmarson A 1982a Beta-receptor blocker

withdrawal. A preoperative problem in general surgery. Acta Anaesthesiologica Scandinavica (suppl) 76: 32–37

Ponten J, Biber B, Bjuro T, Henriksson B A, Hjalmarson A, Lundberg D 1982b Beta-receptor blockade and spinal anaesthesia. Withdrawal versus continuation of long-term therapy. Acta Anaesthesiologica Scandinavica (suppl) 76: 62–69

Pringle S D, MacEwen C J 1987 Severe bradycardia due to interaction of timolol eye drops and verapamil. British Medical Journal 294: 155–156

Prys-Roberts C 1980 Adrenergic mechanisms, agonists and antagonist drugs. In: Circulation in Anaesthesia, Blackwell Scientific, Oxford

Prys-Roberts C 1984 Kinetics and dynamics of beta-adrenoceptor antagonists. In: Pharmacokinetics of Anaesthesia. Blackwell Scientific, Oxford

Seidl D C, Martin D E 1984 Prolonged bradycardia after neostigmine administration in a patient taking nadolol. Anesthesia and Analgesia 63: 365–367

Slogoff S, Keats A S, Ott E 1978 Preoperative propranolol therapy and aortocoronary bypass operations. Journal of the American Medical Association 240: 1487–1490

Smulyan H, Weinberg S E, Howanitz P J 1982 Continuous propranolol infusion following abdominal surgery. Journal of the American Medical Association 247: 2539–2542

Villers D, Pinaud M L J, Bourin M, Frison B, Souron R J, Nicolas F M 1984 Propranolol postoperative maintenance by continuous intravenous infusion. Anesthesiology 60: 594–598

CALCIUM CHANNEL BLOCKERS

A heterogenous group of drugs which interfere with calcium flux across cell membranes, and which may be used in the treatment of angina, hypertension, supraventricular arrhythmias, cerebral artery vasospasm and hypertrophic cardiomyopathy. Individual drugs produce variable effects on AV conduction, myocardial contractility and vascular smooth muscle.

In the ischaemic myocardium, oxygen consumption is decreased by reductions in heart rate and myocardial contractility. Oxygen supply to ischaemic muscle is increased by coronary vasodilatation, prevention of coronary spasm, and reduction in diastolic wall tension. As with beta blockers, their sudden withdrawal prior to surgery may increase ischaemia or provoke angina.

Calcium antagonists have certain advantages over beta blockers, in that they do not exacerbate obstructive airway disease, or peripheral vascular disease.

VERAPAMIL

1. Use:
Angina, hypertension, supraventricular tachycardia and hypertrophic cardiomyopathy. Produces systemic and coronary vasodilatation, but causes some impairment of AV conduction and moderate myocardial depression.
2. Route:
Oral/i.v.

3. Half-life:
5–10 hours.
4. Side-effects:
Flushing and constipation. After i.v. verapamil, hypotension, heart block and transient asystole may occur.
5. Interactions:
With beta blockers to cause hypotension and conduction defects. With quinidine to cause hypotension.
6. Contraindications:
Hypotension, severe bradycardia, sick sinus syndrome, first- and second-degree AV block and decompensated heart failure.

DILTIAZEM

1. Use:
Angina. Produces both systemic and coronary vasodilatation. Although it has less effect than verapamil on AV conduction, the heart rate is often slowed.
2. Route:
Oral.
3. Half-life:
4–6 hours.
4. Side-effects:
Bradycardia, first-degree heart block and ankle oedema.
5. Interactions:
With beta blockers and digoxin.
6. Contraindications:
Bradycardia, first- and second-degree heart block, sick sinus syndrome and in women of childbearing age.

NIFEDIPINE

1. Use:
Hypertension, angina and Raynaud's disease. Causes systemic and coronary vasodilatation, without myocardial depression or AV conduction impairment.
2. Route:
Oral.
3. Half-life:
3–5 hours.
4. Side-effects:
Flushing, and oedema of the lower limbs.
5. Interactions:
Postural hypotension with beta blockers and other antihypertensives.
6. Contraindications:
In women of childbearing age.

NICARDIPINE

1. Use:

Angina and hypertension. Primary action is that of systemic and coronary vasodilatation. Does not depress left ventricular function and in fact may cause a reflex improvement in pump activity. AV conduction is not impaired.

2. Route:

Oral.

3. Half-life:

1–2 hours.

4. Side-effects:

Dizziness, flushing and lower limb oedema.

5. Interactions:

Nicardipine may increase serum digoxin levels, and cimetidine may increase nicardipine levels.

6. Contraindications:

Severe aortic stenosis.

Potential problems associated with anaesthesia

1. Sudden withdrawal of calcium channel blockers may exacerbate angina.

2. Drug interactions may occur.

a. Volatile agents

Halothane, enflurane and isoflurane are all non-specific calcium antagonists. Animal studies suggested that additive effects might occur in patients during anaesthesia, causing hypotension, either due to peripheral vasodilatation or myocardial depression. Clinical reports suggest that this is so (Schulte-Sasse et al 1984), and particularly in the presence of beta blockers (Fahmy & Lappas 1983). One case of cardiac arrest has been reported with halothane (Moller 1987).

b. Muscle relaxants

Animal experiments have suggested that calcium antagonists can potentiate the effects of neuromuscular blocking agents. This may only become clinically significant if other factors are operative. For example, respiratory failure occurred in a patient with Duchenne muscular dystrophy given i.v. verapamil (Zalman et al 1983). A prolonged block with vecuronium was reported in a patient with renal failure on i.v. verapamil (van Poorten et al 1984).

c. Narcotic analgesics

Marked hypotension was produced in patients on nifedipine and propranolol when given fentanyl (Freis & Lappas 1982).

d. Beta blockers

Severe bradycardia occurred in a patient having verapamil and timolol eye-drops (Pringle & MacEwan 1987). Serious haemodynamic

complications and conduction defects were reported during coronary artery bypass surgery (Hartwell & Mark 1986).
e. Digoxin
Verapamil may precipitate digitalis toxicity by impairing its clearance.
f. Dantrolene
In animals, serious AV conduction defects have occurred when verapamil and dantrolene are given together (Saltzman et al 1984).
3. Despite being used for the treatment of hypertension and angina, calcium antagonists may not prevent the harmful cardiovascular responses to stressful stimuli (Gorven et al 1986).
4. A decrease in lower oesophageal sphincter tone. The clinical significance of this has not as yet been evaluated.
5. Increases in intracranial pressure have been reported, due to cerebral vasodilatation, particularly when the pressure is already raised (Bedford et al 1983).

Management

1. Volatile agents should be used cautiously in patients on calcium channel blockers. Similarly, i.v. verapamil given during anaesthesia may produce significant myocardial depression.
2. Neuromuscular function should be monitored carefully.
3. If i.v. beta blockers are used with verapamil or diltiazem, atropine, isoprenaline, calcium and/or temporary pacing should be available (Jenkins & Scoates 1985).
4. Acute cardiovascular side-effects may occur with i.v. administration of calcium channel blockers. Heart block can be treated with atropine, isoprenaline or a temporary pacemaker. Hypotension and myocardial insufficiency should be treated with inotropic agents such as dopamine or dobutamine, or calcium gluconate 10%, 10 ml.

BIBLIOGRAPHY

Bedford R F, Dacey R, Winn H R, Lynch III C 1983 Adverse impact of a calcium entry-blocker (verapamil) on intracranial pressure in patients with brain tumors. Journal of Neurosurgery 59: 800–802
Fahmy N R, Lappas D G 1983 Interaction of nifedipine, propranolol and halothane in humans. Anaethesiology 59: A39
Freis E S, Lappas D G 1982 Chronic administration of calcium entry blockers and the cardiovascular responses to high doses of fentanyl in man. Anesthesiology 57: A295
Gorven A M, Cooper G M, Prys-Roberts C 1986 Haemodynamic disturbances during anaesthesia in a patient receiving calcium channel blockers. British Journal of Anaesthesia 58: 357–360
Hartwell B L, Mark J B 1986 Combination of beta blockers and calcium channel blockers: cause of malignant perioperative conduction disturbances. Anesthesia and Analgesia 65: 905–907
Jenkins L C, Scoates P J 1985 Anaesthetic implications of calcium channel blockers. Canadian Anaesthetists' Society Journal 32: 436–447
Moller I W 1987 Cardiac arrest following iv verapamil combined with halothane anaesthesia. British Journal of Anaesthesia 59: 522–523
Pringle S D, MacEwen C J 1987 Severe bradycardia due to interaction of timolol eye drops and verapamil. British Medical Journal 294: 155–156

Saltzman I S, Kates R A, Corke B C, Norfleet E A, Heath K R 1984 Hyperkalaemia and cardiovascular collapse after verapamil and dantrolene administration in swine. Anesthesia and Analgesia 63: 473–478

Schulte-Sasse U, Hess W, Markschies-Hornung A, Tarnow J 1984 Combined effect of halothane anesthesia and verapamil on systemic hemodynamics and left ventricular myocardial contractility in patients with ischemic heart disease. Anesthesia and Analgesia 63: 791–798

van Poorten J F, Dhasmana K M, Kuypers R S, Erdmann W 1984 Verapamil and reversal of vecuronium neuromuscular blockade. Anesthesia and Analgesia 63: 155–157

Zalman F, Perloff J K, Durant N N, Campion D S 1983 Acute respiratory failure following intravenous verapamil in Duchenne Muscular Dystrophy. American Heart Journal 105: 510–511

CORTICOSTEROIDS

Equivalent dosages for a given glucocorticoid effect:

Hydrocortisone	100 mg
Cortisone	130 mg
Prednisolone	25 mg
Prednisone	25 mg
Methylprednisolone	20 mg
Betamethasone	4 mg
Triamcinolone	25 mg
Dexamethasone	4 mg

Drugs with mineralocorticoid effects:

Hydrocortisone	weak
Cortisone	weak
Fludrocortisone	strong

Corticosteroid cover for surgery and other stresses

1. Adrenal atrophy is detected 5 days after the onset of glucocorticoid therapy, and if it is given for more than a few weeks, a return to completely normal homeostasis may take up to 1 year (Axelrod 1976). While it is possible to test a patient's response to stress prior to operation, in order to determine which patients will need steroid supplements, in practice this is rarely done. Supplementary steroid cover is generally given to those who have had therapy within the previous year.

2. The rise in cortisol output in normal patients occurs at the start of surgery, and if the surgery is major, it may remain elevated for 3 days. The cortisol output may increase to 150 mg/day, although the maximum possible output from normal adrenals is double that level.

3. For minor surgery, steroid supplements are only required for 1 day. For major surgery, they are usually needed for 3 days, and possibly longer if serious complications arise.

4. If oral supplements are not possible, the most appropriate regimen is either:

    a. Hydrocortisone i.m. 100 mg 6-hourly, or

    b. Hydrocortisone infusion: 400 mg over 24 hours, in either dextrose 5% or saline 0.9%.

BIBLIOGRAPHY

Axelrod L 1976 Glucocorticoid therapy. Medicine 55: 39–65

DIGOXIN

1. Use:
Control of the ventricular response rate to supraventricular arrhythmias such as atrial fibrillation and atrial flutter, and AV nodal re-entry tachycardia. Treatment of cardiac failure.

2. Action:
Prolongation of conduction time and the refractory period of the AV node. Reduction of ventricular refractoriness.

3. Route:
Oral/i.v./i.m.

4. Half-life:
33–38 hours. One daily dose is therefore sufficient.

5. Therapeutic blood level:
Blood taken 6 hours after the last dose should be in the range 1.3–2.5 ng/ml.

6. Side-effects:
Digoxin toxicity occurs in up to 10% of hospital admissions on digoxin therapy. Precipitating factors include old age, hypokalaemia, impaired renal function, hypothyroidism, quinidine, amiodarone and verapamil therapy.

7. Interactions:
Amiodarone, quinidine, diltiazem, nicardipine and verapamil all potentiate the effect of digoxin. Diuretics may precipitate toxicity due to hypokalaemia. Suxamethonium and calcium salts can provoke arrhythmias in patients on digoxin.

8. Contraindications:
The treatment of supraventricular arrhythmias due to WPW syndrome.

Digitalis toxicity

1. Toxicity is diagnosed on clinical criteria. Symptoms include fatigue, visual disturbances, muscle weakness, nausea, anorexia, abdominal pains, dizziness, diarrhoea and vomiting. Arrhythmias include ventricular extrasystoles, atrial tachycardia (atrial waves 150–200/min) with AV block, junctional tachycardia, first-, second- and third-degree heart block, bradycardia, ventricular tachycardia, slow ventricular response to AF and sinoatrial block.

2. Drug levels are less helpful in diagnosing toxicity, as certain potentiating factors result in clinical signs of toxicity, even when blood levels are within the therapeutic range. However, toxicity is unlikely at levels <1.5 ng/ml, and likely at those >3.0 ng/ml. Between these levels, the possibility of toxicity exists.

Treatment of digitalis toxicity

1. Stop the digoxin preparation.

2. Correct hypokalaemia.

3. Among the drugs recommended for treatment of digitalis toxicity are phenytoin, lignocaine and beta blockers.

4. Temporary cardiac pacing.

5. n.b. Cardioversion is dangerous in digitalis toxicity.

6. In the severe case, where the usual treatment fails, digoxin-specific antibody fragments (Fab fragments, Digibind, Wellcome Medical Division) may be considered. At present this treatment is reserved for life-threatening manifestations of toxicity only. (See manufacturer's literature for details of treatment.) Improvement in signs and symptoms begins within 30 minutes.

BIBLIOGRAPHY

Jones M, Hawker F, Duggin G, Falks M 1987 Treatment of severe digoxin toxicity with digoxin specific antibody fragments. Anaesthesia and Intensive Care 15: 234–236

DIURETICS AND POTASSIUM REPLACEMENT

1. Oral potassium replacement:

A maximum of 15 g (195 mmol) in 24 hours for potassium depletion.

2. Intravenous replacement:

Add potassium chloride 1.5 g to dextrose 5%, 500 ml or sodium chloride 0.9%, and infuse over 2–3 hours.

The maximum rate of infusion should be 40 mmol given over 2 hours, or 240 mmol/24 h. If high rates of infusion are necessary, continuous ECG monitoring is required, and serum potassium levels should be checked regularly.

FENFLURAMINE

Used for the treatment of obesity, fenfluramine is related in structure to adrenaline and amphetamine, but without the CNS-stimulating effects of amphetamines. Interaction with halothane may occur (Bennett & Eltringham 1977). Cardiovascular collapse and pulmonary oedema occurred in a patient during dental anaesthesia with halothane. Subsequent studies on rabbits suggested that in some animals, the combination of fenfluramine and halothane decreased cardiac activity, and that the effect was unlike that seen with adrenaline. In view of the formation of active metabolites, it was suggested that the danger of interaction with halothane continued for a week after cessation of therapy.

Interaction with MAOIs can occur.

BIBLIOGRAPHY

Bennett J A, Eltringham R J 1977 Possible dangers of anaesthesia in patients receiving fenfluramine. Anaesthesia 32: 8–13

LITHIUM

Used in acute mania associated with manic depressive illnesses. Therapeutic range: 0.8–1.2 mmol/l, toxic levels > 2.0 mmol/l.

Problems associated with lithium therapy

1. The decrease in renal function normally associated with surgery may cause lithium accumulation and toxicity. Signs of lithium intoxication include nausea, vomiting, diarrhoea, muscle weakness, tremor, slurred speech, sleepiness, confusion, T-wave depression and QRS widening. Increasing blood levels cause convulsions and coma (Havdala et al 1979).
2. If lithium therapy is stopped for a prolonged period during surgery, acute mania may occur (Schou & Hippus 1987).
3. Lithium may produce polyuria. Dehydration therefore occurs readily, and may precipitate toxicity.
4. Lithium may prolong the action of neuromuscular blocking drugs by inhibiting the presynaptic synthesis of acetylcholine.
5. Changes in blood levels can occur in association with haemodialysis.
6. Lithium may produce a neutrophil leucocytosis.
7. Thiazide diuretics interact with lithium, such that the half-life is prolonged (Kerry et al 1980).

Management

1. Lithium should be stopped 48–72 hours before elective surgery. This will prevent potential toxicity, or interactions with muscle relaxants.
2. It should be started again as soon as possible after the operation, provided that renal function, fluid and electrolyte balance are normal.

3. Lithium may cause polyuria. Thus fluid restriction can cause dehydration. Intravenous fluids should be given during preoperative starvation, vomiting or unconsciousness.

4. Toxicity should be treated by stopping lithium and giving i.v. saline 0.9%, 2 litres in 6 hours. Excretion of lithium can be increased with mannitol, but loop and thiazide diuretics must not be given.

BIBLIOGRAPHY

Havdala H S, Borison R L, Diamond B I 1979 Potential hazards and applications of lithium in anesthesiology. Anesthesiology 50: 534–537
Kerry R J, Ludlow J M, Owen G 1980 Diuretics are dangerous with lithium. British Medical Journal 281: 371
Schou M, Hippus H 1987 Guidelines for patients receiving lithium treatment who require major surgery. British Journal of Anaesthesia 59: 809–810

MONAMINE OXIDASE INHIBITORS

1. Use

Despite being the cause of a number of serious, and occasionally fatal, drug interactions, monoamine oxidase inhibitors (MAOI) are still used for the treatment of depression unresponsive to other types of therapy.

2. Action

They form an irreversible complex with monoamine oxidase (MAO), which is one of the enzymes responsible for the breakdown of biogenic amines. It is now known that there are two types of MAO, the differentiation being made on substrate preference. Type A selectively deaminates serotonin, noradrenaline and dopamine. Type B tends to deaminate tyramine and phenethylamine (Michaels et al 1983). As a result of treatment with MAOIs there is a considerable increase in the stable and mobile pools of noradrenaline in the adrenergic neurones.

In addition, MAO is found in neurones where dopamine and 5-hydroxytryptamine act as transmitters, and is also present in hepatic microsomes and in the intestine where it breaks down amines. Enzymes other than MAO are additionally inhibited, and the hepatic metabolism of many drugs, other than amines, is thus affected.

3. Indirect effects of MAOIs

Ingestion or administration of indirect-acting sympathomimetic amines will cause immediate release of catecholamines from nerve endings, resulting in a severe hypertensive response. Drugs whose metabolism is in part dependent on MAO will have a longer, and presumably a more profound, action.

4. Onset and cessation of effect

The onset of therapeutic effect is slow, as is the cessation of action after withdrawal of a MAOI, since new enzyme must be manufactured. The effects of tranylcypromine wear off more quickly than those of phenelzine.

5. Interactions

Occasionally, serious adverse reactions, or even death, may occur as a result of drug interactions. Drugs involved have included pethidine, indirect-acting amines and tricyclic antidepressants. A severe hypermetabolic state in a young man receiving an MAOI/tricyclic combination, which terminated in a fatal disseminated intravascular coagulation, has been reported (Tackley & Tregaskis 1987). Agitation and hypertension may occur when levodopa is given. Potentiation of the effects of all the direct-acting amines occurs.

6. Currently used preparations

Monoamine oxidase inhibitors in current use in the UK inhibit both type A and type B monamine oxidase.

Marplan = isocarboxazid
Nardil = phenelzine
Parnate = tranylcypromine
Parstelin = tranylcypromine and trifluoperazine

7. Selective inhibition

The discovery of two different forms of MAO, A and B, has increased interest in the possible development of a safer, selective inhibitor.

Potential anaesthetic problems

1. Serious interactions occur with pethidine and dextromethorphan (which is present in Actifed linctus, Cosylan syrup and Lotussin linctus). Two different types of reaction with pethidine have been described (Stack et al 1988). Excitation may occur, with hyperpyrexia, agitation, headache, hypo- or hypertension, fits and coma. In addition there may be a depressive effect which produces hypotension, respiratory depression and coma.

Phenoperidine and fentanyl are both chemically related to pethidine, and phenoperidine is metabolized to norpethidine. Although the manufacturer's literature on fentanyl suggests that it is contraindicated in patients receiving MAOIs, no interactions with fentanyl have been documented (Michaels et al 1983) and this author has used it without complications. The use of epidural fentanyl has also been described (Youssef & Wilkinson 1988).

2. Interaction with indirect-acting sympathomimetic amines, which function by releasing endogenous catecholamines. Large amounts of catecholamines will have accumulated in stores in the CNS and nerve endings, during the period of treatment with MAOIs. A severe hypertensive response may occur during sympathetic stimulation and fatalities have been recorded in some patients who have accidentally taken sympathomimetics. Drugs which may interact include amphetamines, methylphenidate, fenfluramine, ephedrine and levodopa.

3. An increase in effect and the duration of action of narcotic analgesics and thiopentone may occur, due to the effect of MAOIs on microsomal enzyme systems in the liver. There is little reliable information in the literature about this.

4. There will be an enhanced response to the direct-acting sympathomimetics, adrenaline, noradrenaline, isoprenaline and dopamine.

Management

1. The initial decision to be made is whether or not to stop the MAOI for 2–3 weeks before surgery. Even 2 weeks after stopping therapy, there may be residual effects, particularly with phenelzine. With tranylcypromine the period required is less than this (Michaels et al 1983). In the case of emergency surgery, there is no choice. However, even with elective surgery there are arguments in favour of continuing the MAOI. If antidepressants are stopped for a long period, the danger of suicide exists. However, if the decision is made to continue therapy, certain drugs must be avoided, while others should be administered with caution.

2. If MAOIs are continued, pethidine, metaraminol, ephedrine and amphetamine are absolutely contraindicated. Dopamine has an indirect as well as direct sympathomimetic effect, and if required, should be given cautiously, in reduced doses.

3. If major analgesics are needed, morphine is probably the best choice. It must be given with caution, and the dose titrated against the effect. Buprenorphine may also be used. Animal studies, comparing pethidine and buprenorphine, showed that those rabbits given an MAOI/pethidine combination had severe hypertension, hyperpyrexia and agitation, and a 50% mortality. Those receiving buprenorphine with an MAOI had no adverse reactions (Mackenzie & Frank 1988).

4. If direct-acting sympathetic agents are required, they should be given very cautiously, as receptor sensitivity has been reported.

BIBLIOGRAPHY

Mackenzie J E, Frank L W 1988 Influence of pretreatment with a monoamine oxidase inhibitor (phenelzine) on the effects of buprenorphine and pethidine in the conscious rabbit. British Journal of Anaesthesia 60: 216–221

Michaels I, Serrins M, Shier N Q, Barash P G 1983 Anesthesia for cardiac surgery in patients receiving monoamine oxidase inhibitors. Anesthesia and Analgesia 63: 1041–1044

Stack C G, Rogers P, Linter S P K 1988 Monamine oxidase inhibitors and anaesthesia. British Journal of Anaesthesia 60: 222–227

Tackley R M, Tregaskis B 1987 Fatal disseminated intravascular coagulation following a monoamine oxidase inhibitor/tricyclic interaction. Anaesthesia 42: 760–763

Youssef M S, Wilkinson P A 1988 Epidural fentanyl and monoamine oxidase inhibitors. Anaesthesia 43: 210–212

TRICYCLIC ANTIDEPRESSANTS
(TCAD)

Members of this group of drugs, used for the treatment of depression, block the reuptake of noradrenaline by adrenergic nerve terminals.

Increased levels of circulating noradrenaline occur. In patients receiving TCAD therapy, adrenergic responses tend to be enhanced, as there is interference with the normal mechanism of termination.

Potential problems during anaesthesia

1. Interactions with catecholamines
The effects of exogenous adrenaline and noradrenaline on the circulation will be potentiated causing severe arrhythmias and hypertension.
2. Interactions with anaesthetic agents
Reports concerning the possible dysrhythmogenic effects of TCAD treatment are conflicting. An increased incidence of ventricular arrhythmias was reported in dogs on acute and chronic imipramine therapy, receiving pancuronium and halothane. It was suggested that this combination be avoided (Edwards et al 1979). However, only short- as opposed to long-term treatment with TCAD increased halothane-adrenaline arrhythmias (Spiss et al 1984). In dogs on chronic therapy, there was no increase in arrhythmic and adrenergic responsiveness during halothane anaesthesia, despite five-fold increases in circulating noradrenaline. It has been suggested that 'down regulation' of beta adrenergic receptors may occur with chronic therapy.
3. Interactions between tricyclics and MAOIs
This combination is occasionally used therapeutically and fatal reactions have been reported (Tackley & Tregaskis 1988). An acute hypermetabolic state may occur, with dystonic reactions and alterations in conscious level.

Management

1. Avoid the use of adrenaline, noradrenaline and isoprenaline. Should a vasopressor be required, felypressin or methoxamine can be used.
2. If drugs with a potential to produce tachycardia or arrhythmias, such as halothane and pancuronium are used, the ECG should be monitored closely.

BIBLIOGRAPHY

Edwards R P, Miller R D, Roizen M F, Ham J, Way W L, Lake C R, Roderick L 1979 Cardiac response to imipramine and pancuronium during anesthesia with halothane or enflurane. Anesthesiology 50: 421–425
Spiss C K, Smith C M, Maze M 1984 Halothane-epinephrine arrhythmias and adrenergic responsiveness after chronic imipramine administration in dogs. Anesthesia and Analgesia 63: 825–828
Tackley R M, Tregaskis B 1987 Fatal disseminated intravascular coagulation following a monoamine oxidase inhibitor/tricyclic combination. Anaesthesia 42: 760–763

3

Perioperative Drugs

ANALGESICS AND ANTAGONISTS

ALFENTANIL

Action

Short-acting narcotic analgesic. Peak effect 90 seconds. Duration of analgesia 5–10 minutes. Half-life 1.5–1.8 hours.

Presentation

500 μg/ml   2 ml and 10 ml ampoules.
100 μg/ml   5 ml ampoules.
5 mg/ml   1 ml ampoules.

Dosage

a. Spontaneous respiration: 200–500 μg given slowly over 30 seconds, then supplementary doses of up to 250 μg each 4–5 minutes.
b. Ventilated patients: a loading dose of 30–50 μg/kg and then either supplements of 15 μg/kg or an infusion of 0.5–1 μg/kg/min.
Infusion for longer procedures:
Loading dose of 50–100 μg/kg then a maintenance infusion.
Discontinue 30 minutes before the end of surgery.

Conversion table for infusions: Recommended maintenance infusion rates in μg/kg/min converted to ml/h; concentration, alfentanil 500 μg/ml

Body weight in kg	Maintenance infusion rates in μg/kg/min	
	0.7	0.8
40	3.4	3.8
45	3.8	4.3
50	4.2	4.8
55	4.6	5.3
60	5.0	5.8
65	5.5	6.2
70	5.9	6.7
75	6.3	7.2
80	6.7	7.7
85	7.2	8.2
90	7.6	8.6
95	8.0	9.1
100	8.4	9.6
105	8.8	10.1
110	9.2	10.6
115	9.7	11.0
120	10.1	11.5

Side-effects

Respiratory depression of peak effect in 1–2 minutes and duration 5 minutes, bradycardia, transient hypotension, muscle rigidity, nausea and vomiting.

Contraindications

Interactions may occur with MAOIs.

FENTANYL

Action

Short acting synthetic opioid analgesic. Duration of action 20–30 minutes with 100 μg, and 1 hour with a 500 μg bolus. Half-life 3.5–4 hours, but prolonged with high doses.

Presentation

50 μg/ml   2 ml and 10 ml ampoules.

Dosage

Intraoperative:
a. Spontaneous respiration
Adults 0.5–3 μg/kg, with supplements of 0.5–1 μg/kg.
Children 3–5 μg/kg, with supplements of 1 μg/kg.
b. Assisted ventilation
1–50 μg/kg, the high dose giving analgesia for 4–6 hours. The requirement depends upon the duration of the procedure and the use of other agents.
Postoperative:
Continuous infusion of 100 μg/h for postoperative pain relief has been described (Duthie & Nimmo 1985). However, in order to achieve a steady state, the infusion was started 2 hours before surgery, and an additional 100 μg bolus given during surgery. Some patients required additional morphine i.m..

Side-effects

Respiratory depression. High doses may produce increases in muscle tone with glottic closure, such that the patient is difficult to ventilate. With such doses, late recurrence of respiratory depression may also occur after apparent recovery. Nausea and vomiting. Bradycardia, responsive to atropine.

Contraindications

Although the manufacturers recommend its avoidance with MAOIs, its uneventful use, both i.v. and for epidural anaesthesia has been reported (Michaels et al 1984, Youssef & Wilkinson 1988).

MORPHINE

Action

Opiate analgesic producing euphoria, and drowsiness. Reduces arterial and venous tone, decreasing venous return to the heart. Half-life 2.5–4 hours.

Presentation

10 mg/ml, 15 mg/ml, 30 mg/ml in 1 ml and 2 ml ampoules

Dosage

a. Intraoperative
High-dose morphine 1–4 mg/kg may be used during anaesthesia for cardiac surgery (Bovill et al 1984).
b. Postoperative analgesia
i.m.: 0.15–0.3 mg/kg.
i.v.: Up to a similar total dose, but divided into incremental doses of 2.5 mg i.v. at 5-minute intervals until desired effect achieved.
i.v. infusion: Morphine 10 mg added to 50 ml diluent to give a solution of 0.2 mg/ml, infused at about 12.5 ml/h, and titrated against the effect. An initial loading dose will be needed. The effect of an infusion must be carefully monitored, as the requirement for analgesia in individual patients is very variable, as is the degree of respiratory depression and sedation produced.

Side-effects

Respiratory depression 2–5 minutes after i.v. injection, cough suppression, hypotension, bradycardia, histamine release, chest wall rigidity and occasionally hypertension.

Contraindications

Respiratory failure.

PETHIDINE

Action

Synthetic narcotic analgesic, with minimal euphoric action. Atropine-like activity. Half-life 2.5–4 hours.

Presentation

50 mg/ml   1 ml and 2 ml ampoules.
10 mg/ml   5 ml and 10 ml ampoules.

Dosage

Postoperative analgesia
i.m.: 1–1.5 mg/kg.
i.v.: Up to the same total dose, in 10–25 mg increments.
infusion: Pethidine 100 mg added to 50 ml diluent to give 2 mg/ml, infused at about 12.5 ml/h, and titrated against effect. An initial loading dose will be required. The effect of an infusion must be carefully monitored.

Side-effects

Respiratory depression, histamine release, tachycardia, depression of myocardial contractility and hypotension, delayed gastric emptying, nausea and vomiting. Pethidine can produce physical dependence.

CNS excitation may sometimes occur with repeated or high-dose pethidine, or in patients with renal failure. With increasing doses of pethidine, a longer-acting, active metabolite, norpethidine, may accumulate. Norpethidine causes CNS excitation, and the onset of twitching and irritability has been linked to elevated ratios of norpethidine to pethidine (Szeto & Inturrisi 1977). If norpethidine toxicity occurs the use of naloxone may worsen the situation by antagonizing the depressant effects of pethidine (Armstrong & Bersten 1986).

Precautions

Decreased clearance may occur during halothane anaesthesia or when renal function is reduced. The use of naloxone in acute pethidine toxicity has exacerbated convulsions (Inturrisi & Umans 1983).

Contraindications

In patients receiving monoamine oxidase inhibitors. Two types of reaction have been described (Stack et al 1988). Excitation may occur, with hyperpyrexia, agitation, headache, hypo- or hypertension, fits and coma. In addition, there may be a depressive effect, which produces hypotension, respiratory depression and coma (see also Section 2 MAOI).

PHENOPERIDINE

Action

Analgesia, respiratory depression. Onset of action 2–3 minutes. Duration 45–60 minutes, although some analgesia will persist longer. Chemically related to pethidine.

Presentation

1 mg/ml   2 ml and 10 ml ampoules

Dosage

> Intraoperative analgesia
> **a.** Spontaneous respiration:
> Adults: 0.5–1 mg (7–15 µg/kg), then 0.5 mg each 40–60 minutes.
> Children: 30–50 µg/kg.
> **b.** Assisted ventilation:
> Adults: 2–5 mg (30–70 µg/kg), then 1 mg (15 µg/kg) as required.
> Children: 100–150 µg/kg.

Side-effects

Respiratory depression, bradycardia, muscle rigidity, nausea and vomiting.

Caution

In liver disease.

Contraindications

Patients on MAOIs (see Pethidine).

NALOXONE

Action

A competitive opiate antagonist, reversing both analgesia and respiratory depression. Its affinity for different opiate receptors is variable (Smith & Pinnock 1985). Naloxone can also produce partial reversal of stimulation-induced analgesia. Experimental work and clinical reports have shown that the overall effect of naloxone administration is more complex than was originally thought. Both have provided increasing evidence of a link between the endogenous opioid peptide and the catecholamine systems. Increases in heart rate, systolic blood pressure, cardiac index and myocardial oxygen consumption have been shown after reversal of opiates with low-dose naloxone (Desmonts et al 1978). Naloxone can produce pressor effects in septic shock and hypovolaemia (Peters et al 1981), while noradrenaline release in a patient with a phaeochromocytoma occurred with high doses (10 mg) of naloxone, although not with a normal dose (Mannelli et al 1983).

Length of action

Naloxone is short acting, with reversal of opiate-induced respiratory depression lasting only about 30 minutes.

Use

Reversal of opiate induced respiratory depression. Treatment of acute opiate toxicity.

3

Presentation

400 µg/ml   1 ml ampoule, 10 ml vial.
20 µg/ml   2 ml ampoule (for neonatal use).

Dosage

Adults:
   i.v.: 100–200 µg (1.5–3 µg/kg) slowly, monitoring blood pressure and
   pulse rate.
   infusion: 2 mg naloxone in 500 ml dextrose 5% or saline 0.9%
   (4 µg/ml). Infuse according to response.
Neonates: either 10 µg/kg i.v., i.m. or s.c. and repeat after 2–3 minutes
or give single i.m. dose of 200 µg.

Side-effects

Naloxone was originally thought to possess no side-effects. As a result, high-dose opiate techniques were sometimes devised, following which reversal with naloxone would be routine. Unfortunately, a few cases have occurred in which naloxone opiate reversal has been associated with a state of acute central adrenergic stimulation resulting in serious cardiovascular complications. Pre-existing hypertension or ischaemic heart disease were thought to be predisposing factors. However, some incidents have involved apparently healthy patients. Pulmonary oedema has occurred in a patient with pre-existing cardiac disease (Flacke et al 1977), and also in fit young men (Taff 1983, Prough et al 1984). Ventricular fibrillation (Cuss et al 1984), severe hypertension and multiple atrial ectopics (Azar & Turndorf 1979) have also been reported. Fatal reactions occurred in two fit young women after elective surgery, one of whom had a cardiac arrest and the other pulmonary oedema (Andree 1980).

Precautions

   a. Naloxone should only be given when absolutely necessary. The
   practice of giving large doses of opiates and then routinely reversing

them is inappropriate. Particular caution should be employed in patients with hypertension or myocardial ischaemia. If it is essential that naloxone be given, it should be diluted and given in increments, while monitoring the blood pressure.

b. Naloxone is short acting, therefore a recurrence of respiratory depression may be expected with long acting analgesics, or in the case of opiate overdose.

c. Naloxone has been reported to exaggerate convulsions in cases of pethidine overdose.

d. It can also produce acute withdrawal symptoms in opiate addicts.

DOXAPRAM

Action

A general cerebrospinal stimulant. At low doses a non-specific antagonist of respiratory depression, acting via peripheral chemoreceptors Increases tidal volume rather than rate. There is a narrow margin between stimulation of respiration and convulsive doses. Doxapram increases oxygen consumption. Duration of action is approximately 10 minutes.

Use

Occasionally it may be useful as a short-term measure to stimulate respiration, but in general there is little indication for its use. Although it has been recommended during recovery from anaesthesia, the side-effects make its use undesirable. Treatment with IPPV is more appropriate. It has no place in the treatment of poisoning.

Presentation

20 mg/ml   5 ml ampoule.
2 mg/ml   premixed in 500 ml dextrose 5%.

Dosage

i.v.: bolus of 1–1.5 mg/kg.
infusion: 0.5–4 mg/min of a 2 mg/ml soln.
Maximum total dose 4 mg/kg

Side-effects

Mild hypertension and tachycardia. During recovery from anaesthesia it may be associated with a hyperactive state, with agitation, sweating, muscle twitching, tonic clonic convulsions, confusion, extrasystoles and vomiting.

Precautions

Oxygen should be given if doxapram is used. If combined with aminophylline, it may produce agitation and muscle twitching. Potentiation can occur with MAOIs.

Contraindications

Severe hypertension, coronary artery disease, status asthmaticus, thyrotoxicosis, upper respiratory tract obstruction and epilepsy.

3

BIBLIOGRAPHY

Andree R A 1980 Sudden death following naloxone administration. Anesthesia and Analgesia 59: 782–788

Armstrong P J, Bersten A 1986 Normeperidine toxicity. Anesthesia and Analgesia 65: 536–538

Azar I, Turndorf H 1979 Severe hypertension and multiple atrial premature contractions following naloxone administration. Anesthesia and Analgesia 58: 524–525

Bovill J G, Sebel P S, Stanley T H 1984 Opioid analgesics in anesthesia: with special reference to their use in cardiovascular anesthesia. Anesthesiology 61: 731–755

Cuss F M, Colaco C B, Baron J H 1984 Cardiac arrest after reversal of the effects of opiates with naloxone. British Medical Journal 288: 363–364

Desmonts J M, Bohm G, Couderc E 1978 Hemodynamic responses to low doses of naloxone after narcotic-nitrous oxide anaesthesia Anesthesiology 49: 12–16

Duthie D J R, Nimmo W S 1987 Adverse effects of opioid analgesic drugs. British Journal of Anaesthesia 59: 61–77

Flacke J W, Flacke W E, Williams G D 1977 Acute pulmonary edema following naloxone reversal of high-dose morphine anesthesia. Anesthesiology 47: 376–378

Inturrisi C E. Umans J G 1983 Pethidine and its active metabolite, norpethidine. In: Opiate analgesia. Clinics in Anesthesiology W B Saunders, Philadelphia

Mannelli M, Maggi M, Defeo M L, Cuomo S, Forti G, Moroni F, Giusti G 1983 Naloxone administration releases catecholamines. New England Journal of Medicine 308: 654–655

Michaels I, Serrins M, Shier N Q, Barash P G 1984 Anesthesia for cardiac surgery in patients receiving monoamine oxidase inhibitors. Anesthesia and Analgesia 63: 1041–1044

Peters W P, Johnson M W, Friedman P A, Mitch W E 1981 Pressor effect of naloxone in septic shock. Lancet i: 529–532

Prough D S, Roy R, Bumgarner J, Shannon G 1984 Acute pulmonary edema in healthy teenagers following conservative doses of naloxone. Anesthesiology 60: 485–486

Smith G, Pinnock C 1985 Naloxone – paradox or panacea. British Journal of Anaesthesia 57: 547–549

Stack C G, Rogers P, Linter S P K 1988 Monoamine oxidase inhibitors and anaesthesia. British Journal of Anaesthesia 60: 222–227

Szeto H H, Inturrisi C E, Houde R, Saal S, Cheigh J, Reidenberg M M 1977 Accumulation of normeperidine, an active metabolite of meperidine in patients with renal failure or cancer. Annals of Internal Medicine 86: 738–741

Taff R H 1983 Pulmonary edema following naloxone administration in a patient without heart disease. Anesthesiology 59: 576–577

Youssef M S, Wilkinson P A 1988 Epidural fentanyl and monoamine oxidase inhibitors. Anaesthesia 43: 210–212

ANTIARRHYTHMICS

In general, if rhythm disturbances appear for the first time in the perioperative period, the initial search should be for a precipitating cause

3

associated with either the surgery or anaesthesia. Correction of this is usually all that is required. Antiarrhythmics will rarely be needed intraoperatively. Causes include:

1. General problems
Hypoxia, hypercarbia, metabolic and electrolyte abnormalities, light anaesthesia, or manoeuvres which stimulate the output of catecholamines. Endotracheal intubation, ophthalmic, oral surgery, thoracic or neurosurgical procedures.

2. Drugs
Accidental overdosage with local anaesthetics. Absorption of adrenaline during surgical infiltration. The use of halothane in the presence of hypercarbia or adrenaline. Suxamethonium in patients with neuromuscular disease. Digitalis toxicity. The use of naloxone for opiate reversal.

3. Pre-existing cardiac disease
Ischaemic, congenital or rheumatic heart disease, cardiomyopathy, mitral valve prolapse, WPW or the prolonged Q–T syndromes.

4. Rare causes
Undiagnosed phaeochromocytoma, thyrotoxicosis, carcinoid syndrome, malignant hyperpyrexia, and drug or solvent abuse.

BRETYLIUM

Action

A class II adrenergic neurone blocking drug, with class III antiarrhythmic activity. It prolongs the action potential and produces pharmacological defibrillation. It is a vasodilator.

Use

A second-line treatment for serious ventricular arrhythmias, especially VT and VF unresponsive to lignocaine, or refractory to defibrillation. It may be the first-line drug for VF or VT associated with bupivacaine overdose (Kasten & Martin 1985).

Presentation

50 mg/ml   2 ml ampoule.

Half-life

7–10 hours.

Dosage

i.v.: 5–10 mg/kg. Repeat after 1–2 hours if necessary.
Onset of action may take 20–40 minutes.

Caution

Hypersensitivity to infused catecholamines may occur.

Side-effects

May produce marked hypotension and bradycardia.

Contraindications

Should not be used as a primary treatment of ventricular arrhythmias, nor for those induced by digoxin.

DIGOXIN

Action

Acts on the AV node and junctional tissues. The refractory periods of the AV node and His bundle are prolonged, and conduction time increased. Thus, the ventricular response to supraventricular arrhythmias is slowed, and the time for diastolic filling lengthened. However, myocardial excitability (capacity to respond to a stimulus) and automaticity (capacity to initiate beats) is increased. Vagal stimulation also occurs. Digoxin has a positive inotropic effect on the failing myocardium, without an increase in oxygen consumption.

Onset of action

After parenteral administration, occurs within 10 minutes, with a maximum effect at 2 hours.

Use

Atrial fibrillation or atrial flutter. Cardiac failure.

Presentation

250 μg/ml   2 ml ampoule.

Half-life

35–48 hours.

Dosage

i.v.: 0.5–1 mg slowly or by infusion diluted in sodium chloride 0.9% or dextrose 5%.

Caution

Digoxin can itself produce arrhythmias, in a dose related manner (see Section 2: Digoxin). Toxicity can be precipitated by hypokalaemia.

Side-effects

Rapid i.v. injection can produce vasoconstriction or reduce coronary artery blood flow.

Contraindications

It should not be used parenterally if a cardiac glycoside has been given during the preceding 2 weeks. It is contraindicated in supraventricular arrhythmias due to WPW syndrome or digitalis toxicity.

DISOPYRAMIDE

Action

Membrane stabilisation. Reduces automaticity of pacemaker cells and excitability of myocardium. It slows conduction in the bundle of His and increases the atrial and ventricular refractory periods.

Use

Supraventricular and ventricular arrhythmias, and supraventricular arrhythmias associated with WPW syndrome.

Presentation

10 mg/ml   5 ml ampoule.

Half-life

5–8 hours.

Dosage

Loading dose of 2 mg/kg to a maximum of 150 mg slowly over 5 minutes, followed by maintenance infusion of 5–7 μg/kg/min. Add disopyramide 500 mg to 450 ml saline 0.9% or dextrose 5% to give a dilution of 1000 μg/ml.

Caution

May cause torsade de pointes ventricular tachycardia (see Section 4). The maximum recommended dose is 300 mg in the first hour and 800 mg within 24 hours.

Reduce the dose if renal function is impaired.

Side-effects

Hypotension, anticholinergic effects, atrioventricular block.

Contraindications

Heart block, shock and uncompensated cardiac failure.

3

LIGNOCAINE

Action

A class IB membrane-stabilizing agent. It shortens the time taken for repolarization.

Use

First-line drug for prevention and treatment of ventricular tachyarrhythmias. Prophylaxis against arrhythmias during endotracheal intubation.

Presentation

20 mg/ml in 5 ml for i.v. injection.
200 mg/ml in 5 ml for dilution.
Premixed infusions of 1 mg/ml and 2 mg/ml in 500 ml and 1000 ml dextrose 5%.

Half-life

1–2 hours.

Concentration

If dilution is required, add 1 g or 2 g to 500 ml diluent to give 2 mg/ml or 4 mg/ml respectively.

Dose

Prophylaxis against intubation arrhythmias: A bolus of 1 mg/kg before induction.
Treatment of ventricular arrhythmias: bolus of 1 mg/kg (50–100 mg) slowly, followed by a maintenance infusion of 4 mg/min for 30 minutes, 2 mg/min for 2 hours, then 1 mg/min.
Therapeutic blood level 2–5 μg/ml.

Caution

Lignocaine has negative inotropic effects. The toxic and therapeutic levels are close, therefore observe for toxicity. Features include paraesthesia, drowsiness, tinnitus and muscle twitching (see Section 4: Local anaesthetic toxicity). It is metabolized by the liver (70% on the first passage), and therefore dependent on hepatic blood flow. Halothane decreases lignocaine metabolism. Particular caution is needed in liver failure and cardiac failure.

Side-effects

Dizziness, confusion, convulsions, hypotension.

Contraindications

AV block and cardiac decompensation. Malignant hyperpyrexia.

VERAPAMIL

Action

A calcium channel blocker, it reduces AV and SA node action potentials, prolongs AV nodal refractoriness and decreases the ventricular response rate to atrial impulses.

Use

Paroxysmal supraventricular tachycardia. Atrial fibrillation and flutter, by slowing ventricular response rate.

Presentation

2.5 mg/ml   2 ml ampoule.

Half-life

5–7 hours

Dosage

5–10 mg with ECG monitoring. A further 5 mg after 5 minutes.

Caution

Interactions may occur with digoxin or beta blockers. Bradycardia or asystole can be produced by i.v. verapamil. Tachyarrhythmias involving accessory pathways, such as the WPW syndrome, may sometimes be worsened.

Side-effects

Hypotension, bradycardia, heart block, asystole.

Interactions

With beta blockers, digoxin and dantrolene sodium to prolong
conduction time. With class I drugs, to cause myocardial depression. With
volatile agents to produce hypotension or a prolongation of the effects
of muscle relaxants.

3

Contraindications

Bradycardia, sick sinus syndrome, first- and second-degree AV block
and heart failure.

BIBLIOGRAPHY

Carson I W, Lyons S M, Shanks R G 1979 Anti-arrhythmic drugs. British Journal of
    Anaesthesia 51: 659–670
Davies D W, Camm A J 1987 Individual antiarrhythmic drugs. In: Anaesthesia review 4.
    Churchill Livingstone, Edinburgh
Kasten G W, Martin S T 1985 Bupivacaine cardiovascular toxicity. Comparison of
    treatment with bretylium and lidocaine. Anesthesia and Analgesia 64: 911–916
Wellens H J J, Brugada P, Penn O C 1987 The management of preexcitation syndromes.
    Clinical Cardiology 257: 2325–2333

INTRAVENOUS SEDATIVE AND ANAESTHETIC AGENTS

DIAZEPAM

Presentation

5 mg/ml   2 ml ampoule.

Dosage

For premedication: 0.1–0.2 mg/kg.
For sedation: 0.1–0.3 mg/kg over 2–4 minutes.
For cardioversion: 0.2–0.6 mg/kg slowly.

Caution

Dose requirements vary greatly, and the degree of sedation necessary
for procedures such as cardioversion is difficult to judge. It has a long
half-life (20–70 hours) and produces active metabolites
(desmethylflunitrazepam, oxazepam, temazepam). High blood levels recur
at 6–8 hours due to enterohepatic circulation. Cumulation may occur
when it is used for sedation in intensive care.

Side-effects

Respiratory depression.

ETOMIDATE

Presentation

2 mg/ml   10 ml ampoule.

Dosage

Normal induction: 0.3 mg/kg.
High-risk patients: 0.1 mg/kg over 3 minutes.

Length of action

6–8 minutes.

Advantages

Good cardiovascular stability. It rarely causes anaphylactoid reactions.

Side-effects

Muscle movements. Pain on injection. Etomidate may adversely affect pituitary-adrenal function (Owen & Spence 1984). Increased death rates from infection were reported in patients receiving i.v. etomidate for sedation in intensive care. Prolonged infusions were shown to produce reversible suppression of adrenocortical response due to mitochondrial enzyme inhibition. The effect and clinical significance of a single dose of etomidate or an infusion limited to the duration of anaesthesia alone is under debate (Owen & Spence 1984, Yeoman et al 1984, Boidin 1986, Diago et al 1988).

Caution

Do not use as a prolonged continuous infusion.

KETAMINE

Presentation

1% solution   10 mg/ml.
5% solution   50 mg/ml.
10% solution   100 mg/ml.

Induction

    a. i.m. 10 mg/kg
    Onset of action 3–4 minutes.
    Duration 12–25 minutes.
    b. i.v. 1–2 mg/kg over 1 minutes.
    Duration 5–10 minutes.
    Increments of 0.5 mg/kg.

Maintenance infusion

Depends on adjuvants. Reports vary from 20–175 µg/kg/min.

Caution

With repeated anaesthetics, tolerance may occur.

Side-effects

Hypertension, tachycardia, hallucinations, emergence delirium,
increased muscle tone with tonic and clonic movements, and nystagmus.
Can be minimized with a benzodiazepine premedication.

Contraindications

Hypertension, eclampsia or pre-eclampsia.

METHOHEXITONE

Presentation

For preparation of a 1% solution: 100 mg powder for reconstitution in
10 ml; 500 mg powder for reconstitution in 50 ml; 2.5 g powder for
reconstitution in 250 ml.

Induction

1–1.5 mg/kg.

Side-effects

Pain on injection, excitatory phenomena.

Contraindications

Porphyria, barbiturate hypersensitivity, children with epilepsy.

MIDAZOLAM

Presentation

2 mg/ml   5 ml ampoule.
5 mg/ml   2 ml ampoule.

Dosage

Sedation: 0.07 mg/kg.
Induction of anaesthesia:
     With an opiate premedicant   0.2 mg/kg, elderly 0.1 mg/kg.
     Without a premedicant   0.3 mg/kg, elderly 0.2 mg/kg.
The dose should be titrated against the effect.

Half-life

1.5–2.5 hours.
Normally, produces no active metabolites. However, in a few patients the half-life is greatly prolonged, to over 10 hours, possibly due to abnormal metabolites. The ability of critically ill patients to metabolize midazolam may also be impaired, such that cumulation occurs (Shelly et al 1987).

Advantages

Shorter acting than diazepam. No active metabolites.

Side-effects

May cause respiratory and cardiovascular depression with 0.15 mg/kg, or with a lower dose in elderly patients.

PROPOFOL

Presentation

10 mg/ml   20 ml ampoule.

Dosage

For induction: <55 years   2–2.5 mg/kg.
                 >55 years   1.5–2 mg/kg.

Guide to induction doses with propofol (10 mg/ml).

Propofol 10 mg/ml	Body weight (kg)				
	50 kg	60 kg	70 kg	80 kg	90 kg
Fit adults up to 55 yr (2–2.5 mg/kg)	10–12.5 ml	12–15 ml	14–17.5 ml	16–20 ml	18–22.5 ml
Over 55 yr (1.5–2 mg/kg)	7.5–10 ml	9–12 ml	10.5–14 ml	12–16 ml	13.5–18 ml

3

Maintenance

a. Incremental dosage
2.5–5.0 ml (25–50 mg) according to response.
b. Continuous infusion
6–12 mg/kg/h.

Propofol in ml/h by body weight (rate of 6–12 mg/kg/h)

Body weight (kg)	50	60	70	80	90
Propofol (ml/h)	30–60	36–72	42–84	48–96	54–108

Caution

Inject slowly (max. rate 4 ml/10 s). More slowly in less fit patients. Care with elderly patients, or in presence of hypovolaemia, cardiovascular, hepatic or renal impairment.

Side-effects

Pain on injection, hypotension.

THIOPENTONE SODIUM (2.5% soln)

Presentation

2.5 g powder for reconstitution with 100 ml.
500 mg powder for reconstitution with 20 ml.

Dosage

Induction: 4–7 mg/kg.

Caution

Thiopentone should be given with care in hypovolaemia, cardiovascular, respiratory and hepatic disease, muscular dystrophies, myasthenia gravis and myxoedema.

Side-effects

Respiratory depression, reduction in cardiac output, venous dilatation, damage from extravasation or intra-arterial injection.

Contraindications

Porphyria, cardiac tamponade and barbiturate hypersensitivity.

BIBLIOGRAPHY

Boidin M P 1986 Can etomidate cause an Addisonian crisis? Acta Anaesthesiologia Belgica 37: 165–170
Diago M C, Amado J A, Otero M, Lopez-Cordovilla J J 1988 Anti-adrenal action of a subanaesthetic dose of etomidate. Anaesthesia 43: 644–645
Langley M S, Heel B C 1988 Propofol. A review of its pharmacodynamic and pharmacokinetic properties and use as an intravenous anaesthetic. Drugs 35: 334–372
Owen H, Spence AA 1984 Etomidate. British Journal of Anaesthesia 56: 555–557
Shelly M P, Mendel L, Park G R 1987 Failure of critically ill patients to metabolise midazolam. Anaesthesia 42: 619–626
Yeomans P M, Fellows I W, Byrne A J, Selby C 1984 The effect of anaesthetic induction using etomidate upon pituitary-adreno cortical function. British Journal of Anaesthesia 56: 1291–1292

INOTROPIC AGENTS AND SYMPATHOMIMETICS

Inotropic agents and vasoactive drugs (see also Vasodilators) should be given with extreme caution, and their haemodynamic effects monitored closely. Although these notes summarize the general properties of individual drugs, their effect on a particular patient will depend upon the state of the myocardium, the peripheral circulation and the presence of localized myocardial ischaemia (Scallan et al 1979). The action of a drug in a clinical situation may not be the same as that seen experimentally. In the latter, studies may have been done on isolated myocardial preparations, on an intact animal, or on a normal myocardium. By contrast, patients requiring inotropic support often have poor myocardial function and regional ischaemia. In an ischaemic heart, the overall effects of drugs on the coronary circulation, and the balance between myocardial oxygen demand and availability, are crucial.

Unmonitored and uncontrolled polypharmacy can be extremely hazardous. Before drugs are used to treat an apparently failing circulation, haemodynamic monitoring should be instituted. The next step involves restoration of vascular volume, and correction of arterial hypoxia, hypercarbia, acid base and electrolyte disturbances. Drug treatment should only be instituted after this has been completed.

Effects of stimulation at different adrenergic receptor subtypes

Beta₁ receptor

Increases myocardial contractility, cardiac conduction, excitability and automaticity, and produces coronary artery vasodilatation, renin release and relaxation of intestinal muscle.

Beta₂ receptor

Results in peripheral vasodilatation, bronchodilatation, glycogenolysis, uterine relaxation (of the pregnant uterus), insulin secretion, prejunctional release of noradrenaline, and tremor. Increases cardiac automaticity.

Alpha₁ receptor

Produces vasoconstriction, platelet aggregation, bronchoconstriction, pupillary dilatation and insulin suppression.

Alpha₂ receptor

Produces presynaptic inhibition of adrenergic nerve transmission. The distinction between the alpha receptor types is more complex than was previously thought (Langer & Hicks 1984).

ADRENALINE

Action

Stimulation of peripheral alpha, and beta₂ receptors, and cardiac beta₁ receptors. In low doses (0.01–0.05 μg/kg/min), adrenaline produces mainly beta stimulation. With higher doses (0.2–0.35 μg/kg/min), alpha₁ effects predominate to produce peripheral vasoconstriction and a reduction in renal blood flow. Increases in cardiac contractility occur. There is a rise in systolic and initially a fall in diastolic pressure. The pulse rate may rise little, as the cardiac chronotropic effects are opposed by reflex slowing secondary to the rise in blood pressure. When given during anaphylactoid reactions, adrenaline inhibits mast cell degranulation, supports the circulation and causes bronchodilatation.

Use

a. A bolus in cardiopulmonary resuscitation for asystole.
b. A first-line treatment in anaphylactoid reactions.

c. A bolus for initial treatment of anaphylaxis. In view of its brevity of action, an infusion may subsequently be required. After a bolus has been given, or an infusion terminated, secondary hypotension may occur, as the beta effects persist longer than the alpha effects.
d. Treatment of bronchospasm.

Presentation

1 in 1000 (1 mg/ml)	0.5 ml and 1 ml ampoules and disposable syringes.
1 in 10000 (100 μg/ml)	in 10 ml syringe.

Dosage

i.v. bolus: 0.5–1 mg undiluted in an emergency, or preferably give a diluted solution (100 μg/ml) 3–5 μg/kg and repeat if necessary.
Infusion: Dilute 5 mg adrenaline into 500 ml solution to make a 10 μg/ml soln. Give 0.01–0.05 μg/kg/min initially, increasing up to a maximum of 0.5 μg/kg/min. Above this marked vasoconstriction may occur.

Precautions

Should be given preferably via a central vein, because of the risks of peripheral gangrene with a prolonged infusion. Caution in anaphylactoid reactions, when the patient has been receiving halothane, as VF may occur.

Side-effects

Increases in heart rate, cardiac arrhythmias, reduced renal blood flow and peripheral gangrene.

NORADRENALINE

Action

Predominantly alpha$_1$ and alpha$_2$ effects, but with beta$_1$ inotropic effects. Causes peripheral vasoconstriction, thus decreasing blood flow to kidney, liver and muscle. A bradycardia occurs, as the baroreceptor reflex in response to hypertension predominates over the beta inotropic effects.

Use

Its clinical use is limited to the emergency treatment of acute hypotension.

Presentation

2 mg/ml   2 ml and 4 ml ampoules.
200 µg/ml   2 ml ampoule.

Dilution

4 mg noradrenaline in 500 ml dextrose 5% or dextrose/saline solution to give 8 µg/ml.

Dosage

0.05–0.07 µg/kg/min.

Side-effects

Marked vasoconstriction due to the predominant alpha$_1$ stimulation. Necrosis may occur at the site of injection. Serious cardiac arrythmias.

Contraindications

Myocardial infarction, pregnancy and halothane anaesthesia.

ISOPRENALINE

Action

A selective beta$_1$ and beta$_2$ adrenergic agonist. It increases cardiac output and rate, and decreases peripheral vascular resistance by vasodilatation, particularly in skeletal muscle beds. Is a direct coronary artery dilator. It relaxes smooth muscle, especially bronchial.

Use

When circulatory failure and bradycardia are associated. Treatment of bradycardia due to drugs such as beta blockers. The emergency treatment of Stokes–Adams attacks in complete heart block. Sometimes used in torsade de pointes atypical ventricular tachycardia (see Section 4).

Presentation

20 µg/ml   10 ml syringe.
200 µg/ml   1 ml ampoule.
1 mg/ml   2 ml ampoule.

Dilution

4 mg isoprenaline added to 500 ml solution to give 8 µg/ml.

Dosage

0.01–0.1 µg/kg/min.

Precautions

Caution in patients with ischaemic heart disease and when treating torsade de pointes ventricular tachycardia (Martinez 1987).

Side-effects

Tachycardia, cardiac arrhythmias and hypotension. Peripheral vasodilatation reduces aortic diastolic pressure, and coronary artery filling may be impaired.

Contraindications

Acute coronary artery disease and patients prone to VF.

DOPAMINE

Action

A central neurotransmitter and a noradrenaline precursor. Dopamine has a positive inotropic action, with effects on alpha and beta adrenergic, and dopaminergic receptors. At low doses it stimulates renal cortical and mesenteric blood flow. Glomerular flow rate and natriuresis are improved. With medium doses, an increase in cardiac output and arterial pressure occurs. There is also an improvement in coronary artery blood flow. At high dosage, vasoconstrictor effects predominate, secondary to alpha stimulation, and produce an effect similar to that of noradrenaline. Its effects are in part due to release of noradrenaline from endogenous stores.

Use

Myocardial failure, with a need for improved renal blood flow. It may be used in conjunction with a direct-acting vasodilator. Inotropic support for organ donor management.

Presentation

40 mg/ml   5 ml ampoule.
40 mg/ml   5 ml, 10 ml and 20 ml vials.
160 mg/ml   5 ml ampoule.
Intravenous infusions in dextrose 5%:
0.8 mg/ml, 1.6 mg/ml and 3.2 mg/ml.

Dilution

Either use premixed infusion, or add dopamine 800 mg to a 500 ml solution to give a concentration of 1.6 mg/ml.

Diluent

Dextrose 5%, saline 0.9% or Hartmann's solution.

Dosage

1–5 μg/kg/min dilates the renal and mesenteric vascular beds.
5–15 μg/kg/min has a direct inotropic effect on the myocardium with a further increase in urine output.
20–60 μg/kg/min exerts alpha adrenergic stimulation of peripheral blood vessels which further increases blood pressure, but reduces organ perfusion.

Dose chart for infusion of dopamine solution of 1.6 mg/ml

Body weight (kg)	Dose in μg/kg/min									
	1	2	5	10	15	20	30	40	50	60
	Approx infusion rate in ml/h									
40	1	3	7	15	23	30	45	60	75	90
50	2	4	9	19	28	37	56	75	94	112
60	2	5	11	23	35	45	67	90	112	135
70	3	5	13	26	40	52	78	105	131	157
80	3	6	15	30	45	60	90	120	150	180
90	3	7	17	34	51	67	101	135	168	202
100	4	7	19	37	56	75	112	150	187	225
110	4	8	21	41	62	82	124	165	206	247
120	5	9	23	45	68	90	135	180	225	270

Precautions

Hypovolaemia must be corrected, before using dopamine. Careful monitoring is required. In patients with peripheral vascular disease, observe closely for signs of vasoconstriction. A large vein should be used, and extravasation prevented. Patients treated with MAOIs or TCADs will require reduced doses. Dopamine is inactivated by sodium bicarbonate solutions.

Side-effects

Tachycardia and arrhythmias.

Contraindications

Phaeochromocytoma and tachyarrhythmias.

DOBUTAMINE

Action

A synthetic drug with positive inotropic effects. Less tachycardia is produced than by other sympathomimetics, due to primarily beta$_1$ effects. There is a lesser increase in myocardial oxygen demands than with other catecholamines. Its action is complex, probably due to it being a racemic mixture of *d*- and *l*-isomers which have differing effects. Cardiac contractility is increased, but few arrhythmias produced. It has a direct effect on beta$_1$ receptors, and indirect effect on alpha$_1$ and alpha$_2$ receptors. However, there are minimal effects on the peripheral vascular circulation, possibly because the actions of the two isomers on the peripheral vessels counterbalance each other (Colucci et al 1986). Unlike dopamine, it has no dopaminergic effects to produce a selective increase of renal cortical blood flow, although it may increase urine output secondary to improvements in cardiac output. Noradrenaline is not released from endogenous stores.

Use

Inotropic support for low output cardiac failure associated with septic or cardiogenic shock. It can be used in myocardial infarction and cardiomyopathies, and may be particularly appropriate where there is a tachycardia and a high peripheral resistance. Can be used with a dopamine infusion or with vasodilators.

Presentation

250 mg of powder for preparation of an infusion.
An intravenous solution of 12.5 mg/ml in 20 ml for dilution.

Dilution

Add dobutamine 500 mg to 500 ml diluent to give a concentration of 1000 μg/ml.

Diluent

Sodium chloride 0.9%, dextrose 5% or Hartmann's solution. Use within 24 hours of preparation.

Dosage

2.5–10 μg/kg/min. Rarely, up to 40 μg/kg/min.

Dosage chart for a dobutamine solution of 1000 µg/ml

Body weight (kg)	Dose in µg/kg/min			
	2.5	5.0	7.5	10.0
	Approx infusion rate in ml/h			
40	6	12	18	24
50	7	15	22	30
60	9	18	27	36
70	10	21	31	42
80	12	24	36	48
90	13	27	40	54
100	15	30	45	60
110	16	33	49	66
120	18	36	54	72

3

Precautions

Correct hypovolaemia first. Close monitoring is required. In acute myocardial infarction, tachycardia may increase ischaemia. Care should be taken with use in hypertrophic subaortic stenosis, where outlet obstruction may be worsened.

Side-effects

May increase the ventricular rate in patients with atrial fibrillation.

Contraindications

Marked obstruction to cardiac ejection.

SALBUTAMOL

Action

A selective beta$_2$ adrenergic receptor agonist with minimal beta$_1$ effects. Predominantly beta effects on the bronchi and uterus. Directly dilates the coronary vessels. In high doses the vasodilator effects decrease both systemic vascular resistance and left ventricular filling pressure. An improvement in cardiac output can occur in patients with heart failure.

Use

A bronchodilator for patients with asthma. Suppression of premature labour. Occasionally used for treatment of heart failure, or acute circulatory failure where there is a high peripheral resistance.

Presentation

50 μg/ml   5 ml ampoule.
500 μg/ml   1 ml ampoule.
1 mg/ml   5 ml ampoule.

Dilution

Infusion: add salbutamol 5 mg to 500 ml diluent to give 10 μg/ml.

Diluent

Sodium chloride 0.9% or dextrose 5%.

Dosage

i.v.: 250 μg (4 μg/kg) slowly. Repeat if necessary.
Infusion: 0.05–0.5 μg/kg/min. For status asthmaticus.

Precautions

When given for acute asthma, oxygen should be administered at the same time. Salbutamol may produce ketoacidosis and an increase in blood glucose in diabetics, particularly those receiving steroids.

Side-effects

Mild hypotension and tachycardia. Pulmonary oedema has been associated with the use of salbutamol for suppression of labour (see Section 1: Pulmonary oedema).

Contraindications

When premature labour is associated with pre-eclamptic toxaemia or antepartum haemorrhage.

PHENYLEPHRINE

Action

A selective direct-acting alpha$_1$ agonist producing a rise in blood pressure due to constriction of most vascular beds, and a reflex bradycardia. Coronary blood flow is increased, but there is pulmonary vasoconstriction and an increase in PAP. A single i.v. dose lasts for about 20 minutes. It has a mild beta$_2$ bronchodilator effect.

Use

May be used for its pressor action in combination with an inotrope after cardiac surgery. Can be used in the treatment of hypotension due to spinal anaesthesia, if the heart rate is above 90/min. The accompanying reduction in placental blood flow makes it not appropriate for use in obstetrics. It is useful in conditions where the heart is normal, but the peripheral circulation disturbed, such as in autonomic dysfunction due to the Shy–Drager syndrome. By utilizing the reflex bradycardia, it has been used to treat tachycardia in WPW syndrome. Phenylephrine provides an alternative to adrenaline as a local vasoconstrictor for LA infiltration.

Presentation

10 mg/ml   1 ml ampoule.

Dilution

i.v. use: Dilute to 10 ml.
Infusion: add phenylephrine 10 mg to 500 ml solution to give 20 μg/ml.

Diluent

Dextrose 5%.

Dosage

i.v.: a single dose of 0.1–0.5 mg slowly each 15 minutes.
Infusion: 0.1–0.5 μg/kg/min, adjusted according to response.

Precautions

Care in patients with hypertension. Phenylephrine sensitizes the heart to the effects of catecholamines.

Side-effects

Hypertension and bradycardia.

Contraindications

Severe coronary artery disease.

METARAMINOL

Action

A sympathomimetic similar to noradrenaline, with indirect and direct effects. It has alpha$_1$ adrenergic stimulating properties, but with some beta effects on cardiac contractility. Systolic and diastolic blood pressure, and the force of myocardial contraction are increased. There may be a reflex bradycardia. If this is treated with atropine, marked increases in cardiac output can occur.

Onset of action 1–2 minutes.
Maximum effect at 10 minutes.
Duration of action, 20–80 minutes.

Use

Treatment of acute hypotension due to loss of vasoconstrictor tone, for example, during spinal anaesthesia. It may be useful as a temporizing measure while fluid replacement is organized.

Presentation

10 mg/ml   1 ml ampoule.

Dilution

15–100 mg added to 500 ml diluent to give 30–200 μg/ml.

Diluent

Sodium chloride 0.9% or dextrose 5%. Use within 24 hours.

Dosage

An undiluted i.v. injection should not be given, unless life saving, in which case 0.05–0.5 ml should be given using a 1 ml syringe for accuracy. Alternatively 10 mg can be diluted to 10 ml and 0.5–5 ml given.
Infusion: 30–200 μg/ml. Adjust according to the effect.

Precautions

Select a large vein, especially in patients with vascular disease. Use with caution in patients on digoxin, and in those with hypertension and coronary artery disease.

Side-effects

Reduced renal blood flow. Reflex bradycardia. Pulmonary vasoconstriction. Tissue necrosis.

Contraindications

Contraindicated with halothane anaesthesia or MAOIs.

3

METHOXAMINE

Action

A direct-acting alpha$_1$ agonist, similar to phenylephrine. Produces an increase in blood pressure and a reflex bradycardia. It has beta blocking effects, which reduces the incidence of ventricular arrhythmias. Peripheral vasoconstriction results in increased peripheral resistance, and a decrease in renal blood flow. Its effect lasts for 60–90 minutes.

Use

Acute treatment of hypotension, due to vasodilatation, caused by hypotensive agents. Hypotension due to spinal anaesthesia, particularly if the pulse rate is above 90/min (but not in obstetrics due to decrease in uterine blood flow). It is the drug of choice for correcting peripheral vasodilatation in hypertrophic cardiomyopathy. It has occasionally been used for treatment of SVT, although more suitable drugs are now available.

Presentation

20 mg/ml   1 ml ampoule.

Dosage

i.v.: 2–5 mg at a rate not exceeding 1 mg/min

Precautions

Hypertension, thyrotoxicosis and vascular disease.

Side-effects

Bradycardia, hypertension, renal artery constriction and reduced GFR.

Contraindications

Severe coronary artery disease and severe hypertension. Patients receiving MAOIs.

3

EPHEDRINE

Action

A mixed direct- and indirect acting alpha and beta adrenergic stimulator, which releases catecholamines at receptor sites and delays their breakdown. It has inotropic and chronotropic effects, and causes venous constriction, thus improving venous return. There is no arteriolar constriction, and peripheral resistance is not usually increased. It raises systolic blood pressure and increases pulse pressure. It causes bronchodilatation and CNS stimulation. Duration of action 30–40 minutes. Its effects are similar to those of adrenaline, but of longer duration because it is not broken down by catechol-*O*-methyltransferase.

Use

Treatment of hypotension due to spinal and epidural anaesthesia. It is the drug of choice in obstetrics, as it is not a pure alpha agonist and does not decrease uterine blood flow.

Presentation

30 mg/ml   1 ml ampoule.

Dosage

i.v.: 3 mg. Repeat if necessary.

Cautions

Tachyphylaxis occurs.

Side-effects

Tachycardia and increase in myocardial irritability.

Contraindications

Severe coronary artery disease.

BIBLIOGRAPHY

Colucci W S, Wright R F, Braunwald E 1986 New positive inotropic agents in the treatment of congestive heart failure. New England Journal of Medicine 314: 290–299
Langer S Z, Hicks P E 1984 Physiology of the sympathetic nerve endings. British Journal of Anaesthesia 56: 689–700
Martinez R 1987 Torsade de pointes: atypical rhythm, atypical treatment. Annals of Emergency Medicine 16: 878–884

Scallan M J H, Gothard J W W, Branthwaite M A 1979 Inotropic agents. British Journal of
   Anaesthesia 51: 649–658
Smith L D R, Oldershaw P J 1984 Inotropic and vasopressor agents. British Journal of
   Anaesthesia 56: 767–780

LOCAL ANAESTHETIC INFORMATION
(see also Section 4: LOCAL ANAESTHETIC TOXICITY)

3

AMETHOCAINE

A potent ester type of local anaesthetic, only used topically in
ophthalmic surgery in the UK. In North America it is used for spinal
anaesthesia.

Maximum safe dose

1.5 mg/kg.

BENZOCAINE

Low potency and low toxicity. Used only topically in the UK.

Presentation

Benzocaine lozenge 10 mg and compound benzocaine lozenge 100 mg.

Use

To provide topical anaesthesia for the mouth and tongue prior to
bronchoscopy or endoscopy.

BUPIVACAINE

A long-acting amide type of local anaesthetic. The margin between CNS
and cardiac toxicity is less than with lignocaine. Pregnant patients seem to
be more susceptible.

For further discussion see Section 4: Local anaesthetic toxicity.

Presentation

a. A heavy solution for spinal anaesthesia: bupivacaine 0.5% (5
mg/ml) and glucose 80 mg/ml in 4 ml ampoules.
b. Bupivacaine plain. 0.25% (2.5 mg/ml) in a 10 ml ampoule.
c. Bupivacaine plain. 0.5% (5 mg/ml) in a 10 ml ampoule.
d. Bupivacaine plain. 0.75% (7.5 mg/ml) in a 10 ml ampoule.

e. Bupivacaine 0.25% (2.5 mg/ml) with adrenaline 1 in 200 000 (5 μg/ml) in a 10 ml ampoule.
f. Bupivacaine 0.5% (5 mg/ml) with adrenaline 1 in 2000 000 (5 μg/ml) in a 10 ml ampoule.

Maximum safe dose

Up to 2 mg/kg of the plain solution in any 4-hour period (30 ml of 0.5%, or 60 ml of 0.25%), or 3 mg/kg with adrenaline.

Dosages in spinal anaesthesia
Spinal anaesthesia with bupivacaine 0.5% in 8% dextrose (heavy)

	Sitting	Supine	Sitting	Supine
	3 ml		4 ml	
Onset to max effect (min)	15–20	15–20	15–20	15–20
Max spread (mean)	T8–10	T4–5	T6–8	T4–5
Duration thoracic (h)	1–1.5	2	1.5–2	2–2.5
Duration lumbar (h)	4	3.5	4.5	4

Toxicity and treatment

See Section 4: Local anaesthetic toxicity.

Contraindications

a. Bupivacaine should not be used for intravenous regional anaesthesia.
b. Bupivacaine 0.75% is not recommended for use in obstetric anaesthesia.

CHLOROPROCAINE

An ester with a rapid onset of action and low toxicity. Not available in the UK but used in North America.

COCAINE

A toxic local anaesthetic agent with vasoconstrictor properties. Used topically in ENT surgery, mainly for these vasoconstrictor effects. When cocaine paste or cocaine solutions are used for nasal preparation, it is difficult to estimate the dose actually given by the surgeon. It is not uncommon for signs of mild toxicity to be seen during anaesthesia.

Maximum safe dose

Recommendations for topical analgesia vary. Nasal application should probably be limited to 1.5 mg/kg.

Toxicity

Myocardial toxicity, respiratory depression, ventricular fibrillation, convulsions, coma and death (see Section 1: Cocaine abuse).

ETIDOCAINE

An amide derivative of lignocaine. Its action has a fast onset and lasts longer than lignocaine. Motor effects are more pronounced than sensory. Used in North America, but not generally in the UK at present.

Maximum safe dose

4 mg/kg plain solution.

LIGNOCAINE

An amide-linked local anaesthetic, metabolized in the liver. Its toxicity is reduced, and its action is prolonged, by adding adrenaline to the solution. It is also used for the treatment and prophylaxis of ventricular arrhythmias.

Presentation

Lignocaine 0.5% (5 mg/ml) in 10 ml, 20 ml and 50 ml ampoules.
Lignocaine 1.0% (10 mg/ml) in 2 ml, 10 ml, 20 ml and 50 ml ampoules.
Lignocaine 1.5% (15 mg/ml) for epidural use in a 25 ml ampoule.
Lignocaine 0.5% with adrenaline 1 in 200 000 (5 μg/ml) in a 50 ml vial.
Lignocaine 1% with adrenaline 1 in 200 000 (5 μg/ml) in 10 ml, 20 ml and 50 ml vials.
Lignocaine 2% (20 mg/ml) in 5 ml, 20 ml and 50 ml vials.
Lignocaine 2% with adrenaline 1 in 200 000 (5 μg/ml) in 20 ml and 50 ml vials.

Maximum safe dose

Lignocaine plain: 3 mg/kg.
Lignocaine with adrenaline: 7 mg/kg.

| | Lignocaine concentration | | | | |
	0.5%	1%	1.5%	2%	4%
			Maximum safe dose		
Plain:	40 ml	20 ml	14 ml	10 ml	4 ml
With adrenaline:	100 ml	50 ml	30 ml	25 ml	

Dosage for treatment of arrhythmias

See Antiarrhythmics.

Toxicity

See Section 4: Local anaesthetic toxicity.

MEPIVACAINE

An amide type of local anaesthetic with a profile similar to that of lignocaine. Fast onset with intermediate potency and duration of action. Not available in the UK.

Maximum safe dose

5 mg/kg.

PRILOCAINE

An amide type of local anaesthetic, similar in profile to lignocaine, but with a slightly longer duration of action, and lower toxicity. It has no vasodilator action.

Presentation

Prilocaine 0.5% (5 mg/ml) in 20 ml and 50 ml vials.
Prilocaine 1.0% (10 mg/ml) in 20 ml and 50 ml vials.
Prilocaine 0.5% preservative free, single dose, 50 ml vial (also prilocaine 3% with felypressin, and prilocaine 4%, both for dental use)

Maximum safe dose

Prilocaine plain: 5–6 mg/kg.
Prilocaine with adrenaline: 8 mg/kg.

Toxicity

Doses above 600 mg may cause methaemoglobinaemia (see Section 1: Methaemoglobinaemia).

PROCAINE

An ester type of local anaesthetic of slow onset of action, and short duration, rarely used in the UK. In malignant hyperpyrexia susceptible (MHS) patients, procaine may be useful for local anaesthetic infiltration. It may also be used to treat arrhythmias during an MH episode. It was originally used for the treatment of acute episodes of MH, prior to the introduction of dantrolene. However, although animal models and in vitro experiments showed inhibition of MH contractures with procaine, it was ineffective once the contractures were established. Procaine was also ineffective in porcine models, when treatment with dantrolene was effective. Safe clinical doses may not produce sufficient tissue concentrations.

Presentation

Procaine 2% (20 mg/ml)   2 ml ampoule

Maximum safe dose

15 mg/kg (up to 1 g, or procaine 0.5%, 200 ml).

MUSCLE RELAXANTS

ALCURONIUM

Presentation

5 mg/ml   2 ml ampoule.

Dosage

Adults: 0.2–0.3 mg/kg initial; 0.05 mg/kg repeat.
Children: 0.125–0.2 mg/kg initial; 0.05 mg/kg repeat.

ATRACURIUM

Atracurium is metabolized by Hofmann degradation and alkaline ester hydrolysis, so its elimination half-life is independent of hepatic and renal function. Laudanosine, a metabolite of atracurium, is a CNS stimulant. Increased plasma laudanosine concentrations have been found to occur in renal failure, but no gross evidence of CNS stimulation was seen (Fahey et al 1985).

Presentation

10 mg/ml   2.5 ml and 5 ml ampoules.

Dosage

Adult: 0.3–0.6 mg/kg, repeat doses of 0.1–0.2 mg/kg.
Children (over the age of 1 month): 0.5 mg/kg, repeat doses of 0.1–0.2 mg/kg.

Continuous infusion

Use an initial paralysing dose, followed by an infusion of 0.005–0.01 mg/kg/min (0.3–0.6 mg/kg/h).

Diluent

Sodium chloride 0.9%, is the most suitable, and can be used for 24 hours. Spontaneous degradation occurs more readily when other solutions are used for dilution.

Preparation of a solution of 5 mg/ml

For use in a syringe pump make up a solution of 5 mg/ml, by diluting the volume of atracurium required with an equal volume of the diluent.

Atracurium infusion dosage chart (5 mg/ml)

Body weight (kg)	Dosage in mg/kg/h			
	0.3	0.4	0.5	0.6
	Infusion rate in ml/hr			
10 kg	0.6	0.8	1.0	1.2
20 kg	1.2	1.6	2.0	2.4
30 kg	1.8	2.4	3.0	3.6
40 kg	2.4	3.2	4.0	4.8
50 kg	3.0	4.0	5.0	6.0
60 kg	3.6	4.8	6.0	7.2
70 kg	4.2	5.6	7.0	8.4
80 kg	4.8	6.4	8.0	9.6
90 kg	5.4	7.2	9.0	10.8
100 kg	6.0	8.0	10.0	12.0

PANCURONIUM

Presentation

2 mg/ml   2 ml ampoule

Dosage

Adult: 0.05–0.1 mg/kg, repeat doses of 0.01–0.02 mg/kg.
Child: 0.06–0.1 mg/kg, repeat doses of 0.01–0.02 mg/kg.
Neonate: 0.03–0.04 mg/kg, repeat doses of 0.01–0.02 mg/kg.

Caution

The elimination half-life is prolonged in renal failure.

d-TUBOCURARINE

Presentation

10 mg/ml   1.5 ml ampoule.

Dosage

Adult: 0.3–0.5 mg/kg, repeat doses of 0.1 mg/kg.
Child: 0.3–0.5 mg/kg, repeat doses of 0.1 mg/kg.
Neonate: 0.25 mg/kg, repeat doses of 0.1 mg/kg.
Premature: 0.125 mg/kg, repeat doses of 0.05 mg/kg.

Caution

The elimination half-life is prolonged in renal failure.

VECURONIUM

Presentation

10 mg for dilution in 5 ml (2 mg/ml).

Dosage

Adult: 0.08–0.1 mg/kg, repeat doses of 0.03–0.05 mg/kg.
Child: 0.08–0.1 mg/kg, repeat doses of 0.03–0.05 mg/kg.
Infusion: 0.05–0.08 mg/kg/h.

Caution

The elimination half-life is slightly prolonged in renal failure.
Bradycardia may occur, especially when used with fentanyl.

BIBLIOGRAPHY

Fahey M R, Rupp S M, Canfell C et al 1985 Effect of renal failure on laudanosine
    excretion in man. British Journal of Anaesthesia 57: 1049–1051

PLASMA REPLACEMENT AND PLASMA SUBSTITUTES

DEXTRAN 70 in 0.9% saline

Use

Short-term volume expansion. Prophylaxis against DVT.

Type

Glucose polymer.

Content

Dextran 60 g/l, sodium 154 mmol/l, chloride 154 mmol/l.

Colloid osmotic pressure

268 mmH$_2$O

Molecular weight

Number average 35 200, weight average 70 000.

Half-life

12 hours.

Haemostasis

Infusions of >20 ml/kg may reduce factor VIII levels. Dextran interferes with cross-matching.

Reactions

In a prospective study, dextran 70 was associated with an incidence of anaphylactoid reactions of 0.069% (Ring & Messmer 1977). Another prospective study involving its use at Caesarean section and in major gynaecology surgery, suggested that the risk of dextran 70 treatment exceeded the risks of thromboembolism (Paull 1987). Dextran reactions, even mild ones, are often associated with a marked metabolic acidosis (Ljungstrom & Renck 1987).

Caution

A maximum of 2.5 l/day. Care in renal insufficiency and cardiac failure.

GELOFUSINE

Use

Short-term volume expansion

Type

Succinyl gelatin

Content

Gelatin 40 g/l, sodium 154 mmol/l, chloride 125 mmol/l, potassium <0.4 mmol/l, calcium <0.4 mmol/l.

Colloid osmotic pressure

465 mmH$_2$O.

Molecular weight

Number average 22 600, weight average 35 000.

Half-life

4 hours.

Haemostasis

Only a dilutional effect. Does not interfere with grouping and cross-matching.

Reactions

A low incidence.

HAEMACCEL

Use

Short-term volume expansion.

Type

A urea-linked gelatin, polygeline.

Content

Polygeline 35 g/l, sodium 145 mmol/l, chloride 145 mmol/l, potassium 5.1 mmol/l, calcium 6.25 mmol/l.

Colloid osmotic pressure

350–390 mmH$_2$O.

Molecular weight

Number average 24 500, weight average 35 000.

Half-life

5 hours.

Haemostasis

Only a dilutional effect. Does not interfere with grouping and cross-matching.

Reactions

Low, but twice the incidence of that of succinylated gelatin. Fatalities have been reported (Barratt & Purcell 1988).

Caution

The high calcium content may cause clotting of citrated blood. Wash through with normal saline, when given before or after blood. Take care with patients on digoxin. Infusion limit of 2 litres in 24 hours.

HESPAN (hetastarch)

Use

Short-term volume expansion.

Content

Hetastarch 60 g/l, sodium 154 mmol/l, chloride 154 mmol/l.

Type

6% solution of hydroxyethyl starch in 0.9% saline.

Colloid osmotic pressure

Equivalent to 5% albumin.

Molecular weight

Number average 70 000, weight average 450 000.

Half-life

17 days, 30% taken up by reticuloendothelial system.

Reactions

Few, slightly higher than gelofusine and dextran 70.

Cautions

Renal failure or cardiac failure. Maximum recommended dose, 1.5 l/day.

PLASMA PROTEIN FRACTION

Use

Hypoproteinaemia after burns, replacement fluid in plasma exchange, pump priming on CPB, and haemorrhagic shock.

Content

Human serum albumin 43–50 g/l, sodium and chloride variable, but approx 140 mmol/l, potassium <2 mmol/l.

Molecular weight

Number average 69 000, weight average 69 000.

Haemostasis

No effect. Dilutional with large volumes.

Reactions

0.014% incidence (Ring & Messmer 1977). Incidence, between that of gelofusine and hetastarch.

Caution

Severe anaemia and cardiac failure.

SALT-POOR ALBUMIN SOLUTION

Use

Severe hypoproteinaemia due to hepatic, renal and gastrointestinal disease and severe pre-eclamptic toxaemia. It is active oncotically. Within 15 minutes of administration, three times the volume of fluid given is drawn from the tissues into the circulation.

Content

Human serum albumin 200 g/l, sodium 130 mmol/l, potassium <1 mmol/l.

Presentation

20% (20 g/100 ml) in 100 ml vial.

Dosage

For treatment of hypoproteinaemia, 200–300 ml, at a rate not exceeding 100 ml in 30–45 minutes. In cases of hypertension or cardiac insufficiency, dilute with 200 ml dextrose 10% and give at 100 ml/h.

Precautions

Do not use when the patient is dehydrated. In hypovolaemia, additional fluid must be given. Watch for pulmonary oedema.

BIBLIOGRAPHY

Barratt S, Purcell G J 1988 Refractory bronchospasm following 'Haemaccel' infusion and bupivacaine epidural anaesthesia. Anaesthesia and Intensive Care 16: 208–211
Brozovic B 1986 Blood and blood products. Hospital Update 12: 445–458
Drugs and Therapeutics Bulletin 1987 Plasma substitutes: the choice during surgery and intensive care. 25: 37–39
Ljungstrom K–G, Renck H 1987 Metabolic acidosis in dextran-induced anaphylactic reactions. Acta Anaesthesiologica Scandinavica 31: 157–160
Paull J 1987 A prospective study of dextran-induced anaphylactoid reactions in 5745 patients. Anaesthesia and Intensive Care 15: 163–167
Ring J, Messmer K 1977 Incidence and severity of anaphylactoid reactions to colloid volume substitutes. Lancet 1: 466–469
Rudowski W J 1980 Evaluation of modern plasma expanders and blood substitutes. British Journal of Hospital Medicine 23: 389–399
Saddler J M, Horsey P J 1987 The new generation gelatins. Anaesthesia 42: 998–1004

VASODILATORS

DIAZOXIDE

Action

A direct acting vasodilator, predominantly arteriolar. The resultant hypotension and decrease in peripheral vascular resistance induces a tachycardia, which may be prevented by the concomitant use of beta blockers. There is an increase in myocardial oxygen consumption.

Use

Acute severe hypertension which is refractory to other therapy, or control of blood pressure in pre-eclampsia during labour.

Onset of action

3–5 minutes.

Duration of action

4–18 hours.

Presentation

300 mg in 20 ml (15 mg/ml).

Dosage

i.v.: 150–300 mg given over 1 minute in a supine patient.
Can be repeated up to three times in 24 hours.

Precautions

Monitor blood sugar levels.

Side-effects

Hyperglycaemia – each injection causing a transient rise in the blood
sugar of 10%. During labour it may cause a delay in the second stage.
Tachycardia.

Contraindications

Severe coronary artery disease or left ventricular failure.

HYDRALAZINE

Action

A direct-acting vasodilator, predominantly arteriolar. Hypotension and a
fall in peripheral vascular resistance induces a tachycardia, which may be
prevented by the concomitant use of beta blockers. There is an increase
in myocardial oxygen consumption.

Use

Acute hypertension, control of blood pressure in pre-eclampsia, during
labour.

Onset of action

3–6 minutes.

Duration of action

3–8 hours.

Presentation

20 mg in powder form for dilution.

Dilution

i.v. use: dissolve in 1 ml of water, then further dilute with 10 ml 0.9% sodium chloride and give slowly over 20 minutes. Repeat after 30 minutes if necessary.
Infusion: dissolve 20 mg powder in 1 ml water, then add to 500 ml 0.9% sodium chloride.

Precautions

In hepatic or renal insufficiency.

Side-effects

Tachycardia, hypotension, flushing.

Contraindications

Myocardial ischaemia or left ventricular failure. Constrictive pericarditis.

ISOSORBIDE DINITRATE

Action

A venous and arterial vasodilator, which reduces both preload and afterload.

Use

Treatment of left ventricular failure or severe angina.

Presentation

Isosorbide dinitrate as 1 mg/ml (0.1%), in 10 ml, 50 ml and 100 ml volumes.

Dilution

Remove from the diluent an equivalent volume prior to the addition of the undiluted isosorbide dinitrate. To prepare 500 ml of a 100 μg/ml solution, withdraw and discard 50 ml from the original 500 ml of diluent and then add isosorbide dinitrate 50 mg (50 ml).

Diluent

Saline 0.9% or dextrose 5%. The resulting solution is compatible with glass and polyethylene infusion packs (Boots Polyfusor) or syringes, and polyethylene tubing.

Infusion rate

Isosorbide dinitrate 0.5–2.0 μg/kg/min.

Precautions

Close monitoring of pulse and blood pressure is required. Due to loss of activity, the drug is incompatible with the usual infusion bags and administration sets made of PVC.

Contraindications

Cardiogenic shock, hypotension, hypovolaemia, severe anaemia, head injury and cerebral haemorrhage.

NITROGLYCERIN (glyceryl trinitrate) infusion

Action

A direct venous and arterial vasodilator, with venous dilatation predominating. The main effect is on capacitance vessels, so it decreases preload to a much lesser extent than afterload. Myocardial work load and oxygen consumption are reduced. Improvement of coronary artery flow occurs, which appears to be independent of the state of the arteries. It is a pulmonary vasodilator.

Use

Controlled hypotension during surgery, acute hypertensive crisis, critical myocardial ischaemia producing unstable angina and left ventricular failure. Control of hypertensive response to intubation in severe pre-eclampsia (Hood et al 1985).

Presentation

Nitrocine: 1 mg/ml (0.1%), in 10 ml ampoules, 50 ml bottle.
Nitronal: 1 mg/ml, 5 ml and 25 ml ampoules and 50 ml vials.
Nitroglycerin: 5 mg/ml (0.5%) in 5 ml and 10 ml vials.

Dilution

Exchange the required volume of nitroglycerin with an equal volume of the diluent, e.g. 50 mg nitroglycerin (1 mg/ml soln) into 450 ml of diluent to give 100 μg/ml.

Diluent

Dextrose 5% or 0.9% sodium chloride. Compatible with glass bottles and polyethylene infusion packs.

Infusion rate

The rate required depends upon the type of infusion bag and giving set used. Sets made from PVC absorb a certain quantity of nitroglycerin and higher doses may be required than those needed when low absorption polyethylene sets are used. There is therefore a range of recommended of dosages, from both the literature and the manufacturers.
The general principles are:

a. The dose required usually ranges from 5 μg/min to 200 μg/min.

b. Close monitoring of the patient's response is required.

c. With low absorption polyethylene sets, or glass or plastic syringes, start at a rate of 5 μg/min. With PVC sets an initial rate would be 10 μg/min.

d. Increments of 5–10 μg/min should be made at 3–5-minute intervals. When a response is seen, the dose increase should be reduced and the interval between increments increased.

e. Higher doses may be needed for controlled hypotension during surgery, than for treatment of heart failure or unstable angina.

Conversion table for nitroglycerin, from μg/min to ml/h

Nitroglycerin concentration (μg/ml)				
100	200	300	400	Infusion (ml/h)
	Required dosage in μg/min			
5	10	15	20	3
10	20	30	40	6
20	40	60	80	12
30	60	90	120	18
40	80	120	160	24
50	100	150	200	30
60	120	180	240	36
70	140	210	280	42
80	160	240	320	48
90	180	270	360	54
100	200	300	400	60
110	220	330	440	66
120	240	360	480	72
130	260	390	520	78
140	280	420	560	84
150	300	450	600	90

Precautions

If the infusion apparatus is made of PVC, due to absorption, losses of up to 40% of the dose of nitroglycerin may occur. Pulse and blood pressure should be monitored closely to assess the patient's response. An initial rise in intracranial pressure occurs, especially in the presence of intracranial hypertension.

Contraindications

Hypovolaemia or severe hypotension, anaemia, cerebral haemorrhage and nitrate hypersensitivity.

SODIUM NITROPRUSSIDE

Action

a. Cardiovascular
A direct-acting vascular smooth muscle relaxant. Blood pressure is lowered by producing arterial and venous vasodilatation. The hypotension may be accompanied by a baroreceptor-induced tachycardia, particularly in young patients. Cardiac output may be unchanged or increased. In patients with heart failure, a decrease in preload and afterload improves cardiac output. Increased coronary blood flow may occur, with an improvement in myocardial oxygenation, or it may be unchanged due to a reduction in myocardial metabolic requirements. If, however, there is severe coronary artery disease, a 'steal' phenomenon may occur, in which blood flow in normal vessels is increased, but at the expense of those in ischaemic areas. Pulmonary artery and right atrial pressures are also reduced. Sodium nitroprusside impairs the pulmonary vascular response to hypoxia, so increased inspired oxygen concentrations are required (D'Oliveira et al 1981).

b. Cerebrovascular
Dilatation of cerebral vessels occurs, with an increase in cerebral blood flow. This shifts cerebral autoregulation to the left, and permits lower mean arterial pressures to be used more safely. However, the resultant increase in cerebral blood volume and pressure is undesirable in the presence of a raised intracranial pressure. As with the coronary vessels, cerebral 'steal' may compromise focal ischaemic areas of the brain.

c. Metabolic
Sodium nitroprusside is short acting, as a result of rapid conversion first to cyanide and then thiocyanate. If the maximum safe dose is exceeded, cyanide or thiocyanate toxicity can occur. Some nitroprusside is broken down within the RBC to produce an unstable nitroprusside. Five cyanide ions are released. One combines with methaemoglobin to form cyanmethaemoglobin. Other ions are broken down by rhodanase, a mitochondrial enzyme system present in the liver and kidneys. Some cyanide may also inactivate cytochrome oxidase, causing tissue cyanide toxicity. Thiocyanate has a long half-

life, and is itself toxic. Certain patients are resistant to the effects of sodium nitroprusside, and this state has been associated with the formation of free cyanide. It is in this group of patients that toxicity is most likely to occur.

Use

a. Production of deliberate hypotension during surgery.
b. Situations where there is a raised venous pressure and a high peripheral resistance. Reduction in afterload after myocardial infarction or severe cardiac failure.
c. Control of a hypertensive crisis in an untreated patient or control of hypertension in a patient already on antihypertensives.

Presentation

50 mg powder for reconstitution with 2 ml of dextrose solution provided.

Dilution

This solution should be then diluted in dextrose 5%, sodium chloride 0.9% or Hartmann's solution, either 500 ml or 1000 ml, to give solutions of 100 μg/ml and 50 μg/ml respectively.

Infusion rate

A starting rate of 0.3–1.0 μg/kg/min. Onset of action is in 2–5 minutes, the effect wearing off rapidly once the infusion is stopped. In acute situations, such as the induction of hypotension during surgery, a maximum of 1.5 μg/kg/min is recommended. For heart failure this limit is increased to 6 μg/kg/min and for a hypertensive crisis, to 8 μg/kg/min.

Maximum safe dose

The recommended dose for hypotensive anaesthesia is a total dose not exceeding 1.5 mg/kg.

For longer term use in the ITU, the onset of cyanide toxicity may be suggested by the development of a metabolic acidosis, raised lactate and lactate/pyruvate ratios, and a raised mixed venous blood content (Tinker & Michenfelder 1976).

Prophylactic treatment has been advised when sodium nitroprusside is being given close to its maximum safe dose. Either sodium thiosulphate or hydroxocobalamin can be used (Krapez et al 1981, Ivankovich et al 1982).

Precautions

Protect the solution from light by wrapping in a material such as aluminium foil. If the colour exceeds a faint brown tint, or becomes bluish, it should not be used. Care should be taken not to exceed the maximum safe dose. If during surgery the patient appears resistant to the hypotensive effect, it is safer to use an alternative technique.

3

Toxic effects

If the administration of nitroprusside overloads the capacity of the metabolic system, toxicity occurs. Should plasma cyanide concentration rise above 8 μg/dl, there may be tachycardia and arrhythmias, sweating, hyperventilation and severe metabolic acidosis. Marked hypotension and a failure of the blood pressure to return to normal within 2–10 minutes of stopping the infusion, suggests toxicity. Deaths have been reported, all of which involved large doses of nitroprusside, often accompanied by an apparent resistance to its action. In the treatment of cardiac failure, if the duration of the infusion exceeds 3 days, plasma thiocyanate levels should be monitored (Tinker & Michenfelder).

Methaemoglobinaemia may occasionally produce cyanosis.

Treatment of overdosage

Stop the infusion. Give sodium thiosulphate 25 ml of 50% solution (12.5 g) in dextrose 5%, 50 ml over 10 minutes.

Contraindications

Patients with compensatory hypertension such as coarctation of the aorta. Liver function impairment or malnutrition.

BIBLIOGRAPHY

D'Oliveira M, Sykes M K, Chakrabarti M K, Orchard C, Keslin J 1981 Depression of hypoxic pulmonary vasoconstriction by sodium nitroprusside and nitroglycerine. British Journal of Anaesthesia 53: 11–18
Hood D D, Dewan D M, James F M, Floyd H M, Bogard T D 1985 The use of nitroglycerine in preventing the hypertensive response to tracheal intubation in severe pre-eclampsia. Anesthesiology 63: 329–332
Ivankovich A D, Braverman B, Shulman M, Klowden A J 1982 Prevention of nitroprusside toxicity with thiosulphate in dogs. Anesthesia and Analgesia 61: 120–126
Krapez J R, Vesey C J, Adams L, Cole P V 1981 Effects of cyanide antidotes used with sodium nitroprusside infusions; sodium thiosulphate and hydroxocobalamin given prophylactically to dogs. British Journal of Anaesthesia 53: 793–803
Tinker J H, Michenfelder J D 1976 Sodium nitroprusside. Anesthesiology 45: 340–354

4

Perioperative Emergency Conditions

ADDISONIAN CRISIS OR ACUTE ADRENOCORTICAL INSUFFICIENCY

(see also Section 1)

4

An extremely rare cause of perioperative cardiovascular collapse. It may be due to primary adrenocortical disease or secondary to withdrawal of chronic steroid therapy.

Although rare, it must not be overlooked. An unrecognized and untreated Addisonian crisis can be fatal. The preoperative diagnosis is difficult to make in patients with mild clinical disease, and yet it is these whose adrenal cortex may be incapable of responding to the stresses of anaesthesia and surgery.

Presentation

1. Acute cardiovascular collapse during surgery can occur under a wide variety of circumstances:

a. Cardiac arrest during appendicectomy in a 15-year-old girl responded to cardiac massage, saline and bicarbonate (Salam & Davies 1974). She was subsequently found to have a normal resting blood cortisol, but no response to adrenal stimulation.

b. An acute Addisonian crisis associated with a serum sodium of 106 mmol/l, was deliberately provoked by a patient who stopped his own steroid therapy and then cut his neck and wrists (Smith & Byrne 1981).

c. Severe perioperative hypotension occurred in a young man with an acute abdominal emergency, despite administration of fluids and inotropic agents (Hertzberg & Schulman 1985). An improvement in his condition only took place when steroids were given. His postoperative complications included myocardial infarction and pericarditis. A subsequent adrenal stimulation test indicated Addison's disease.

d. Patients with adrenocortical insufficiency may be subfertile. Cardiovascular collapse occurred in a young woman undergoing infertility investigations under general anaesthesia (personal communication). Sudden death occurred a week later, in a period of steroid withdrawal, during adrenocortical investigations.

2. There may be a history of steroid therapy within the previous 12 months. Adrenocortical atrophy is detectable 5 days after the onset of glucocorticoid therapy, and if it is given for more than a few weeks, a return to completely normal homeostasis may take up to 1 year (Axelrod 1976).

Management

1. Hydrocortisone hemisuccinate i.v. 200 mg, followed by an infusion of

hydrocortisone 400 mg in either dextrose 5% or saline 0.9%, to be given over 24 hours.
2. Saline 0.9% i.v., 1 litre rapidly initially, and then more slowly.
3. Dextrose 10% i.v. to correct hypoglycaemia.
4. Subsequently, the presumptive diagnosis must be confirmed or refuted with plasma cortisol estimations and adrenal stimulation tests. Prior to these, the hydrocortisone should be changed to dexamethasone, which does not register in plasma cortisol assays.

BIBLIOGRAPHY

Axelrod L 1976. Glucocorticoid therapy. Medicine 55: 39–65
Hertzberg L B, Schulman M S 1985. Acute adrenal insufficiency in a patient with appendicitis during anesthesia. Anesthesiology 62: 517–519
Salam A A, Davies D M 1974. Acute adrenal insufficiency during surgery. British Journal of Anaesthesia 46: 619–622
Smith M G, Byrne A J 1981. An Addisonian crisis complicating anaesthesia. Anaesthesia 36: 681–684

AIR EMBOLISM

When a patient is in an upright position, air inadvertently entering the venous system will normally be carried to the right side of the heart, where it localizes initially at the junction of the right atrium and the superior vena cava. Some air may remain in the upper part of the right atrium, while the rest is carried through the tricuspid valve and into the pulmonary artery. Small amounts of air are filtered by the pulmonary capillaries. Larger amounts cause pulmonary artery outflow obstruction and a fall in cardiac output. Air embolism can occur in any situation in which there is an open vein and a subatmospheric pressure.

Recent concern has focused on the subject of 'paradoxical' air embolism (Clayton et al 1985). At postmortem, 20–35% of all patients have a 'probe patent' foramen ovale. In such a patient, if the RAP were to exceed the LAP, venous air could theoretically enter the systemic circulation. Haemodynamic studies have shown that in the sitting position, the interatrial pressure gradient can become reversed (Perkins-Pearson et al 1982). It has been suggested that, if the incidence of air embolism in the upright position is 30–40%, and that of patent foramen ovale is 20–35%, 1 in 10 patients operated on in this position could have conditions predisposing to the entry of air into the systemic circulation (Gronert et al 1979). This 'paradoxical' air embolism might account for a number of cases of air embolism, in which Doppler changes occurred without $ETCO_2$ changes, where ST segment or QRS changes suggested entry of air into the coronary arteries, or where there were postoperative clinical signs of cerebral air embolism. The possibility of a transpulmonary route for access of venous air to the systemic circulation has also been postulated.

Presentation

1. Type of surgery

The reported incidence of air embolism depends on the monitoring techniques employed. The Doppler method is particularly sensitive and capable of detecting extremely small emboli. With this technique, an incidence of up to 58% has been reported in patients having posterior fossa or cervical disc surgery in the sitting position. Using new echocardiographic techniques, 66% of infants undergoing craniectomy in the supine position have been reported to have echocardiographic evidence of venous air embolism (Harris et al 1987). Emboli can also occur when large veins are opened in head and neck operations, if there is a head-up tilt. In hip arthoplasty, Doppler evidence of air embolism has been reported in 30% of patients immediately following the insertion of the femoral cement. There was an accompanying drop in blood pressure in only 4% (Michel 1980). Air may also enter the uterine sinuses in up to 40% of Caesarean deliveries. Massive emboli are however rare, and most likely to occur in the hypovolaemic patient with placenta praevia, or abruption (Younker et al 1986). The increasing use of CVP lines has been associated with a number of incidents of accidental introduction of air (Seidelin et al 1987).

2. Factors affecting clinical signs

The effects of air embolism depend on the rate of entry and quantity of air, the differences between the venous and atmospheric pressure, and the percentage of nitrous oxide being adminstered. Animal research indicates that 0.5 ml/kg/min can produce symptoms. The entry of large boluses of air has been associated with the insertion of central venous lines, especially when the head-down position was not used and if the CVP was low. Experiments have shown that with a pressure difference of 5 cmH_2O, as much as 100 ml air/s can be drawn in through a 2 mm needle. The concomitant administration of nitrous oxide effectively increases the volume of air drawn into the bloodstream. A concentration of 50% N_2O produces an effective increase of 200% and 75% N_2O one of 400%.

3. Site or timing of air entry

In neurosurgical procedures, air enters most frequently via veins held open by the neck muscles, or those in the dura, venous sinuses or bone. In hip surgery, emboli can occur when cement is inserted into the femoral shaft. Of 79 cases of air embolism associated with central venous lines, the majority involved technical problems (Seidelin et al 1987). One-third happened during catheter insertion and death occurred in 32% of the cases reported.

4. Clinical signs of air embolism

These may include a hissing sound from the wound, hypotension, arrhythmias, cyanosis, or changes in respiratory pattern in a spontaneously breathing patient. However, with adequate monitoring, subclinical air entry should be detected before many of these signs occur.

Diagnosis

1. A precordial Doppler produces the earliest signs of air embolism, but is very sensitive. The use of an oesophageal Doppler has been described. The diagnosis may be confirmed by aspiration through a right heart catheter, which should have been placed high in the right atrium.
2. A fall in $ETCO_2$ occurs before clinical signs, but will not necessarily change as quickly, or as much, if a paradoxical air embolus has also occurred.
3. Later signs of significant emboli include a 'mill wheel' murmur, arrhythmias, hypotension, a fall in oxygen saturation, and increases in CVP or in PAWP.
4. The occurrence of paradoxical air embolism is difficult to prove unless a neurosurgeon observes air in small cerebral arteries. However, its possibility may be suggested by the ECG changes of ST elevation or depression, or cardiac arrest. Monitored changes of cerebral function have been attributed to cerebral emboli. Localization of air in the cardiac chambers using two-dimensional transoesophageal echocardiography has been reported, but at present this is primarily of research interest (Cucchiara et al 1984).

Management

1. **a.** In neurosurgery

   Identify the site of access and prevent further entry. Cover or flood the wound. Compress the neck to show open veins. Deal surgically with the open vein or apply bone wax, if appropriate. While aspiration of air from a right heart catheter may have a diagnostic role, its therapeutic value is doubtful.

   b. Central venous lines

   To prevent air embolism during insertion of a central venous line, it is important that the patient is in a head-down position. Occlusion of the catheter after insertion, and use of a three-way tap when disconnecting infusion sets, will reduce the risks.
2. If the entry of a large amount of air occurs, cardiopulmonary resuscitation may be required. Place the patient in a head-down position to reduce pulmonary outflow obstruction.
3. It has been suggested the morbidity and mortality is such that the sitting position should no longer be used for neurosurgical procedures. However, an analysis of 554 cases showed that with careful patient selection, monitoring, and anaesthetic and surgical skills, this can be minimized (Matjasko et al 1985).
4. An inflatable neck tourniquet, which could be used to identify venous bleeding points during the incision through muscle and bone, has been described (Sale 1984).

4

BIBLIOGRAPHY

Clayton D G, Evans P, Williams C, Thurlow A C 1985 Paradoxical air embolism during neurosurgery. Anaesthesia 40: 981–989

Cucchiara R F, Nugent M, Seward J B, Messick J M 1984 Air embolism in upright neurosurgical patients: detection and localisation by two-dimensional transesophageal echocardiography. Anesthesiology 60: 353–355

Gronert G A, Messick J M Jr, Cucchiara R F, Michenfelder J D 1979 Paradoxical air embolism from a patent foramen ovale. Anesthesiology 50: 548–549

Harris M M, Yemen T A, Davidson A, Strafford M A, Rowe R W, Sanders S P, Rockoff M A 1987 Venous air embolism during craniectomy in supine infants. Anesthesiology 67: 816–819

Matjasko J, Petrozza P, Cohen M, Steinberg P 1985 Anesthesia and surgery in the seated position: analysis of 554 cases. Neurosurgery 17: 695–702

Michel R 1980 Air embolism in hip surgery. Anaesthesia 35: 858–862

Perkins-Pearson N, Marshall W, Bedford R 1982. Atrial pressures in the seated position. Anesthesiology 57: 493–497

Sale J P 1984 Prevention of air embolism during sitting neurosurgery. Anaesthesia 39: 795–799

Seidelin P H, Stolarek I H, Thompson A M 1987 Central venous catheterisation and fatal air embolism. British Journal of Hospital Medicine 38: 438–439

Younker D, Rodriguez V, Kavanagh J 1986 Massive air embolism during Cesarean section. Anesthesiology 65: 77–79

AMNIOTIC FLUID EMBOLISM
(see Section 1)

ANAPHYLACTOID REACTIONS TO INTRAVENOUS AGENTS

A general term for a clinical event which either threatens life or disrupts the course of an operation. It is a multisystem response to a drug, or drug combination, to which the patient may or may not have been previously exposed. The term anaphylactoid does not explain the mechanism. Usually, the type of reaction may only be elucidated subsequently, by evaluation of history, immunology and, if appropriate, skin testing. Unfortunately more than one drug may have been given immediately prior to the reaction. The collection of blood samples for immunological studies should start as soon as possible after the event. Understanding the mechanism of the reaction is important for the subsequent management of the patient.

There appears to be an increase in the number of these reactions (Stoelting 1983). It has been estimated that, in the UK, the incidence lies between 5000 and 10 000 per annum, and that there may be as many as 100 deaths per year (Watkins 1985). Reactions occur more frequently in women than in men. An analysis of 154 serious cases in France showed that 70% occurred in women (Laxenaire et al 1985).

1. Drugs producing reactions
   a. Induction agents

Thiopentone causes more reactions than either methohexitone or etomidate. Etomidate is considered to be 'immunologically safe' (Watkins 1983), and a low incidence of anaphylactoid reactions has been reported.

b. Muscle relaxants

Produce a surprising number of anaphylactoid responses and may be involved in up to 50% of reactions occurring during anaesthesia. In decreasing order of frequency, those reported to have been involved in anaphylactoid reactions were: suxamethonium, alcuronium, atracurium, tubocurarine, pancuronium, vecuronium and gallamine (Watkins 1985). At the time of Watkins' study, pancuronium was in very common use, yet rarely involved. Subsequently, the use of either vecuronium or atracurium (despite the incidence of local histamine release) has been suggested as being relatively safe in patients with allery or atopy.

Controversy exists about the potential for cross-reactivity between muscle relaxants, based on common quaternary or tertiary ammonium ions (Baldo 1986, Watkins 1987). Confusion may also occur with intradermal testing because neuromuscular blockers can cause skin histamine release, even at dilutions of 1:1000 or 1:10 000 (Watkins & Nimmo 1985).

c. Plasma expanders (see also Section 3)

Anaphylactoid reactions to colloid volume substitutes have been studied (Ring & Mesmer 1977) and the dextrans were shown to have the highest incidence. A study of 50 dextran-induced reactions showed that a metabolic acidosis had occurred in all the severe reactions, and also frequently in the less severe ones (Ljungstrom & Renck 1987). A technique of hapten administration (dextran 1) prior to the use of dextran has been reported to have dramatically reduced the number of serious reactions in Sweden (Ljungstrom et al 1988).

d. X-ray contrast media

Adverse systemic reactions to contrast media occur in 5% of patients (Goldberg 1984). The majority receiving intravenous contrast media have an increased serum osmolality, a decreased haematocrit and a subsequent osmotic diuresis. In addition, some patients will develop an actual anaphylactoid response, usually within 2 minutes of the injection. There may be nausea and vomiting, cardiovascular collapse, upper airway obstruction, bronchospasm and hypoxia. The newer contrast media are likely to be much safer in this respect.

e. Local anaesthetic agents

The differentiation between anaphylactoid and toxic reactions is difficult. However, the incidence of true allergy is probably very low (Incaudo et al 1978).

f. Antibiotics

Penicillin produces a high incidence of anaphylactic reactions, a proportion of which are fatal. IgE is frequently involved (Sogn 1984).

4

Up to 8% of patients allergic to penicillin also react to cephalosporins. All intraoperative antibiotics should be given slowly, having been diluted into 50–250 ml of fluid (Levy 1986). Requests that they are given at induction of anaesthesia should be resisted. If a reaction occurs, there may be major difficulty in identifying the drug responsible.

2. Types of reactions

Some immunologists believe that non-specific anaphylactoid reactions are more common than immune-mediated ones, and that skin testing is only of value where clinical and laboratory evidence strongly favours immune involvement (Watkins & Nimmo 1985). This view is not shared by other workers (Fisher 1984). In general the immune-mediated response tends to be more severe, and is more likely to result in death.

a. Type I hypersensitivity response

A true anaphylactic or allergic response, which depends upon previous exposure to the drug. On the first occasion, lymphocytes produce specific IgE antibodies which become attached to the membrane of mast cells and basophils. A second exposure results in cross-linkages between these primed cells, changes in the cell membrane, and mast cell and basophil degranulation. Mediators such as histamine and leukotriene C are released from mast cells, causing some or all of the pharmacological effects associated with anaphylactic reactions. Complement is not involved. IgE involvement is most common, IgG may be concerned and C4 is consumed. Disappearance of basophils is said to be highly indicative of a type I reaction (Watkins 1987). This type of reaction may occur after multiple exposures to thiopentone and, although uncommon, can be fatal.

b. Complement-mediated reaction

This classical reaction can occur on initial exposure to the drug. Activation of C1-C9, the complement cascade, occurs and C4 and C3 are consumed. C3a and C5a (anaphylatoxins) are mast cell degranulators. Once again chemical mediators are released.

c. Alternate complement pathway

Activation of this results in direct conversion of C3, C3a once again being released. Again, a previous exposure is not necessary. Reactions to cremophor-containing drugs were frequently of this type.

d. Non-immune anaphylactoid responses

These are common and it may be difficult to identify the drug responsible. Chemical mediators are released as a result of a direct or an indirect effect on mast cells and basophils. The diagnosis is generally one of exclusion. No IgE changes occur, and complement C3 and C4 are not consumed. It has been suggested that this reaction may occur on exposure to a particular group of drugs, such as muscle relaxants, when they share common molecular characteristics (Baldo 1986).

There may be predisposing factors such as chronic atopy, complement abnormalities or a history of regular exposure to the particular drug. The greater the amount of drug and the more rapid its administration, the more severe the reaction is likely to be.
e. Miscellaneous
In some cases a similar response may be due to drug interactions, or drug overdose. Rarely, it is secondary to an unexpected pathology, such as a hormone-secreting tumour.

Presentation

1. Cutaneous
Include flushing and urticaria and may cause significant fluid depletion. The development of a 1 mm layer of subcutaneous fluid over the whole body is approximately equivalent to a loss of 1.5 litres of extracellular volume.
2. Cardiovascular
Feature most commonly and vary in severity from moderate hypotension to total cardiovascular collapse. Hypotension is due to release of histamine (and other vasoactive peptides), which causes widespread capillary vasodilatation and increased capillary permeability. Changes in heart rate or rhythm accompany the hypotension. ECG changes were analysed in 186 cases (Fisher 1986). A supraventricular tachycardia developed in 153 (82%), and this was acompanied by ST elevation in a further eight patients. The remaining arrhythmias included asystole, rapid AF and ventricular fibrillation. Arrhythmias other than SVT tended to be associated with pre-existing cardiac disease. This was so in 24 out of 26 patients with heart disease, whereas 151 out of the 160 patients without cardiac disease had SVT alone. The four episodes of VF came from both groups and were usually associated with the administration of adrenaline in the presence of halothane.
3. Bronchospasm
Was noted to have occurred in 39% of cases studied in France (Laxenaire et al 1985). It is serious and can be responsible for deaths, secondary to cerebral hypoxia.
4. Glottic oedema
May occur occasionally.
5. Gastrointestinal
Immediately after recovery from the reaction, the patient may complain of abdominal pain, diarrhoea or vomiting. This may be secondary to hyperperistalsis and oedema of the gut.
6. Miscellaneous
Other effects include AV conduction defects, coagulation disorders and leucopenia.

Management

1. Resuscitation

a. Stop administration of the suspected drug and turn off all inhalational agents. There is no place for these in the treatment of anaphylactoid bronchoconstriction.

b. Administer 100% oxygen and maintain the airway.

c. Give adrenaline i.v., 0.1–0.5 mg (0.1–0.5 ml of 1:1000 soln, or 5 μg/kg) for cardiovascular collapse. For less severe reactions dilute to 1:10 000 and give 0.5–1 ml and repeat as required.

Adrenaline is the drug of first choice in anaphylactoid reactions and should be given early. In view of its brevity of action, in severe reactions an adrenaline infusion may be subsequently required. Additional to its cardiovascular effects, adrenaline inhibits further degranulation of mast cells and basophils, by increasing levels of intracellular AMP. In six out of seven fatal reactions, adrenaline had been given late in the treatment (Fisher 1986). For patients who are on beta blockers, the hypotension does not respond well to adrenaline (Laxenaire et al 1985), and isoprenaline may have to be given in higher than normal doses. In less severe reactions the adrenaline can be diluted and given more slowly. Its effects require close monitoring and caution is essential if halothane has been in use, as VF may be precipitated.

d. Give crystalloid or colloid i.v. to expand the vascular volume. Following analysis of treatment given to 203 cases, it was concluded that colloid was preferable (Fisher 1986).

e. Manage the airway. In the presence of severe laryngeal oedema and failure of intubation, tracheostomy or cricothyroidotomy may be required.

f. Measure pH and blood gases. Marked acidosis may occur and require treatment with sodium bicarbonate (Ljungstrom & Renck 1987).

2. Second-line treatment

a. Antihistamines

Chlorpheniramine i.v. 10–20 mg can be given slowly over 1 minute. Antihistamines occupy cellular H_1-receptor sites and are competitive inhibitors of histamine binding. However, they only partially reverse anaphylactoid responses, as chemicals other than histamine are involved. Also, it may not be possible to achieve complete block of certain histamine receptor sites.

b. Aminophylline

A dose of 250–500 mg (5 mg/kg), given slowly over 20 minutes, may be required if bronchospasm persists. Aminophylline prevents degradation of 3, 5-cyclic AMP, and reduces the release of histamine and arachnidonic acid metabolites. Its effect on respiratory function is not solely that of bronchodilatation.

c. Corticosteroids

There is little place for corticosteroids in the immediate treatment, as their onset of action at a cellular level may take several hours. However, they may be used where the reaction does not quickly resolve and hypotension persists.

3. Investigations
   a. Immediate
      i. As soon as possible, blood samples should be taken for subsequent assessment of the mechanisms of the reaction.

      ii. Additional advice can be obtained from the National Adverse Reactions Advisory Service (Dr John Watkins, Supraregional Protein Reference Unit, Department of Immunology, Royal Hallamshire Hospital, Sheffield S10 2JF, UK. Telephone 0742 766222, Ext. 2837/2058).

      iii. Take two sets of venous blood samples in two EDTA tubes as soon as possible after the start of the reaction. (EDTA stabilizes plasma complement proteins.) Further duplicated samples should be taken at 3 hours, 6 hours, 12 hours and 24 hours.

      iv. The first set should be sent to the local haematology department for Hb, WCC (total and differential), platelet count and haematocrit.

      v. Plasma should be separated from the second set. This should be stored at -20 to $-25°C$ until ready for despatch (without ice) by first class post to the Immunology Laboratory, as soon as the 24-hour collection is complete. Alternatively, some hospitals may have their own facilities for performing complement and immunoglobulin levels.

      vi. Detailed documentation should accompany the samples. This will include a full record of the incident, the agents and batch numbers, details of previous administration of these substances and relevant history, such as allergies and atopy.

      vii. Other similar, but more complex protocols exist, arising from recommendations by a joint European workshop in Nancy (Laxenaire et al 1983).

If these samples have been taken correctly, it should be possible to resolve the mechanism of the reaction. Should the results of immunological testing indicate, by changes in IgE and disappearance of basophils, an immune reaction, then skin testing is appropriate. If, as more frequently happens, the reaction involves neither IgE nor complement, then the offending drug may be more difficult to identify.

   b. Subsequent
      i. Skin testing with drugs at low dilutions, 6 weeks after the initial reaction. A regimen for intradermal testing has been described, with recommendations on drug dilutions (Fisher 1984). This should preferably be undertaken by someone experienced in the technique. However, controversy exists over the indications for skin testing and its reliability if used indiscriminately. Some believe

that it is appropriate when there is clinical and laboratory evidence of an immune response, but not when there is direct histamine release (Watkins & Nimmo 1985), whereas others recommend it routinely (Fisher 1984). There is also debate as to whether cross-reactivity, based on common quaternary or tertiary ammonium ions, occurs between muscle relaxants. Detection of serum IgE antibodies which reacted with more than one relaxant has been reported (Baldo & Fisher 1983).

ii. The basophil degranulation test, or measurement of basophil histamine release (Withington et al 1987).

iii. RAST test. This radioallergosorbent test involves the use of commercially prepared antigen to detect drug-specific antibodies. At present the usefulness of this test is limited, both by the availability of preparations, and by the occurrence of false-positive and false-negative results.

4. Communication of information

a. Report the reaction to the Committee on Safety of Medicines via the Yellow Card system.

b. Inform the patient of the results of investigations. Issue a warning card or suggest a Medic Alert bracelet.

c. Document the results clearly in the patient's notes.

d. Inform the general practitioner.

5. Management of subsequent anaesthetics

a. If the reaction is shown to be immune mediated and the drug is identified by skin testing, then this drug should not be used again. In an immune-mediated reaction, there is no place for the use of i.v. test doses, as even minute amounts of a drug may prove fatal.

b. If the reaction is non-specific, then future anaesthetics should be conducted using drugs considered to be relatively safe, while avoiding those known to produce reactions more readily. Currently, drugs with the fewest reports of serious problems are fentanyl, etomidate, vecuronium, pancuronium and atracurium. Further advice can be obtained from the National Adverse Reactions Advisory Service. If closely repeated anaesthetics are required in the same patient, consideration should be given to varying the techniques and drugs used. All drugs should be given slowly.

c. Pretreatment with H_1 and H_2 antagonists has been recommended. However, as other mediators are also involved, this does not guarantee freedom from a response.

BIBLIOGRAPHY

Baldo B, Fisher M McD 1983 Detection of serum IgE antibodies that react with alcuronium and tubocurarine after life-threatening reactions to muscle relaxants. Anaesthesia and Intensive Care 11: 194–197

Baldo B A 1986 Cross-reactions of neuromuscular blocking drugs and anaphylactoid reactions. Anaesthesia 41: 550–551

Clarke R S J, Dundee J W, Garrett R T, McArdle G K, Sutton J A 1975 Adverse reactions to intravenous anaesthetics. A survey of 100 reports. British Journal of Anaesthesia 47: 575–585

Fisher M M 1984 Intradermal testing after anaphylactoid reactions to anaesthetic drugs. Practical aspects of performance and interpretation. Anaesthesia and Intensive Care 12: 115–120

Fisher M McD 1986 Clinical observations on the pathophysiology and treatment of anaphylactic cardiovascular collapse. Anaesthesia and and Intensive Care 14: 17–21

Goldberg M 1984 Systemic reactions to intravascular contrast media. Anethesiology 60: 46–56

Incaudo G, Schatz M, Patterson R, Rosenberg M, Yammamoto F, Hamburger R N 1978 Administration of local anesthetics to patients with a history of prior adverse reaction. Journal of Allergy and Clinical Immunology 61: 339–345

Laxenaire M–C, Moneret-Vautrin D A, Watkins J 1983 Diagnosis of the causes of anaphylactoid anaesthetic reactions. A report of the recommendations of the joint Anaesthetic and Immunoallergological Workshop, Nancy, France: 19 March 1982 Anaesthesia 38: 147–148

Laxenaire M–C, Moneret-Vautrin D–A, Vervloet D 1985 The French experience of anaphylactoid reactions. International Anesthesiology Clinics 23: 145–160

Levy J H 1986 Anaphylactic reactions in anesthesia and intensive care. Butterworths, Guildford

Ljungstrom K–G, Renck H 1987 Metabolic acidosis in dextran-induced anaphylactic reactions. Acta Anaesthesiologica Scandinavica 31: 157–160

Ljungstrom K–G, Renck H, Hedin H, Richter W, Wiholm B–E 1988 Hapten inhibition and dextran anaphylaxis. Anaesthesia 43: 729–732

Ring J, Messmer K 1977 Incidence and severity of anaphylactoid reactions to colloid volume substitutes. Lancet i: 466–469

Sogn D D 1984 Penicillin allergy. Journal of Allergy and Clinical Immunology 74: 589–593

Stoetling R K 1983 Allergic reactions during anesthesia. Anesthesia and Analgesia 62: 341–356

Watkins J, Thornton J A, Clarke R S J 1979 Adverse reactions to iv agents. British Journal of Anaesthesia 51: 469

Watkins J 1983. Etomidate: an 'immunologically safe' anaesthetic agent. Anaesthesia 38 (suppl): 34–38

Watkins J 1985 Adverse anaesthetic reactions. An update from a proposed national reporting and advisory service. Anaesthesia 40: 797–800

Watkins J, Nimmo W S 1985 'Allergic' drug reactions during anaesthesia. Anaesthesia 40: 813–814

Watkins J 1987 Investigation of allergic and hypersensitivity reactions to anaesthetic agents. British Journal of Anaesthesia 59: 104–111

Withington D E, Leung K B P, Bromley L, Scadding G K, Pearce F L 1987 Basophil histamine release. Anaesthesia 42: 850–854

ANGIONEUROTIC OEDEMA

A general term applied to the development of acute oedema in the subcutaneous or submucous tissues. Anaesthetic assistance may be sought during an attack, when oedema of the lips, tongue or larynx may cause respiratory problems. Angio-oedema may be due to release of histamine, or a number of other vasoactive substances such as the bradykinins, prostaglandins or leukotrienes. The development of oedema may be:

a. Part of a general anaphylactoid or anaphylactic reaction to a drug, bite, sting or the ingestion of a substance.

b. A manifestation of hereditary angioneurotic oedema, a familial condition due to a deficiency of C1 esterase inhibitor (see Section 1: Hereditary angioneurotic oedema).

c. Due to an acquired form of C1 esterase inhibitor deficiency which usually occurs in association with a B-lymphocyte malignancy (see Section 1: C1 Esterase inhibitor deficiency).

Presentation

1. There may be a history of a predisposing factor. This can be ingestion of food or a drug, an infection, bite or sting, a family history of angio-oedema, or a B-lymphocytic malignancy.

2. Oedema of subcutaneous tissue may occur on its own, or be accompanied by hypotension.

Management

1. If the angio-oedema is part of an anaphylactic or anaphylactoid reaction, see appropriate section.

> **a.** Give adrenaline i.v. or i.m., 0.1–0.5 mg depending on the severity.
> **b.** If the condition is severe and involves the glottis, an airway should be established, either by intubation, cricothyroidotomy or tracheostomy.
> **c.** Second-line treatment includes i.v. fluids, chlorpheniramine i.v. 10–20 mg, and steroids.

2. Hereditary angio-oedema, or acquired C1 esterase inhibitor deficiency. These do not respond to adrenaline or antihistamines, but to replacement of the deficient inhibitor by either:

> **a.** An infusion of fresh frozen plasma. There is a risk that the additional presence of C2 and C4 may initially cause a deterioration, but this objection appears to be largely theoretical.
> **b.** Purified C1 esterase inhibitor can be obtained from the Scottish Blood Transfusion Service, or from Immuno Ltd (Rye Lane, Dunton Green, Sevenoaks, Kent TN14 5HB. UK, telephone 0732 458101).

ARRYTHMIAS

The diagnosis and treatment of certain cardiac arrhythmias can on occasions be complex and may require cardiological expertise. However, during anaesthesia a cardiologist may not be available immediately, therefore the anaesthetist needs a basic working knowledge of the common abnormalities and their likely causes. There is often a correctable surgical or anaesthetic precipitating factor, so the need for complex antiarrhythmic therapy in theatre is unusual.

If the use of an antiarrhythmic is contemplated, careful thought should be given to possible interactions. In the presence of anaesthetic agents, or preoperative drug therapy, the i.v. administration of potent cardiac drugs can precipitate serious side-effects. The anaesthetist must be aware of these and be prepared to treat complications should they arise. However, on occasions, the urgent treatment of a life-threatening arrhythmia may be essential.

In general, if rhythm disturbances appear for the first time in the perioperative period, the initial search should be for a precipitating cause, associated with either the surgery or anaesthesia.

Predisposing factors

1. General problems
Hypoxia, hypercarbia, metabolic and electrolyte abnormalities, light anaesthesia, or manoeuvres which stimulate the output of endogenous catecholamines.
2. Drug causes
Accidental overdose with local anaesthetics, absorption of adrenaline during surgical infiltration or pre-existing medication with drugs such as digoxin.
3. Pre-existing cardiac disease
Ischaemic heart disease, congenital heart disease, cardiomyopathy, WPW, mitral valve prolapse or the prolonged QT syndromes.
4. Rare causes
Undiagnosed thyrotoxicosis, phaeochromocytoma, carcinoid syndrome, 'athlete's heart', malignant hyperpyrexia, and drug or solvent abuse.

Presentation

1. Atrial fibrillation
Fast chaotic atrial activity, irregular fibrillation waves of 350–600/min best seen in V1. An irregular ventricular response of 100–200/min and varying AV conduction. Only if AF is associated with AV block is the ventricular rate regular. Causes include ischaemic, hypertensive and rheumatic heart disease, thyrotoxicosis, sick sinus syndrome, alcohol abuse and atrial septal defect. Transient AF may occur during an acute toxic illness. Patients are at risk from systemic embolism.
2. Atrial flutter
Regular atrial rate of 250–350/min with saw-toothed flutter waves, which are best seen in leads II, III, AVF and VI. There may be a 2 : 1 or 3 : 1 AV block. The ventricular rate is also regular, varying from 125–350 b.p.m. Causes are similar to those for AF.
3. Atrial tachycardia with AV block
P waves are visible but often inverted in leads II, III and AVF. The atrial rate is regular at 120–250/min, with a fixed or varying degree of AV block. Ventricular activity is usually normal, but occasionally bundle

branch block occurs. Most often associated with digitalis toxicity, but can be due to ischaemic heart disease, cardiomyopathy or sick sinus syndrome.

4. Paroxysmal supraventricular tachycardia (AV nodal re-entrant tachycardia)

Ventricular rate regular at 130–250/min. No normal P waves seen, but inverted ones follow the QRS complex. Normal ventricular activity, sometimes with BBB. Often occurs in the absence of cardiac disease, but can be associated with WPW or Ebstein's anomaly. An abrupt onset of palpitations may cause hypotension, syncope, chest pain, polyuria and, if it persists, occasionally heart failure occurs.

5. Atrial ectopic beats

A premature, abnormal-shaped or sometimes inverted, P wave, best shown in V1. The QRS is usually normal and there is no compensatory pause after the ectopic. The next beat occurs exactly one sinus cycle after the ectopic, thus resetting the cycle. Atrial ectopics are frequently benign, but if they occur with heart disease, they may presage AF.

6. Ventricular ectopic beats

A widened bizarre-shaped QRS, without a preceding ectopic P wave. There is a short interval between a normal beat and the ectopic, followed by a compensatory pause before the next normal beat. If the ectopic falls early onto the T wave of the previous contraction (R on T), then ventricular tachycardia or fibrillation may be precipitated. Causes include ischaemic heart disease, cardiomyopathies, digoxin toxicity and valvular disease. However, the cause may not be obvious.

7. Ventricular fibrillation

An incoordinate contraction of ventricular myocardial fibres associated with loss of consciousness and an absence of cardiac output.

8. Ventricular tachycardia (see also Torsade de pointes)

A rapid ventricular rhythm of 120–250/min, lasting for at least three or more beats, with abnormal-shaped complexes. Evidence of separate atrial activity occurring at a slower rate, with P waves dissociated from ventricular complexes, helps to distinguish it from supraventricular tachycardia. If in doubt, the distance between any visible P waves may be shown to be mathematically related. R waves occur only in V1 and the QRS width is >140 ms.

Problems

1. The presenting arrhythmia may cause hypotension and a reduction in cardiac output. Ventricular fibrillation and occasionally ventricular tachycardia, cause circulatory arrest.

2. Myocardial ischaemia may be provoked.

3. If there is pre-existing left-sided heart disease, there may be cardiac decompensation and pulmonary oedema.

4. The arrhythmia may precipitate a more serious or fatal one, such as ventricular tachycardia or ventricular fibrillation.

Management

1. Atrial fibrillation

Digoxin slows the ventricular response rate to atrial activity. Verapamil will slow the ventricular rate. In AF of acute onset, direct current cardioversion will result in sinus rhythm.

2. Atrial flutter

Verapamil and digoxin may not control the ventricular rate. Cardioversion may be successful in reverting flutter to sinus rhythm. Atrial pacing can be tried.

3. Atrial tachycardia with AV block

Stop digoxin, correct any hypokalaemia and give lignocaine i.v. 1 mg/kg. Should this fail, direct current cardioversion or rapid atrial pacing may be tried. If the patient is not already on digoxin, treatment with this may control the ventricular rate.

4. Paroxysmal supraventricular tachycardia

Carotid sinus massage or a Valsalva manoeuvre to increase vagal tone (for details see Autonomic dysfunction). Pressure should be exerted by two fingers over the carotid artery at the level of the thyroid cartilage. Verapamil i.v. 5–10 mg is usually successful, but should not be given if the patient is on beta blockers. Digoxin, propranolol, quinidine, procainamide, disopyramide and cardioversion can also be used.

5. Atrial ectopic beats

No treatment is usually necessary, unless they are very frequent, or are associated with cardiac disease. In such a case digoxin may help.

6. Ventricular ectopic beats

In general no treatment is needed, unless they are frequent, or of the early R on T type. A lignocaine infusion or a beta blocker may then be needed.

7. Ventricular fibrillation

A single precordial blow can be tried, otherwise defibrillation is required. If the heart is resistant to defibrillation then prior treatment with bretylium tosylate i.v. 400 mg may raise the fibrillation threshold.

8. Ventricular tachycardia (see also Torsade de pointes)

The urgency and method of treatment depends upon the degree of haemodynamic impairment. In the presence of shock, direct current cardioversion is required. Where there is no marked hypotension, or for short episodes of tachycardia, drug treatment can be used. Lignocaine is the drug of first choice. If this fails, disopyramide, flecainide or mexiletine can be used.

BRONCHOSPASM
(see also Section 1: Asthma)

In a large study of anaesthesia, an incidence of bronchospasm of 0.17% was reported. It was usually triggered in susceptible patients by mechanical stimuli (Olsson 1987). Other causes include anaphylactoid reactions, inhalation of gastric contents, and rarely, certain hormone-secreting tumours.

Presentation

1. Predisposing factors to intraoperative bronchospasm include asthma, obstructive airways disease, respiratory infection and tracheal intubation. It is most likely to occur during airway manipulation in a patient who has previously exhibited a capacity for airway constriction.
2. Bronchospasm may be one manifestation of an anaphylactoid reaction. Other signs such as flushing, urticaria, hypotension and tachycardia should be sought.
3. It may be due to silent inhalation of gastric contents. This may have been associated with intubation difficulties.
4. In rare hormone-secreting tumours, such as carcinoids, flushing and hypotension may additionally occur.

Management

1. Bronchospasm is frequently associated with intubation or airway manipulation, in a patient with a history of bronchitis, asthma or wheezing. Its incidence can be significantly reduced by preoperative preparation, avoidance of intubation during light anaesthesia and the use of topical or i.v. lignocaine (Kingston & Hirshman 1984). Despite these measures, if it still occurs, an attempt should be made to deepen the anaesthetic, using an inhalational agent and oxygen. Halothane, enflurane and isoflurane are all effective at reversing antigen-induced bronchospasm. However, halothane sensitizes the heart to the effect of exogenous and endogenous catecholamines. In addition, it interacts with aminophylline to produce arrhythmias. Isoflurane, therefore, is probably the best choice.
2. A bronchodilator, such as aminophylline 5 mg/kg over 10–15 minutes or a salbutamol infusion 5–20 μg/min can be given.
3. If the clinical situation suggests an anaphylactoid reaction, then adrenaline i.m. or i.v. is the treatment of choice.
4. If there is evidence of gastric inhalation, appropriate treatment should be instituted. (See Mendelson's Syndrome).

BIBLIOGRAPHY

Kingston H G G, Hirshman C A 1984 Perioperative management of the patient with asthma. Anesthesia and Analgesia 63: 844–855
Olsson G L 1987 Bronchospasm during anaesthesia. A computer-aided incidence study of 136 929 patients. Acta Anaesthesiologica Scandinavica 31: 244–252

CARCINOID SYNDROME
(see also Section 1)

Less than 25% of patients with carcinoid tumours have carcinoid syndrome. The majority of patients with the syndrome have liver metastases. Exceptions are the tumours whose venous drainage bypasses the liver. Flushing and hypertension have occurred during anaesthesia in the absence of metastases (Jones & Knight 1982). They were thought to be due to manipulation of the tumour itself. Preoperative features include flushing, diarrhoea, wheezing and valvular lesions of the heart. The patient may present unexpectedly during anaesthesia with cardiovascular or respiratory complications due to secretion of vasoactive chemical mediators such as serotonin, bradykinins, prostaglandins or histamine.

4

Presentation

1. Release of hormones from carcinoid tissue may occur as a result of certain stimuli during anaesthesia and surgery. These include intubation, tumour handling, hypotension, and catecholamine release.
2. Serotonin is known to cause hyperkinetic states of hypertension, tachycardia and certain sorts of flushing. Bradykinins may produce hypotension, increased capillary permeability, oedema, flushing and bronchospasm. Other vasoactive peptides such as histamine and prostaglandins may be involved, but their part in the syndrome has not as yet been elucidated.
3. Serious reactions during anaesthesia have included severe hypertension which responded to ketanserin (Casthely et al 1986), cardiovascular collapse which responded to a somatostatin analogue (Marsh et al 1987), severe bronchospasm (Miller et al 1980) and facial oedema (Lippmann & Cleveland 1973).

Management

1. The use of a number of different antiserotoninergic drugs has been reported during attempts to treat complications arising during anaesthesia. These include methotrimeprazine i.v. 2.5 mg (Mason & Steane 1976), cyproheptadine i.v. 1 mg (Solares et al 1987), ketanserin i.v. 10 mg over 3 minutes and an infusion of 3 mg/h (Fischler et al 1983, Casthely et al 1986). The choice is often governed by availability of the drug.
2. Somatostatin analogues have been found to inhibit the release of active mediators from carcinoid tumours. The use of octreotide (100 µg i.v., Sandostatin, Sandoz SMS 201–995) for pre- and intraoperative treatment during excision of metastatic carcinoid tumours has been

reported (Roy et al 1987), and in one case where cardiovascular collapse occurred it was life saving (Marsh et al 1987).

3. Antibradykinin drugs include aprotinin (infusion of 200 000 kiu in 250 ml saline) and corticosteroids. However, there have been variable reports of their effectiveness in treating complications.

4. The role of histamine is uncertain. Flushing was successfully blocked in a patient with a gastric carcinoid using a combination of H_1 and H_2 antagonists (Roberts et al 1979).

BIBLIOGRAPHY

Casthely P A, Jablons M, Griepp R B, Ergin M A, Goodman K 1986 Ketanserin in the preoperative and intraoperative management of a patient with carcinoid tumour undergoing tricuspid valve replacement. Anesthesia and Analgesia 65: 809–811

Fischler M, Dentan M, Westerman M N, Vourc'h G, Freitag B 1983 Prophylactic use of ketanserin in a patient with carcinoid syndrome. British Journal of Anaesthesia 55: 920

Jones R M, Knight D 1982 Severe hypertension and flushing in a patient with a non-metastatic carcinoid tumour. Anaesthesia 37: 57–59

Lippmann M, Cleveland R J 1973 Anesthetic management of a carcinoid patient undergoing tricuspid valve replacement. Anesthesia and Analgesia 52: 768–771

Marsh H M, Martin J K, Kvols L K et al 1987 Carcinoid crisis during anesthesia: successful treatment with a somatostatin analogue. Anesthesiology 66: 89–91

Mason R A, Steane P A 1976 Carcinoid syndrome: its relevance to the anaesthetist. Anaesthesia 31: 228–242

Miller R, Boulukos P A, Warner R R P 1980 Failure of halothane and ketamine to alleviate carcinoid syndrome-induced bronchospasm during anesthesia. Anesthesia and Analgesia 59: 621–623

Roberts L J II, Marney S R Jr, Oates J A 1979 Blockade of the flush associated with metastatic gastric carcinoid by combined histamine H1 and H2 receptor antagonists. New England Journal of Medicine 300: 236–238

Roy R C, Carter R F, Wright P D 1987 Somatostatin, anaesthesia, and the carcinoid syndrome. Anaesthesia 42: 627–632

Solares G, Blanco E, Pulgar S, Diago C, Ramos F 1987 Carcinoid syndrome and intravenous cyproheptadine. Anaesthesia 1987; 42: 989–992

CARDIAC TAMPONADE
(see also Section 1)

Can occur when a pericardial effusion, or a collection of blood within the pericardial cavity, restricts cardiac filling during diastole by the effect of external pressure. At the point at which the pericardium becomes no longer distensible, small volume increases result in a rapid increase in intrapericardial pressure. There is a fixed decreased diastolic volume of both ventricles. Induction of anaesthesia may cause cardiovascular collapse.

Presentation

1. Causes include malignancy (which may present as a large mediastinal mass), recent cardiac surgery, trauma, closed cardiac massage, intracardiac injection, CVP line or pacemaker insertion, and anticoagulant therapy.

2. In the presence of one of the above predisposing factors, a raised CVP, rapid low volume pulse, hypotension, and reflex peripheral arterial and venous vasoconstriction, may arouse suspicions of tamponade, particularly if respiratory distress is accentuated in the supine position.
3. Pulsus paradoxicus. Normally on inspiration there is a slight fall in systolic pressure. In cardiac tamponade this fall is accentuated, usually to >10 mmHg, and sometimes even to >20 mmHg. Pulsus paradoxicus is easily detected by palpation, but may be measured by an auscultation method (Lake 1983). Using a sphygmomanometer, the cuff pressure should first be reduced until the sound is intermittent, then deflation continued until all beats are heard. The difference between the two pressures is then measured.
4. Tamponade presented with cardiovascular collapse on induction of anaesthesia in a young boy with a mediastinal mass (Keon 1981). At postmortem, a large lymphoma was found to have enveloped the heart and infiltrated the pericardium.

Diagnosis

If the fluid collection is >250 ml, the CXR may show an enlarged globular cardiac outline, the border of which may be straight or even convex. The right cardiophrenic angle is less than 90°. The lung fields are clear. Reduced cardiac pulsation may be detected on fluoroscopy. Echocardiography is the most reliable method of diagnosis (Horgan 1987).

Management

1. Monitor direct arterial and central venous pressures.
2. Minimize factors which worsen the haemodynamic situation.
These include:
    a. An increase in intrathoracic pressure
    If ventilation is already being undertaken, for example after cardiac surgery, then PEEP should be avoided as it further reduces cardiac output, especially at slow rates of ventilation (Mattila et al 1984).
    b. A low intravascular volume
    Maintain the blood volume with i.v. fluids, according to the haemodynamic responses.
    c. A decreased myocardial contractility
    Dopamine may have a favourable effect on haemodynamics, even in the presence of severe tamponade (Mattila et al 1984).
3. Relief of tamponade
If possible, needle pericardiocentesis, with or without catheter insertion, should be performed under local anaesthetic, with ECG and radiological screening and facilities for emergency thoracotomy. The subxiphoid approach can be used in which the needle enters the angle between the xiphisternum and the left costal margin, and is aimed towards the left shoulder. An alternative apical approach can be made through the fifth

intercostal space on the left side (Lake 1983). In either case a soft catheter should be introduced using a Seldinger wire technique, to avoid perforating the myocardium as the fluid or blood is aspirated. Safety may be increased by use of a sterile ECG lead attached to the needle.

BIBLIOGRAPHY

Cobbe S M 1980 Pericardial effusions. British Journal of Hospital Medicine 23: 250–255
Horgan J H 1987 Cardiac tamponade. British Medical Journal 295: 563
Keon T P 1981 Death on induction of anaesthesia for cervical node biopsy. Anesthesiology 55: 471–472
Lake C L 1983 Anesthesia and pericardial disease. Anesthesia and Analgesia 62: 431–443
Mattila I, Takkunen O, Mattila P, Harjula A, Mattila S, Merikallio E 1984 Cardiac tamponade and different modes of ventilation. Acta Anaesthesiologica Scandinavica 28: 236–240

4

DISSEMINATED INTRAVASCULAR COAGULATION
(DIC)

A general term for a derangement of the coagulation process, in which activation of the clotting system results in consumption of platelets and clotting factors, and subsequent overactivation of the fibrinolytic system (Preston 1982). Clinically evident DIC, which presents with bleeding, usually only occurs in critically ill patients.

The occurrence of DIC signals an underlying disease. Therefore the mortality in patients with severe DIC, reported to be as high as 65–85%, is usually a function of the precipitating condition, rather than the DIC itself.

The original stimulus may be tissue damage, toxin production or a drug reaction. Initially there may be just local fibrin deposition at the sites of endothelial damage, thromboplastin or phospholipid release. This can produce mild abnormalities of laboratory tests, without overt clinical problems. On rare occasions, and if the underlying cause is not removed, a pathological state of widespread fibrin deposition can develop, with consumption of clotting factors and secondary fibrinolysis. A wide variety of disease processes can be responsible for the initiating stimulus of a severe DIC, and treatment should be directed towards the correction of this in the first instance. Some doubt has been cast on the role and extent of microvascular thrombosis and organ infarction in the condition (Mant & King 1979). In their series of 47 patients with severe DIC, the mortality was 85%. At autopsy, microvascular thrombosis and organ infarction was found to be uncommon. DIC was only a contributing factor in a quarter of the deaths, and was considered by the authors to be a preterminal event.

Presentation

1. Predisposing factors include Gram-negative septicaemia, malignancy, trauma, surgery, burns, amniotic fluid embolism, pre-eclamptic toxaemia, placental abruption, intrauterine death, fat embolism, malignant hyperpyrexia, late midtrimester abortion (White et al 1983), and drug interactions (Tackley & Tregaskis 1987).
2. The clinical picture is that of widespread oozing from a variety of previously damaged sites, such as wounds, puncture sites or incisions. More clinically serious bleeding may occur from the gastrointestinal tract, the lungs or the uteroplacental bed.
3. The patient is often shocked and acidotic, and proceeds to develop hypoxia and respiratory distress.
4. Coagulation tests basically show evidence of consumption of coagulation factors and platelets, and increased fibrinolysis. The findings are therefore of prolonged one-stage prothrombin time, partial thromboplastin time, thrombin clotting time and usually thrombocytopenia. There is reduced fibrinogen level and increased fibrin degradation products.

Management

1. Early involvement of a haematologist is essential.
2. The diagnosis and treatment, if possible, of the underlying cause, such as infection, retained placenta, etc.
3. The treatment of other abnormalities such as hypoxia, acidosis, electrolyte imbalance and renal failure.
4. Correction of clinically significant abnormalities of haemostasis, as a temporizing measure, with the hope that the initial pathological process might be arrested. On a haematologist's advice, the following may be required:
  a. Fresh frozen plasma.
  b. Cryoprecipitate, especially if hypofibrinogenaemia is present.
  c. Platelet concentrates.
Coagulation tests should be repeated to assess the progress of the condition and its treatment.
5. There is considerable disagreement about the advisability of using of heparin. In a detailed study of 47 patients, heparin was rarely found to be beneficial, and was often suspected of being the cause of severe bleeding (Mant & King 1979). Again, haematological advice is essential.

BIBLIOGRAPHY

Mant M J, King E G 1979 Severe, acute disseminated intravascular coagulation. American Journal of Medicine 67: 557–563
Preston F E 1982 Disseminated intravascular coagulation. British Journal of Hospital Medicine 28: 129–137
Tackley R M, Tregaskis B 1987 Fatal disseminated coagulation following a monoamine oxidase inhibitor/tricyclic interaction. Anaesthesia 42: 760–763

White P F, Coe V, Dworsky W A, Margolis A 1983 Disseminated intravascular coagulation following midtrimester abortions. Anesthesiology 58: 99–101

GLYCINE ABSORPTION
(see TURP SYNDROME)

HIGHER OXIDES OF NITROGEN POISONING

In 1967, an incident occurred in which a batch of nitrous oxide, contaminated with impurities, was used for anaesthesia in the south west of England (Clutton-Brock 1967). Three cases of poisoning occurred, and two of the patients died. The impurities included nitric oxide, nitrogen dioxide and carbon monoxide. A clinical picture of respiratory damage, similar to that produced by a severe acid aspiration syndrome, and circulatory failure, was produced.

Presentation

1. Intense cyanosis occurs due to a combination of methaemoglobinaemia, which reduces the oxygen-carrying capacity of the blood, and arterial desaturation due to pulmonary oedema.
2. The onset of tachypnoea, tachycardia and respiratory distress.
3. Hypotension and circulatory failure. Nitrates and nitrites relax smooth muscle and cause vasodilatation.
4. Respiratory and metabolic acidosis. Nitrogen dioxide dissolves in body fluids to produce nitrous and nitric acids. Lactic acidosis also occurs due to tissue hypoxia.

Diagnosis

Crude testing: moistened starch iodide paper is placed in a large syringe, into which 15 ml of the suspect nitrous oxide and 5 ml of oxygen is drawn. If contamination of >30 parts/10^6 is present, then the starch iodide paper will turn blue within 10 minutes.

Management

1. Give 100% oxygen. IPPV and PEEP may be required.
2. Insert a radial artery cannula and take serial samples for blood gases, acid base status and oxygen content. Estimate the haemoglobin and methaemoglobin levels.
3. Attempt to convert the methaemoglobin using methylene blue 1–2 mg/kg. This should be titrated against blood levels of methaemoglobin, as excess methylene blue can in itself cause methaemoglobinaemia, as well as a haemolytic anaemia.

4. Hypotension should be treated with a vasopressor, such as methoxamine or noradrenaline, both of which have specific peripheral smooth muscle effects. Other cardiovascular support may be required.
5. Antibiotics, parenteral steroids and bronchodilators have been suggested for the pneumonitis (Prys-Roberts 1967).
6. In a severe case, specific treatment with dimercaprol has been recommended (Prys-Roberts 1967).

BIBLIOGRAPHY

Clutton-Brock J 1967 Two cases of poisoning by contamination of nitrous oxide with higher oxides of nitrogen. British Journal of Anaesthesia 39: 388–392
Prys-Roberts C 1967 Principles of treatment of poisoning by higher oxides of nitrogen. British Journal of Anaesthesia 39: 432–439

4

LOCAL ANAESTHETIC TOXICITY

Local anaesthetic toxicity may occur if the maximum safe dose is exceeded, or if transient high blood levels are achieved by accidental intravenous injection, or rapid absorption from an inflamed or vascular area.

During the last decade, certain aspects of local anaesthetic practice have been a source of concern and debate. An early problem concerned the use of bupivacaine for intravenous regional anaesthesia. Several deaths occurred in the UK, some in young people, and followed the use of this technique by accident and emergency medical staff.

Three main factors might have contributed to the fatalities – the equipment, the drugs or the people using them (Heath 1982). In unfamiliar hands, accidental deflation of an automatic tourniquet can occur before the local anaesthetic has become fixed. Inappropriately high doses of the drug may be given. Standard resuscitation procedures in casualty may be inadequate. The difficulties experienced in resuscitation when collapse did occur raised the possibility that bupivacaine might be cardiotoxic. A combination of these factors was possible. Bupivacaine is now no longer recommended for intravenous regional anaesthesia in the UK.

Over the last few years, increasing amounts of clinical and experimental evidence have indeed suggested that the two longer-acting local anaesthetics, bupivacaine and etidocaine, may possess cardiotoxic properties.

Some controversy still exists, as severe lactic and respiratory acidosis has also been shown to accompany the convulsions (Moore et al 1980). A series of reports of deaths, chiefly associated with obstetric anaesthesia, and the subsequent evidence presented to the FDA (Albright 1979, Reiz &

Nath 1986), led to the withdrawal of bupivacaine 0.75% for obstetric use in the USA. There was some disquiet about this decision, as few of the clinical reports of these deaths had appeared in the national anaesthetic literature. In the UK, the manufacturers now state that the 0.75% solution is contraindicated in obstetric anaesthesia, and that bupivacaine should not be used at all for intravenous regional anaesthesia.

Presentation

1. Causative factors include administration of a local anaesthetic in doses exceeding the toxic levels, the sudden release of a normal dose into the circulation or the injection of small amounts into an artery supplying the brain. The arterial concentration, and in particular the proportion of blood going to the brain, is important in acute toxicity. Toxicity is therefore likely to be worst in a hypovolaemic or shocked patient (Scott 1986). The threshold for CNS toxicity with lignocaine is $5 \mu g/ml$, which is close to the therapeutic dose for treatment of ventricular extrasystoles.

2. Symptoms of toxicity include lightheadedness, circumoral tingling, numbness of the tongue, a metallic taste, tinnitus, visual disturbances, anxiety and restlessness. Convulsions and apnoea may follow.

3. The combination of apnoea and convulsions leads to hypoxia, respiratory and metabolic (in particular lactic) acidosis. With drugs such as lignocaine, it had been accepted that a wide margin existed between CNS and cardiovascular toxicity. However, the situation with bupivacaine appears to be different, in that following convulsions, hypotension, serious ventricular arrhythmias or cardiac arrest have been reported. Resuscitation had proved to be particularly difficult or impossible (Albright 1979, Prentiss 1979). Successful resuscitation has however been reported on occasions (Davis & de Jong 1982, Mallampati et al 1984). In late pregnancy the associated problems of aortocaval occlusion and supine resuscitation cannot be ignored.

4. In the cases of bupivacaine and etidocaine, the margin between CNS and cardiac toxicity does appear to be narrower than that with lignocaine. The cardiac effects of bupivacaine do not appear to be attributable solely to hypoxia and acidosis, and may be in part related to differences in myocardial uptake of the drug (Morishima et al 1985).

5. There is now clinical and experimental evidence to suggest that pregnant patients are particularly vulnerable to bupivacaine toxicity (Morishima et al 1983). While the combination of severe lactic acidosis and hypoxia during convulsions was felt to be sufficient to account for the resuscitation difficulties (Moore & Bonica 1985), even these authors now admit that the evidence in favour of cardiac toxicity is increasing. Severe ventricular arrhythmias occurred with bupivacaine in pregnant sheep, even when the acidosis was rapidly corrected (Marx 1984).

6. Physical injury may sometimes result from local anaesthetic toxicity.

Convulsions caused posterior dislocation of the shoulder in two cases, after bupivacaine injection during sacral and epidural anaesthesia respectively (Pagden et al 1986).

Prophylaxis

1. Do not exceed the maximum safe dose for the particular local anaesthetic being used.
2. With epidural anaesthesia there is no foolproof method of ensuring that intravascular or subarachnoid injection has not occurred.
3. All injections should be given slowly and the dose should be fractionated. Where a large volume of local anaesthetic is required, a rate not exceeding 1 ml/s and the use of a 10 ml rather than a 30 ml syringe has been recommended (Moore & Bonica 1985).
4. Aspiration for blood and CSF should always be performed. However, a negative test does not ensure safe placement of the epidural catheter.
5. The use of a test dose is controversial. It has been suggested that for a single test dose of local anaesthetic to be of value in signalling the possibility of an i.v. or subarachnoid injection, it must contain a dose of local anaesthetic sufficient to rapidly produce evidence of spinal anaesthesia, plus 0.015 mg adrenaline. Thus a systemic tachycardia will give warning of an accidental intravascular injection (Moore & Batra 1981). This means the use of 3 ml of local anaesthetic containing 1 :200 000 adrenaline. However, there are doubts about the safety of using adrenaline in obstetric patients. It was found to decrease uterine blood flow in up to 50% of pregnant ewes, sometimes with signs of fetal distress (Hood et al 1986). The heart rate in the pregnant patient is so variable that its reliability has also been called into question (Leighton et al 1987).
6. The patient's mental state should be continuously assessed throughout the injection, usually by engaging her in active conversation. Each subsequent dose of local anaesthetic should be considered as if it were a test dose.
7. The immediate availability of resuscitation equipment and experienced personnel.

Management

The method by which the convulsions are controlled is arguable, and depends partly upon the experience of the attendant.

1. Oxygenation and control of convulsions
   a. Suxamethonium will immediately control convulsions, and allow oxygen to be given by bag and mask ventilation, prior to intubation. During local anaesthetic-induced convulsions, severe hypoxia, hypercarbia and lactic acidosis occur simultaneously. Lactic acid production stops immediately after administration of suxamethonium.

Rapid intubation is permitted, no myocardial depression occurs and its effects wear off rapidly (Moore & Bonica 1985).

b. Thiopentone 150–200 mg has been advocated in preference to suxamethonium, on the grounds that suxamethonium is unsafe unless given by someone capable of managing a paralysed patient, and may result in an awake, intubated patient (Scott 1986).

c. Diazepam 2–5 mg has also been recommended. However it takes several minutes to become effective, during which time the convulsions continue and acidosis progresses. It is a long-acting drug and it has respiratory-depressant properties.

2. Cardiac resuscitation

May be required with a massive local anaesthetic overdose or if bupivacaine has been used. ECG monitoring may show bradycardia, asystole, ventricular tachycardia or ventricular fibrillation.

a. Cardiac massage must be sustained and effective, as bupivacaine remains longer in the myocardium than lignocaine.

b. Hypoxia and acidosis must be corrected rapidly.

c. If ventricular fibrillation occurs, defibrillation may not be successful on the first occasion.

d. Ventricular tachycardia is treated. The ventricular tachycardia threshold has been tested during bupivacaine toxicity in dogs (Kasten & Martin 1985). Bretylium raised the ventricular tachycardia threshold, whereas lignocaine was either ineffective or further lowered it. It was noted that bupivacaine prolonged the Q–T interval and produced a ventricular tachycardia similar to that of a torsade de pointes atypical VT. Bretylium tosylate 5–10 mg/kg (diluted to 10 mg/ml with 5% dextrose or normal saline) can be given slowly over 8–10 minutes, with ECG observation.

e. Hypotension may need to be treated with inotropes or vasopressors.

BIBLIOGRAPHY

Albright G A 1979 Cardiac arrest following regional anesthesia with etidocaine or bupivacaine. Anesthesiology 51: 285–287

Davis N L, de Jong R H 1982 Successful resuscitation following massive bupivacaine overdose. Anesthesia and Analgesia 61: 62–64

Heath M 1982 Deaths after intravenous regional anaesthesia. British Medical Journal 285: 913–914

Hood D D, Dewan D M, James F M 1986 Maternal and fetal effects of epinephrine in gravid ewes. Anesthesiology 64: 610–613

Kasten G W, Martin S T 1985 Bupivacaine cardiovascular toxicity. Comparison of treatment with bretylium and lignocaine. Anesthesia and Analgesia 64: 911–916

Leighton B, Norris M, Sosis M, Epstein R, Chayen B, Larijani G E 1987 Limitations of epinephrine as a marker of intravascular injection in laboring women. Anesthesiology 66: 688–691

Mallampati S R, Liu P L, Knapp R M 1984 Convulsions and ventricular tachycardia from bupivacaine with epinephrine: successful resuscitation. Anaesthesia and Analgesia 63: 856–859

Marx G F 1984 Cardiotoxicity of local anesthetics – the plot thickens. Anesthesiology 60: 3–5

Moore D C, Batra M S 1981 The components of an effective test dose prior to epidural block. Anesthesiology 55: 693–696

Moore D C, Bonica J J 1985 Convulsions and ventricular tachycardia from bupivacaine with epinephrine: successful resuscitation – congratulations. Anesthesia and Analgesia 64: 844–845

Moore D C, Crawford R D, Scurlock J E 1980 Severe hypoxia and acidosis following local anesthetic-induced convulsions. Anesthesiology 53: 259–260

Morishima H O, Pedersen H, Finster M et al 1983 Is bupivacaine more cardiotoxic than lignocaine? Anesthesiology 59S: A409

Morishima H O, Pedersen H, Finster M et al 1985 Bupivacaine toxicity in pregnant and non-pregnant ewes. Anesthesiology 63: 134–139

Pagden D, Halaburt A S, Wirpszor R, Karyn A 1986 Posterior dislocation of the shoulder complicating regional anaesthesia. Anesthesia and Analgesia 65: 1063–1065

Prentiss J E 1979 Cardiac arrest following regional anaesthesia with etidocaine or bupivacaine. Anesthesiology 51: 285–287

Reiz S. Nath S 1986 Cardiotoxicity of local anaesthetic agents. British Journal of Anaesthesia 58: 736–746

Scott D B 1986 Toxic effects of local anaesthetic agents on the central nervous system. British Journal of Anaesthesia 58: 732–735

MALIGNANT HYPERPYREXIA
(see also Section 1)

Presentation

1. Failure to relax after suxamethonium. Muscle rigidity after suxamethonium is an abnormal reaction (Ellis & Halsall 1984). It may be an early sign of MH, although other muscular disorders, such as the myotonic or muscular dystrophies, can be responsible. Susceptibility to MH was identified in about half of a group of 77 patients, investigated after an episode of isolated masseter rigidity (Rosenberg & Fletcher 1986). (see also Masseter muscle rigidity).

2. An increasing tachycardia temperature, and the appearance of ventricular ectopic beats.

3. Tachypnoea occurs in a spontaneously breathing patient and there is an increased requirement for muscle relaxants in the paralysed patient. Both states are due to stimulation of respiration by rising $PaCO_2$ levels and a metabolic acidosis. When a capnograph is in use, an increased $ETCO_2$ may be the earliest sign of MH (Thomas et al 1987). In the later stages, cyanosis occurs, due to a massive increase in oxygen consumption, and to ventilation perfusion defects.

4. A severe metabolic acidosis develops. In the earlier reports of fulminating MH, an arterial pH of less than 7.0 was not uncommon. Severe acidosis (or possibly hyperkalaemia) may have been responsible for the cases in which sudden 'unexpected' death occurred in the operating theatre.

5. Rigidity of some, but not necessarily all, groups of muscles. Although a non-rigid group has been described, it is not yet certain whether this is a different biochemical process, or an earlier stage of the same process. A contracture of the muscle actually takes place and if the process is not

aborted, oedema, and subsequent ischaemia, of the muscle can develop.
6. Myoglobin and potassium may be released in large quantities,
sometimes resulting in massive myoglobinuria and renal failure. The
serum CPK can be elevated to exceed 100 000 iu/l.
7. Disseminated intravascular coagulation may occur in advanced cases,
possibly secondary to thromboplastin release.
8. Cerebral and pulmonary oedema may develop.

Management

If an unexpected intraoperative diagnosis of MH is made, the treatment
required will depend upon the severity of the reaction at the time of
diagnosis. The patient's susceptibility, the promptness of the diagnosis
and hence the dose of the triggering agent received, are important factors
(Gronert 1980). With a short exposure and a rapid diagnosis the
syndrome may be aborted by the first measure alone:

1. Stop the use of all MH trigger agents. Terminate surgery if possible.
Observe ECG and capnograph. Estimate blood gases.
2. Delegate one person to prepare dantrolene sodium, 1 mg/kg.
3. Record core temperature, pulse rate and blood pressure every 5
minutes.
4. Hypercarbia should be treated with hyperventilation, acidosis with
sodium bicarbonate 2–4 mmol/kg, and oxygenation maintained.
5. Send venous samples for electrolytes, calcium and CPK.
6. Give dantrolene sodium i.v. 1 mg/kg and repeat, up to 10 mg/kg.
7. If the syndrome is severe, treat symptomatically. Institute cooling and
treat hyperkalaemia if necessary.
8. Save the first urine sample for myoglobin estimation. Measure urine
output. If there is obvious myoglobinuria, give i.v. fluids, with mannitol or
frusemide to reduce the possibility of renal failure.
9. The use of steroids is controversial. They may be indicated in the
severe case, particularly if there is cerebral oedema.
10. Repeat the CPK at 24 hours.
11. Treat DIC if necessary.
12. The half-life of dantrolene is only 5 hours, therefore if retriggering
occurs in the first 24 hours, it may need to be repeated.

BIBLIOGRAPHY

Ellis F R, Halsall P J 1984 Suxamethonium spasm, British Journal of Anaesthesia 56:
    381–384
Gronert G A 1980 Malignant hyperthermia. Anesthesiology 53: 395–423
Rosenberg H, Fletcher J E 1986 Masseter musle rigidity and malignant hyperthermia
    susceptibility. Anaesthesia and Analgesia 65: 161–164
Thomas D W, Dev V J, Whitehead M J 1987 Malignant hyperpyrexia and isoflurane.
    British Journal of Anaesthesia 59: 1196–1198

MASSETER MUSCLE RIGIDITY
(MMR)

Severe rigidity involving the masseter muscle may occasionally occur after the administration of suxamethonium, with or without an inhalational agent. The rigidity can last several minutes, and may be such that the jaw can barely be opened. Intubation may temporarily be impossible, although ventilation on a mask is usually feasible. It is more likely to happen in young patients. All cases have some rhabdomyolysis, as evidenced by a rise in CPK. The masseter spasm may be associated with ventricular arrhythmias and myoglobinuria.

4

Most authors agree that masseter muscle rigidity is an abnormal reaction and that a significant proportion of patients in whom MMR develops will be susceptible to malignant hyperpyrexia (MHS). The masseter muscle is known to contain a unique form of myosin. This may explain the localization of the spasm to the jaw muscles (Fletcher 1987).

1. MMR associated with malignant hyperpyrexia
The exact percentage of MMR patients found subsequently to be MH susceptible (MHS) varies with the studies reported. One claimed an incidence of 100% in 15 patients (Schwartz et al 1984). However, the diagnosis of MH was made on the basis of a sarcoplasmic reticulum calcium uptake test. This has not been accepted as diagnostic by a number of workers in the field, and an incidence as high as this has therefore been disputed (Ellis & Halsall 1986).

Using caffeine and halothane contracture tests, other workers have found the incidence to be between 40% and 60%. Nearly 50% of 77 patients who had developed MMR after suxamethonium were found to be MHS using these tests (Rosenberg & Fletcher 1986). Another study reported four out of six boys with isolated MMR to be MHS (Flewellen & Nelson 1984).

Muscle rigidity, not necessarily of the masseter alone, is a common feature in MH episodes. It appeared in about 80% of MHS patients studied by Britt and Kalow (1970). In 31 out of 75 patients, MH episodes with muscle rigidity occurred after the use of suxamethonium. In another study of 147 patients found to be MHS after referral for investigation (Ellis & Halsall 1984), 65% had responded to suxamethonium with muscle spasm. In 5% of these MHS patients, the suxamethonium spasm was the only sign of MHS.

The onset of MMR may therefore allow early diagnosis of MH and cessation of the triggering agents.
2. MMR not associated with malignant hyperpyrexia
Further investigations of the group of patients with MMR who were shown not to be susceptible to malignant hyperthermia (MHN), revealed a small number who had some other myopathy. These included

Duchenne and Becker muscle dystrophies and myotonia congenita. The
remainder must be assumed to have an abnormal reaction to
suxamethonium.

3. Incidence of masseter muscle 'spasm' in children

Two studies claim that masseter spasm occurs in as many as 1% of
children after halothane induction followed by suxamethonium
administration (Schwartz et al 1984, Carroll 1987). The discrepancy
between these figures, and the 50% incidence of MHS with MMR, is
difficult to explain. A difference in definition of MMR may contribute
(Rosenberg 1987). MMR is a situation in which the jaw can hardly be
opened, even with considerable effort by the anaesthetist. This situation,
which is rare, must be differentiated from a mere increase in muscle tone,
which is common among children (van der Spek et al 1987).

Presentation

1. Administration of suxamethonium is associated with a degree of
rigidity of the jaw muscles, such that the patient's mouth can hardly be
opened. It may last several minutes and result in intubation difficulty.

2. Peripheral muscles are usually flaccid, and there is no response to
nerve stimulation.

3. The episode may be accompanied by tachycardia or ventricular
arrhythmias.

4. Pyrexia can develop subsequently, or the patient may be apyrexial.

5. CPK will be raised, and myoglobinuria may occur, within the first 24
hours.

6. Muscle pains, stiffness and occasionally weakness may last for
several days.

7. 40–60% of patients may proceed to MH, although this may not be
immediately clinically obvious.

Management

1. If a patient develops MMR after suxamethonium, all MH trigger
agents should be stopped. The patient can usually be ventilated with
oxygen by mask. A second dose of suxamethonium should not be given.
The patient should be assumed to be potentially at risk from MH, until
proved otherwise.

2. If the surgery is elective, postponement has been advocated, as even
in the absence of an overt MH episode, significant rhabdomyolysis may
occur (Rosenberg 1987). Other authors have suggested that surgery
might be continued with close metabolic and acid base monitoring and
only stopped if signs suggest an abnormal metabolic response (Gronert
1988). The former approach is recommended. Difficulties may arise should
signs of MH occur after surgery has been started.

3. If surgery is urgent, a N_2O/narcotic analgesic/relaxant technique should be used, and carbon dioxide, temperature and biochemistry closely monitored. Some authors believe that, in addition, dantrolene 2.5 mg/kg should be given (Flewellen & Nelson 1982). This has not been completely accepted.

4. Postoperative CPK levels should be done. In all patients with MMR, the CPK will be elevated. However, in one of the studies, levels above 20 000 u occurred only in patients found to be MHS, or in MHN patients with muscle dystrophy (Rosenberg & Fletcher 1986).

5. If frank myoglobinuria occurs, intravenous fluids and an osmotic diuretic should be given. Renal function requires monitoring.

6. All patients should be investigated subsequently, to exclude MHS. Those who are shown to be MHS should subsequently only have non-triggering anaesthetics.

7. Those who have experienced an episode of masseter rigidity following suxamethonium, but on testing are found to be MHN, can receive inhalational agents for subsequent anaesthetics. However, they should not be given suxamethonium again and the patient should be given a warning card to this effect. Muscle biopsy on relatives of these patients is said to be unnecessary, as there is no evidence that suxamethonium muscle rigidity is inherited (Rosenberg 1988).

8. The results of investigations should be clearly conveyed to the patients and recorded in the notes.

BIBLIOGRAPHY

Britt B A, Kalow W 1970 Malignant hyperthermia: a statistical review. Canadian Anaesthetists' Society Journal 17: 293–315

Carroll J B 1987 Increased incidence of masseter spasm in children with strabismus anaesthetised with halothane and succinylcholine. Anesthesiology 67: 559–561

Ellis F R, Halsall P J 1984 Suxamethonium spasm. A differential diagnostic conundrum. British Journal of Anaesthesia 56: 381–384

Ellis F R, Halsall P J 1986 Improper diagnostic test may account for high incidence of malignant hyperthermia associated with masseter spasm. Anesthesiology 64: 291

Fletcher R 1987 4th International Hyperpyrexia Workshop. Report of a meeting. Anaesthesia 42: 206

Flewellen E H, Nelson T E 1982 Masseter spasm induced by succinylcholine in children: contracture testing for malignant hyperthermia: report of 6 cases. Canadian Anaesthetists' Society Journal 29: 42–49

Flewellen E H, Nelson T E 1984 Halothane-succinylcholine induced masseter spasm: indicative of malignant hyperthermia susceptibility? Anesthesia and Analgesia 63: 693–697

Gronert G A 1988 Management of patients in whom trismus occurs following succinylcholine. Anesthesiology 68: 653–654

Rosenberg H 1987 Trismus is not trivial. Anesthesiology 67: 453–455

Rosenberg H 1988 Clinical presentation of malignant hyperthermia. British Journal of Anaesthesia 60: 268–273

Rosenbert H, Fletcher J E 1986 Masseter muscle rigidity and malignant hyperthermia susceptibility. Anesthesia and Analgesia 65: 161–164

Schwartz L, Rockoff M A, Koka B V 1984 Masseter spasm and anesthesia: incidence and implications. Anesthesiology 61: 772–775

van der Spek A F L, Fang W B, Ashton-Miller J A, Stohler C S, Carlson D S, Schork M A 1987 The effect of succinylcholine on mouth opening. Anesthesiology 67: 459–465

MENDELSON'S SYNDROME, ACID ASPIRATION SYNDROME

A syndrome which follows pulmonary aspiration of acid gastric contents. Gastric fluid, particularly that with a pH of 2.5 or less, causes chemical damage to the alveolar epithelium and the capillary endothelium. As a result of permeability changes, fluid and protein leak from the capillaries into the alveoli and interstitial spaces, causing pulmonary oedema and hypoxia. This leakage is enhanced by increases in pulmonary artery pressure. It is particularly, but not exclusively, associated with obstetric anaesthesia and is more likely to occur in cases in which intubation difficulties have been encountered.

4

Presentation

1. Regurgitation and aspiration may be obvious at induction, or it may pass unnoticed, particularly if intubation problems are encountered. Under the latter circumstances, signs may be delayed for several hours. The syndrome has been reported to follow the aspiration of as little as 25 ml of acid.
2. Unexplained bronchospasm may occur during the anaesthetic. In the absence of a history of asthma, aspiration should be suspected.
3. Postoperatively, tachycardia, tachypnoea, cyanosis and respiratory difficulty may develop.
4. CXR may be normal initially, but can progress from patchy pulmonary infiltration, most commonly in the basal or perihilar regions, to signs of gross pulmonary oedema.
5. If significant inhalation has occurred, serial blood gases will show a deterioration in oxygenation. A decreasing PaO_2 and a metabolic acidosis will occur.

Management

1. The patient should be placed in a head-down position and the pharynx or endotracheal tube sucked out. There is little place for bronchoscopy unless solid pieces of food have been inhaled.
2. If inhalation has occurred or is suspected, treatment should be aggressive. The endotracheal tube should be kept in situ and IPPV and PEEP instituted. The aim of treatment is to provide respiratory support until pulmonary function returns to normal. A policy of waiting for deterioration may prove to be disastrous.
3. The advisability of using high-dose steroids remains controversial. One view is that there is little evidence to support their use, and that if infection occurs, there may also be interference with tissue immunity. High-dose steroids were of no benefit in treating pneumonitis induced in

rabbits (Wynne et al 1979). On the contrary, a clinical impression has been gained that, in man, their use for a 72-hour period may limit the extent of damage (Zorab 1984).

4. If the inhaled material is obviously contaminated, then antibiotics can be given. Otherwise they should be reserved for the presence of proven infection, and the appropriate antibiotic used to which the organism is sensitive.

5. Bronchodilators may be given for bronchospasm. Aminophylline i.v. 5 mg/kg over 10–15 minutes, can be followed by an infusion of 0.5 mg/kg/h.

6. Occasionally dopamine 5–20 μg/kg/min may be required for inotropic support.

4

BIBLIOGRAPHY

Wynne J W, Reynolds J C, Hood I, Auerbach D, Ondrasick J 1979 Steroid therapy for pneumonitis in rabbits by aspiration of foodstuffs. Anesthesiology 51: 11–19
Zorab J S M 1984 Pulmonary aspiration. British Medical Journal 288: 1631–1632

PHAEOCHROMOCYTOMA
(see also Section 1)

Patients with unsuspected phaeochromocytoma may undergo anaesthesia for routine surgical or obstetric procedures. The danger of this situation is underlined by the results of a study of 54 patients in whom tumours were shown at autopsy. These had been clinically unsuspected prior to the event leading to death, or were only diagnosed postmortem (Sutton et al 1981). One-third of these patients had died suddenly during, or immediately after, minor operations for unrelated conditions. Death was associated with either hypotensive or hypertensive crises.

Severe complications may occur with remarkable rapidity. If disaster is to be averted, the anaesthetist must be aware of the possibility of the diagnosis, the detailed pharmacology of the condition, and the correct method of treatment. Tachycardia treated blindly with beta blockers may result in extreme hypertension. Patients are at risk from cerebral haemorrhage, encephalopathy, pulmonary oedema, myocardial infarction, ventricular fibrillation or renal failure. Phaeochromocytoma during pregnancy carries a particularly bad prognosis. A maternal mortality of 48%, and a fetal mortality of 55% have been reported (Mitchell et al 1987).

The commonest preoperative clinical features are episodes of headache, pallor, palpitations, and sweating. Patients may have an unusually labile blood pressure and a pressor response to the induction of anaesthesia.

Presentation

1. Severe hypertension or severe hypotension during the perioperative period (Sutton et al 1981, Wooster & Mitchell 1981, Bittar 1979, 1982, Jones & Hill 1981).

2. Tachyarrhythmias. A patient with an abdominal mass, high output left ventricular failure and hypertension underwent laparotomy. Severe cardiovascular instability was treated with practolol and phentolamine. Massive blood loss was reduced by means of sodium nitroprusside. Direct arterial and pulmonary artery pressure monitoring assisted cardiovascular control. Subsequent histology confirmed a phaeochromocytoma (Darby & Prys-Roberts 1976).

3. Acute pulmonary oedema may present unexpectedly. A 43-year-old man with a history of attacks of sweating and palpitations, was admitted to ITU with pulmonary oedema and shock (Blom et al 1987). He was treated with IPPV and cardiovascular monitoring. Biochemistry indicated a predominantly adrenaline-secreting phaeochromocytoma.

4. Phaeochromocytomas presenting in pregnancy are associated with a high mortality. The condition may be forgotten, or misdiagnosed as pre-eclampsia. Tachycardia and gross pulmonary oedema occurred on extubation at the end of a Caesarean section in a patient with pre-eclampsia (personal communication). Death occurred 3 days later, and the diagnosis was only made at autopsy.

5. An acute abdominal emergency. Haemorrhagic necrosis of the tumour mimicked an acute abdominal emergency in two cases (Jones & Durning 1985). One patient developed pulmonary oedema after induction and surgery was abandoned. The second developed a tachycardia of 180/min and an unrecordable BP during surgery. Both died postoperatively.

Management

1. Incidental surgery in a patient with an undiagnosed phaeochromocytoma carries a high mortality. The patient's best chance of survival lies in the early recognition of the condition, cessation of the proceedings, and admission to an ITU for haemodynamic monitoring (Smith et al 1978).

2. Phentolamine, phenoxybenzamine and sodium nitroprusside have all been used to control hypertension. The use of magnesium sulphate in a pregnant patient has been reported (James et al 1988). Magnesium is known to inhibit catecholamine release from the adrenal medulla, to decrease the sensitivity of the alpha adrenergic receptors to catecholamines and to cause vasodilatation. A bolus of magnesium sulphate i.v. 4 g over 15 minutes was used, followed by an infusion of 1.5 g/h.

3. If hypotension occurs, phenylephrine or dopamine have been suggested as the most appropriate agents to use (Roizen et al 1982).

4. Beta blockers should only be used to treat a tachycardia after alpha blockers have been given.

BIBLIOGRAPHY

Bittar D A 1979 Innovar-induced hypertensive crises in patients with pheochromocytoma. Anesthesiology 50: 366–369
Bittar D A 1982 Unsuspected phaeochromocytoma. Canadian Anaesthetists' Society Journal 29: 183–184
Blom H J, Karsdorp V, Birnie R, Davies G 1987 Phaeochromocytoma as a cause of pulmonary oedema. Anaesthesia 42: 646–650
Darby E, Prys-Roberts C 1976 Unusual presentation of phaeochromocytoma. Management of anaesthesia and cardiovascular monitoring. Anaesthesia 31: 913–916
James M F M, Huddle K R L, Owen A D, van der Veen B W 1988 Use of magnesium sulphate in the anaesthetic management of phaeochromocytoma in pregnancy. Canadian Journal of Anaesthesia 35: 178–182
Jones D J, Durning P 1985 Phaeochromocytoma presenting as an acute abdomen: report of two cases. British Medical Journal 291: 1267–1269
Jones R M, Hill A B 1981 Severe hypertension associated with pancuronium in a patient with a phaeochromocytoma. Canadian Anaesthetists' Society Journal 28: 394–396
Mitchell S Z, Freilich J D, Brant D, Flynn M 1987 Anesthetic management of pheochromocytoma resection during pregnancy. Anesthesia and Analgesia 66: 478–480
Roizen M F, Horrigan R W, Koike M et al 1982 A prospective randomised trial of 4 anaesthetic techniques for resection of pheochromocytoma. Anesthesiology 57: A43
Smith D S, Aukburg S M, Levitt J D 1978 Induction of anesthesia in a patient with undiagnosed pheochromocytoma. Anesthesiology 49: 368–369
Sutton M St J, Sheps S G, Lie J T 1981 Prevalence of clinically unsuspected pheochromocytoma. Mayo Clinic Proceedings 56: 354–360
Wooster L, Mitchell R I 1981 Unsuspected phaeochromocytoma presenting during surgery. Canadian Anaesthetists' Society Journal 28: 471–474

PNEUMOTHORAX

An air-containing space within the pleural cavity which communicates with the bronchial tree. It may cause compression and collapse of lung tissue, resulting in atelectasis and intrapulmonary shunting. During anaesthesia a pneumothorax may increase in size, either due to diffusion of nitrous oxide, or secondary to positive pressure ventilation. Conversion to a tension pneumothorax will cause compression of mediastinal structures. In the absence of treatment this can result in cardiovascular collapse and death. Bilateral pneumothorax may occasionally occur during anaesthesia.

Presentation

1. Factors predisposing to the development of a pneumothorax include:
   a. Chronic bronchitis and emphysema.
   b. Congenital lung cysts
   A rise in tension within the cyst, due to rapid diffusion of nitrous oxide, may cause it to rupture.
   c. Fractured ribs

With or without surgical emphysema.

d IPPV

Particularly with high inspiratory pressures. This has occurred, secondary to pulmonary barotrauma, as a result of ventilator dysfunction (Hilton & Clement 1983).

e. Jet ventilation techniques

Unilateral pneumothorax occurred as a result of the catheter being placed in the left main bronchus (Chang et al 1980). High alveolar pressures may be achieved with laryngeal obstruction of only brief duration.

f. Cystic fibrosis

Pneumothorax is a common complication of cystic fibrosis in adults. It tends to be recurrent, and may be difficult to treat (Penketh et al 1982, Robinson & Branthwaite 1984).

g. In neonates

May occur in association with tracheo-oesophageal fistula, diaphragmatic hernia (Diaz 1987) and during prolonged ventilation for RDS.

h. Surgical procedures

Including nephrectomy, cervical sympathectomy and rib resection.

i. Local anaesthetic procedures

Such as supraclavicular or interscalene brachial plexus, stellate ganglion or intercostal blocks.

j. Subclavian venous cannulation

Fatalities have been reported due to bilateral pneumothorax during attempted subclavian venous cannulation (Schapira & Stern 1967).

k. In association with laparoscopy

Bilateral pneumothoraces which required urgent treatment (Doctor & Hussain 1973), and a transient pneumothorax which spontaneously resolved, and was probably due to nitrous oxide (Batra et al 1983), have been reported in association with laparoscopy.

l. Endotracheal intubation

Subcutaneous emphysema and pneumothorax resulted from accidental oesophageal intubation and perforation (Johnson & Hood 1986).

2. Clinical signs

If the patient is being ventilated, there will be a decreased compliance, difficulty in ventilation, hyperresonance on percussion and diminished movement of one side of the chest. If unrelieved, it may progress to signs of mediastinal shift, cyanosis, tachycardia and hypotension. Further progression may lead to cardiovascular collapse and death.

Diagnosis

1. Clinical

Decreased chest movement on one side, with absent breath sounds, hyperresonance, tracheal shift, a fall in oxygen saturation and eventual frank cyanosis.

2. If time and the clinical situation permits, confirmation is by CXR.

Management

1. Stop nitrous oxide administration.
2. Immediately insert a chest drain

In an emergency, when the patient is on IPPV, a 12 gauge needle can be inserted into the second intercostal space in order to relieve the tension. An Argyle-type catheter and introducer can then be inserted at leisure into the second intercostal interspace, anteriorly, in the midclavicular line and connected to an underwater seal drain.

Alternatively the fifty interspace can be used, in the anterior axillary line, posterior to pectoralis major.

BIBLIOGRAPHY

Batra M S, Driscoll J J, Coburn W A, 1983 Evanescent N$_2$O pneumothorax after laparoscopy. Anesthesia and Analgesia 62: 1121–1123
Chang J–L, Bleyaert A, Bedger R 1980 Unilateral pneumothorax following jet ventilation during general anesthesia. Anesthesiology 53: 244–246
Diaz J 1987 Tension pneumoperitoneum-pneumothorax during repair of congenital diaphragmatic hernia. Anesthesia and Analgesia 66: 577–580
Doctor N H, Hussain Z 1973 Bilateral pneumothorax associated with laparoscopy. Anaesthesia 28: 75–81
Hilton P J, Clement J A 1983 Surgical emphysema resulting from ventilator malfunction. Anaesthesia 38: 342–345
Johnson K G, Hood D D 1986 Esophageal perforation associated with endotracheal intubation. Anesthesiology 64: 281–283
Penketh A, Knight R K, Hodson M E, Baten J C 1982 Management of pneumothorax in adults with cystic fibrosis. Thorax 37: 850–853
Robinson D A, Branthwaite M A 1984 Pleural surgery in patients with cystic fibrosis. A review of anaesthetic management. Anaesthesia 39: 655–659
Schapira M, Stern W Z 1967 Hazards of subclavian vein cannulation for central venous pressure monitoring. Journal of the American Medical Association 201: 327–329

PULMONARY OEDEMA
(see also Section 1)

Acute pulmonary oedema occurring in the perioperative period can be broadly divided into two groups; that of cardiogenic, and of non-cardiogenic, origin. There are some cases in which the aetiology may not be clear cut, and a number of factors may contribute. Broadly, one of two basic abnormalities may occur to produce pulmonary oedema. The first is an increase in the gradient between hydrostatic and colloid osmotic pressure across the pulmonary capillary wall. The second is an increase in pulmonary capillary permeability.

1. Increased pulmonary hydrostatic pressure may be secondary to:
  a. Increase in right atrial pressure, or preload (due to fluid retention or fluid overload).
  b. Decreased myocardial contractility (due to myocardial infarction or a cardiomyopathy).
  c. Increase in left atrial pressure, e.g. in mitral stenosis.
  d. Increased afterload (due to severe hypertension, peripheral vasoconstriction, an anatomical or a pathological obstruction).
2. Increased capillary permeability may be due to:
  a. Pulmonary aspiration of acid gastric contents.
  b. Air, gas or amniotic fluid embolism.
  c. Allergic reactions to drugs or blood products.
  d. Higher oxides of nitrogen.
  e. Pneumonias and septicaemias.
  f. Shock lung or ARDS.

There are a number of specific types of non-cardiogenic pulmonary oedemas whose mechanisms have not been completely elucidated, but which may present in the perioperative period. These include neurogenic pulmonary oedema, oedema associated with the relief of severe upper airway obstruction, the therapeutic use of beta$_2$ sympathomimetics for premature labour or naloxone for opiate antagonism, and pulmonary oedema associated with gas or fluid embolism.

These conditions will be considered separately, as the treatment required may be different.

Differentiation between cardiogenic and permeability pulmonary oedema

1. History. In many cases the diagnosis will be obvious. There may be a history of a previous myocardial infarction, episodes of cardiac failure, hypertension or valvular heart disease. The sudden onset of an arrhythmia, such as atrial fibrillation, may cause acute cardiac decompensation. In the absence of one of these causes, the presence of a precipitating factor for non-cardiogenic oedema should be sought.
2. Clinical examination. In general, the physical signs are similar. In both there will be tachycardia, cool peripheries, respiratory distress, frothy sputum, cyanosis and basal and parasternal crepitations. In primary cardiac disease there may be obvious cardiac enlargement, murmurs or an arrhythmia. A third sound may point to a cardiac cause.
3. CXR may show cardiac enlargement in addition to the pulmonary oedema.
4. ECG may show evidence of infarction, an arrhythmia or chamber hypertrophy.
5. In difficult cases, measurement of PAP and PCWP may be contributory.

6. Measurement of protein levels in pulmonary oedema fluid. This can only be done where there is copious, uncontaminated fluid for sampling (see Section 1: Pulmonary oedema).

CARDIOGENIC PULMONARY OEDEMA

In a patient with cardiac disease, this may occur at any time in the perioperative period.

1. In the preoperative period it presents as a sudden onset of dyspnoea, tachycardia, a third heart sound (gallop rhythm), sweating and hyper- or hypotension, with bilateral basal or parasternal crepitations on auscultation. It is most likely to occur in a patient with known ischaemic, hypertensive or rheumatic heart disease. It may be associated with overenthusiastic fluid therapy prior to emergency surgery, or the onset of an arrhythmia such as AF.
2. Pulmonary oedema is relatively rare intraoperatively, as IPPV and the decreased peripheral vascular resistance during anaesthesia tend to oppose the hydrostatic forces and reduce the afterload. Early signs are tachycardia, decreased compliance and reduced oxygen saturation. The patient may try to breathe against the ventilator. In severe cases, pulmonary oedema fluid may emerge from the endotracheal tube.
3. In the postoperative period a combination of factors may tip a patient from borderline, into florid pulmonary oedema, usually within the first half hour of the recovery period. The main factor is the redistribution of fluid from the peripheral into the pulmonary circulation. Peripheral vasoconstriction may be due to pain or cold, coinciding with the effects of the anaesthetic wearing off. In addition, i.v. fluids administered during the operation may compound the problem.

Management

1. If the patient is conscious, he should be placed in an upright position and oxygen administered. If not IPPV should be continued or started.
2. Morphine i.v., 2 mg increments at 2-minute intervals, up to a total of 10 mg. This reduces preload by venodilatation, and relieves agitation.
3. Frusemide i.v. or i.m. 20–50 mg, especially if there is fluid overload. Acute venodilatation and a subsequent diuresis results.
4. A vasodilator, such as isosorbide dinitrate, nitroglycerin, or nitroprusside may be used. An isosorbide dinitrate infusion (diluted) can be given at a rate of 2–10 mg/h.
5. If the patient is in fast AF, control of the heart rate with verapamil or digoxin is required. With ECG control, verapamil 5–10 mg i.v. given slowly.
   n.b. Verapamil i.v. is contraindicated if the patient is taking beta blockers.

PULMONARY OEDEMA ASSOCIATED WITH SEVERE UPPER AIRWAY OBSTRUCTION

A well-recognized complication of acute airway obstruction, and in over 50% of the reported cases, the onset of clinical pulmonary oedema followed the relief of the obstruction (Barin et al 1986).

Presenting problems

1. The onset of pulmonary oedema is preceded by an episode of severe upper respiratory tract obstruction. Recognized causes include laryngeal spasm or oedema (Barin et al 1986), epiglottitis (Galvis et al 1980), malignancy and attempted strangulation.
2. Relief of the obstruction is usually accompanied by the outpouring of large amounts of pink frothy oedema fluid. There is cyanosis and respiratory distress.

Diagnosis

1. Bilateral basal crepitations are heard on auscultation.
2. CXR shows diffuse pulmonary oedema. The heart size is usually normal.
3. Blood gases show a large arterial/alveolar PO_2 difference.

Management

1. Give oxygen, either via a mask or an endotracheal tube. A review of the literature showed that at the time of intubation or soon after more than 50% of patients had a PO_2 of <8 kPa (Barins et al 1986).
2. IPPV or PEEP may be required to improve oxygenation. A pneumothorax may occur as a complication of this.
3. The use of diuretics has been suggested. However, in cases where intracardiac pressures have been measured, these have not in general been found to be elevated (Weissman et al 1984).

BIBLIOGRAPHY

Barin E S, Stevenson I F, Donnelly G L 1986 Pulmonary oedema following acute upper airway obstruction. Anaesthesia and Intensive Care 14: 54–57
Galvis A G, Stool S E, Bluestone C D 1980 Pulmonary edema following relief of acute upper airway obstruction. Annals of Otology, Rhinology and Laryngology 89: 124–128
Weissman C, Damask M C, Yang J 1984 Noncardiogenic pulmonary edema following laryngeal obstruction. Anesthesiology 60: 163–165

PULMONARY OEDEMA ASSOCIATED WITH BETA₂SYMPATHOMIMETICS FOR PREMATURE LABOUR

Presenting problems

1. Drugs thought to be linked with this type of pulmonary oedema are terbutaline, ritodrine, isoxuprine, salbutamol and fenoterol.

2. Pulmonary oedema has been reported with oral, subcutaneous and intravenous routes of administration. The duration of treatment prior to its onset varied widely, as did the rates of infusion and the total dose given (Hawker 1984 a,b). In the four cases which had haemodynamic monitoring, three had a normal or low PAP.

3. Patients were frequently in a positive fluid balance of at least 1 litre.

4. Corticosteroids and indomethacin had often been given in conjunction with tocolytics. Both can cause fluid retention.

5. General anaesthesia, or the administration of ergometrine, may precipitate pulmonary oedema.

Diagnosis

1. A history of a sudden onset of dyspnoea, cyanosis and expectoration of pink frothy sputum, during or after the suppression of premature labour with beta$_2$ tocolytics. There is usually pre-existing tachycardia and the patient is in positive fluid balance.

2. On auscultation bilateral basal crepitations are heard. CXR shows pulmonary oedema, and blood gases will indicate hypoxia.

Management

1. The justification for the use of tocolytics should be considered before instituting such treatment. Observe the patient throughout for the development of a positive fluid balance. A persistent tachycardia during therapy may be a warning sign of impending pulmonary oedema.

2. If evidence of early pulmonary occurs, the infusion should be stopped.

3. Oxygen should be administered and, if necessary, IPPV established.

4. Diuretics are required.

BIBLIOGRAPHY

Hawker F 1984 Pulmonary oedema associated with beta$_2$-sympathomimetic treatment of premature labour. Anaesthesia and Intensive Care 12: 143–151

Hawker F 1984 Five cases of pulmonary oedema associated with beta$_2$-sympathomimetic treatment of premature labour. Anaesthesia and Intensive Care 12: 159–171

NEUROGENIC PULMONARY OEDEMA

A rare complication associated with intracranial damage, which may be due to head injury, tumour or cerebrovascular accident.

Presentation

1. The patient (often a young adult or child who is unconscious after a head injury) develops sudden dyspnoea, cyanosis, marked tachycardia or bradycardia, and hypertension.

2. Clinical signs of intense peripheral vasoconstriction occur, with pallor, sweating and cold extremities.

3. If the patient is intubated, profuse frothy pink pulmonary secretions will pour out of the endotracheal tube. If the patient is ventilated, there will be a sudden decrease in lung compliance, and, unless fully paralysed, the patient will attempt to breathe against the ventilator. Oxygen saturation decreases rapidly.

Management

1. Maintenance of oxygenation
If not already instituted, IPPV with a high inspired oxygen is required. PEEP may be needed.

2. Manoeuvres to reduce the intracranial pressure, if raised.

a. $PaCO_2$ should be kept around 3–4 kPa. A $PaCO_2$ of 3.4 kPa reduces cerebral blood flow by 33%.

b. An infusion of thiopentone.

c. Surgical decompression, if necessary.

d. High-dose steroids. Dexamethasone is often used, but its value is doubtful.

3. Reduction of peripheral vasoconstriction.

a. Diuretics will assist by reducing the overall blood volume, especially if crystalloid solutions have been used for resuscitation. Frusemide 2 mg/kg may be used. Mannitol is usually only indicated prior to surgical decompression, as it may cause a subsequent rebound increase in intracranial pressure.

b. Alpha adrenergic blockers such as phenoxybenzamine 0.5–2 mg/kg in 300 ml 5% dextrose as an infusion have been advocated on the grounds that the syndrome is thought to be due to massive sympathetic discharge (Loughnan et al 1980). Other drugs which have been suggested are droperidol i.v. 200–300 μg/kg or phentolamine infusion 30 μg/kg/min.

c. Vasodilators, such as sodium nitroprusside 1–8 μg/kg/min as a short-term infusion, have been advocated to reduce peripheral vascular resistance. Direct arterial monitoring is essential.

4. Occasionally inotropic support may be required. Isoprenaline and dobutamine are both suitable, as neither has alpha adrenergic receptor-stimulating properties.

5. Control of fits with benzodiazepines or thiopentone.

BIBLIOGRAPHY

Loughnan P M, Brown T C K, Edis B, Klug G L 1980 Neurogenic pulmonary oedema in man: aetiology and management with vasodilators based upon haemodynamic studies. Anaesthesia and Intensive Care 8:65–71

PULMONARY OEDEMA ASSOCIATED WITH NALOXONE REVERSAL OF OPIATES

Pulmonary oedema is one of a number of cardiovascular complications which have occasionally been reported following the reversal of opiates with naloxone. It is thought to be due to profound stimulation of the CNS, similar to that occurring in neurogenic pulmonary oedema.

Presentation

Acute pulmonary oedema has occurred, in close association with the administration of naloxone to reverse the effect of opiates in the recovery period. It was first described in a 70-year-old man following cardiac surgery in which high-dose morphine was used (Flacke et al 1977). In view of the patient's pre-existing cardiac state, this might not be considered to be remarkable. However, pulmonary oedema also occurred after small doses of naloxone in two fit young men (Prough et al 1984).

BIBLIOGRAPHY

Flacke J W, Flacke W E, Williams S G D 1977 Acute pulmonary edema following naloxone reversal of high-dose morphine anesthesia. Anesthesiology 47: 376–378
Prough D S, Roy R, Bumgarner J, Shannon G 1984 Acute pulmonary edema in healthy teenagers following conservative doses of iv naloxone. Anesthesiology 60: 485–486

SUXAMETHONIUM APNOEA
(see also Section 1: PLASMA CHOLINESTERASE DEFICIENCY ABNORMALITY)

Prolonged apnoea and neuromuscular blockade may occur following the administration of suxamethonium, either due to the presence of a genetic variant of plasma cholinesterase, or due to low levels of the normal enzyme.

Presentation

1. Spontaneous respiration fails to return after the giving of suxamethonium in a normal clinical dosage.
2. The patient may have a known family history of plasma cholinesterase abnormalities.
3. A low level of the normal enzyme may result from a number of pathological causes. These include severe liver disease, tetanus, malnutrition, renal failure, malignant disease, Huntington's chorea and collagen disorders.
4. Iatrogenic causes include radiotherapy, renal dialysis, plasmapheresis, cardiac bypass, cytotoxic drugs, ecothiopate eye-drops, oral contraceptives, propanidid, neostigmine, chlorpromazine, pancuronium and exposure to organophosphorus compounds (Whittaker 1980).

Diagnosis

Confirm complete neuromuscular blockade with a peripheral nerve stimulator. During the return of neuromuscular function there will be signs of a phase II block, with fade in response to train-of-four stimulation.

Management

1. Continue IPPV until adequate respiration is re-established. Maintain light anaesthesia to reduce distress.
2. After full recovery, a detailed anaesthetic, family and drug history should be taken from the patient.
3. A clotted blood sample should be taken for plasma cholinesterase activity, dibucaine and fluoride numbers. This may be sent to the Cholinesterase Research Unit, Royal Postgraduate Medical School, Hammersmith Hospital, London W12 0HS (Whittaker & Britten 1987).
4. The results should be given to the patient, and a warning card issued, if applicable. Investigation of other close relatives may be suggested.

BIBLIOGRAPHY

Whittaker M 1980 Plasma cholinesterase variants and the anaesthetist. Anaesthesia 35: 174–197
Whittaker M, Britten J J 1987 Phenotyping of individuals sensitive to suxamethonium. British Journal of Anaesthesia 59: 1052–1055

THYROTOXIC CRISIS OR STORM

The abrupt onset of symptoms of a severe hypermetabolic state associated with the output of thyroxine, in a patient with pre-existing thyroid disease. This is a clinical, not a bichemical diagnosis. It may occur in a patient with occult thyroid disease, in whom a crisis may be precipitated by an acute medical, traumatic or surgical problem. It can also occur in treated thyrotoxic patients following thyroidectomy, either if there is inadequate preoperative control (Jamison & Done 1979), or if antithyroid therapy has been discontinued too early in the postoperative period.

While the onset of the crisis is most likely to occur in the postoperative period, intraoperative problems have been described. A thyroid crisis can also be concealed by the use of beta blockers (Jones & Solomon 1981). Beta blockers only affect the peripheral effects on beta adrenergic receptors, not the output of thyroid hormone or the thyroid hormone tests.

Presentation

1. Intraoperative tachycardia or atrial fibrillation (Robson 1985), ventricular tachycardia and cardiac arrest (Peters et al 1981).

2. A hypermetabolic state which may resemble malignant hyperpyrexia (Murray 1978, Peters et al 1981, Stevens 1983). Respiratory and metabolic acidosis occurs, with increased oxygen consumption.

3. Intraoperative pulmonary oedema has been described. This may present as cyanosis, tachycardia and respiratory distress. It is due to a combination of increased cardiac output, tachycardia or atrial fibrillation, mild hypertension, increased red cell mass and raised blood volume. A case was reported in which an undiagnosed thyrotoxic patient with a fractured hip developed pulmonary oedema, pyrexia and tachycardia during surgery (Stevens 1983). This state was diagnosed and treated as malignant hyperpyrexia. The true diagnosis was only made during postoperative investigations.

4. The sudden onset of confusion or mania.

5. Postoperatively it can present with pyrexia, tachycardia, agitation, nausea, vomiting, abdominal pain, diarrhoea, jaudice, hepatomegaly, dehydration and infection.

6. It may also occur in an adequately prepared toxic patient in whom therapy is stopped too soon postoperatively, or where the thyrotoxicosis is being treated with propranolol alone (Eriksson et al 1977).

Management

1. Antithyroid drugs

   a. Carbimazole 60–120 mg or propylthiouracil 600–1200 mg, given orally or if necessary, by nasogastric tube. This usually starts to act within 1 hour of administration.

   b. Potassium or sodium iodide acts immediately to inhibit further release of thyroid hormone.

2. Beta blockers

Propranolol oral 20–80 mg 6-hourly, or i.v. 1–5 mg 6-hourly.

3. Active cooling.

4. IPPV and muscle paralysis if necessary.

5. Steroids

Hydrocortisone i.v. 100 mg 6-hourly.

6. Fluid i.v. (including dextrose).

7. Dantrolene has been used to treat a child with thyroid storm who failed to respond to conventional treatment (Christensen & Nissen 1987). Although dantrolene successfully controlled the hypermetabolic state, the patient subsequently died from respiratory and renal failure.

BIBLIOGRAPHY

Christensen P A, Nissen L R 1987 Treatment of thyroid storm in a child with dantrolene. British Journal of Anaesthesia 59: 522–526

Erikkson M, Rubenfeld S, Garber A J, Kohler P O 1977 Propranolol does not prevent thyroid storm. New England Journal of Medicine 296: 263–264

Jamison M H, Done H J 1979 Postoperative thyrotoxic crisis in a patient prepared for thyroidectomy with propranolol. British Journal of Clinical Practice 33: 82–83

Jones D K, Solomon S 1981 Thyrotoxic crisis masked by treatment with beta blockers. British Medical Journal 283: 659

Murray J F 1978 Hyperpyrexia of uncertain origin. British Journal of Anaesthesia 50: 387–388

Peters K R, Nance P, Wingard D W 1981 Malignant hyperthyroidism or malignant hyperthermia? Anesthesia and Analgesia 60: 613–615

Robson N J 1985 Emergency surgery complicated by thyrotoxicosis and thyrotoxic periodic paralysis. Anaesthesia 40: 27–31

Stevens J J 1983 A case of thyrotoxic crisis that mimicked malignant hyperthermia. Anesthesiology 59: 263

4

TORSADE DE POINTES
(see also Section 1)

An atypical paroxysmal ventricular tachycardia associated with delayed repolarization of the ventricles. It is frequently drug induced, but may also occur with metabolic abnormalities.

Presentation

1. The patient may complain of episodes of palpitations, faintness or fatigue. Sudden death may occur.

2. ECG shows paroxysms of an atypical ventricular tachycardia in which the QRS complexes vary in form and amplitude, and the axis of the complexes twists around the baseline. During periods of ordinary sinus rhythm there is a prolonged Q–Tc of >0.44 second or an uncorrected Q–T interval of >0.5 second. Immediately before the onset on the event there is a characteristic 'long-short' sequence (Raehl et al 1985) in which a premature ectopic is followed by a long pause, then a second premature ectopic initiates the torsade de pointes.

3. Predisposing factors.

a. Any disease that causes prolongation of the Q–T interval such as the Romano-Ward, Jervell and Lange-Nielsen syndromes or familial ventricular tachycardia.

b. Metabolic abnormalities
Including hypokalaemia, hypomagnesaemia and hypocalcaemia. It has been suggested that hypomagnesaemia should be considered in any patient with a combination of gastrointestinal losses and torsade de pointes (Ramee et al 1985).

c. Drug induced
A number of drugs, some of which prolong myocardial repolarization, have been reported to precipitate torsade de pointes. These include amiodarone, disopyramide, lidoflazine, prenylamine, procainamide, propranolol, quinidine, sotalol, amitriptyline,

imipramine, maprotiline, thioridazine, trifluoperazine, vasopressin and diuretics (Raehl et al 1985).
d. Following surgery involving right block dissection of the neck (Otteni et al 1983).

Diagnosis

Torsade de pointes can be differentiated from polymorphous ventricular tachycardia by the long Q–Tc and the 'long–short' initiating sequence.

Management

1. Stop any potentially causative drug.
2. Avoid the use of class I antiarrhythmics, or any of those already mentioned.
3. Correct potential metabolic causes such as hypokalaemia, hypocalcaemia or hypomagnesaemia.
4. Defibrillation, if VF occurs.
5. Atrial or ventricular pacing may be required until the Q–Tc is normal. The duration of pacing required will depend upon the half-life of the precipitating drug.
6. Isoprenaline may increase the heart rate and therefore shorten the Q–T interval. A dose of 1–2 μg/min has been recommended. However, this is a potentially dangerous treatment and should be used with caution. Contraindications to its use include myocardial ischaemia and hypertensive heart disease (Raehl et al 1985).
7. Occasionally bretylium (Raehl et al 1985), lignocaine, or magnesium sulphate (Ramee et al 1985, Martinez 1987) have been reported to be effective.

BIBLIOGRAPHY

Martinez R 1987 Torsade de pointes: atypical rhythm, atypical treatment. Annals of Emergency Medicine 16: 878–884
Otteni J C, Pottecher R T, Bronner G, Flesch H, Diebolt J R 1983 Prolongation of the Q–T interval and sudden cardiac arrest following right radical neck dissection. Anesthesiology 59: 358–361
Raehl C L, Patel A K, LeRoy M 1985 Drug-induced torsade de pointes. Clinical Pharmacy 4: 675–690
Ramee S R, White C J, Svinarich J T, Watson T D, Fox R F 1985 Torsade de pointes and magnesium deficiency. American Heart Journal 109: 164–167

TOTAL SPINAL ANAESTHESIA

A syndrome of central neurological blockade. It occurs when a volume of local anaesthetic solution intended for epidural anaesthesia enters the subarachnoid space and ascends to the cervical region. This results in cardiovascular collapse, phrenic nerve paralysis and unconsciousness. Deaths have occasionally been reported.

Accidental total spinal analgesia may occur in association with the original epidural, or subsequently following a top-up dose, due to accidental puncture of the dura by the epidural cathether.

Presentation

1. Cardiovascular collapse usually takes place immediately after the epidural injection, although delays of up to 45 minutes have been reported (Woerth et al 1977). There is severe hypotension due to blockade of the sympathetic outflow. Occasionally cardiac arrest occurs.

   Three cases of total spinal anaesthesia have been reported after epidural injections of local anaesthetic were given into the interspace adjacent to an inadvertent dural perforation (Hodgkinson 1981). All three incidents occurred when the patients were in active labour. It was postulated that frequent uterine contractions can result in some of the local anaesthetic solution being forced through a puncture hole into the subarachnoid space.

2. Rapidly increasing paralysis involves the respiratory muscles, resulting in apnoea and hypoxia.

3. The pupils become dilated and consciousness is lost.

4. Apnoea may vary from 20 minutes to 6 hours, unconsciousness from 25 minutes to 4 hours, while full recovery of sensation may take up to 9 hours (Gillies & Morgan 1973). The lengths of time vary with the agent, the dose and volume of local anaesthetic given. Bupivacaine lasts longer than lignocaine.

Management

1. Precautions should be taken to prevent the occurrence of total spinal anaesthesia. A test dose of local anaesthetic is recommended. The injection of 3 ml of the local anaesthetic containing adrenaline 1 : 200 000, followed by an adequate pause, to assess the effects, has been suggested (Moore & Batra 1980). The use of this during labour is controversial (see Local anaesthetic toxicity). It has been recommended that if dural puncture occurs during active labour when a Caesarean section is required, then further attempts should not be made. Either a spinal or a general anaesthetic should be employed as an alternative (Hodgkinson 1981). Others claim never to have seen this complication, and challenge the advice (Crawford 1983).

2. If an accidental total spinal does occur, a non-pregnant patient should be turned supine, tilted head down and the legs elevated to encourage venous return. The pregnant patient should be tilted in the lateral position to prevent aortocaval compression (Rees & Willis 1988).

3. The lungs should be inflated with oxygen.

4. A pressor agent such as ephedrine i.v. in 5–10 mg increments up to 30 mg. Adrenaline 0.1–0.5 mg may occasionally be required but should preferably be avoided in patients in labour.

5. Intravenous fluids should be infused rapidly.

6. An endotracheal tube can then be inserted. IPPV may have to be continued for up to 2 hours, depending upon the local anaesthetic and the volume used.

BIBLIOGRAPHY

Crawford J S 1983 Collapse after epidural injection following inadvertent dural perforation. Anesthesiology 59: 78–79
Gillies I D S, Morgan M 1973 Accidental total spinal analgesia. Anaesthesia 28: 441–445
Hodgkinson R 1981 Total spinal block after epidural injection into an interspace adjacent to an inadvertent dural perforation. Anesthesiology 55: 593–595
Moore D C, Batra M S 1981 The components of an effective test dose prior to epidural block. Anesthesiology 55: 693–696
Rees G A D, Willis B A 1988 Resuscitation in late pregnancy. Anaesthesia 43: 347–349
Woerth S D, Bullard J R, Alpert C C 1977 Total spinal anesthesia. A late complication of epidural anesthesia. Anesthesiology 47: 380–381

4

TURP SYNDROME

A syndrome which may occur during transurethral resection of the prostate, in which large quantities of the glycine 1.5% irrigating fluid are absorbed into the general circulation through open prostatic venous sinuses. Glycine 1.5% is a non-electrolytic, slightly hypotonic solution (2.1% would be isotonic) which on absorption is mainly confined to extracellular fluid (ECF). Plasma sodium levels are decreased by more than that which would be caused by an equivalent volume of water alone. In general, the amount absorbed depends upon the number and size of prostatic venous sinuses opened, the length of exposure and the hydrostatic pressure of the irrigating fluid. Absorption studies suggest an average rate of 20 ml/min, but as much as 87 ml/min has been reported (Alexander et al 1986). Risk factors for the development of a severe syndrome include a long resection time, a large prostate, profuse bleeding from open prostatic veins, and pre-existing hyponatraemia.

In some centres, isotonic dextrose is used as the irrigating fluid. In a study of 22 patients, dextrose was found to give a significantly greater fall in plasma sodium than glycine and some patients developed severe hyperglycaemia (Allen et al 1981). Several deaths due to the syndrome have been reported (Aasheim 1973, Osborn et al 1980, Rhymer et al 1985).

Presentation

1. The patient is usually undergoing a TURP and glycine 1.5% is being used as an irrigating fluid. It has also been described during percutaneous ultrasonic lithotripsy (Sinclair et al 1985).

2. The time of onset is variable. In one case a grand mal fit occurred

4

during spinal anaesthesia after only 15 minutes of resection (Hurlbert & Wingard 1979). There were no warning signs despite the plasma sodium having fallen to 104 mmol/l. Absorption of glycine may continue beyond the resection time into the postoperative period.

3. Initially there is an increase in systolic blood pressure and a widening of pulse pressure. This is followed by bradycardia, hypotension and occasionally cardiac arrest (Charlton 1980). Other ECG abnormalities, including nodal rhythm and U waves, have been reported. Blood loss may mask the initial hypertensive phase.

4. Pulmonary oedema may occur (Aasheim 1973, Allen et al 1981). The patient can present with respiratory distress and cyanosis in the postoperative period (Rhymer et al 1985).

5. Cerebral oedema may result in mental confusion and fits. Five cases were reported in which visual disturbances occurred. These were thought to be due to the effects of glycine on the retinal synapses (Ovassapian et al 1982). Delayed awakening from anaesthesia has been reported (Roesch et al 1983).

6. Profound hyponatraemia can occur, plasma sodium levels of 102–105 mmol/l often being reported. In one fatal case, the plasma sodium, after more than 5 hours' resection, was 83 mmol/l. The sodium level does not necessarily correlate with the amount of fluid absorbed since the presence of glycine enhances the hyponatraemia. In a study of 372 prostatectomies, 15% of patients had plasma sodium levels below 125 mmol/l. All had clinical evidence of hyponatraemia (Shearer & Standfield 1981). In contrast, other authors claimed to have seen patients with levels of 104 mmol/l, without clinical signs (Allen et al 1981).

7. Decreased serum osmolality usually occurs, but the degree is very variable.

8. The syndrome is likely to present earlier in a conscious patient undergoing spinal anaesthesia than in one having a general anaesthetic. Restlessness, confusion, headache, nausea and retching may herald its onset. Convulsions have been reported. During general anaesthesia, detection may be delayed, particularly if the initial hypertensive phase is masked by blood loss.

9. The extent to which high levels of glycine and its metabolites contribute to the CNS effects of the syndrome is the subject of continuing discussion. Products of glycine metabolism include serine, ammonia, oxalate and glycolate. Glycine (and to a lesser extent serine) is known to be an inhibitory neurotransmitter in the brain, spinal cord and retina, with a similar action to GABA on chloride channels.

Although early reports indicated that ammonia accumulation was not a problem, in one case, delayed recovery from anaesthesia was associated with a blood ammonia level of 500 μmol/l (Roesch et al 1983). It was suggested that some patients may be more vulnerable to ammonia production and toxicity than others.

Twenty-four-hour urinary oxalate and glycolate levels were studied in three patients, who were selected from a total of 34 patients, on the basis of hyponatraemia the morning after surgery (Fitzpatrick et al 1981). Urinary levels of oxalate and glycolate were high in all three patients and oxalate continued to be excreted for up to 2 weeks.

Diagnosis

1. Plasma sodium. Values as low as 83 mmol/l have been reported.
2. Plasma osmolality may be reduced.
3. Hb and haematocrit levels are decreased.
4. Plasma glycine levels are high (N = 176–332 μmol/l). The results of glycine level estimations may take several days to become available, and are therefore not of immediate use. Levels as high as 8000 μmol/l have been reported.
5. Blood ammonia may be raised (N = 11–35 μmol/l). In the patient with delayed recovery from anaesthesia, the blood ammonia was 500 μmol/l.
6. When isotonic dextrose was used as the irrigating fluid, one patient developed a blood glucose of 61.8 mmol/l (Allen et al 1981).
7. Urinary oxalate (N = 0.1–0.5 mmol/24 h) and glycolate levels (N = 0.10–0.35 mmol/24 h) may be elevated.

Management

1. Prophylaxis and anticipation
    a. Prostatic resection time should, in general, be limited to 1 hour. However, one case of convulsions and a sodium of 104 mmol/l developed after only 15 minutes (Hurlbert & Wingard 1979).
    b. Irrigating pressure should be kept to about 60–70 cmH$_2$O, and certainly should never be allowed to go above 100 cmH$_2$O.
    c. Sodium-free i.v. solutions should not be used during prostatic resection.
    d. Postoperatively, the bladder irrigation fluid should be changed from glycine to saline.
2. Treatment of hyponatraemia
This is controversial. Recommendations range from no treatment at all, to saline 0.9%, hypertonic saline, mannitol, loop diuretics and peritoneal dialysis. Those who have reservations about the use of active therapy observed that some patients with a sodium of 104 mmol/l were asymptomatic, and that spontaneous correction of hyponatraemia normally occurred within 12–24 hours. In addition, rapid correction of hyponatraemia is potentially dangerous due to osmotic gradients which may occur and result in cerebral damage (Arieff 1986, Sterns 1986). However, a number of deaths associated with the syndrome have been reported, and in the elderly patient, cardiac arrhythmias, convulsions,

pulmonary and cerebral oedema are dangerous complications.

a. Each case must be dealt with individually in conjunction with a knowledge of the patient's clinical state, his cardiovascular and respiratory status, and the biochemical results.

b. If active therapeutic correction of the hyponatraemia is required, it should be carried out with extreme caution. Saline 0.9% is usually sufficient, perhaps with the addition of a loop diuretic. However, a loop diuretic is less effective in dilutional hyponatraemia, and has the disadvantage of causing the loss of sodium in addition to water. If the serum osmolality is very low, hypertonic saline may be required. A plasma sodium correction rate of not more than 2 mmol/l/h has been suggested.

c. Prophylactic IPPV and ITU monitoring is essential, at least until the plasma sodium and hypervolaemia is corrected, if the hyponatraemia is severe. This will prevent hypoxia, minimize the effects of cerebral oedema or convulsions, and allow detection and treatment of cardiac arrhythmias.

3. Calcium and inotropic agents may be required. The routine use of calcium gluconate 10% 10 ml, has been recommended for this syndrome and in particular where cardiovascular collapse has occurred.

4. Coagulation studies should be performed in the presence of persistent bleeding and hyponatraemia. Dilutional abnormalities are the most frequent, although DIC may also occur. Defects should be appropriately treated.

5. Urinary volumes should be maintained postoperatively, to prevent the deposition of calcium oxalate in the urinary tract.

BIBLIOGRAPHY

Aasheim G M 1973 Hyponatraemia during transurethral surgery. Canadian Anaesthetists' Society Journal 20: 274–280

Alexander J P, Polland A, Gillespie I A 1986 Glycine and transurethral resection. Anaesthesia 41: 1189–1195

Allen P R, Hughes R G, Goldie D J, Kennedy R H 1981 Fluid absorption during transurethral resection. British Medical Journal 282: 740

Arieff A I 1986 Hyponatremia, convulsions, respiratory arrest and permanent brain damage after elective surgery in healthy women. New England Journal of Medicine 314: 1529–1535

Charlton A J 1980 Cardiac arrest during transurethral prostatectomy after absorption of 1.5% glycine. Anaesthesia 35: 804– 806

Fitzpatrick J M, Kasidas G P, Rose G A 1981 Hyperoxaluria following glycine irrigation for transurethral prostatectomy. British Journal of Urology 53: 250–252

Hatch P D 1987 Surgical and anaesthetic considerations in transurethral resection of the prostate. Anaesthesia and Intensive Care 15: 203–211

Hurlbert B J, Wingard D W 1979 Water intoxication after 15 minutes of transurethral resection of the prostate. Anesthesiology 50: 355–356

Osborn D E, Rao P N, Greene M J, Barnard J 1980 Fluid absorption during transurethral resection. British Medical Journal 281: 1549–1550

Ovassapian A, Joshi C W, Brunner E A 1982 Visual disturbances: an unusual symptom of transurethral prostate resection reaction. Anesthesiology 57: 332–334

Rhymer J C, Bell T J, Perry K C, Ward J P 1985 Hyponatraemia following transurethral resection of the prostate. British Journal of Urology 57: 450–452

Roesch R P, Stoelting R K, Lingeman J E, Kahnoski R J, Backes D J, Gephardt S A 1983

Ammonia toxicity resulting from glycine absorption during a transurethral resection of the prostate. Anesthesiology 58: 577–579

Shearer R J, Standfield N J 1981 Fluid absorption during transurethral resection. British Medical Journal 282: 740

Sinclair J F, Hutchison A, Baraza R, Telfer A B M 1985 Absorption of 1.5% glycine after percutaneous ultrasonic lithtripsy for renal stone disease. British Medical Journal 291: 691–692

Sterns R H, Riggs J E, Schochet S S Jr 1986 Osmotic demyelination syndrome following correction of hyponatraemia. New England Journal of Medicine 314: 1535–1542

4

Miscellaneous Problems

CARDIOPULMONARY RESUSCITATION
(CPR)

A. CARDIAC RESUSCITATION IN THE ADULT

1. ECG shows ventricular tachycardia without output, or ventricular fibrillation

a. Defibrillate with 180 J within 30 seconds of collapse.

b. If this fails, start CPR and repeat defibrillation, first with 180 J, then with 360 J.

c. Give lignocaine i.v. slowly, 50–100 mg, to raise the VF threshold. This may be followed by an infusion of lignocaine:

    4 mg/min for 30 minutes then

    2 mg/min for 2 hours then

    1 mg/min.

Use premixed infusion bags of lignocaine 0.1% (1 mg/ml) in glucose, or lignocaine 0.2% (2 mg/ml) in glucose. Alternatively add lignocaine 1 g to dextrose 5%, 500 ml to give a 2 mg/ml solution.

d. Defibrillate with 360 J.

e. Give adrenaline 1 : 10 000 i.v., 5–10 ml (0.5–1 mg).

f. Defibrillate with 360 J.

h. Give sodium bicarbonate i.v. 1 mmol/kg (n.b. Do not mix with calcium and do not allow the solution to extravasate).

i. If conversion fails, or a spontaneous pulse reverts to VF or VT, then consider the use of bretylium tosylate i.v. 400 mg.

2. ECG shows asystole

a. Start cardiopulmonary resuscitation.

b. Give atropine i.v. 0.6–2 mg.

c. Give adrenaline 1:10 000 i.v., 5–10 ml (0.5–1 mg) and repeat each 2–5 minutes.

d. After 2 minutes of circulatory arrest give sodium bicarbonate i.v., 1 mmol/kg.

e. Sodium bicarbonate 0.5 mmol/kg can be repeated empirically every 10–15 minutes, or preferably according to arterial pH measurements.

f. Isoprenaline 100 μg, then an infusion of 4 μg/min. A solution 8 μg/ml is made by adding isoprenaline 4 mg to dextrose 5% 500 ml.

3. Electromechanical dissociation (ECG complexes present but no generation of a cardiac output).

a. Consider and correct possible causes. These include hypovolaemia, cardiac tamponade, tension pneumothorax or a drug effect.

b. Give adrenaline 1 : 10 000, 5–10 ml (0.5–1 mg).

c. Give isoprenaline i.v. 100 μg then an infusion of 4 μg/min.

d. Give calcium gluconate 10%, 10 ml.

4. Summary of resuscitation drug therapy and indications

a. Asystole of cardiac origin:
Adrenaline, atopine.
b. Asystole of non-cardiac origin:
Adrenaline, atropine, calcium.
c. Electromechanical dissociation:
Adrenaline, isoprenaline, calcium.
d. Ventricular fibrillation (fine):
Adrenaline and defibrillation.
e. Ventricular fibrillation (coarse):
Lignocaine and defibrillation, bretylium, disopyramide.
f. Ventricular tachycardia (no output):
Lignocaine and defibrillation.
g. Ventricular tachycardia (with output):
Lignocaine.
h. Torsade de pointes atypical ventricular tachycardia:
See Section 4: Torsade de pointes.

5. Role of bicarbonate and calcium in resuscitation

Bicarbonate is not necessary in the early stages of an arrest, particularly if defibrillation is successful, or if the output from ECM is effective. The first dose should only be given after 10–15 minutes and further administration controlled by acid base samples. A metabolic alkalosis must be avoided. Calcium increases muscle spasticity and oxygen requirements in the ischaemic heart and may worsen coronary artery spasm. In an arrest of cardiac origin it should therefore be avoided. It may be of use in asystole of non-cardiac origin, particularly in the presence of a metabolic cause such as hyperkalaemia, hypocalcaemia and dilutional hyponatraemia. It is a second-line drug for electromechanical dissociation.

6. Routes of administration of resuscitation drugs
  a. Intravenous:
  Drugs should preferably be given via a central vein to avoid thrombophlebitis in peripheral veins.
  b. Intracardiac:
  An effective route, but may cause myocardial damage.
  c. Intratracheal:
  Administration of drugs by this route is still controversial (Greenbaum 1987). It is suitable for adrenaline, atropine, lignocaine or naloxone, when each is diluted to 10 ml, but blood levels achieved may be unreliable (Quinton et al 1987). The possibility of introducing foreign bodies exists. Bicarbonate and calcium are NOT suitable for intratracheal use.

7. Defibrillation technique
  a. One paddle should be placed to the right of the upper sternum, just below the clavicle, the other to the apex of the heart. Contact is achieved with electrode jelly, or impregnated pads. Use special paddles for children and infants (see Paediatric resuscitation).

b. Remove any trinitrate patches from chest wall.

c. Charge the defibrillator to 180 J.

d. All personnel must be warned to stand back and avoid any contact with the patient during defibrillation.

e. Discharge the shock, by pressing appropriate button(s) on paddles.

B. RESUSCITATION IN PREGNANCY

A number of factors contribute to problems encountered in the resuscitation of the pregnant patient and modifications to the conventional treatment of cardiac arrest are needed. The differences in management are necessitated by the altered cardiovascular physiology in the pregnant patient, and by the presence of the fetus. Effective ECM must be combined with a lateral tilt to reduce aortocaval compression. Crucial decisions may have to be made on the possible therapeutic benefits and ethical considerations of immediate Caesarean section, and the question of initiating open cardiac massage at an early stage. The maturity of the fetus is also important. Prior to 24–26 weeks, primarily maternal considerations operate. After this, the question of fetal viability enters the equation.

1. Altered maternal cardiovascular physiology

Changes include an increase in cardiac output, vascular volume and oxygen consumption. The volume distribution of blood flow is altered, such that about 25% goes to the uterus. In the later stages of pregnancy, a key factor contributing to resuscitation difficulties at cardiac arrest is aortocaval compression by the gravid uterus, when the patient is supine. This may markedly decrease venous return, in addition to reducing arterial blood flow to the uterus and kidneys. The contribution of aortocaval compression to poor outcome was stressed in reports on bupivacaine toxicity (Marx 1982), and in the death of a patient with sickle cell trait, when insufficient lateral tilt was applied during Caesarean section (Anaesthetic Advisory Committee 1987).

2. Special considerations in CPR in late pregnancy

a. Relief of aortocaval compression

This is a crucial factor influencing outcome and can be achieved by:

i. Maintenance of a lateral tilt

This is essential, but hampers effective cardiac massage. A head-down position, with a wedge under one buttock, and manual displacement of the uterus by an assistant, have been suggested. A special resuscitation wedge for pregnant patients has also been described (Rees & Willis 1988). It is 100 cm long, inclined at an angle of 27° and has a fixed side piece to retain the patient during external cardiac massage.

ii. Immediate Caesarean section

Maternal survival without neurological deficit has been accomplished by this method of relieving compression (Marx 1982).

Even if fetal death has occurred, this may be an effective therapeutic manoeuvre (Lindsay & Hanson 1987). Successful outcome for both mother and child has been reported after 'postmortem' Caesarean section (DePace et al 1982). A paediatrician should therefore form part of the resuscitation team.

b. Open cardiac massage

Should be seriously considered, if a satisfactory circulation has not been achieved after 15 minutes of closed cardiac massage (Lee et al 1986).

c. Drug therapy

May require modification in the pregnant patient. Both acidosis and the administration of adrenaline cause reductions in uterine blood flow. Treatment with bicarbonate at a stage earlier than usual has therefore been recommended. The use of adrenaline should be delayed if possible (Lee et al 1986).

C. PAEDIATRIC RESUSCITATION

1. Causes of cardiac arrest in infants and children

a. Hypoxia, secondary to ventilatory failure or upper respiratory tract obstruction.

b. Secondary to hypovolaemia.

c. A result of sudden infant death syndrome.

d. Secondary to septicaemia.

e. Associated with congenital heart disease.

2. Paediatric endotracheal tube sizes

	Diameter (mm)	Length of oral tube (cm)
Premature	2.5–3.0	11
Newborn	3.5	12
1 yr	4.0	13
2 yr	4.5	14
4 yr	5.0	15
6 yr	5.5	17
8 yr	6.0	19
10 yr	6.5	20
12 yr	7.0	21
14 yr	7.5	22

3. Drugs for paediatric resuscitation

Adrenaline:

0.1 ml/kg i.v. of a 1 : 10 000 dilution.

Used for asystole, bradycardia, ventricular fibrillation. Injection should be via a central vein or intracardiac.

Atropine:

0.01 mg/kg i.v.

Used for bradycardia or AV block.

Bicarbonate (sodium):
1 mmol/kg i.v.
Used for metabolic acidosis. Do not overcorrect the acidosis. Ensure adequate ventilation.
Calcium chloride:
1 ml/5 kg of a 10% solution i.v.
Used for asystole.
Dexamethasone:
1 mg in infants, 8 mg in adolescents.
Dextrose:
1 ml/kg of a 50% solution.
Used for neonatal hypoglycaemia.
Inotropic agents:
Can be used for situations when the perfusion is poor but the electrical activity good.
   a. Dopamine: 5–20 μg/kg/min.
   b. Isoprenaline: 0.1–0.5 μg/kg/min.
Lignocaine:
0.5 mg/kg.
Used for ventricular tachycardia.
Mannitol:
0.5–1 g/kg infusion over 20 minutes.
Used to improve urinary output.
Naloxone:
0.01 mg/kg i.v., i.m. or s.c.
Used for reversal of respiratory depression due to opiates.

4. Paediatric defibrillation
Only use special paediatric electrodes. They should be positioned so that the heart lies between the two electrodes:
Positive electrode: left midclavicular line, at xiphoid level.
Negative electrode: right of sternum, second rib level.

   a. Infants:
   Neonate to age 3 years
   Paddles 4.5 cm diameter

      Defibrillator charge for infants:
      1.5 kg   premature   3–6 J
      3.5 kg   neonate   7–14 J
        7 kg   6 months   14–28 J
       10 kg   1 year   20–40 J
       15 kg   3 years   30–60 J

   b. Children
   Aged 3–15 years
   Paddles 8.0 cm diameter

Defibrillator charge for children:

15 kg	3 years	30–60 J
20 kg	5 years	40–80 J
22 kg	7 years	45–90 J
30 kg	10 years	60–120 J
50 kg	15 years	100–200 J

D. NEONATAL RESUSCITATION

1. Apgar scoring for assessment at 1 minute and 5 minutes
   a. Appearance:
      0 = blue, pale
      1 = body pink, peripheries blue
      2 = Pink all over
   b. Heart rate:
      0 = absent
      1 = <100/min
      2 = >100/min
   c. Reflex irritability on stimulation of the soles of the feet:
      0 = no response
      1 = some movement
      2 = a cry
   d. Muscle tone
      0 = flaccid, limp
      1 = some flexion
      2 = good flexion
   e. Respiratory effort
      0 = absent
      1 = irregular respiration
      2 = strong cry

Assessment on total scoring:
0–3 = severe depression
4–6 = moderate depression
7–10 = good state

2. Normal birth
   a. Aspirate mucus from the mouth.
   b. Dry the skin and reduce heat loss by covering body and head.
   c. Fit name-bands and complete identification procedures.
3. Moderate depression of the neonate
   a. Give 100% oxygen.
   b. Stimulate the feet and dry the skin.
   c. If there is a bradycardia of <100/min or breathing is inadequate, perform IPPV with bag and mask until improvement occurs.

d. If there is no improvement, perform laryngoscopy, intubate and treat as for severe neonatal depression.

4. Severe depression of the neonate

a. Ventilate with 100% oxygen using a bag and mask.

b. Perform pharyngeal suction, laryngoscopy and endotracheal intubation.

c. If there is a bradycardia of <100/min, start ECM, at a rate of 120/min, with fingers behind the chest and thumbs over the lower third of the sternum.

d. Drug therapy should be given via the umbilical artery or vein. A useful technique to achieve rapid catheterization of the umbilical artery has been described (Cole and Rolbin 1980). This must be performed within 15 minutes of birth, before the onset of arterial spasm. It can subsequently be used for blood sampling, drug and fluid administration and aortic pressure monitoring.

   i. Sodium bicarbonate 1 mmol/kg, then according to the acid base state.

   ii. Dextrose 0.5–2 g/kg for hypoglycaemia.

   iii. Adrenaline: up to 0.05 mg/kg may be required for the acidotic neonate, and 0.01 mg/kg for the non-acidotic one.

   iv. Naloxone i.v. 0.01 mg/kg (or 0.02 mg/kg i.m.), but only if the mother has received opiate analgesia. Naloxone is short acting, so depression may recur after 30 minutes.

BIBLIOGRAPHY

Anaesthesia Advisory Committee to the Chief Coroner of Ontario 1987 Intraoperative death during Caesarean section in a patient with sickle cell trait. Canadian Journal of Anaesthesia 34: 67–70

Baskett P J F 1985 Towards better resuscitation. British Journal of Hospital Medicine 34: 345–350

Bembridge M, Lyons G 1988 Myocardial infarction in the third trimester of pregnancy. Anaesthesia 43: 202–204

Bray R J 1985 The management of cardiac arrest in infants and children. British Journal of Hospital Medicine 34: 72–81

Cole A F D, Rolbin S H 1980 A technique for rapid catheterisation of the umbilical artery. Anesthesiology 53: 254–255

DePace N L, Betesh J S, Kotler M N 1982 'Postmortem' Cesarean section with recovery of both mother and offspring. Journal of the American Medical Association 248: 971–973

Greenbaum R 1987 Down the tube. Anaesthesia 42: 927–928

Lee R V, Rodgers B D, White L M, Harvey R C 1986 Cardiopulmonary resuscitation of pregnant women. American Journal of Medicine 81: 311–318

Lindsay S L, Hanson G C 1987 Cardiac arrest in near-term pregnancy. Anaesthesia 42: 1074–1077

Lissauer T 1980 Paediatric emergencies. Cardiorespiratory arrest. Hospital Update 6: 1067–1077

Marx G F 1982 Cardiopulmonary resuscitation of late-pregnant women. Anesthesiology 56: 156

Quinton D N, O'Byrne G, Aitkenhead A R 1987 Comparison of endotracheal and peripheral venous adrenaline in cardiac arrest. Lancet i: 828–829

Rees G A D, Willis B A 1988 Resuscitation in late pregnancy. Anaesthesia 43: 347–349

Safar P, Bircher N G 1988 Cardiopulmonary cerebral resuscitation. W B Saunders, Philadelphia

DIAGNOSIS OF BRAIN DEATH

1. Certification

Two doctors, clinically independent of each other, are required for certification; one a consultant, the other either a consultant or a senior registrar. Both should have expertise in brain death diagnosis, and neither should be a member of the transplant team. A formal checklist should be used.

2. Preconditions

a. 'Does the patient suffer from a condition that has led to irremediable brain damage?'

b. 'What was the time of onset of unresponsive coma?'

c. 'Have potentially reversible causes for the patient's condition been adequately excluded?' In particular:

  i. depressant drugs.

  ii. neuromuscular blocking drugs.

  iii. hypothermia.

  iv. metabolic or endocrine disturbances.

3. Tests for absence of brain stem function

a. 'Do the pupils react to light?'

Pupils should be fixed and dilated. Sudden changes in light intensity should not cause any response.

b. 'Are there corneal reflexes?'

c. 'Is there eye movement on caloric testing?'

The slow injection of 20 ml ice-cold water in turn into each auditory canal, free of blood or wax, should not produce any eye movements.

d. 'Are there motor responses in the cranial nerve distribution, in response to stimulation of the face, limbs or trunk?'

Somatic stimulation, such as firm supraorbital or eye pressure, should not produce any motor response.

e. 'Is there a gag reflex?'

If the test is practicable.

f. 'Is there a cough reflex?'

There should be no response to the passage of a suction catheter down the endotracheal tube.

g. 'Have the recommendations concerning testing for apnoea been followed?'

h. 'Were any respiratory movements seen?'

The test for apnoea is very important (Rudge 1988). A sufficiently high $PaCO_2$ must be produced to cause respiratory stimulation, but not at the expense of hypoxia. It has been suggested that the initial $PaCO_2$ should be 6 kPa, and that the period of apnoea must be sufficient to produce a further rise of 6.66 kPa, confirmed by blood gases estimation. Prior to the test, 100% oxygen should be given for

5

15 minutes. At the end of this time, the patient should be disconnected from the ventilator, and oxygen 6 l/min insufflated using a narrow catheter which is passed down the endotracheal tube. Observation of the patient for any signs of respiratory movement must continue for 10 minutes, after which the patient is reconnected to the ventilator.

4. Confirmatory testing

Brain death can only be conclusively established when the criteria have been satisfied on two successive occasions. The interval between testing will depend on the original condition. Patients with possible drug overdosage or hypothermia may require a longer period of observation. In the case of drug toxicity, blood levels of the relevant drug may be required.

5 MANAGEMENT OF THE BRAIN DEAD DONOR FOR ORGAN HARVEST

1. General criteria of suitability
   a. A diagnosis of brain stem death has been made.
   b. No damage has been sustained by the organ to be harvested.
   c. No sepsis or systemic infection is present.
   d. No malignancy, except in the case of a proven primary brain tumour.
   e. No prolonged period of hypotension.
   f. HIV negative, HBV negative, no slow virus disease.
   g. No i.v. drug abuse.
   h. Consent has not been refused by relatives, coroner or equivalent legal officer.
   i. No juvenile onset diabetes mellitus.
2. Guidelines for suitability for specific organ harvest
   a. Kidney
      i. Age range: 2–70 years.
      ii. No hepatic or renal damage, no history of hypertension.
      iii. A good urinary output (>0.5 ml/kg/h).
      iv. HLA compatibility.
   b. Liver
      i. Age range: 4 months–65 years.
      ii. No clinical liver damage, no history of alcohol abuse.
      iii. Normal liver function tests.
      iv. Gall bladder must be present.
      v. Normal gross appearance of the liver.
   c. Pancreas
      i. Age range: 15–50 years.
      ii. Normal serum amylase.
      iii. No diabetes mellitus.

d. Heart or heart/lung

    i. Age: Male <40 years.

          Female <45 years.

    ii. No heart disease, chronic lung disease, hypertension or myocardial trauma. For lung transplant, only non-smokers are acceptable.

    iii. No prolonged cardiac arrest period, a stable cardiovascular system requiring minimal or no inotropic support.

    iv. No abnormality of the heart. The lungs should be normal on clinical examination.

    v. ECG and CXR normal.

    vi. A short ventilatory period of <24 hours, to reduce risk of infection.

    vii. Size compatibility with the potential recipient.

3. Preliminary intensive care management

a. Discussion with relatives

The patient may have carried a signed donor consent card. If not, the relatives should be approached by an experienced, and preferably senior member of staff, to obtain their views. Even if the patient has signed a donor card, discussion with the relatives is appropriate and their feelings must be considered. (For further discussion and medicolegal details, see DHSS Cadaveric Organs for Transplantation 1983.) Donor confidentiality should be maintained unless the relatives indicate otherwise. All details of discussions should be recorded in the patient's case records.

b. Discussion with the coroner

The coroner, or equivalent officer, need only be approached if the case would normally be reported to him because of the circumstances leading to the patient's death. Under such circumstances, the procedures set out by the local coroner must be followed.

c. Discussion with the transplant team

Contact should be made early with the regional transplant coordinator or the transplant team, giving the details listed below. At this stage it must be clearly indicated whether or not consent from the relatives has already been obtained.

d. Profile of the donor

    i. The transplant centre will require information on the medical history and cause of brain stem death, age, sex, height and weight of patient.

    ii. Blood should be taken for ABO grouping, HLA typing, HIV and HBV status.

    iii. The results of recent investigations, where appropriate for the organs being taken, will be needed. These may include electrolytes and urea, full blood count, liver function tests, serum amylase, a 12 lead ECG, a recent CXR and blood gases.

e. Maintenance of physiological homeostasis of donor

i. Continued respiratory support

Should aim to maintain a PaO_2 of 10 kPa and a PCO_2 of 5 kPa. The reduction in CO_2 production by brain-dead patients may necessitate the addition of a dead space to the respiratory circuit. PEEP may be required to maintain oxygenation, especially in the case of heart/lung donors.

ii. Blood presure

In order to maintain the systolic BP >90 mmHg, inotropic support, with a dopamine infusion of not more than 10 μg/kg/min, may be required. The lowest possible dose should be used to avoid the alpha adrenergic effects, which occur at doses above 10 μg/kg/min. Drugs with alpha$_1$ adrenergic effects should not be used, as they may compromise vital organ blood flow. This could subsequently impair the function of the transplanted organ.

iii. Vascular volume

The CVP should be maintained at 5–10 cm H_2O with gelatin or PPF, or with blood, should there be a continuing blood loss, to keep the Hb >8 g/dl. If diabetes insipidus is present, desmopressin (DDAVP) i.v. or i.m., 0.5–2 μg 6-hourly is given. Desmopressin is preferable to vasopressin, as it has no vasoconstrictor effect, and is longer acting.

iv. Urinary output

Is monitored and a volume of >0.5 ml/kg/h is maintained. Urinary fluid and electrolyte losses from diabetes insipidus are replaced and the CVP kept in the desired range. If the urine output remains low, a diuretic may be required. Frusemide i.v. 1–2 mg/kg or a frusemide infusion of <4 mg/min, or a mannitol infusion of 0.5 mg/kg can be used. Alpha$_1$ adrenergic agonists are not given because of the accompanying decrease in organ perfusion.

v. Body temperature

Is maintained at 34–36°C to prevent arrhythmias or cardiac arrest. Brain stem death is usually accompanied by a gradual decrease in body temperature. A warming blanket, warm fluids and humidification may be required.

vi. Prevention of infection

Infection must be prevented, so a strict aseptic technique is used for all procedures.

4. Management of the organ donor in the operating theatre

a. Maintenance of monitoring and physiological homeostasis should be continued. Plasma expanders or blood transfusion may be needed to replace blood loss which occurs during dissection. The average blood loss during multiple organ harvesting was found to be 4 units in adults and 2 units in children (Rosenthal 1983).

Direct arterial monitoring is useful, even if inotropic support is not required. It provides access for rapid arterial blood sampling for blood gases during the procedure, should there be any doubt about the suitability of the lungs for harvest. Similarly, a CVP line will enable intraoperative blood samples to be obtained for subsequent immunological testing.

b. Muscle relaxants are required for abdominal relaxation, and to prevent spinal reflexes. There may be haemodynamic responses to surgery which can be alarming to inexperienced staff, but which do not invalidate the diagnosis of brain death (Wetzel et al 1985). Marked increases in systolic and diastolic pressures and heart rate, persisting for up to 25 minutes, can occur in response to skin incision.

Occasionally inhalational agents may be required to control these responses (Kang & Gelman 1987).

c. The exact drug regimen will depend upon the organ(s) being harvested and the individual preferences of the transplant team. The following are commonly required:

i. Broad-spectrum antibiotics, such as flucloxacillin, or cefitoxime and benzyl penicillin, with or without gentamicin.

ii. Phenoxybenzamine i.v. 1 mg/kg prior to removal of the kidneys. This prevents vasoconstriction.

iii. Heparin i.v. 10–15 000 units for adults, but appropriately reduced for children is given, after mobilisation of the viscera but before the organs are excised.

iv. Methylprednisolone may be needed in the case of heart/lung removal.

5. Factors adversely affecting organ survival

Prolonged hypotension, and the use of vasopressors, dopamine and vasopressin, were all found to be factors contributing to the occurrence of tubular necrosis, and hence a decrease in the chance of kidney survival.

BIBLIOGRAPHY

Conference of Medical Royal Colleges and their Faculties in the United Kingdom 1976 Diagnosis of brain death. British Medical Journal 2: 1187–1188
Department of Health and Social Security 1983 Cadaveric organs for transplantation. HMSO, London
Graybar G B, Tarpey M 1987 Kidney transplantation. In: Anesthesia and organ transplantation. W B Saunders, Philadelphia
Grebenik C R, Hinds C J 1987 Management of the multiple organ donor. British Journal of Hospital Medicine 62–65
Jennett B 1981 Brain death. British Journal of Anaesthesia 53: 1111–1119
Kang Y G, Gelman S 1987 Liver transplantation. In Anesthesia and organ transplantation. W B Saunders, Philadelphia
Rolles K 1986 Management of the multiple organ donor. Hospital Update 633–638
Rosenthal J T, Shaw B W Jr, Hardesty R L, Griffith B P, Starzl T E, Hakala T R 1983 Principles of multiple organ procurement from cadaver donors. Annals of Surgery 198; 617–621
Rudge C J 1988 Organising organ donation. British Journal of Hospital Medicine 40: 127–130
Wetzel R C, Setzer N, Stiff J L, Rodgers M C 1985 Hemodynamic responses in brain dead organ donor patients. Anesthesia and Analgesia 64: 125–128

6

Normal Values

BIOCHEMISTRY
plasma or serum data

The biochemical normal values depend upon the techniques used and the individual laboratory. Where there values are particularly variable, space has been left for the insertion of the local range.

6

Constituent	Normal or reference values
ACTH	
ADH	
Adrenaline + noradrenaline	
Adrenaline	
Alanine aminotransferase	5–40 IU/l
Albumin	35–52 g/l
Alcohol legal limit	80 mg/dl
Aldolase	
Aldosterone	
Alkaline phosphatase	Adult 30–130 u/l
	Child 30–300 u/l
	Pregnant 100–300 u/l
Aluminium	
Amino acid nitrogen, fasting	
Amylase	70–300 U/l
Angiotensin-converting enzyme inhibitor	
Angiotensin II	
Anion gap $(Na + K) - (HCO_3 + Cl)$	6–16 mmol/l
Antidiuretic hormone	
Aspartate aminotransferase	5–40 IU/l
Bicarbonate	22–32 mmol/l
Bilirubin	
total	5–20 μmol/l
conjugated	<3.0 μmol/l
Caeruloplasmin	
Calcitonin	
Calcium total	2.15–2.60 mmol/l
Calcium corrected for albumin	2.20–2.55 mmol/l
Carbonic acid	
Carbon dioxide whole blood	4.5–6.0 kPa
C1 esterase inhibitor	
Chloride	98–108 mmol/l
Cholesterol	
Cholinesterase	0.8–1.2 U/ml
dibucaine number	normal approx. 80
	homozygous approx. 20
	heterozygous approx. 60
fluoride number	57–63
Cortisol	165–715 nmol/l
8am-10am	165–715 nmol/l
9pm-midnight	<330 nmol/l
Creatinine	70–125 μmol/l
Creatine kinase	
males	25–170 iu/l
females	25–150 iu/l
Gamma glutamyl transferase	7–50 U/l
Gastrin	

Constituent	Normal or reference values
Glucagon	
Glucose (plasma)	3.3–6.0 mmol/l
Growth hormone	
Hydrogen ion activity (pH)	36–44 nmol/l
	7.36–7.44
Hydroxybutyrate dehydrogenase	
Insulin (fasting)	
Lactate	0.75–1.25 mmol/l
Lactic acid dehydrogenase (total)	240–525 U/l
Lipids (total)	
Luteinizing hormone	
Magnesium	0.7–1.2 mmol/l
Methionine	
Noradrenaline	
Osmolality	275–295 mOsm/kg
Oxygen (whole blood)	11–15 kPa
Pancreatic polypeptide	
Parathyroid hormone	
Phosphatases (acid)	
acid total	0–5 U/l
prostatic fraction	0–1 U/l
Phosphate	0.7–1.4 mmol/l
Phospholipids	
Potassium	3.5–5.3 mmol/l
Protein	
total	62–80 g/l
albumin	35–52 g/l
Pyruvate	
Renin	
recumbent	
ambulant	
Sodium	135–145 mmol/l
Testosterone	
males	
females	
Thyroid-stimulating hormone	0.4–4 mU/l
T4	50–150 nmol/l
	pregnancy 117–258 nmol/l
T3	1–3 nmol/l
Transferrin	
Triglycerides (fasting)	
Urate	male 0.11–0.45 mmol/l
	female 0.12–0.40 mmol/l
Urea	2.5–7.5 mmol/l

HAEMATOLOGICAL VALUES

Bleeding time (Template)	2.5–9.5 min
Coagulation time	5–11 min
Prothrombin time	12–15 s
Partial thromboplastin time (KCCT)	35–42 s
Thrombin clotting time	15–18 s
Prothrombin consumption index	≤20%
Plasma fibrinogen	2.0–4.0 g/l
Euglobulin lysis time	90–240 min

6

Fibrin degradation products	absent or trace
Platelet count	$150\text{--}400 \times 10^9/\mathrm{l}$
ESR (Westergren, 1 h)	male $\leq$10 mm
	female $\leq$20 mm
Serum folate	3–20 μg/l
Red cell folate	160–640 μg/l
Serum B12	160–925 ng/l
Serum iron	13–32 μmol/l
Iron binding capacity	45–70 μmol/l
Serum ferritin	male 20–340 μg/l
	female 15–40 μg/l
Haemoglobin	male 155 $\pm$ 25 g/l
	female 140 $\pm$ 25 g/l
Haematocrit	male 0.47 $\pm$ 0.07
	female 0.42 $\pm$ 0.05
Red cell count	male $5.5 \pm 1 \times 10^{12}/\mathrm{l}$
	female $4.8 \pm 1 \times 10^{12}/\mathrm{l}$
Mean corpuscular volume	86 $\pm$ 10 fl
Mean corpuscular haemoglobin	29.5 $\pm$ 2.5 pg
Mean corpuscular haemoglobin concentration	33 $\pm$ 2 g/dl
Red cell volume	male 30 $\pm$ 5 ml/kg
	female 25 $\pm$ 5 ml/kg
Plasma volume	40–50 ml/kg
Total blood volume	70 $\pm$ 10 ml/kg
Total leucocyte count	$4\text{--}11 \times 10^9/\mathrm{l}$
Neutrophils (40–75%)	$2\text{--}7.5 \times 10^9/\mathrm{l}$
Lymphocytes (20–45%)	$1.5\text{--}4.0 \times 10^9/\mathrm{l}$
Monocytes (2–10%)	$0.2\text{--}0.8 \times 10^9/\mathrm{l}$
Eosinophils (1–6%)	$0.04\text{--}0.4 \times 10^9/\mathrm{l}$
Basophils ($\leq$1%)	$\leq 0.1 \times 10^9/\mathrm{l}$
Reticulocytes (0.2–2%)	$(10\text{--}100 \times 10^9/\mathrm{l})$
Serum haptoglobin	0.3–2.4 g/l
Haemoglobinm A2	1.5–3.2%
Haemoglobin F	0.5–0.8%
Plasma viscosity	1.50–1.72 cp
Serum immunogloulin	
IgG	6–15 g/l
IgA	1–4.5 g/l
IgM	0.5–3.5 g/l

6

THERAPEUTIC BLOOD LEVELS

Digoxin	0.8–2 μg/l
Ethosuximide	40–100 mg/l
Gentamicin	therapeutic peak 5–10 mg/l
	therapeutic trough 0.5–2 mg/l
Lithium	0.8–1.2 mmol/l
	12 h after last dose
Lignocaine	1–5 μg/ml
Phenobarbitone	15–30 mg/l
Phenytoin	10–20 mg/l
Primidone	5—12 mg/l
Salicylate	analgesic <20 mg/l
	antiinflammatory <300 mg/l
Sodium valproate	50–100 mg/l
Theophylline	10–20 mg/l

CARDIOLOGICAL NORMAL VALUES

1. ECG TIMES

Small squares = 0.04 s   Large squares = 0.2 s

P wave	atrial wave	<0.10 s
P–R interval	AV conduction	0.12–0.20 s

(Measured from onset of P wave to onset of QRS.)

QRS time	rapid ventricular depolarisation	0.05–0.10 s
Q–T interval	length of ventricular complex	0.35–0.42 s

(Measured from beginning of Q to the end of the T wave. The Q–T interval decreases with increasing heart rate.)

QTc is the Q–T interval corrected for heart rate

$$QTc = \frac{\text{measured Q–T interval}}{\text{square root of cycle length}}$$

T wave	repolarization	≤0.22 s

6

2. CARDIOVASCULAR PARAMETERS

Pressures	Systolic (mmHg)	Diastolic (mmHg)	Mean (mmHg)
Peripheral venous			6–12
Right atrial pressure			0–7
Right ventricular pressure	14–32	0–7	12–17
Pulmonary arterial pressure	14–32	2–13	8–19
Pulmonary wedge or left atrial			6–14
Left ventricular end diastolic		2–10	8
Arterial pressure	100–150	60–90	80–100

Haemodynamic variables (70 kg)

Cardiac output	5 l/min
Cardiac index	3.2 l/min/m^2
Stroke volume	75 ml
Stroke volume index	50 ml/m^2
Ejection fraction	>0.60
Pulmonary vascular resistance	50–140 dyn. s. cm^{-5}
Systemic vascular resistance	90–1500 dyn. s. cm^{-5}

RESPIRATORY NORMAL VALUES

Predicted peak expiratory flow rate (l/min): men

Age (yr)	Height				
	5ft 3in (160 cm)	5ft 6in (168 cm)	5ft 9in (175 cm)	6ft 0in (183 cm)	6ft 3in (190 cm)
20	570	600	625	655	680
25	575	600	625	655	680
30	560	585	610	640	665
35	545	570	600	625	650
40	535	560	585	610	635
45	525	550	570	600	625
50	510	535	560	585	610
55	500	525	550	575	595
60	490	510	535	560	580
65	475	500	520	545	565
70	465	485	505	530	550
75	450	470	495	515	535
80	440	460	485	505	525

6

Predicted peak expiratory flow rate (l/min): women

Age (yr)	Height				
	4ft 9in (145 cm)	5ft 0in (152 cm)	5ft 3in (160 cm)	5ft 6in (168 cm)	5ft 9in (175 cm)
20	375	400	435	460	490
25	375	400	435	460	490
30	365	390	420	450	480
35	355	380	410	440	470
40	345	370	400	425	460
45	335	360	390	420	450
50	325	350	380	405	435
55	315	340	370	395	425
60	300	330	360	385	415
65	295	320	350	375	405
70	280	310	340	365	395
75	270	300	330	355	385
80	260	290	320	345	375

Forced vital capacity prediction table (in litres): men

Age (yr)	Height				
	5ft 3in (160 cm)	5ft 6in (168 cm)	5ft 9in (175 cm)	6ft 0in (183 cm)	6ft 3in (190 cm)
20	4.17	4.53	4.95	5.37	5.73
25	4.17	4.53	4.95	5.37	5.73
30	4.06	4.42	4.84	5.26	5.62

Forced vital capacity prediction table (in litres): men

Age (yr)	Height				
	5ft 3in (160 cm)	5ft 6in (168 cm)	5ft 9in (175 cm)	6ft 0in (183 cm)	6ft 3in (190 cm)
35	3.95	4.31	4.73	5.15	5.51
40	3.84	4.20	4.62	5.04	5.40
45	3.73	4.09	4.51	4.93	5.29
50	3.62	3.98	4.40	4.82	5.18
55	3.51	3.87	4.29	4.71	5.07
60	3.40	3.76	4.18	4.60	4.96
65	3.29	3.65	4.07	4.49	4.85
70	3.18	3.54	3.96	4.38	4.74
75	3.07	3.43	3.85	4.27	4.63

Forced vital capacity prediction table (in litres): women

Age (yr)	Height				
	4ft 9in (145 cm)	5ft 0in (152 cm)	5ft 3in (160 cm)	5ft 6in (168 cm)	5ft 9in (175 cm)
20	3.13	3.45	3.83	4.20	4.53
25	3.13	3.45	3.83	4.20	4.53
30	2.98	3.30	3.68	4.05	4.38
35	2.83	3.15	3.53	3.90	4.23
40	2.68	3.00	3.38	3.75	4.08
45	2.53	2.85	3.23	3.60	3.93
50	2.38	2.70	3.08	3.45	3.78
55	2.23	2.55	2.93	3.30	3.63
60	2.08	2.40	2.78	3.15	3.48
65	1.93	2.25	2.63	3.00	3.33
70	1.78	2.10	2.48	2.85	3.18
75	1.63	1.95	2.33	2.70	3.03

Forced expiratory volume prediction table (at 1 s in litres): men

Age (yr)	Height				
	5ft 3in (160 cm)	5ft 6in (168 cm)	5ft 9in (175 cm)	6ft 0in (183 cm)	6ft 3in (190 cm)
20	3.61	3.86	4.15	4.44	4.69
25	3.61	3.86	4.15	4.44	4.69
30	3.45	3.71	4.00	4.28	4.54
35	3.30	3.55	3.84	4.13	4.38
40	3.14	3.40	3.69	3.97	4.23
45	2.99	3.24	3.53	3.82	4.07
50	2.83	3.09	3.38	3.66	3.92
55	2.68	2.93	3.22	3.51	3.76
60	2.52	2.78	3.06	3.35	3.61
65	2.37	2.62	2.91	3.20	3.45
70	2.21	2.47	2.75	3.04	3.30
75	2.06	2.31	2.60	2.89	3.14

6

Forced expiratory volume prediction table (at 1 s in litres): women

Age (yr)	Height				
	4ft 9in (145 cm)	5ft 0in (152 cm)	5ft 3in (160 cm)	5ft 6in (168 cm)	5ft 9in (175 cm)
20	2.60	2.83	3.09	3.36	3.59
25	2.60	2.83	3.09	3.36	3.59
30	2.45	2.68	2.94	3.21	3.44
35	2.30	2.53	2.79	3.06	3.29
40	2.15	2.38	2.64	2.91	3.14
45	2.00	2.23	2.49	2.76	2.99
50	1.85	2.08	2.34	2.61	2.84
55	1.70	1.93	2.19	2.46	2.69
60	1.55	1.78	2.04	2.31	2.54
65	1.40	1.63	1.89	2.16	2.39
70	1.25	1.48	1.74	2.01	2.24
75	1.10	1.33	1.59	1.86	2.09

PAEDIATRIC VALUES

Paediatric endotracheal tube sizes

Age	Internal diameter (mm)	Length (cm)	
		Oral	Nasal
Premature	2.5–3.0	11	13.5
neonate	3.5	12	14
1 yr	4.0	13	15
2 yr	4.5	14	16
4 yr	5.0	15	17
6 yr	5.5	17	19
8 yr	6.0	19	21
10 yr	6.5	20	22
12 yr	7.0	21	22
14 yr	7.5	22	23
16 yr	8.0	23	24

Paediatric haemoglobin levels

Newborn	20 g/dl (range 18–22 g/dl)
Second week	17 g/dl
3 months	10–11 g/dl
2 years	11 g/dl
3–5 years	12.5–13.0 g/dl
5–10 years	13.0–13.5 g/dl
> 10 years	14.5 g/dl

Paediatric blood volumes and blood pressure

Age	Weight (kg)	Blood volume (l)	Blood pressure (mmHg)	
			Systolic	Diastolic
Newborn	3.5	0.2	70	45
3 mth	5.0	0.4	70	45
6 mth	7.0	0.52	70	45
9 mth	8.5	0.65	70	45
1 yr	10	0.75	80	60
2 yr	13	0.9	80	60
3 yr	15	1.05	85	60
4 yr	17	1.22	87	60
5 yr	19	1.37	90	60
6 yr	21	1.52	90	60
7 yr	23	1.7	92	62
8 yr	25	1.9	95	62
9 yr	28	2.06	98	64
10 yr	32	2.4	100	65
11 yr			105	65
12 yr			108	67

Paediatric respiratory parameters

Body weight (kg)	MV (ml)	TV (ml)	RR (min)	FGF with 'T' piece to prevent rebreathing	
				Mask	ETT
2	480	14–16	30–45		
3	600	17–24	25–40		
5	875	35		8	6
10	1680	80	21	8	6
15	2400	120		10	7.5
20	3040	160	19	12	9
25	3240	180		14	10.5
30	4080	240	17	14	10.5
35	4160	260		15	11.5
40	4800	320	15	16	12.0
45				17	12.5

Paediatric weight conversion chart

st	lb	kg	st	lb	kg	st	lb	kg
	3	1.36	1	0	6.35	1	11	11.34
	4	1.81	1	1	6.80	1	12	11.79
	5	2.27	1	2	7.26	1	13	12.24
	6	2.72	1	3	7.71	2	0	12.7
	7	3.18	1	4	8.16	2	4	14.5
	8	3.63	1	5	8.62	2	8	16.3
	9	4.08	1	6	9.07	2	12	18.1
	10	4.54	1	7	9.53	3	0	19.1
	11	4.99	1	8	9.98	3	4	20.9
	12	5.44	1	9	10.43	3	8	22.7
	13	5.90	1	10	10.89	3	12	24.5

6

SI FRACTIONS OR MULTIPLES

10^{-1}	deci	d		10^{1}	deca	da
10^{-3}	milli	m		10^{3}	kilo	k
10^{-6}	micro	μ		10^{6}	mega	M
10^{-9}	nano	n		10^{9}	giga	G
10^{-12}	pico	p		10^{12}	tera	T
10^{-15}	femto	f		10^{15}	peta	P
10^{-18}	atto	a		10^{18}	exa	E

PRESSURE CONVERSION CHART

1 mmHg = 1.36 cmH$_2$O = 133.3 N/m^2 = 0.0194 psi
1 mmHg = 0.133 kPa
1 cmH$_2$O = 0.098 kPa = 98.06 N/m^2
1 bar = 760 mmHg = 29.9 inHg = 1 atmosphere absolute
1 kPa = 1 $\times$ 10^3 N/m^2 = 7.5 mmHg = 0.146 psi
1 psi = 6.895 kPa = 51.7 mmHg

GENERAL WEIGHT CONVERSION CHART

st	lb	kg	st	lb	kg	st	lb	kg
2	0	12.7	8	0	50.8	14	0	88.9
2	4	14.5	8	4	52.6	14	4	90.7
2	8	16.3	8	9	54.4	14	8	92.5
2	12	18.1	8	12	56.2	14	12	94.3
3	0	19.1	9	0	57.2	15	0	95.2
3	4	20.9	9	4	59.0	15	4	97.0
3	8	22.7	9	8	60.8	15	8	98.9
3	12	24.5	9	12	62.6	15	12	100.7
4	0	25.4	10	0	63.5	16	0	101.6
4	4	27.2	10	4	65.3	16	4	103.4
4	8	29.0	10	8	67.1	16	8	105.2
4	12	30.8	10	12	68.9	16	12	107.0
5	0	31.8	11	0	69.9	17	0	107.9
5	4	33.6	11	4	71.7	17	4	109.8
5	8	35.4	11	8	73.5	17	8	111.6
5	12	37.2	11	12	75.3	17	12	113.4
6	0	38.1	12	0	76.2	18	0	114.3
6	4	39.9	12	4	78.0	18	4	116.1
6	8	41.7	12	8	79.8	18	8	117.9
6	12	43.5	12	12	81.6	18	12	119.7
7	0	44.5	13	0	82.6	19	0	120.7
7	4	46.3	13	4	84.4	19	4	122.5
7	8	48.1	13	8	86.2	19	8	124.3
7	12	49.9	13	12	88.0	19	12	126.1
						20	00	127.0

A

Appendix

Useful addresses and telephone numbers

Association of Anaesthetists
9 Bedford Square
London WC1B 3RA
01 631 1650

British Medical Association
BMA House
Tavistock Square
London WC1H 9JP
01 387 4499

British Postgraduate Medical Federation
33 Millman Street
London WC1N 3EJ
01 831 6222

Cholinesterase Research Unit
Hammersmith Hospital
Du Cane Road
London W12 0HS
01 743 2030

Clinical Research Centre
Northwick Park
Harrow
Middlesex HA1 3UJ
01 864 5311

College of Anaesthetists
Royal College of Surgeons
35–43 Lincoln's Inn Fields
London WC2A 3PN
01 405 3474

Committee on Safety of Medicines
Market Towers
1 Nine Elms Lane
London SW8 5NQ
01 720 2188

Department of Health and Social Security
Alexander Fleming House
Elephant and Castle
London SE1 6BY
01 407 5522

General Medical Council
44 Hallam Street
London W1N 6AE
01 580 7642

Health and Safety Executive: Medical Division
Baynard's House
1 Chepstow Place
Westbourne Grove
London W2 4TF
01 229 3456

Home Office
50 Queen Anne's Gate
London SW1H 9AT
01 273 3000

H.K. Lewis
Medical and Scientific Lending Library
136 Gower Street
London WC1 6BS
01 387 4282

Malignant Hyperpyrexia Unit
St James' University Hospital
Leeds LS9 7TF
0532 433144

Medical Defence Union
3 Devonshire Place
London W1N 2EA
01 486 6181

Medical Protection Society
50 Hallam Street
London W1
01 637 0541

Medical Research Council
20 Park Crescent
London W1N 4AL
01 636 5422

National Adverse Reactions Advisory Service
Supraregional Protein Reference Unit
Royal Hallamshire Hospital
Sheffield S10 2JF
0742 766222 ext. 2837/2058 or bleep 288

POISONS CENTRES

Belfast
Royal Victoria Hospital
Grosvenor Road

Belfast BT12 6BA
0232 240503

Birmingham
West Midlands Poisons Unit
Dudley Road Hospital
Birmingham B18 7QH
021 5543801 ext. 4109

Cardiff
Llandough Hospital
Penarth
South Glamorgan
0222 709901

Dublin
Jervis Street Hospital
Jervis Street
Dublin 1
0001 745588

Edinburgh
The Royal Infirmary of Edinburgh
Edinburgh EH3 9YW
031 229 2477 ext. 2233

London
New Cross Hospital
Avonley
London SE14 5ER
01 635 9191

Newcastle
Royal Victoria Infirmary
Newcastle upon Tyne NE1 4LP
091 232 5131

Scottish National Blood Transfusion Service
Ellen's Glen Road
Edinburgh EH17 7QT
031 664 2317

Royal College of Surgeons of England
Lincoln's Inn Fields
London WC2A 3PN
01 405 3474

Royal Society of Medicine
1 Wimpole Street
London W1M 8AE
01 408 2119

Welsh Office Health and Social Services Groups
New Crown Buildings
Cathays Park
Cardiff CF1 3NQ
0222 825111

Detailed Contents

The text is laid out as a reference system and as the topics are generally covered in alphabetical order within the various sections a conventional index is unnecessary. Instead a detailed contents list has been included for ease of reference.

SECTION 2 Preoperative drugs 315

SECTION 2 Preoperative drugs 315